D0360030

2012
YEAR BOOK OF
PEDIATRICS®

The 2012 Year Book Series

Year Book of Anesthesiology and Pain Management™: Drs Chestnut, Abram, Black, Gravlee, Lien, Mathru, and Roizen

Year Book of Cardiology®: Drs Gersh, Cheitlin, Elliott, Gold, Graham, and Thourani

Year Book of Critical Care Medicine®: Drs Dellinger, Parrillo, Balk, Dorman, Dries, and Zanotti-Cavazzoni

Year Book of Dermatology and Dermatologic Surgery™: Dr Del Rosso

Year Book of Diagnostic Radiology®: Drs Osborn, Abbara, Elster, Manaster, Oestreich, Offiah, Rosado de Christenson, Stephens, and Walker

Year Book of Emergency Medicine®: Drs Hamilton, Bruno, Handly, Mullin, Quintana, and Ramoska

Year Book of Endocrinology®: Drs Schott, Apovian, Clarke, Eugster, Ludlam, Meikle, Schinner, Schteingart, and Toth

Year Book of Gastroenterology™: Drs Talley, DeVault, Harnois, Murray, Pearson, Philcox, Picco, and Smith

Year Book of Hand and Upper Limb Surgery®: Drs Yao and Steinmann

Year Book of Medicine®: Drs Barker, Garrick, Gersh, Khardori, LeRoith, Seo, Talley, and Thigpen

Year Book of Neonatal and Perinatal Medicine®: Drs Fanaroff, Benitz, Donn, Neu, Papile, Polin, and van Marter

Year Book of Neurology and Neurosurgery®: Drs Klimo and Rabinstein

Year Book of Obstetrics, Gynecology, and Women's Health®: Drs Dungan and Shulman

Year Book of Oncology®: Drs Arceci, Bauer, Chiorean, Gordon, Lawton, Murphy, Thigpen, and Tsao

Year Book of Ophthalmology®: Drs Rapuano, Cohen, Flanders, Fudemberg, Hammersmith, Milman, Myers, Nagra, Nelson, Penne, Pyfer, Sergott, Shields, Talekar, and Vander

Year Book of Orthopedics®: Drs Morrey, Beauchamp, Huddleston, Swiontkowski, and Trigg

Year Book of Otolaryngology-Head and Neck Surgery®: Drs Sindwani, Balough, Franco, Gapany, and Mitchell

Year Book of Pathology and Laboratory Medicine®: Drs Raab, Parwani, Bejarano, and Bissell

Year Book of Pediatrics®: Dr Stockman

Year Book of Plastic and Aesthetic Surgery™: Drs Miller, Gosman, Gurtner, Gutowski, Ruberg, Salisbury, and Smith

2012

The Year Book of
PEDIATRICS®

Editor

James A. Stockman III, MD

President, The American Board of Pediatrics; Clinical Professor of Pediatrics,
University of North Carolina Medical School at Chapel Hill, and Duke
University Medical Center, Durham, North Carolina

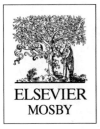

ELSEVIER
MOSBY

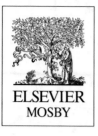

ELSEVIER
MOSBY

Vice President, Continuity: Kimberly Murphy
Editor: Kerry Holland
Production Supervisor, Electronic Year Books: Donna M. Skelton
Electronic Article Manager: Emily Ogle
Illustrations and Permissions Coordinator: Dawn Vohsen

Printed in the United States of America
Transfered to Digital Printing, 2012

Editorial Office:
Elsevier
Suite 1800
1600 John F. Kennedy Blvd.
Philadelphia, PA 19103-2899

International Standard Serial Number: 0084-3954
International Standard Book Number: 978-0-323-08890-9

Table of Contents

Journals Represented

Journals represented in this YEAR BOOK are listed below.

Acta Paediatrica
Annals of Internal Medicine
Archives of Disease in Childhood
Archives of Pediatrics & Adolescent Medicine
British Medical Journal
Blood
Clinical Pediatrics
Epilepsia
Journal of Adolescent Health
Journal of Allergy and Clinical Immunology
Journal of Developmental & Behavioral Pediatrics
Journal of Pediatric Gastroenterology and Nutrition
Journal of Pediatric Hematology/Oncology
Journal of Pediatric Orthopaedics
Journal of Pediatric Surgery
Journal of Pediatrics
Journal of the American Academy of Child and Adolescent Psychiatry
Journal of the American Medical Association
Lancet
New England Journal of Medicine
Pediatric Emergency Care
Pediatric Infectious Disease Journal
Pediatric Research
Pediatrics
Science

STANDARD ABBREVIATIONS

The following terms are abbreviated in this edition: acquired immunodeficiency syndrome (AIDS), cardiopulmonary resuscitation (CPR), central nervous system (CNS), cerebrospinal fluid (CSF), computed tomography (CT), deoxyribonucleic acid (DNA), electrocardiography (ECG), health maintenance organization (HMO), human immunodeficiency virus (HIV), intensive care unit (ICU), intramuscular (IM), intravenous (IV), magnetic resonance (MR) imaging (MRI), ribonucleic acid (RNA), ultrasound (US), and ultraviolet (UV).

NOTE

To facilitate the use of the YEAR BOOK OF PEDIATRICS® as a reference tool, all illustrations and tables included in this publication are now identified as they appear in the original article. This change is meant to help the reader recognize that any illustration or table appearing in the YEAR BOOK OF PEDIATRICS® may be only one of many in the original article. For this reason, figure and table numbers will often appear to be out of sequence within the YEAR BOOK OF PEDIATRICS.®

Introduction

Dedicated to Lee for her 34 years of behind-the-scenes support of the
YEAR BOOK OF PEDIATRICS.

*"Depend upon it ... there comes a time when for every addition of
knowledge you forget something that you knew before. It is of the
highest importance, therefore, not to have useless facts elbowing
out the useful ones."*

Sir Arthur Conan Doyle (1859-1930)

The above expressing the suggestion that the human mind is like a computer's hard drive with only so many terabytes of storage capability, while
not precisely correct, are words of wisdom that have some merit. One
could suggest that Sir Arthur is also saying that it makes sense to be as
efficient as possible in the way we add knowledge to our memory banks,
for while brain capacity may not be fixed, the time in which to acquire
knowledge truly is. The YEAR BOOK OF PEDIATRICS is designed to address
the need for learning in a most efficient way. Articles are chosen for inclusion specifically for the purpose of covering the waterfront of topics that
those providing care to children encounter.

The introductions of several past editions of the YEAR BOOK OF PEDIATRICS
have commented on learnings that this editor has derived from our family's
non-human offspring. This YEAR BOOK'S introduction, being no different,
closes with a very instructive story. In earlier editions, it was noted that
Jordan, the family pug, taught us about the presentation of Cushing's
syndrome and the daily management of one of its complications, diabetes
mellitus. Then there was Theo, also a pug, who at the tender age of
6 months died suddenly. We missed the clue to the cause of his passing until
the performance of a belated literature search. Theo was deaf. Pugs
apparently are a breed that has a much-higher-than-expected prevalence
of a genetically transmitted defect associated with a cardiac ion channel
abnormality. It is highly likely that Theo was unfortunate enough to carry
the gene for the Jervell and Lange-Nielson syndrome (hereditary deafness
and prolonged QT interval syndrome). Riley, our shar-pei, was a different
learning experience. Starting at 9 months of age, she began to have periodic
episodes of high fever, shaking chills, abdominal distention, and swollen
limbs. She was a diagnostic dilemma for her care providers, this editor
included, until investigators from Germany published a report of a line of
shar-peis with inheritance of a gene causing "familial shar-pei fever
(FSF)," the precise animal model of the human disease familial Mediterranean fever (FMF). Riley became well-known in the veterinary and human
medical community as she participated in a number of clinical research protocols for the study of prevention of disease flairs and the development of
amyloidosis, the lethal complication of FSF and FMF. With generous
amounts of colchicine and the excellent care provided by my wife, Lee
(aka "Fourdogmom") to whom this YEAR BOOK is dedicated, Riley lived

happily to an advanced age contrary to the natural history of FSF and was adored by her many extended family members.

Now to Jack, the dalmatian, this past year's source of new medical knowledge. Jack is a grand dog, a foundling, owned by one of our real offspring and her husband and children. No one knows Jack's age, except perhaps for Jack himself, but he is well into the second decade of his life. Early last year, he began to decline over a several-month period. His symptoms included clumsiness followed by staggering and finally inability to stand or walk. It was clear that he could no longer use his hind legs. Prior to this, he was as youthful as the day he was found abandoned in a locked and empty apartment. The guess was that he was experiencing the rapid onset of canine Alzheimer disease. Jack's family reconciled itself to the fact that Jack was likely headed to canine heaven, but Jack, not burdened with any thoughts about an afterlife, struggled on for some weeks without a specific diagnosis. Ultimately, an MRI of the head and spine ordered by extraordinarily knowledgeable consultants at the North Carolina State University College of Veterinary Medicine gave the clue to the origins of what now was a complete quadriplegia: three badly herniated cervical disks. Following expert care that was better than most humans receive, care that included a lengthy course of steroids, spinal cord decompression and fusion, time in an ICU, and a carefully structured rehabilitation program, Jack not only was back on his feet, but he was able to undertake almost all the sorts of physical activity he once enjoyed, including sniffing human and other canine bodily parts. Unfortunately after a short while, however, he became critically ill with a bout of fulminant pancreatitis. The etiology of pancreatitis in dogs is little different than that in humans. In Jack's case, the ultimate cause was likely to have been the steroids that he had been on for weeks. He recovered from the episode of pancreatitis satisfactorily, but there was one more bump in the road that came not long after. One morning Jack was found profoundly lethargic, largely unresponsive, but in no apparent pain. No amount of stimulation was effective in rousing him. He was truly on his way out. This editor, following a cursory examination, proposed a differential diagnosis that included poisoning, uremia, hepatic failure, and the remote possibility that the signs and symptoms were related to an addisonian crisis from the earlier abrupt withdrawal of steroids, a diagnosis that this hematologist had not actually seen before. Iatrogenic Addison's disease was confirmed by diagnostic studies. Amazingly a touch of steroids and hours later, like Lazarus arising from the grave, Jack was barking recriminations at those who had neglected to remember that those who walk on all fours can develop secondary Addison's disease the same as humans.

Yes there is a lot that we can learn from woman's and man's best friend. If Sir Arthur Conan Doyle was correct and you have to make room for one new piece of knowledge, make it a learning experience from a pooch. The one I value the most was acquired from Fritzie, our black lab: the principle of always turning around three times before going to potty. Works like a charm every time.

James A. Stockman III, MD

1 Adolescent Medicine

US Adolescent Nutrition, Exercise, and Screen Time Baseline Levels Prior to National Recommendations

Foltz JL, Cook SR, Szilagyi PG, et al (Univ of Rochester School of Medicine and Dentistry, NY)

Clin Pediatr 50:424-433, 2011

Experts have recommended daily obesity prevention goals: ≥5 fruits/vegetables, <2 hours of screen time, >1 hour of physical activity, and no sugar-sweetened beverages (5-2-1-0). The authors analyzed National Health and Nutrition Examination Survey data for 1999-2002 to determine the proportion of US adolescents (12-19 years) who would have met each goal prior to dissemination of the 5-2-1-0 recommendations. Merely 0.4% would have met all goals; 41% would have met none. Only 9% consumed ≥5 fruits/vegetables, 27% reported <2 hours of screen time, 32% had >1 hour of physical activity, and 14% consumed no sugar-sweetened beverages per day. Demographic subgroups (eg, racial/ethnic minority and lower income) would have been even farther from meeting the goals. Clinicians are likely to encounter adolescents with nutrition, exercise, and screen time behaviors that are far from 5-2-1-0 goals, and can use these guidelines during clinical encounters to counsel adolescents regarding healthier lifestyles (Figs 1 and 2).

▶ It was in 2007 that the American Academy of Pediatrics Expert Committee released its Recommendations on the Prevention, Assessment, and Treatment of Child and Adolescent Overweight and Obesity.[1] This report provided approaches based on the best available evidence. The recommendations were designed to direct physicians to assess nutrition and physical activity health behaviors at all preventive visits. The expert committee also recommended that pediatric weight management and behavioral counseling should include the promotion of nutrition and physical activity and also the application of the 5-2-1-0 mnemonic: 5 or more servings of fruits and vegetables, < 2 hours of screen time (TV, computer, video games), at least 1 hour of physical activity, and no (0) sugar-sweetened beverages. This 5-2-1-0 recommendation offers a simple and succinct message that can be used in both clinical care and community-based health promotion activities. The authors of this report evaluated how adolescent behaviors would have measured up to the 5-2-1-0 goals prior to the dissemination of the 5-2-1-0 message by estimating the proportion of US adolescents who met each criterion based on information in the 1999 to 2002 National Health and Nutrition Examination Survey.

1

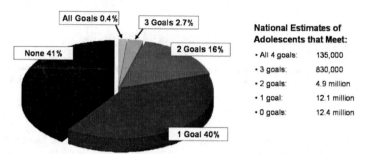

National Estimates of
Adolescents that Meet:

- All 4 goals: 135,000
- 3 goals: 830,000
- 2 goals: 4.9 million
- 1 goal: 12.1 million
- 0 goals: 12.4 million

FIGURE 1.—Percentage of US adolescents, aged 12 through 19 years, who would have met the 5-2-1-0 nutrition and activity goals in 1999-2002. (Reprinted from Foltz JL, Cook SR, Szilagyi PG, et al. US adolescent nutrition, exercise, and screen time baseline levels prior to national recommendations. *Clin Pediatr.* 2011;50:424-433. © 2011 by Clinical Pediatrics. Reprinted by permission of SAGE Publications.)

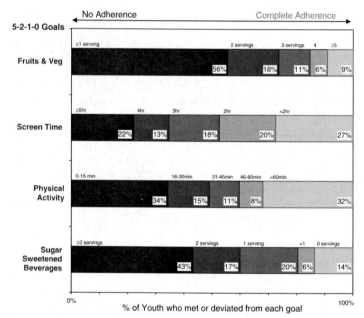

FIGURE 2.—Percentage of US adolescents who would have met each 5-2-1-0 goal in 1999-2002. Each bar represents one of the 5-2-1-0 goals; the degree of meeting the goal is listed above each bar segment. On the bottom is percentage of youth who adhered to or deviated from each goal; the corresponding numerical values are found imbedded in the bar segments. The right segment shows those who fully met the goal; left those who deviated most (eg, 56% ate ≤1 serving of fruits and vegetables, 9% ate ≥5). (Reprinted from Foltz JL, Cook SR, Szilagyi PG, et al. US adolescent nutrition, exercise, and screen time baseline levels prior to national recommendations. *Clin Pediatr.* 2011;50:424-433. © 2011 by Clinical Pediatrics. Reprinted by permission of SAGE Publications.)

Figs 1 and 2 say it all. Virtually no child in 1999 to 2002 would have met all the goals of the 5-2-1-0 set of recommendations. The significant majority (80%) would have met no goal or only 1 goal. Fig 2 demonstrates the percentage of children meeting some of the specifics of each of the 5-2-1-0 goals. The information from this report is critically important because it does provide the best baseline information for telling whether the current aggressive approaches to prevent the onset of obesity are working. These baseline data can guide current clinical, community, and policy interventions as well as provide a benchmark for future studies evaluating adolescent behaviors following the dissemination of the 5-2-1-0 guidelines.

The Society for Adolescent Medicine has changed its name. It is now the Society for Adolescent Health and Medicine and is the society that represents the profession of adolescent medicine specialists. This change represents the commitment of the society to advancing a holistic approach to adolescent well being and recognizes that it takes a variety of unique health services and disciplines coming together to ensure a healthy adolescent and young adult population. The addition of "health" to the name of the organization reflects the desire of the society to change its profile so that it can expand its identity and embrace all the partners that play a role in adolescent health. To read more about the society's name change, see the editorial of D'Angelo.[2]

J. A. Stockman III, MD

References

1. Barlow SE, Expert Committee. Expert committee recommendations regarding the prevention, assessment and treatment of child and adolescent overweight and obesity: summary report. *Pediatrics.* 2007;120:S164-S192.
2. D'Angelo L. Society's name change advances our mission. *J Adolesc Health.* 2010; 47:211.

Compulsive Internet Use: The Role of Online Gaming and Other Internet Applications
van Rooij AJ, Schoenmakers TM, van de Eijnden RJJM, et al (IVO Addiction Res Inst, Rotterdam, The Netherlands; Utrecht Univ, The Netherlands; et al)
J Adolesc Health 47:51-57, 2010

Purpose.—Increasing research on Internet addiction makes it necessary to distinguish between the medium of Internet and its specific applications. This study explores the relationship between time spent on various Internet applications (including online gaming) and Compulsive Internet Use in a large sample of adolescents.

Methods.—The 2007 (N = 4,920) and 2008 (N = 4,753) samples of a longitudinal survey study among adolescents were used, as well as the 2007−2008 cohort subsample (N = 1421). Compulsive Internet Use was predicted from the time spent on the various Internet applications in two cross-sectional multiple linear regression models and one longitudinal regression model in which changes in behavior were related to changes in Compulsive Internet Use.

Results.—In both samples, downloading, social networking, MSN use, Habbo Hotel, chatting, blogging, online games, and casual games were shown to be associated with Compulsive Internet Use. Of these, online gaming was shown to have the strongest association with Compulsive

Internet Use. Moreover, changes in online gaming were most strongly associated with changes in Compulsive Internet Use over time for the longitudinal cohort.

Conclusions.—A clear relationship was shown between online gaming and Compulsive Internet Use. It is further argued that a subgroup of compulsive Internet users should be classified as compulsive online gamers.

▶ No one would have guessed 10 or 15 years ago that a new disorder would be described in the pediatric and adult literature: CIU. CIU stands for compulsive Internet use. If you have not heard the term, you will be hearing it more and more often. The capacity of the Internet for socialization is a primary reason for the excessive amount of time people spend having real-time interactions using e-mail, discussion forums, chat rooms, and online games.

In adults, the strongest predictor of CIU is visitation to sex sites, but at any age, chatting and gaming have also been shown to be strong correlations with CIU. The capacity for socializing plays a significant role in the addictive nature of various Internet applications. Given the suspected role of socializing, it is not at all surprising that the introduction of social interaction and video games has been accompanied by a parallel increase in reported cases of video game addiction. These video games in many cases show structural characteristics of slot machines, which are known to play a role in pathological gambling. Games can contain aural and visual stimuli with rewards, peer group attention and/or approval, the requirement of total concentration, the keeping of the digital score, and incremental rewards for winning, which reinforce these behaviors. One can actually show off one's rewards in a social way in a truly virtual environment. Interestingly, online games frequently demand much more time from the gamer than offline games.

What the study of van Rooij et al does is to contribute knowledge about CIU by specifically exploring the relationship between the various Internet applications (including online and casual games) and CIU in a large sample of adolescents. There is a validated CIU Scale available to study these issues. This scale covers 5 dimensions of behavior addiction including loss of control, preoccupation, withdrawal symptoms, mood modification, and conflict. Although most Internet applications have a social nature, online gaming is the only example that combines a distinct reward structure, an open-ended design, and a strong social component. All this translates into online games being more demanding or addictive in comparison with other Internet applications. You will need to read this report in some detail to understand the methodology used, but the bottom line is that among adolescents, social networking, MSN use, chatting, blogging, online games, and casual games are all associated with CIU. Online gaming, however, is most strongly associated with CIU, confirming the original hypothesis of these authors. There was no relationship between CIU and surfing or simple e-mailing, although surfing is one of the most popular activities on the Internet. Thus, the absence of an association for surfing and the presence of online gaming as the strongest association indicate that there are differences in the addictive potential of the various Internet activities. CIU is more than simply spending a lot of time online since many surfers do this without becoming addicted.

Hopefully it will not be another 10 years before we learn more about the consequences of CIU. Just imagine what it would be like if a whole generation of adolescents became compulsive gamblers as a result of online gaming, the strongest correlate of CIU. There would not be enough slot machines in the world, much less in Las Vegas, to satisfy such an addiction. Internet use is indeed potentially an addiction since a recent survey from Switzerland shows a U-shaped relation between mental health and internet use in teenagers; an increased risk was seen both in teenagers who were heavy users of the internet (for more than 2 hours of the day) and in those who did not use the internet at all.[1]

J. A. Stockman III, MD

Reference

1. Bélanger RE, Akre C, Berchtold A, et al. A U-Shaped association between intensity of internet use and adolescent health. *Pediatrics*. 2011;127:e330-e335.

Adolescence Sleep Disturbances as Predictors of Adulthood Sleep Disturbances—A Cohort Study

Dregan A, Armstrong D (Univ of Surrey, Guildford, UK; King's College, London, UK)
J Adolesc Health 46:482-487, 2010

Purpose.—The present study aimed to estimate whether sleep disturbances in adolescence predicted sleep disturbances in later years.

Method.—Our sample included 7,781 cohort members from the United Kingdom's National Child Development Study. Sleep disturbances at ages 16, 23, 33, and 42 were measured by asking whether cohort members had difficulties in falling/maintaining sleep or waking unnecessarily early in the morning.

Results.—Multivariate regression analyses indicated that sleep disturbance at age 16 was a significant predictor of sleep disturbances at ages 23, 33, and 42. Continuity of a number of risk factors, especially depression, accounted for some of the persistence of sleep disturbances over time but did not explain a significant part of ongoing sleep disturbance.

Conclusions.—Our findings suggest that many sleep disturbances start in adolescence and continue into later years.

▶ In the United Kingdom, there is a very interesting study underway that tracks a number of different characteristics of enrolled individuals over many decades. The United Kingdom-based National Child Development Study (NCDS) has followed up with 17 415 people born in the United Kingdom between March 3 and March 9, 1958. To date, there have been surveys done of these individuals at ages 7, 11, 16, 23, 33, 42, and 46 years of age. Included in the survey have been a number of questions about sleep. The data from Great Britain therefore are important in providing us longitudinal information about the tracking of sleep disturbances over time. Without question, the NCDS data show that sleep disturbance at the age of 16 years is a significant predictor of sleep disturbances at each subsequent tracking period.

If sleep disturbances do in fact persist over time, this might be explained in a number of different ways. First, there may be a genetic cause that is primary and that persists over one's lifetime. Second, a sleep disturbance early in life may simply be a pattern that becomes established and then later engenders sleep disturbances again over decades, perhaps through some underlying physiologic cause or the creation of a behavioral pattern. Alternatively, ongoing sleep disturbances may be secondary to another quite different factor that persists over time and of which sleep disturbance is simply a symptom. Chronic depression is a classic example of the latter since it can produce lifelong sleep disturbances.

The data from the United Kingdom illustrate that sleep disturbances seem to build from age 16. Certainly the extent to which sleep disturbance in adolescence continues into adult life indicates the potential for the development of a chronic problem, which merits early intervention. Depression seems to be the most important underlying factor that can be addressed. Interestingly, the strongest correlation between sleep disturbances and depression seems to occur early in life. The difference in the life-course trajectories for sleep disturbance and depression implies a decreasing specificity of sleep disturbances for depression with age. It is entirely possible that depression in adolescents creates a behavioral pattern of sleep disturbance even if the depression disappears later in life.

There is a lot more that we need to learn about sleep disturbances not only in adulthood but also in childhood and adolescence. We are grateful to Dregan et al for exploring this topic in a serious way. If you want to learn more about adolescent sleep disturbances and the effect of sleep deprivation on perceived health and attractiveness of sleep-deprived people, see the excellent article on this topic by Axelsson et al.[1] Investigators decided to examine whether sleep deprived people would be perceived as less healthy, less attractive, and more tired than after a normal night's sleep. Participants were photographed after a normal night's sleep (8 hours) and after sleep deprivation (31 hours of wakefulness after a night of reduced sleep). The photographs were presented in randomized order and rated by untrained observers. Sleep-deprived people were rated as significantly less healthy, more tired in appearance and definitely less attractive than after a normal night's sleep. While there are no surprises here, the results of this study suggest that humans are in fact sensitive to sleep-related facial cues with potential implications for social and clinical judgments and behavior. We do need our beauty sleep!

J. A. Stockman III, MD

Reference

1. Axelsson J, Sundelin T, Ingre M, Van Someren EJ, Olsson A, Lekander M. Beauty sleep: experimental study on the perceived health and attractiveness of sleep deprived people. *BMJ.* 2010;341:c6614. doi:10.1136/bmj.c6614.

Effects of a Brief Intervention for Reducing Violence and Alcohol Misuse Among Adolescents: A Randomized Controlled Trial

Walton MA, Chermack ST, Shope JT, et al (Univ of Michigan, Ann Arbor)
JAMA 304:527-535, 2010

Context.—Emergency department (ED) visits present an opportunity to deliver brief interventions to reduce violence and alcohol misuse among urban adolescents at risk of future injury.

Objective.—To determine the efficacy of brief interventions addressing violence and alcohol use among adolescents presenting to an urban ED.

Design, Setting, and Participants.—Between September 2006 and September 2009, 3338 patients aged 14 to 18 years presenting to a level I ED in Flint, Michigan, between 12 PM and 11 PM 7 days a week completed a computerized survey (43.5% male; 55.9% African American). Adolescents reporting past-year alcohol use and aggression were enrolled in a randomized controlled trial (SafERteens).

Intervention.—All patients underwent a computerized baseline assessment and were randomized to a control group that received a brochure (n = 235) or a 35-minute brief intervention delivered by either a computer (n = 237) or therapist (n = 254) in the ED, with follow-up assessments at 3 and 6 months. Combining motivational interviewing with skills training, the brief intervention for violence and alcohol included review of goals, tailored feedback, decisional balance exercise, role plays, and referrals.

Main Outcome Measures.—Self-report measures included peer aggression and violence, violence consequences, alcohol use, binge drinking, and alcohol consequences.

Results.—About 25% (n = 829) of screened patients had positive results for both alcohol and violence; 726 were randomized. Compared with controls, participants in the therapist intervention showed self-reported reductions in the occurrence of peer aggression (therapist, −34.3%; control, −16.4%; relative risk [RR], 0.74; 95% confidence interval [CI], 0.61-0.90), experience of peer violence (therapist, −10.4%; control, +4.7%; RR, 0.70; 95% CI, 0.52-0.95), and violence consequences (therapist, −30.4%; control, −13.0%; RR, 0.76; 95% CI, 0.64-0.90) at 3 months. At 6 months, participants in the therapist intervention showed self-reported reductions in alcohol consequences (therapist, −32.2%; control, −17.7%; odds ratio, 0.56; 95% CI, 0.34-0.91) compared with controls; participants in the computer intervention also showed self-reported reductions in alcohol consequences (computer, −29.1%; control, −17.7%; odds ratio, 0.57; 95% CI, 0.34-0.95).

Conclusion.—Among adolescents identified in the ED with self-reported alcohol use and aggression, a brief intervention resulted in a decrease in the prevalence of self-reported aggression and alcohol consequences.

Trial Registration.—clinicaltrials.gov Identifier: NCT00251212.

▶ The underlying principle of this report is to reach a teenager wherever you find them, in this case in the emergency room, in attempting to intervene with adolescents to reduce violence and alcohol misuse. In this report, adolescents receiving emergency services for illness or injury who reported both alcohol use and physical aggression were randomized to receive a brochure, a 35-minute motivational intervention delivered by a therapist or a self-administered animated computer intervention. Almost 6000 patients aged 14 to 18 years were evaluated. Approximately 4000 were eligible for screening. The findings of the study support the efficacy of a brief intervention given by a therapist in decreasing the occurrence of experiencing peer violence in the 3 months following an emergency room visit. In addition, both the therapist and the computer brief interventions were effective at reducing alcohol consequences over 6 months.

An editorial by Saitz and Naimi[1] suggests that the most proven and effective method to reduce youth drinking and alcohol-related violence is to implement population-based strategies such as raising alcohol excise taxes and enforcing minimum legal drinking age laws. The authors of the editorial suggest that unless the findings of Walton et al can be replicated and possibly improved upon, brief interventions for violence prevention in emergency departments may not yield much benefit.

While on the topic of alcohol, a tongue-in-cheek report appeared recently in the *British Medical Journal* examining alcohol's effect on gastric function and the symptoms of drinking wine, black tea, or schnapps with a swiss cheese fondue.[2] These investigators attempted to compare the effects on gastric emptying of drinking white wine or black tea with swiss cheese fondue followed by a shot of cherry schnapps, using a randomized controlled crossover study of 20 healthy adults age 23 to 58. It was concluded that gastric emptying after a swiss cheese fondue is noticeably slower and appetite is suppressed if consumed with higher doses of alcohol. This effect is not associated with dyspeptic symptoms. Black tea has a prokinetic effect, which promotes gastric emptying. By the way, this study was carried out in Switzerland where cheese fondue is a meal served on festive occasions or just when family and friends gather.

J. A. Stockman III, MD

References

1. Saitz R, Naimi TS. Adolescent alcohol use and violence: are brief interventions the answer? *JAMA*. 2010;304:575-577.
2. Heinrich H, Goetzei O, Menne D. Effect on gastric function in symptoms of drinking wine, black tea or schnapps with a swiss cheese fondue: Randomized controlled crossover trial. *BMJ*. 2010;341:c6731. doi:10.1136/bmj.c6731.

Comparison of Teenagers' Early Same-Sex and Heterosexual Behavior: UK Data From the SHARE and RIPPLE Studies
Parkes A, Strange V, Wight D, et al (Univ of Glasgow, UK; Univ of London, UK; et al)
J Adolesc Health 48:27-35, 2011

Purpose.—North American research finds increased sexual risk-taking among teenagers with same-sex partners, but understanding of underlying processes is limited. The research carried out in the United Kingdom compares teenagers' early sexual experiences according to same- or opposite-sex partner, focusing on unwanted sex in addition to risk-taking, and exploring underlying psychosocial differences.

Methods.—Multivariate analyses combined self-reported data from two randomized control trials of school sex education programs (N = 10,250). Outcomes from sexually experienced teenagers (N = 3,766) were partner pressure to have first sex and subsequent regret, and sexual risk measures including pregnancy. Covariates included self-esteem, future expectations, substance use, and communication with mother.

Results.—By the time of follow-up (mean age, 16), same-sex genital contact (touching or oral or anal) was reported by 2.3% of teenagers, with the majority also reporting heterosexual intercourse. A total of 39% reported heterosexual intercourse and no same-sex genital contact. Boys were more likely to report partner pressure (Odds ratio [OR] = 2.56, 95% confidence intervals [CI] = 1.29–5.08) and regret (OR = 2.32; 95% CI = 1.39–3.86) in relation to first same-sex genital contact than first heterosexual intercourse, but girls showed no differences according to partner type. Teenagers with bisexual behavior reported greater pregnancy or partner pregnancy risk than teenagers with exclusively opposite-sex partners (girls, OR = 4.51, 95% CI = 2.35–8.64; boys, OR = 4.43, 95% CI = 2.41–8.14), partially reduced by attitudinal and behavioral differences.

Conclusions.—This UK study confirms greater reporting of sexual risk-taking among teenagers with same-sex partners, and suggests that boys in this group are vulnerable to unwanted sex. It suggests limitations to the interpretation of differences, in terms of psychosocial risk factors common to all adolescents.

▶ This report emanates from the United Kingdom. Although still aiming to account for differences in the behavior and health of youth with and without same-sex relationships, by applying broadly applicable theories of adolescent development and behavior, Parkes et al took a step in the direction of not assuming the developmental primacy of same-sex attraction. Although these investigators did not find that what had been proposed as the core contributors to healthy development measured in their study (eg, quality of communication with parents), they did observe that these contributors are important for sexual minority youth, just as they are from the broader adolescent population. These data are consistent with findings from other investigators examining healthy development among youth with same-sex attractions documenting the fundamental importance of internal and external assets (eg, social competency, familial and extra-familial contexts that offers support, limits, and positive expectations) deemed critical to healthy adolescent development.[1]

The report of Parkes et al extends the evidence based on early same-sex behavior and describes unwanted sex in addition to risk taking. The results confirm the unique vulnerability of teenagers with same-sex partners and suggest limitations to the interpretation of differences using psychosocial risk factors common to all adolescents. This report is confined to the early sexual experiences of a young age group. More research is needed to establish whether the findings from this report extend to subsequent sexual experiences and to those initiating sexual relationships at an older age. Everyone should agree that homophobic bullying and victimization among school-age teenagers remain commonplace not only in the United Kingdom but also in the United States and likely elsewhere as well.

To read more about health disparities in gender minority teens and the health of lesbian, gay, bisexual, and transgender populations, see the excellent editorials that recently appeared in the *Journal of Adolescent Health* and the *Lancet.*[2,3]

J. A. Stockman III, MD

References

1. Benson PL. *All Kids are Our Kids: What Communities Must do to Raise Caring and Responsible Children and Adolescents.* San Francisco, CA: Jossey-Bass Publishers; 1997.
2. Halpern CT. Same-sex attraction and health disparities: Do sexual minority youth really need something different for healthy development? *J Adolesc Health.* 2011; 48:5-6.
3. The health of lesbian, gay, bisexual and transgender populations. *Lancet.* 2011;377:1211.

Criminal-Justice and School Sanctions Against Nonheterosexual Youth: A National Longitudinal Study

Himmelstein KEW, Brückner H (Yale Univ, New Haven, CT)
Pediatrics 127:49-57, 2011

Objective.—Nonheterosexual adolescents are vulnerable to health risks including addiction, bullying, and familial abuse. We examined whether they also suffer disproportionate school and criminal-justice sanctions.

Methods.—The National Longitudinal Study of Adolescent Health followed a nationally representative sample of adolescents who were in grades 7 through 12 in 1994−1995. Data from the 1994−1995 survey and the 2001−2002 follow-up were analyzed. Three measures were used to assess nonheterosexuality: same-sex attraction, same-sex romantic relationships, and lesbian, gay, or bisexual (LGB) self-identification. Six outcomes were assessed: school expulsion; police stops; juvenile arrest; juvenile conviction; adult arrest; and adult conviction. Multivariate analyses controlled for adolescents' sociodemographics and behaviors, including illegal conduct.

Results.—Nonheterosexuality consistently predicted a higher risk for sanctions. For example, in multivariate analyses, nonheterosexual adolescents had greater odds of being stopped by the police (odds ratio: 1.38 [$P < .0001$] for same-sex attraction and 1.53 [$P < .0001$] for LGB self-identification). Similar trends were observed for school expulsion, juvenile arrest and conviction, and adult conviction. Nonheterosexual girls were at particularly high risk.

Conclusions.—Nonheterosexual youth suffer disproportionate educational and criminal-justice punishments that are not explained by greater engagement in illegal or transgressive behaviors. Understanding and addressing these disparities might reduce school expulsions, arrests, and incarceration and their dire social and health consequences.

▶ Much has been written lately about same-sex discriminatory activity at home, in schools, and in the criminal justice system. This report from Connecticut indicates that nonheterosexual adolescents do, in fact, suffer disproportionate punishments by schools and the criminal justice system as well as other youth-serving health and welfare systems that often fail to meet the needs of nonheterosexual adolescents.

There is now sizable literature documenting elevated risk taking and poor health status among youth who have same-sex attractions, experience same-sex sexual relationships, and/or identify themselves as gay, lesbian, or bisexual. These disparities are evident across multiple domains, including substance abuse, sexual risk behaviors, depression, and suicide ideation and attempts. The greater likelihood of experiencing stigma, harassment, victimization and of witnessing and perpetuating violence—and the stress these experiences can cause—are considered to be important contributors to these behavioral and health differences. The suicides of 5 boys aged 13 to 18 years between July and September, 2010, that were apparently the result of antigay bullying and abuse are tragic personal testimonies of the pain and desperation such victimization may inflict.[1]

J. A. Stockman III, MD

Reference

1. Halpern CT. Same-sex attraction and health disparities: do sexual minority youth really need something different for healthy development? *J Adolesc Health*. 2011; 48:5-6.

Use of Social Networking Sites in Online Sex Crimes Against Minors: An Examination of National Incidence and Means of Utilization

Mitchell KJ, Finkelhor D, Jones LM, et al (Univ of New Hampshire, Durham)
J Adolesc Health 47:183-190, 2010

Purpose.—To describe the variety of ways social networking sites (SNSs) are used to facilitate the sexual exploitation of youth, as well as identify victim, offender, and case differences between arrests, with and without a SNS nexus.

Methods.—Mail surveys were sent to a nationally representative sample of over 2,500 local, state, and federal law enforcement agencies in the United States. Follow-up detailed telephone interviews were conducted for 1,051 individual cases ending in an arrest for Internet-related sex crimes against minors in 2006.

Results.—In the United States, an estimated 2,322 arrests (unweighted n = 291) for Internet sex crimes against minors involved SNSs in some way, including an estimated 503 arrests (unweighted n = 93) in cases involving identified victims and the use of SNSs by offenders (the majority of arrests involved undercover operations undertaken by police). SNSs were used to initiate sexual relationships, to provide a means of communication between victim and offender, to access information about the victim, to disseminate information or pictures about the victim, and to get in touch with victim's friends.

Conclusions.—A considerable number of arrests for Internet sex crimes against minors have a SNS nexus to them. The findings support previous claims that prevention messages should target youth behaviors rather than specific online locations where these crimes occur. In targeting behaviors, youth can take this knowledge with them online, regardless of whether they are using SNSs, chat rooms, or instant messaging.

▶ This is an important report showing evidence of significant linkage between social networking sites, such as MySpace and Facebook, and online sex crimes against minors. Well, more than half of teenagers in the United States are currently using social networking sites. The number of adults signed on has rapidly increased as well. If one looks back to 2008, 35% of American adult Internet users had a profile on a social networking site, around 4 times as many as in 2005. It does not take a rocket scientist to deduce that online predators are using personal information from such sites to stalk and commit crimes, sex or otherwise against the youth of our country. Data from 2006 show an estimated 615 arrests for sex crimes involving online meetings between offenders and teenage victims.[1] While this is a small percentage of the thousands of arrests for all sex crimes against teen victims, the number is still worrisome.

The report of Mitchell et al uses data from a national sample of arrests in 2006 for Internet crimes against minors to explore the incidence of such arrests nationally in a 1-year time frame. The investigators also explored the variety of ways social networking sites are used to commit or facilitate sex crimes against minors. Investigators found an estimated 2322 arrests for Internet sex crimes against minors that involved social networking sites in some way. By far, the largest number of social networking site—related arrests ultimately involves police acting in an undercover capacity. The majority of such cases were initiated in chat rooms. A law enforcement presence on social networking sites serves as a deterrent to potential criminals, given the widespread reporting of such surveillance.

J. A. Stockman III, MD

Reference

1. Wolak J, Finkelhor D, Mitchell KJ. *Trends in Arrests of "Online Predators".* Durham, NH: Crimes Against Children Research Center, University of New Hampshire; 2009; 1-10.

Reasons for and Challenges of Recent Increases in Teen Birth Rates: A Study of Family Planning Service Policies and Demographic Changes at the State Level

Yang Z, Gaydos LM (Emory Univ, Atlanta, GA)

J Adolesc Health 46:517-524, 2010

Purpose.—After declining for over a decade, the birth rate in the United States for adolescents aged 15—19 years increased by 3% in 2006 and 1% again in 2007. We examined demographic and policy reasons for this trend at state level.

Methods.—With data merged from multiple sources, descriptive analysis was used to detect state-level trends in birth rate and policy changes from 2000 to 2006, and variations in the distribution of teen birth rates, sex education, and family planning service policies, and demographic features across each state in 2006. Regression analysis was then conducted to estimate the effect of several reproductive health policies and demographic features on teen birth rates at the state level. Instrument variable was used to correct possible bias in the regression analysis.

Results.—Medicaid family planning waivers were found to reduce teen birth rates across all ages and races. Abstinence-only education programs were found to cause an increase in teen birth rates among white and black teens. The increasing Hispanic population is another driving force for high teen birth rates.

Discussion.—Both demographic factors and policy changes contributed to the increase in teen birth rates between 2000 and 2006. Future policy and behavioral interventions should focus on promoting and increasing access to contraceptive use. Family planning policies should be crafted to address the special needs of teens from different cultural backgrounds, especially Hispanics.

▶ The report of Yang and Gaydos from the Department of Health Policy and Management at Emory University provides new information that extends our knowledge from earlier studies that have also examined the impact of state social programs and/or policies on teen birth rates. Currently there is wide variation in rates of teen pregnancy and childbearing. In 2006, for example, the birth rate for Mississippi was 68.4 births per 1000 in the 15- to 19-year-old age group for women. This figure was almost 4 times higher than the birth rate for New Hampshire. As high as these numbers seem, teen births actually declined by 20% in Mississippi in the 15-year period prior to 2006. In New Hampshire, they declined by some 44%. Much of the differences, however, obviously relate to differences in the profile of the populations of these states. Take, for example, Texas and California, states with large minority populations and a rapidly growing Hispanic population. In 1991, both states had sizable rates of teen fertility (78.4 in Texas and 73.8 in California) but have diverged greatly since then, with teen rates by 2006 in Texas being 1.6 times that of California. Between 1991 and 2006, the birth rate in Texas declined by 19%, whereas it declined by 46% in California. To say this differently, California was almost 2.5 times more successful in reducing its teen birth rate than Texas was. Much of these differences between states have to do with state-based policies that were instituted related to teen fertility.

Yang and Gaydos examined differences among states in their declines in teen birth rates between 2000 and 2006. They observed that state Medicaid family planning waivers were associated with lower teen birth rates for every group looked at (younger and older teens and white, black, and Hispanic teens), while state policies favoring abstinence-only programs were associated with higher teen birth rates. Public policies requiring parental consent for abortion and contraceptive conscious laws were associated with higher teen birth rates in certain subgroups but not overall. Social factors such as lower rates of high school graduation and increased religiosity were also associated with increased teen birth rates. An increased proportion of Hispanics in a state was also associated with increased overall teen birth rates.

One can draw a number of conclusions from this new study of Yang and Gaydos. One is that one must look at both social and demographic characteristics of states and state policies when assessing teen fertility rates. Specifically, socioeconomic status, social capital, religious beliefs, racial/ethnic differences, the use of Medicaid waiver, and sex education policies must be examined individually and in aggregate. At the same time, one cannot disassociate social convictions and societal beliefs. For example, socially conservative states are more likely to adopt abstinence-only policies, whereas socially liberal states may be more likely to focus on improved access to contraceptive services. These 2 approaches have widely different outcomes in terms of teen fertility rates.

To read more about what really does and does not make a difference on teen fertility rates, see the excellent editorial on this topic by Santelli and Kirby.[1] Also, see the summary which appeared in a recent *Morbidity and Mortality Weekly Report* dealing with teen pregnancy rates.[2] You will see that in 2009, approximately 410 000 teens aged 15 to 19 years gave birth in the United States and that the teen birth rate remains higher than in other developed countries. However, teen birth rates have actually declined, especially among black and Hispanic teens and in southern states. Fewer high school students are having sexual intercourse, and more sexually active students are using some method of contraception.

J. A. Stockman III, MD

References

1. Santelli J, Kirby D. State policy effects on teen fertility and evidence-based policies. *J Adolesc Health*. 2010;46:515-516.
2. Centers for Disease Control and Prevention (CDC). Vital signs: Teen pregnancy— United States, 1991–2009. *MMWR Morb Mortal Wkly Rep*. 2011;60:414-422.

Recent Changes in the Trends of Teen Birth Rates, 1981–2006

Wingo PA, Smith RA, Tevendale HD, et al (Ctrs for Disease Control and Prevention, Atlanta, GA)
J Adolesc Health 48:281-288, 2011

Purpose.—To explore trends in teen birth rates by selected demographics.

Methods.—We used birth certificate data and joinpoint regression to examine trends in teen birth rates by age (10–14, 15–17, and 18–19 years) and race during 1981–2006 and by age and Hispanic origin during 1990–2006. Joinpoint analysis describes changing trends over successive segments of time and uses annual percentage change (APC) to express the amount of increase or decrease within each segment.

Results.—For teens younger than 18 years, the decline in birth rates began in 1994 and ended in 2003 (APC: −8.03% per year for ages 10–14 years; APC: −5.63% per year for ages 15–17 years). The downward trend for 18- and 19-year-old teens began earlier (1991) and ended 1 year later (2004) (APC: −2.37% per year). For each study population, the trend was approximately level during the most recent time segment, except for continuing declines for 18- and 19-year-old white and Asian/Pacific Islander teens. The only increasing trend in the most recent time segment was for 18- and 19-year-old Hispanic teens. During these declines, the age distribution of teens who gave birth shifted to slightly older ages, and the percentage whose current birth was at least their second birth decreased.

Conclusions.—Teen birth rates were generally level during 2003/2004–2006 after the long-term declines. Rates increased among older Hispanic teens. These results indicate a need for renewed attention to effective teen pregnancy prevention programs in specific populations.

▶ The United States has the highest teen birth rate in the developed world. In 2006, the birth rate for 15- to 19-year-olds was 41.9 births per 1000 females. Other countries with high rates include New Zealand (28.1 in 2006) and the United Kingdom (26.7 in 2004). At the other end of the spectrum, teen birth rates were less than 7 per 1000 females in Korea, Japan, Switzerland, and the Netherlands. Similar low numbers are seen in Sweden and Italy. If one scratches the surface a bit, however, one will see that teen birth rates here in the United States have declined substantially throughout the 1990s and early 2000s from a high of 61.8 births per 1000 females in 1991 to a historic low of 40.5 in 2005. Explanations for this decline have included delayed age at the initiation of sexual intercourse and improved contraception. Induced abortion and fetal loss rates for teens actually declined during this time period.

Wingo et al used birth certificate data to examine trends in teenage birth rates by specific age groups, race, and by looking at other selected demographics. The data show that the greatest declines were seen for 18- and 19-year-old white and Asian/Pacific Islander teens. An increasing trend was actually seen for 18- to 19-year-old Hispanic teens. Also, there was a shift to a slightly older age for first birth in teens.

Lipman et al have examined the young adult outcomes of children born to teen mothers.[1] The authors compared children of nonteen mothers and the young adult children of teen mothers. Clearly the latter experienced poor overall life outcomes. The adverse effects were statistically significant in the areas of education, life satisfaction, and personal income for young adults born to teen mothers. While there are no surprises here, the Lipman et al report provides clear documentation of the problem of giving birth early in one's life in our current society.

One of the bright spots about teen birth rates relates to the fact that teens are more and more frequently using contraceptives. Indeed, condoms are easier to obtain, particularly in New York City. If you need a condom in a hurry, just pop out your iPhone and search New York City's Health Department database and you will find information on over 1000 locations where free condoms can be obtained. The health department has launched an app for both iPhones and Android phones for this purpose. New York distributes on average some 3 million free condoms each month.

J. A. Stockman III, MD

Reference

1. Lipman EL, Georgiades K, Boyle MH. Young adult outcomes of children born to teen mothers: effects of being born during their teen or later years. *J Am Acad Child Adolesc Psychiatr.* 2011;50:232-241.

How Are Restrictive Abortion Statutes Associated With Unintended Teen Birth?

Coles MS, Makino KK, Stanwood NL, et al (Univ of Rochester, NY)
J Adolesc Health 47:160-167, 2010

Purpose.—Legislation that restricts abortion access decreases abortion. It is less well understood whether these statutes affect unintended birth. Given recent increases in teen pregnancy and birth, we examined the relationship between legislation that restricts abortion access and unintended births among adolescent women.

Methods.—Using 2000–2005 Pregnancy Risk Assessment Monitoring System data, we examined the relationship between adolescent pregnancy intention and policies affecting abortion access: mandatory waiting periods, parental involvement laws, and Medicaid funding restrictions. Logistic regression controlled for individual characteristics, state-level factors, geographic regions, and time trends. Subgroup analyses were done for racial, ethnic, and insurance groups.

Results.—In our multivariate model, minors in states with mandatory waiting periods were more than two times as likely to report an unintended birth, with even higher risk among blacks, Hispanics, and teens receiving Medicaid. Medicaid funding restrictions were associated with higher rates of unwanted birth among black teens. Parental involvement laws were associated with a trend toward more unwanted births in white minors and fewer in Hispanic minors.

Conclusions.—Mandatory waiting periods are associated with higher rates of unintended birth in teens, and funding restrictions may especially affect black adolescents. Policies limiting access to abortion appear to affect the outcomes of unintended teen pregnancy. Subsequent research should clarify the magnitude of such effects, and lead to policy changes that successfully reduce unintended teen births.

▶ Whether you are pro-life or pro-choice, the information from this report will be important in understanding how legislative statutes affect teen births. Minors living in states with mandatory waiting periods prior to abortion will experience a more than 2-fold increased likelihood of giving birth to a child that in the definition of this report was mistimed or unwanted. Also noted was an increased likelihood of mistimed and unwanted births among certain minority groups in states with Medicaid funding restrictions on abortion.

This report is among the first to investigate the relationship between pregnancy intention and restrictive abortion statutes. Obviously those who are pro-choice will interpret the data to mean that restrictive statutes result in more unintended births and recognize that such statutes encourage the greater likelihood of carrying a baby to term.

The July 31, 2010, edition of *The Lancet* contained a film review of 12th & Delaware. This was a film directed by Rachel Grady and Heidi Ewing that aired as an HBO film broadcast on August 2 and August 5, 2010. The film describes 2 women and their relationship with a pro-life and pro-choice pair of clinics. Candice opened a Women's World health clinic on the corner of 12th & Delaware in a nondescript Florida neighborhood. Anne and her colleagues across the street have opened the Pregnancy Care Center supported by a religious entity seeking to persuade women not to have abortions. The directors of the film did not insert themselves into the abortion debate. By showing the inner workings of the 2 clinics and by portraying Candice and Anne as 3-dimensional women with solid convictions and emotional investment in the respective causes, 12th & Delaware likely comes as close to a balanced portrayal of abortion as one will probably see here in our country. The most poignant aspects of the film, however, are the portrayals of the individual women who come to the clinics and who reach, for whatever reason, the decisions that they make. The film review itself was written by Danielle Ofri from the Department of Medicine, New York University School of Medicine in New York City.[1]

J. A. Stockman III, MD

Reference

1. Ofri D. Film review. Abortion: the view from both sides of the street. *Lancet.* 2010;376:321.

Induced First-Trimester Abortion and Risk of Mental Disorder

Munk-Olsen T, Laursen TM, Pedersen CB, et al (Aarhus Univ, Denmark; et al)
N Engl J Med 364:332-339, 2011

Background.—Concern has been expressed about potential harm to women's mental health in association with having an induced abortion, but it remains unclear whether induced abortion is associated with an increased risk of subsequent psychiatric problems.

Methods.—We conducted a population-based cohort study that involved linking information from the Danish Civil Registration system to the Danish Psychiatric Central Register and the Danish National Register of Patients The information consisted of data for girls and women with no record of mental disorders during the 1995−2007 period who had a first-trimester induced abortion or a first childbirth during that period. We estimated the rates of first-time psychiatric contact (an inpatient admission or outpatient visit) for any type of mental disorder within the 12 months after the abortion or childbirth as compared with the 9-month period preceding the event.

Results.—The incidence rates of first psychiatric contact per 1000 person-years among girls and women who had a first abortion were 14.6 (95% confidence interval [CI], 13.7 to 15.6) before abortion and 15.2 (95% CI, 14.4 to 16.1) after abortion. The corresponding rates among girls and women who had a first childbirth were 3.9 (95% CI, 3.7 to 4.2) before delivery and 6.7 (95% CI, 6.4 to 7.0) post partum. The relative risk of a psychiatric contact did not differ significantly after abortion as compared with before abortion (P=0.19) but did increase after childbirth as compared with before childbirth (P<0.001).

Conclusions.—The finding that the incidence rate of psychiatric contact was similar before and after a first-trimester abortion does not support the hypothesis that there is an increased risk of mental disorders after a first-trimester induced abortion. (Funded by the Susan Thompson Buffett Foundation and the Danish Medical Research Council).

▶ This is an important report. Many have suggested over the years that having an induced abortion can result in lingering mental health problems on the part of a woman who has decided to have that abortion. Studies done to date in this regard, however, have had a number of limitations, including small and self-selected study samples, low response, and high dropout rates during the follow-up period as well as the lack of control for potential confounders and inadequate measures of exposure and outcome variables. Many of the studies did not control for the other stressors that a pregnant woman may have been under at the time they had to make a decision about obtaining an abortion.

Munk-Olsen et al have attempted to address the deficiencies of prior reports, suggesting a link between induced abortion and mental health problems by designing a cohort study involving national registry data to assess the risk of first psychiatric contact after first-trimester induced abortion, as compared with the period before the event. Data from the Danish Civil Registration

System were used for this purpose. There are no private psychiatric hospitals in Denmark. The registry contains information on all admissions to psychiatric inpatient facilities in that country. The database for all admissions has been computerized since 1969. The psychiatric registry holds information on more than 725 000 persons. It should be noted that induced abortions became legal in Denmark in 1973. Any woman (aged 18 years or older) can have a termination of a pregnancy within the first 12 weeks' gestation. Permission from parents or legal guardians is required for pregnant girls younger than 18 years. The Danish National Registry of Patients includes information on all induced abortions performed in Denmark, except abortions performed by practicing specialists at private clinics, which are extremely small in number. The study population in this report consisted of girls and women born in Denmark between 1962 and 1993 who were alive and had no history of a mental disorder, defined as inpatient psychiatric contact 9 months before a first-ever induced abortion or first childbirth.

During the period from 1995 to 2007, a total of 8620 girls and women had a first-time first-trimester induced abortion. The incidence rates of psychiatric contacts were 14.6 per 1000 person-years before abortion and 15.2 per 1000 person-years postabortion. During the same study period, a total of 280 930 girls and women gave birth to their first live-born child. Of these girls and women, 790 had a first-time psychiatric contact within the 9 months preceding delivery, as did 1916 from 0 to 12 months postpartum. The incidence rate of psychiatric contacts was 3.9 per 1000 person-years before childbirth and 6.7 per 1000 person-years after childbirth. The risk of a psychiatric contact did not differ significantly before and after abortion, but the risk after childbirth was significantly greater than the risk before childbirth.

In summary, in Denmark, where termination of pregnancy is legal and freely available until the 12th week of gestation, there is no significant increase in the incidence of psychiatric contact in the 12 months after a first-trimester abortion as compared with the 9-month period before the abortion. The incidence of psychiatric contact was higher among girls and women who underwent an abortion than among those who underwent delivery, but this relationship was evident before the abortion or childbirth occurred. On the basis of these results, it seems likely that girls and women having induced abortions constitute a population with a somewhat higher psychiatric morbidity to begin with. The authors of this report chose to view this as a selection phenomenon rather than a causal association because the observed difference in psychiatric morbidity between girls and women having abortions and girls and women delivering antedated the abortion or delivery.

For those who are interested in this topic, it would be worthwhile to read this report in detail. You will see summaries of data from New Zealand and from the US National Longitudinal Survey of Youth. Both these studies suggested a higher risk of mental illness in girls and women undergoing abortion. The investigators from Denmark reviewed these 2 studies in detail and noted methodologic problems associated with the study design of these 2 reports. You should be your own judge, however, in interpreting all the data that are available on this topic. That said, the study from Denmark does seem to be bulletproof in terms of rigor and the accuracy of the study design itself.

J. A. Stockman III, MD

Changes in Ambulatory Health Care Use During the Transition to Young Adulthood

Callahan ST, Cooper WO (Vanderbilt Univ Med Ctr, Nashville, TN)
J Adolesc Health 46:407-413, 2010

Purpose.—To identify changes in ambulatory health care use during the transition from adolescence to young adulthood.

Methods.—We analyzed data from health care encounters for adolescents (13–18 year olds) and young adults (19–24 year olds) in the National Ambulatory Medical Care Surveys or National Hospital Ambulatory Medical Care Surveys from 1997 through 2004. We present bivariate analysis of visit characteristics (including clinician specialty and health care setting, primary reason for the visit, and expected source of payment) for young adults as compared with those for adolescents, using weights provided by the National Center for Health Statistics to make national estimates.

Results.—Adolescents and young adults used similar number of health care visits annually; however, a greater proportion of ambulatory care for young adults was delivered in emergency departments as compared with adolescents (20% vs. 14%; $p < .001$), a smaller proportion was delivered to males (27% vs. 46%; $p < .001$), and a smaller proportion was covered by private health insurance (58% vs. 67%, respectively; $p < .001$). Among young adults, preventive care was listed as the reason for 40% of non–emergency department visits for females, whereas it accounted for only 10% of visits for males.

Conclusions.—Significant changes in ambulatory health care use occur during young adulthood. Improving health care during the transition to adulthood will necessitate attention to health care research and delivery agendas that are relevant to the young adult population.

▶ It is hard to believe, but it is true: based on information from this report, young adults are actually worse off than adolescents in terms of the type of care they receive in the US health care system. Using data from the National Ambulatory Care and National Hospital Ambulatory Care Surveys, Callahan et al document the changing pattern of health care use when adolescents (aged 13-18 years) enter adulthood (19-24 years). Even though the 2 groups represent similar numbers of annual visits, there are major differences in the settings in which care is received, the reasons for visits, the physician specialties providing care, and the sources of payment for the services received. Young adults as opposed to adolescents receive a significantly greater proportion of their ambulatory care in emergency departments, a larger portion of their care is not covered by insurance, and gender differences become more apparent in all areas of health care use. Obstetricians/gynecologists provide more of the care to young adult females than any other specialist, and preventive care is the major reason for this nonemergency care. The increase in preventive care for young adult females when compared with adolescent females is related to the increase in care for reproductive health. Again, no surprise. However, young adult men tell a totally different story. General or adult medicine physicians deliver most of their care, with preventive care being the least likely reason for a visit and with acute problems dominating the reasons for seeking care.

In an editorial that accompanied this report, Irwin tells us about 5 crucial factors that emerge from the data of the report by Callahan et al: (1) insurance matters, (2) primary care specialists change, (3) males have greater barriers to accessing primary care than females, (4) clinical guidelines need to be developed to improve the quality and content of care that young adults receive, and (5) young adulthood remains a missed opportunity for preventive interventions.[1] In our country, young adults are twice as likely to be uninsured than any other age segment of our population. This is largely secondary to the loss of private or public coverage that they held as children, fewer opportunities for traditional employment-based coverage, and the inability to purchase health insurance independently. Most young adults will have time during which they do not have insurance, leading them not to seek care when they need it and to high rates of emergency department use. Data from the surveys mentioned show that 1 in 3 visits of the young adult to an emergency room turns out not to be covered by any form of insurance. When young adults do receive care, they do so with care providers who, by and large (with the exception of the American College of Obstetricians and Gynecologists), do not have clinical guidelines available for the management of this age group. Without specific age guidelines for screening and anticipatory guidance for young adults aged 21 years and older, clinicians may not know what should be included in an annual preventive visit. The American Academy of Pediatrics Bright Futures does provide preventive care guidelines but only through the 21st year of life.

Young adulthood should be thought of as a critical point in one's life cycle, a time where the bird has been kicked from the nest, a time during which the young adult should be beginning to assume responsibility for his/her own care and also developing a relationship with a primary care provider. If the young adult does not seize this opportunity, he or she may well drift deeper into adulthood with no roots in the health care system. It is time for our family medicine and general internal medicine colleagues to delve more deeply into the problem of the transitional age patient. Yes, these care providers are inundated with the elderly who need care, but an ounce of preventive care at an early age can go a long way in mitigating against many adult diseases.

With other commentaries in this section discussing the transition from adolescence into adulthood and commenting frequently on birth rates and sexual activity in teens, we close with a question about sexuality this in the opposite end of the age spectrum: the elderly. The question is, how important is sex considered to be by men aged 75 to 95 years? The answer to this query comes from an extensive study reported by Hyde et al.[2] A total of 2783 men provided data on sexual activity. Sex was considered at least somewhat important by 48.8%. In the prior 12 months, 30.8% had had one sexual encounter. Of the latter, 56.5% were satisfied with the frequency of activity whereas 43.0% had less sex than preferred. Increasing age, partner's lack of interest, partner's physical limitations, osteoporosis, prostate cancer, diabetes, antidepressant use, and beta blocker use were independently associated with decreased signs of sexual activity. In a longitudinal analysis, higher testosterone levels were associated with increased odds of being sexually active. By age group, 42% of men 75 to 79 years of age indicated that sex was not at all important; this percentage rose to 58% in those 80 to 84, 70% in those 85 to 89, and 82% in those 90 to 95.

J. A. Stockman III, MD

References

1. Irwin CE Jr. Young adults are worse off than adolescents. *J Adolesc Health.* 2010; 46:405-406.
2. Hyde Z, Flicker L, Hankey GJ, et al. Prevalence of sexual activity and associated factors in men age 75-95 years. *Ann Intern Med.* 2010;153:693-702.

2 Allergy and Dermatology

Nanofiltered C1 Inhibitor Concentrate for Treatment of Hereditary Angioedema

Zuraw BL, Busse PJ, White M, et al (Univ of California, San Diego; Mt. Sinai School of Medicine, NY; Inst for Asthma and Allergy, Wheaton, MD; et al)
N Engl J Med 363:513-522, 2010

Background.—Hereditary angioedema due to C1 inhibitor deficiency is characterized by recurrent acute attacks of swelling that can be painful and sometimes life-threatening.

Methods.—We conducted two randomized trials to evaluate nanofiltered C1 inhibitor concentrate in the management of hereditary angioedema. The first study compared nano-filtered C1 inhibitor concentrate with placebo for treatment of an acute attack of angioedema. A total of 68 subjects (35 in the C1 inhibitor group and 33 in the placebo group) were given one or two intravenous injections of the study drug (1000 units each). The primary end point was the time to the onset of unequivocal relief. The second study was a crossover trial involving 22 subjects with hereditary angio edema that compared prophylactic twice-weekly injections of nanofiltered C1 inhibitor concentrate (1000 units) with placebo during two 12-week periods. The primary end point was the number of attacks of angioedema per period, with each subject acting as his or her own control.

Results.—In the first study, the median time to the onset of unequivocal relief from an attack was 2 hours in the subjects treated with C1 inhibitor concentrate but longer than 4 hours in those given placebo (P = 0.02). In the second study, the number of attacks per 12-week period was 6.26 with C1 inhibitor concentrate given as prophylaxis, as compared with 12.73 with placebo (P<0.001); the subjects who received the C1 inhibitor concentrate also had significant reductions in both the severity and the duration of attacks, in the need for open-label rescue therapy, and in the total number of days with swelling.

Conclusions.—In subjects with hereditary angioedema, nanofiltered C1 inhibitor concentrate shortened the duration of acute attacks. When used for prophylaxis, nanofiltered C1 inhibitor concentrate reduced the frequency of acute attacks. (Funded by Lev Pharmaceuticals; ClinicalTrials.gov numbers, NCT00289211, NCT01005888, NCT00438815, and NCT00462709.)

▶ Hereditary angioedema is an autosomal dominant disorder. It is a fairly rare disorder. It has been estimated that its prevalence ranges anywhere from 1 in 10 000 to 1 in 50 000 live births. The clinical presentation is that of episodic, nonpruritic, localized, subcutaneous and submucosal swelling. The attacks of edema can involve the larynx, oropharynx, face, gastrointestinal (GI) tract, extremities, and/or genitalia. Death can result from respiratory obstruction. Attacks can occur unpredictably and may persist for several days. When the GI tract is affected, it can result in severe pain, vomiting, and diarrhea. More than 1 patient has been operated on unnecessarily. These attacks, when they do occur, generally do not respond to antihistamines, steroids, or epinephrine.

Just less than half a century ago, hereditary angioedema was linked to a deficiency of the plasma inhibitor of the first component of complement (C1 inhibitor). It is a serine protease inhibitor that inactivates target proteases by irreversible binding. Several mutations have been described to cause hereditary angioedema. All of them result in low plasma levels of C1 inhibitor (type 1 disease), while a few produce inactive protein and normal plasma levels (type 2 disease). To date, treatments have been designed to restore normal C1 inhibitor levels through direct replacement, stimulation of C1 inhibitor synthesis, or reduced C1 inhibitor consumption (protease inhibitors). Androgens can directly stimulate C1 inhibitor biosynthesis in some cases. Androgens and protease inhibitors are used primarily for prophylaxis but are frequently ineffective or have excessive side effects of continuous use. For these reasons, replacement with plasma-derived C1 inhibitor has been preferred as part of the management of acute attacks for several decades now. A purified C1 inhibitor was first licensed more than 30 years ago in Europe. It was never approved in the United States because of concerns about possible transmission of viruses, particularly hepatitis C virus. Deaths in Europe are rare, but in the United States, death rates from hereditary angioedema have remained high despite other forms of aggressive management.

The report of Zuraw et al tells us about 2 randomized trials that have evaluated nanofiltered C1 inhibitor concentrate as part of the management of hereditary angioedema. The use of nanofiltration, along with pasteurization of the product used in this study is stated to have provided an additional level of safety against enveloped and nonenveloped viruses and new infectious agents such as prions. The data from this report document that during acute attacks nanofiltered C1 inhibitor concentrate significantly reduces the time to relief of symptoms, when compared with placebo. Also, when used for prophylaxis, C1 inhibitors significantly reduce the frequency of acute attacks when compared with placebo.

Subjects with hereditary angioedema who are at high risk for acute attacks do require prophylactic treatment as used in Europe. Short-term prophylaxis is routinely given before dental procedures or other situations likely to precipitate an attack. Data to date suggest that C1 inhibitor replacement in the form of either fresh frozen plasma or C1 inhibitor concentrate is effective for this purpose.

It was only in 2009 that the FDA approved the use of a pasteurized C1 inhibitor as part of the management of hereditary angioedema in the United States. Since then, efforts have been made to further reduce the risk of virus transmission. Nanofiltration in addition to heat inactivation hopefully will eliminate most viruses. Under development now is a recombinant C1 inhibitor. It is questionable whether this synthetic product will be needed since concern about the safety of plasma-derived products has largely been resolved. Also available is a relatively new agent, ecallantide, a 60-amino acid protein that also shows effectiveness in recent clinical trials.[1] This agent was also approved by the FDA for treatment of acute attacks in 2009. This agent works as a specific kallikrein inhibitor.

Chances are that one will not have a patient with hereditary angioedema in one's practice, given the infrequency of this disorder. However, it is one that we should be aware of in the differential diagnosis of severe attacks of angioedema. It has only been within the last few years in the United States that effective agents have become available for the management of acute attacks of hereditary angioedema. Thus far, 3 agents have been approved by the FDA (the third agent is icatibant, also a kinin inhibitor). Thus far, only nanofiltered C1 inhibitor concentrate has been tested for prophylactic usage.

In this commentary, we conclude with an observation having to do with accidental autoinjection of epinephrine. Obviously, people carry "epi" injectors if they are at risk for severe allergic reactions including anaphylaxis. A retrospective cohort of 365 cases reported to 6 poison centers in the United States over a 6-year period found that everyone who came to the attention of care providers who had this problem recovered completely and no substantial systemic effects were reported. Only 23% of those followed up had actually required any vasodilatory treatment.[2]

J. A. Stockman III, MD

References

1. Cicardi M, Levy RJ, McNeil DL, et al. Ecallantide for the treatment of acute attacks in hereditary angioedema. *N Engl J Med*. 2010;363:523-531.
2. Muck A, Bebarta V, Borys D, Morgan DL. Six years of epinephrine digital injections: absence of significant local or systemic effects. *Ann Emerg Med*. 2010;56: 270-274.

Exposure to Environmental Microorganisms and Childhood Asthma
Ege MJ, for the GABRIELA Transregio 22 Study Group (Univ Children's Hosp Munich, Germany; et al)
N Engl J Med 364:701-709, 2011

Background.—Children who grow up in environments that afford them a wide range of microbial exposures, such as traditional farms, are protected from childhood asthma and atopy. In previous studies, markers of microbial exposure have been inversely related to these conditions.

Methods.—In two cross-sectional studies, we compared children living on farms with those in a reference group with respect to the prevalence of asthma and atopy and to the diversity of microbial exposure. In one study — PARSIFAL (Prevention of Allergy — Risk Factors for Sensitization in Children Related to Farming and Anthroposophic Lifestyle) — samples of mattress dust were screened for bacterial DNA with the use of single-strand conformation polymorphism (SSCP) analyses to detect environmental bacteria that cannot be measured by means of culture techniques. In the other study — GABRIELA (Multidisciplinary Study to Identify the Genetic and Environmental Causes of Asthma in the European Community [GABRIEL] Advanced Study) — samples of settled dust from children's rooms were evaluated for bacterial and fungal taxa with the use of culture techniques.

Results.—In both studies, children who lived on farms had lower prevalences of asthma and atopy and were exposed to a greater variety of environmental microorganisms than the children in the reference group. In turn, diversity of microbial exposure was inversely related to the risk of asthma (odds ratio for PARSIFAL, 0.62; 95% confidence interval [CI], 0.44 to 0.89; odds ratio for GABRIELA, 0.86; 95% CI, 0.75 to 0.99). In addition, the presence of certain more circumscribed exposures was also inversely related to the risk of asthma; this included exposure to species in the fungal taxon eurotium (adjusted odds ratio, 0.37; 95% CI, 0.18 to 0.76) and to a variety of bacterial species, including *Listeria monocytogenes*, bacillus species, corynebacterium species, and others (adjusted odds ratio, 0.57; 95% CI, 0.38 to 0.86).

Conclusions.—Children living on farms were exposed to a wider range of microbes than were children in the reference group, and this exposure explains a substantial fraction of the inverse relation between asthma and growing up on a farm. (Funded by the Deutsche Forschungsgemeinschaft and the European Commission.)

▶ This is another report suggesting that it is far better to have had multiple exposures very young in life than not when it comes to the development of allergies. Specifically, environmental exposure to microorganisms has been repeatedly found to be inversely related to the manifestations of atopic diseases such as asthma and hay fever. Studies from around the world have verified this.

The report of Ege et al underscores the fact that if you live in a home where the buffalo roam (metaphorically speaking), you are far better off allergy wise. Their investigation took place in Europe and demonstrated that children growing up on farms in central Europe were significantly protected from asthma and atopy. Needless to say, children so exposed grew up surrounded by fungi and bacteria. The data support the idea that the greater diversity of microbial exposure among children who live on farms is associated with protection from the development of asthma. Even living indoors, children born and bred on farms were exposed to a greater variety of microbes than children who did not live on farms. The authors of this report speculate about how the diversity of microbial stimuli might be protective against asthma. They suggest that microorganisms could trigger the innate immune system through pattern recognition receptors. Activation of several such receptors has been found in children exposed to farming environments. It is also suggested that environmental exposure to a broad range of microorganisms may prevent colonization of the lower airways with harmful bacteria, which has been associated with an increased risk of asthma among children and adults.

Obviously, being raised on a farm is not common for most citizens on American shores. There is, however, a lot to be learned from the information provided by the report of Ege et al. It will be interesting to see how useful this information is to city dwellers. Should young ones encased in the shadows of high rises be farmed out for the summer months to reduce the prevalence of asthma and hay fever later in life? Good question. If it is not possible to go to summer camp or spend time on a farm, the alternative is to get a dog for your child and do that very early in life. A recent report by Epstein et al notes that the relationship between skin test result positivity to dog or cat at 1, 2, or 3 years of age and eczema at 4 years of age depends on whether the child lived with a dog or cat during the first year of life.[1] In their examination of eczema in this cohort, the investigators reported that exposure to a dog in the home was protective of asthma at 2 and 3 years of age, approximately halving the risk. The relationship of a positive skin test result and eczema with respect to exposure to a cat is exactly the opposite. Children who have lived with a cat during the first year of life and who have a skin test result positive for cat allergen have more than 13-fold increased risk of eczema by 4 years of age. Needless to say, cats are proof positive that the maker did not intend for everything created to have a useful (or any) purpose.

J. A. Stockman III, MD

Reference

1. Epstein TG, Bernstein DI, Levin L, et al. Opposing effects of cat and dog ownership and allergic sensitization on eczema and atopic birth cohort. *J Pediatr.* 2011; 158:265-271.

Use of beclomethasone dipropionate as rescue treatment for children with mild persistent asthma (TREXA): a randomised, double-blind, placebo-controlled trial

Martinez FD, Chinchilli VM, Morgan WJ, et al (Univ of Arizona, Tucson; Penn State Hershey College of Medicine, PA; et al)
Lancet 377:650-657, 2011

Background.—Daily inhaled corticosteroids are an effective treatment for mild persistent asthma, but some children have exacerbations even with good day-to-day control, and many discontinue treatment after becoming asymptomatic. We assessed the effectiveness of an inhaled corticosteroid (beclomethasone dipropionate) used as rescue treatment.

Methods.—In this 44-week, randomised, double-blind, placebo-controlled trial we enrolled children and adolescents with mild persistent asthma aged 5—18 years from five clinical centres in the USA. A computer-generated randomisation sequence, stratified by clinical centre and age group, was used to randomly assign participants to one of four treatment groups: twice daily beclomethasone with beclomethasone plus albuterol as rescue (combined group); twice daily beclomethasone with placebo plus albuterol as rescue (daily beclomethasone group); twice daily placebo with beclomethasone plus albuterol as rescue (rescue beclomethasone group); and twice daily placebo with placebo plus albuterol as rescue (placebo group). Twice daily beclomethasone treatment was one puff of beclomethasone (40 μg per puff) or placebo given in the morning and evening. Rescue beclomethasone treatment was two puffs of beclomethasone or placebo for each two puffs of albuterol (180 μg) needed for symptom relief. The primary outcome was time to first exacerbation that required oral corticosteroids. A secondary outcome measured linear growth. Analysis was by intention to treat. This study is registered with clinicaltrials.gov, number NCT00394329.

Results.—843 children and adolescents were enrolled into this trial, of whom 288 were assigned to one of four treatment groups; combined (n=71), daily beclomethasone (n=72), rescue beclomethasone (n=71), and placebo (n=74)—555 individuals were excluded during the run-in, according to predefined criteria. Compared with the placebo group (49%, 95% CI 37—61), the frequency of exacerbations was lower in the daily (28%, 18—40, p=0·03), combined (31%, 21—43, p=0·07), and rescue (35%, 24—47, p=0·07) groups. Frequency of treatment failure was 23% (95% CI 14—43) in the placebo group, compared with 5·6% (1·6-14) in the combined (p=0·012), 2·8% (0—10) in the daily (p=0·009), and 8·5% (2—15) in the rescue (p=0·024) groups. Compared with the placebo group, linear growth was 1·1 cm (SD 0·3) less in the combined and daily arms (p<0·0001), but not the rescue group (p=0·26). Only two individuals had severe adverse events; one in the daily beclomethasone group had viral meningitis and one in the combined group had bronchitis.

Interpretation.—Children with mild persistent asthma should not be treated with rescue albuterol alone and the most effective treatment to prevent exacerbations is daily inhaled corticosteroids. Inhaled corticosteroids as rescue medication with albuterol might be an effective step-down strategy for children with well controlled, mild asthma because it is more effective at reducing exacerbations than is use of rescue albuterol alone. Use of daily inhaled corticosteroid treatment and related side-effects such as growth impairment can therefore be avoided.

▶ This report is an important one and adds useful information to our knowledge about the management of children with mild persistent asthma. It also reflects on 2 essential and related challenges that continue to exist in the treatment of childhood asthma. One involves what the best strategy is for discontinuing treatment in children with well-controlled mild asthma but who are still at risk for exacerbations. The second challenge involves whether there is a treatment regimen that will decrease the risk of exacerbations in children with mild disease to a greater extent than is achieved with daily inhaled corticosteroids. In children with mild persistent asthma, guidelines recommend the daily use of inhaled corticosteroids in low doses as the preferred treatment for the control of symptoms and asthma exacerbations. For children whose illness is well controlled with such treatment, no studies have established the optimum period for which treatment should be maintained. Guidelines suggest weaning or withdrawal (step-down) of treatment after asthma control is achieved and maintained but with no clear evidence to support these recommendations.

The report of Martinez et al gives us information from a study known as rescue treatment for children with mild persistent asthma (TREXA). This study was undertaken in 5 clinical centers in the United States to establish whether their continuation of daily inhaled corticosteroids in children with well-controlled mild persistent asthma is associated with an increased risk of exacerbations and whether the use of beclomethasone plus albuterol for relief, with or without concomitant use of daily beclomethasone, provides better protection against exacerbations than does a rescue strategy that uses albuterol alone. TREXA was a 44-week randomized double-blind trial. The conclusions of the trial observed that compared with treatment with only albuterol as rescue, daily beclomethasone reduces the risk for a first exacerbation by about 50%, whereas rescue beclomethasone decreased this risk by more than one-third, but this effect was not significant. Treatment failures were substantially decreased in both groups that used daily beclomethasone and in the rescue beclomethasone group. These results suggest that rescue beclomethasone can lower the risk of exacerbations and treatment failures but to a lesser extent than does daily beclomethasone. Treatment failure occurred in nearly a quarter of participants in the placebo group receiving rescue albuterol as the only active treatment. This finding emphasizes the fact that discontinuation of inhaled steroids in children with well-controlled mild persistent asthma substantially increases the risk of asthma exacerbations.

The results of this study suggest that continuation of maintenance inhaled steroids may be necessary in a large percentage of children with mild asthma. Continuation of maintenance inhaled corticosteroids is often resisted and seldom followed by the affected children or by their parents. Moreover, studies of long-term inhaled steroid use have shown that individuals who have received such daily treatment, even in low doses, have had less linear growth than youngsters who receive placebo treatment. Such drawbacks of steroid treatment necessitate the search for alternative treatments for mild persistent asthma. For an absolutely superb review of the management of severe asthma in children, see the commentary of Bush and Saglani.[1]

Do you know the latest new trigger for asthma? The answer is that it appears to be Facebook. Everyone knows that Facebook is a social networking website, one launched in February 2004. As of mid-2010, it had already garnered more than 500 million active users. Recently described was the case of an 18-year-old man for whom Facebook use seemed to be a trigger for asthmatic attack.

This teenager had well controlled asthma except when logging onto Facebook. It turns out the teen had a social relationship with a girlfriend that was facilitated by Facebook entry. Unfortunately this fella was "dumped," but he did succeed in changing his Facebook name and becoming a "friend" to this prior girlfriend once again. His mother noted, however, that he would wheeze when signing onto Facebook and asked him to measure his peak expiratory flow before and after Internet login. His flow rates were 20% decreased over baseline as he logged in each time.[2]

The prior paragraph indicates that Facebook and social networks in general are a brand new source of psychological stress capable of triggering asthmatic exacerbations. Remember the term, "Facebook Asthma," for you may soon see it in your own practice if you have not already.

J. A. Stockman III, MD

References

1. Bush A, Saglani S. Management of severe asthma in children. *Lancet.* 2010;376: 814-825.
2. D'Amato G, Liccardi G, Cecchi L, Pelligrino F, D'Amato M. Facebook: A new trigger for asthma? *Lancet.* 2010;376:1740.

Randomized Trial of Omalizumab (Anti-IgE) for Asthma in Inner-City Children

Busse WW, Morgan WJ, Gergen PJ, et al (Univ of Wisconsin School of Medicine and Public Health, Madison; Univ of Arizona College of Medicine, Tucson; Natl Inst of Allergy and Infectious Diseases, Bethesda, MD; et al)
N Engl J Med 364:1005-1015, 2011

Background.—Research has underscored the effects of exposure and sensitization to allergens on the severity of asthma in inner-city children. It has also revealed the limitations of environmental remediation and guidelines-based therapy in achieving greater disease control.

Methods.—We enrolled inner-city children, adolescents, and young adults with persistent asthma in a randomized, double-blind, placebo-controlled, parallel-group trial at multiple centers to assess the effectiveness of omalizumab, as compared with placebo, when added to guidelines-based therapy. The trial was conducted for 60 weeks, and the primary outcome was symptoms of asthma.

Results.—Among 419 participants who underwent randomization (at which point 73% had moderate or severe disease), omalizumab as compared with placebo significantly reduced the number of days with asthma symptoms, from 1.96 to 1.48 days per 2-week interval, a 24.5% decrease (P<0.001). Similarly, omalizumab significantly reduced the proportion of participants who had one or more exacerbations from 48.8 to 30.3% (P<0.001). Improvements occurred with omalizumab despite reductions in the use of inhaled glucocorticoids and long-acting beta-agonists.

Conclusions.—When added to a regimen of guidelines-based therapy for inner-city children, adolescents, and young adults, omalizumab further improved asthma control, nearly eliminated seasonal peaks in exacerbations, and reduced the need for other medications to control asthma. (Funded by the National Institute of Allergy and Infectious Diseases and Novartis; ClinicalTrials.gov number, NCT00377572.)

▶ This is an important and powerful report, and it comes none too soon. Asthma rates have been surging around the globe over the past 30 or more years. For a long time, researchers thought they had a reasonable explanation of what might be fueling the increase: the world we live in is just a little too clean. According to this hygiene hypothesis, exposure in early childhood to infectious agents programs the immune system to mount differing highly effective defenses against disease-causing viruses, bacteria, and parasites. Better sanitary conditions, the theory goes, deprive the immune system of this training so that for reasons that are still unclear, the body pounces on harmless particles, such as dust and ragweed, as if they were deadly threats. The resulting allergic reaction leads to the classic signs of asthma.

Although a lot of data support the hygiene hypothesis for allergies, the same cannot be said for asthma, however. Contrary to expectations, asthma rates have skyrocketed in urban areas in the United States that are not particularly clean. Moreover, the big increase in asthma rates in developed countries did not kick off until the 1980s, well after general sanitary conditions in richer parts of the world had improved. This collapse of the hygiene hypothesis as a general explanation for the startling jump in asthma rates has led scientists to a new realization: Asthma is much more complex than anyone had previously appreciated, and it may not even be a single disease. Studies now suggest that only about half of asthma cases have any allergic component at all.[1] The short answer to the question of why asthma rates have increased is "we do not know."

The report of Busse et al tells us about how effective immunoglobulin E (IgE)—targeted treatment can be as part of the management of significantly ill children with asthma. Omalizumab is a specifically designed anti-IgE. As we see in this report, adding anti-IgE therapy to the routine care of inner-city children, adolescents, and young adults with asthma that is known to be allergic does result in a significant and clinically meaningful decrease in asthma-related symptoms. It is effective at all levels of asthma severity, but it is not recommended for mild asthma. Interestingly, this study does provide strong proof of concept that the allergic component of asthma is a key factor in the expression of asthma itself.

Chances are you will be hearing a lot more about the use of anti-IgE as part of the management of asthma in children. It is an important breakthrough.

J. A. Stockman III, MD

Reference

1. Greenwood V. Why are asthma rates soaring? *Scientific American.* 2011;304: 32-33.

A randomized controlled study of peanut oral immunotherapy: Clinical desensitization and modulation of the allergic response

Varshney P, Jones SM, Scurlock AM, et al (Duke Univ Med Ctr, Durham, NC; Univ of Arkansas for Med Sciences, Little Rock)
J Allergy Clin Immunol 127:654-660, 2011

Background.—Open-label oral immunotherapy (OIT) protocols have been used to treat small numbers of patients with peanut allergy. Peanut OIT has not been evaluated in double-blind, placebo-controlled trials.

Objective.—To investigate the safety and effectiveness of OIT for peanut allergy in a double-blind, placebo-controlled study.

Methods.—In this multicenter study, children ages 1 to 16 years with peanut allergy received OIT with peanut flour or placebo. Initial escalation, build-up, and maintenance phases were followed by an oral food challenge (OFC) at approximately 1 year. Titrated skin prick tests (SPTs) and laboratory studies were performed at regular intervals.

Results.—Twenty-eight subjects were enrolled in the study. Three peanut OIT subjects withdrew early in the study because of allergic side effects. During the double-blind, placebo-controlled food challenge, all remaining peanut OIT subjects (n = 16) ingested the maximum cumulative dose of 5000 mg (approximately 20 peanuts), whereas placebo subjects (n = 9) ingested a median cumulative dose of 280 mg (range, 0-1900 mg; $P < .001$). In contrast with the placebo group, the peanut OIT group showed reductions in SPT size ($P < .001$), IL-5 ($P = .01$), and IL-13 ($P = .02$) and increases in peanut-specific IgG_4 ($P < .001$). Peanut OIT subjects had initial increases in peanut-specific IgE ($P < .01$) but did not show significant change from baseline by the time of OFC. The ratio of forkhead box protein 3 (FoxP3)^{hi} : FoxP3^{intermediate} CD4+ CD25+ T cells increased at the time of OFC ($P = .04$) in peanut OIT subjects.

Conclusion.—These results conclusively demonstrate that peanut OIT induces desensitization and concurrent immune modulation. The current study continues and is evaluating the hypothesis that peanut OIT causes long-term immune tolerance.

▶ Food allergy is common. In high-income countries, the prevalence in children runs anywhere from 3% to 7% and 1% to 2% in adults. A recent systematic review in the United States disappointingly concluded that "the evidence of the prevalence, diagnosis, management, and prevention of allergies is voluminous, diffuse, and critically limited by the lack of uniformity for the diagnosis of a food allergy, severely limiting conclusions about best practices for management and prevention."[1] One problem in this regard is the breadth of conditions included and the varied definitions of food allergy. The National Institute of Allergy and Infectious Diseases has recently provided us with new US guidelines for the diagnosis and management of food allergy.[2]

Fortunately, as a subset of food allergy, peanut allergy is much more easily identified, defined, and understood. Peanut allergy is one of the most common forms of food allergy, with about 3 million Americans reporting allergy to peanuts or tree nuts. Its prevalence seems to be increasing. Peanut and tree nut allergy account for the significant majority of life-threatening or fatal allergic reactions to foods. Unlike other forms of food allergy, peanut allergy is often life long. By and large, the only treatment options have been strict peanut avoidance and ready access to epinephrine. TNX-901, a humanized monoclonal antibody that prevents binding of immunoglobulin E (IgE) to high affinity receptors on mast cells and basophils has been found to increase the threshold of peanut protein—inducing symptoms in patients with food allergy from less than 1 peanut to almost 11 peanuts.[3] When therapeutic administration of anti-IgE was first reported for this purpose several years back, the thought was that this would hold great promise. However, the prohibitive cost of the use of monoclonal antibodies limits this approach to the management of such a common problem.

What Varshney et al have done is to tell us about the use of allergen immunotherapy as part of the management of peanut allergy. Allergen immunotherapy, an allergen-specific treatment, refers to the administration of increasing amounts of an allergen to individuals with IgE-mediated allergy to diminish the response to the substance on subsequent encounters. Traditional subcutaneous immunotherapy with peanut extract has been studied but has an unacceptably high rate of systemic reactions. On the other hand, peanut oral immunotherapy (OIT) does appear to be relatively safe if performed in a supervised medical setting by trained personnel. In the report of Varshney et al, subjects aged 1 to 16 years with peanut allergy received OIT with peanut flour or placebo. The desensitization protocol was quite intricate. On the initial day of desensitization, the peanut-allergic patient was admitted to a research unit with appropriate emergency medications available. Miniscule amounts of peanut protein were administered, and the amount doubled every 30 minutes until 6 mg of peanut protein were given or the patient began to have symptoms. The highest tolerated dose was the starting dose for the next phase, the buildup phase, which was given in the research unit the following day. Subjects who could tolerate only miniscule amounts of peanut protein were withdrawn from the study. The maximally tolerated dose then was given daily at home followed then by a second buildup phase with the subject returning every 2 weeks for approximately 42 weeks of dose escalations until a 4000 mg maintenance was reached that was subsequently maintained at home. Eighty-four percent of subjects completed 1 year of peanut OIT treatment. Sixteen percent were unable to complete the protocol. All 16, however, were able to tolerate up to 20 peanuts at one sitting. Control subjects who did not go through the program were able to tolerate at best 1 peanut.

The authors of this report concluded that when performed by experienced investigators in an appropriate setting under strict supervision, peanut OIT is a safe allergen-specific therapy effective in inducing desensitization and providing protection against accidental exposure with ongoing therapy. Immunologic changes suggest downregulation of the allergic response. After 1 year of being on the therapeutic protocol, the patients who responded successfully appear to have minimal problems with peanut exposure. Obviously it is necessary to see what the long-term outcomes are in terms of immune tolerance. Nonetheless, the news here is extremely good for those who are willing to commit themselves to a very rigorous desensitization protocol. For more on this topic of food allergy and emerging guidelines on diagnosis and management, see the excellent editorial by Voelker.[4]

J. A. Stockman III, MD

References

1. Schneider C, Newberry SJ, Riedl MA, et al. Diagnosing and managing common food allergies: a systematic review. *JAMA*. 2010;303:1848-1856.
2. Boyce JA, Assa'ad A, Burks AW, et al. Guidelines for the diagnosis and management of food allergy in the United States: summary of the NIAID-sponsored expert panel report. *J Allergy Clin Immunol*. 2010;126:1105-1118.
3. Leung DY, Sampson HA, Yunginger JW, et al. Effect of anti-IgE therapy in patients with peanut allergy. *N Engl J Med*. 2003;348:986-993.
4. Voelker R. Experts hope to clear confusion with first guidelines to tackle food allergy. *JAMA*. 2011;305:457.

The Prevalence of Infections With *Trichophyton tonsurans* in Schoolchildren: the CAPITIS Study

Abdel-Rahman SM, Farrand N, Schuenemann E, et al (Children's Mercy Hosp and Clinics, Kansas City, MO; Score 1 for Health, Kansas City, MO; et al)
Pediatrics 125:966-973, 2010

Background.—Although *Trichophyton tonsurans* has become the leading cause of tinea capitis in the United States, reported infection rates vary widely, and prevalence estimates for the pediatric population at large remain poorly characterized.

Methods.—A prospective, cross-sectional, surveillance study of children attending kindergarten through fifth grade in 44 schools across the bi-state (Kansas/Missouri), Kansas City metropolitan area was conducted. Fungal cultures were collected from all participants, and molecular analyses were used to characterize the patterns of infection within the population.

Results.—Of 10 514 children (age: 8.3 ± 1.9 years) examined for the presence of *T tonsurans* on their scalps, 6.6% exhibited positive cultures. Infection rates at participating schools ranged from 0% to 19.4%, exceeding 30% at a given grade level in some schools. Black children demonstrated the highest rates of infection (12.9%), with prevalence estimates for the youngest members of this racial group approaching 18%. Infection rates for Hispanic (1.6%) and white (1.1%) children were markedly lower. A single genetic strain of *T tonsurans* was identified in only 16.6% of classrooms, whereas each child harbored a unique genetic strain in 51.4%.

Conclusions.—We report a large-scale, citywide, surveillance study of *T tonsurans* infection rates among children in primary school in a metropolitan area. The striking prevalence rates and genetic heterogeneity among the fungal isolates confirm the relatively large degree to which

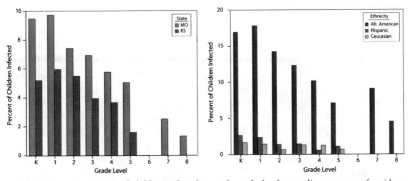

FIGURE 1.—Proportions of children infected at each grade level according to state of residence (A) and ethnicity (B). (Reproduced with permission from *Pediatrics*, Abdel-Rahman SM, Farrand N, Schuenemann E, et al. The prevalence of infections with *trichophyton tonsurans* in schoolchildren: the CAPITIS study. *Pediatrics*. 2010;125:966-973. Copyright © 2010 The American Academy of Pediatrics.)

this pathogen has become integrated into metropolitan communities (Fig 1).

▶ There was a time in the early part of the last century when if a child had tinea capitis, he or she was banned, excluded, and otherwise ostracized from the rest of his or her peers, at least until the condition was well in hand in terms of treatment. If you were born in the first half of the last century, you may well have had your scalp irradiated or the skin might undergo epilation. If you were an immigrant entering this country at Ellis Island, you might even be turned around and sent back to your native country. Borrowing that, you were often detained until the scalp condition was adequately managed.

The introduction of griseofulvin in the late 1950s resulted in an unparalleled reduction in the number of *Microsporum*-associated infections and consequently overall decreases in the active number of cases of tinea capitis. In the interval period of time, we have seen the niche resulting from the control of *Microsporum*-associated infections filled by *Trichophyton tonsurans*, an organism that is decidedly more challenging to screen for and treat. Despite the evolution of newer orally administered antimycotic agents, there has been little decline in infection rates and *T tonsurans* is now the principal agent of tinea capitis here in this country.

To date, prevalence estimates for the pediatric population with respect to *T tonsurans* have been poorly characterized—thus the value of the report of Abdel-Rahman et al who tell us about the Citywide Assessment of the Prevalence of Infections with *Trichophyton tonsurans* in Schoolchildren. The latter study represents a prospective cross-sectional evaluation of children attending kindergarten through fifth grade in Kansas and Missouri metropolitan areas. Some 44 primary schools participated in the investigation. All were visited over a 4-month period ending in January 2009. Children enrolled in this study had cultures taken over their entire scalp for isolation of fungal DNA. Fig 1 shows the proportions of children infected at each grade level according to state of residence and ethnicity. We see that more than 1 in 20 children residing in the greater Kansas City metropolitan area harbored *T tonsurans* on their scalps. The chance of recovering this fungus was more than 10 times greater in African American children compared with their non-African descent peers.

This report also yielded some other very interesting information. Since there are varying genotypes of *T tonsurans*, it was possible in this study to look at the genetic diversity of the populations studied. In fewer than 20% of classrooms, infections were of a single genetic strain and type. Although the finding of high-frequency strain types in the same classroom might be expected to arise by chance, the finding that low-frequency strain types were also implicated in those classrooms supports a role for direct transmission of strains between children in the classroom setting. In more than one-half of the classrooms, however, a different strain type was observed for each infected child, which is consistent with the profile of endemic infection. On the basis of these observations, the theory that infections among school-age children arise from an index case may not be entirely accurate. In this primary school population, infections seem to reflect a mixture of both small epidemics and stable endemic disease.

Please note that this study did not distinguish between children with symptomatic tinea capitis, carriers without symptoms, and children who might have transiently acquired the fungus from other children. That having been stated, previous investigations from these same researchers suggest that the vast majority (> 89%) of children are persistent carriers of this pathogen. Also, these investigators have confirmed that carriage persists throughout primary school suggesting a significantly large population likely to experience recurrent infections and the need for repeated treatment as well as an equally large population capable of serving as a vector of transmission to other children. The authors of this report argue strongly that preventative strategies are necessary to minimize the acquisition of *T tonsurans* in metropolitan African American communities if we are to regain control of this infection in the United States.

Recent data now tell us the best ways to deal with head lice. Suffocating head lice in old days required parents to smear on petroleum jelly, mayonnaise, butter, or olive oil on the heads of Sally or Johnny who had scalp lice. The tactic was to smother the critters. It did not work uniformly well because the lice reflexively are capable of closing their spiracles, the tiny holes through which they breathe, and many lice would therefore survive treatment. Benzyl alcohol lotion 5% (Ulesfia®) is said to stun the lice into opening their spiracles, thereby asphyxiating them. Double-blind trials were done comparing the lotion containing the active drug and plain lotion applied twice (on days 1 and 7). On day 8, the test drug had a 91% success rate compared with 28% in the control group, but on day 14 the success rates dropped to 28% and 16% respectively. Needless to say, this is not a success rate to cheer about. In fact, the only happy critters were the lice themselves. They were intoxicatingly happy.[1]

J. A. Stockman III, MD

Reference

1. Meinking TL, Villar ME, Vicaria M, et al. The Clinical Trials Supporting Benzyl Alcohol Lotion 5% (Ulesfia™): A Safe and Effective Topical Treatment for Head Lice (Pediculosis Humanus Capitis). *Pediatr Dermatol.* 2010;27:19-24.

Cost effectiveness of home ultraviolet B phototherapy for psoriasis: economic evaluation of a randomised controlled trial (PLUTO study)
Koek MBG, Sigurdsson V, van Weelden H, et al (Univ Med Ctr Utrecht, Netherlands; et al)
BMJ 340:c1490, 2010

Objective.—To assess the costs and cost effectiveness of phototherapy with ultraviolet B light provided at home compared with outpatient ultraviolet B phototherapy for psoriasis.

Design.—Cost utility, cost effectiveness, and cost minimisation analyses performed alongside a pragmatic randomised clinical trial (the PLUTO study) at the end of phototherapy (mean 17.6 weeks) and at one year after the end of phototherapy (mean 68.4 weeks).

Setting.—Secondary care, provided by a dermatologist in the Netherlands.

Participants.—196 adults with psoriasis who were clinically eligible for narrowband (TL-01) ultraviolet B phototherapy were recruited from the dermatology departments of 14 hospitals and were followed until the end of phototherapy. From the end of phototherapy onwards, follow-up was continued for an unselected, consecutive group of 105 patients for one year after end of phototherapy.

Interventions.—Ultraviolet B phototherapy provided at home (intervention) and conventional outpatient ultraviolet B phototherapy (control) in a setting reflecting routine practice in the Netherlands. Both treatments used narrowband ultraviolet B lamps (TL-01).

Main Outcome Measures.—Total costs to society, quality adjusted life years (QALYs) as calculated using utilities measured by the EQ-5D questionnaire, and the number of days with a relevant treatment effect ($\geq 50\%$ improvement of the baseline self administered psoriasis area and severity index (SAPASI)).

Results.—Home phototherapy is at least as effective and safe as outpatient phototherapy, therefore allowing cost minimisation analyses (simply comparing costs). The average total costs by the end of phototherapy were €800 for home treatment and €752 for outpatient treatment, showing an incremental cost per patient of €48 (95% CI €−77 to €174). The average total costs by one year after the end of phototherapy were €1272 and €1148 respectively (difference €124, 95% CI €−155 to €403). Cost utility analyses revealed that patients experienced equal health benefits—that is, a gain of 0.296 versus 0.291 QALY (home *v* outpatient) by the end of phototherapy (difference 0.0052, −0.0244 to 0.0348) and 1.153 versus 1.126 QALY by one year after the end of phototherapy (difference 0.0267, −0.024 to 0.078). Incremental costs per QALY gained were €9276 and €4646 respectively, both amounts well below the normally accepted standard of €20 000 per QALY. Cost effectiveness analyses indicated that the mean number of days with a relevant treatment effect was 42.4 versus 55.3 by the end of phototherapy (difference −12.9, −23.4 to −2.4). By one year after the end of phototherapy the number of days with a relevant treatment effect were 216.5 and 210.4 respectively (6.1,

−41.1 to 53.2), yielding an incremental cost of €20 per additional day with a relevant treatment effect.

Conclusions.—Home ultraviolet B phototherapy for psoriasis is not more expensive than phototherapy in an outpatient setting and proved to be cost effective. As both treatments are at least equally effective and patients express a preference for home treatment, the authors conclude that home phototherapy should be the primary treatment option for patients who are eligible for phototherapy with ultraviolet B light.

Trial Registration.—Current Controlled Trials ISRCTN83025173 and Clinicaltrials.gov NCT00150930.

▶ While this report emanates from the Netherlands, the data would likely equally apply to the situation in the United States. Koek et al examined the cost-effectiveness of home-based ultraviolet B phototherapy for the management of psoriasis, a disorder that affects both children and adults. Examined were the incremental costs to society for home treatment and the quality of adjusted life years. Included in the analysis were not only the cost of home treatment but also the cost of absences from work by adults. The bottom line is that this study clearly shows that home ultraviolet B phototherapy is at least as effective and as safe as outpatient-based phototherapy for psoriasis, and if one looks carefully at the numbers, the cost savings are quite dramatic.

So why is this report important? Many individuals with psoriasis, mostly adults, have gravitated to tanning centers for treatment of their condition as an inexpensive alternative to medically administered phototherapy. Properly done, the benefits are equivalent. The other alternative, of course, that is relatively inexpensive in comparison to medical therapy is to rent, lease, or perhaps even buy and share home ultraviolet B phototherapy units. The rub here in the United States, of course, is that the current health care legislation adds a significant tax to the use of nonmedically administered ultraviolet B phototherapy.

The intent of the tax on sunbed use in the United States makes a lot of sense, but there have been unintended consequences for those who use this as a form of therapy for the management of dermatologic conditions. It is not yet clear whether the added tax cost is reducing the use of such units. Data from overseas suggest that as many as 6% of teenagers in Europe use sunbeds. The percentage rises to 50% in girls aged 15 to 17 years in certain parts of England.[1] It should be noted that some dermatologists are recommending home phototherapy not only for psoriasis but also for atopic eczema, desensitization treatment of photodermatoses, and a variety of other conditions.

Are you aware of the potential benefits of the application of beetle juice? It appears that dermatologists are now applying this product to plantar warts. Recently described was a young lady who had the topical application of beetle juice followed several days later by the application of salicylic acid tape for a 1-week period of time. Topical salicylic acid used alone had failed previously. The combination of beetle juice and salicylic acid worked like a charm. The active ingredient in beetle juice is cantharidin, which is a toxic terpenoid secreted by many species of male blister beetles and is used by the beetle to protect female eggs from predators. If you decide to use it, it should be used only topically and appears to be effective by blistering and eventually destroying the infected skin.[2]

J. A. Stockman III, MD

References

1. Sunbed use in children aged 11-17 in England: face to face. *BMJ.* 2010;340:c877.
2. Beetle juice to the rescue. *Pediatr Infect Dis J Newsletter.* 2011;30:A9-A10. doi:10. 1097/01.inf.0000395260.04385.b5.

Prospective Study of Spinal Anomalies in Children with Infantile Hemangiomas of the Lumbosacral Skin

Drolet BA, Chamlin SL, Garzon MC, et al (Med College of Wisconsin, Milwaukee; Northwestern Univ Feinberg School of Medicine, Chicago, IL; Columbia Univ, NY; et al)
J Pediatr 157:789-794, 2010

Objective.—To prospectively evaluate a cohort of patients with infantile hemangioma in the midline lumbosacral region for spinal anomalies to determine the positive predictive value of infantile hemangioma for occult spinal anomalies and to make evidence-based recommendations for screening.

Study Design.—A multicenter prospective cohort study was performed at 9 Hemangioma Investigator Group sites.

Results.—Intraspinal abnormalities were detected in 21 of 41 study participants with a lumbosacral infantile hemangioma who underwent a magnetic resonance imaging evaluation. The relative risk for all patients with lumbosacral infantile hemangiomas for spinal anomalies was 640 (95% confidence interval [CI], 404-954), and the positive predictive value of infantile hemangioma for spinal dysraphism was 51.2%. Ulceration of the hemangioma was associated with a higher risk of having spinal anomalies. The presence of additional cutaneous anomalies also was associated with a higher likelihood of finding spinal anomalies; however, 35% of the infants with isolated lumbosacral infantile hemangiomas had spinal anomalies, with a relative risk of 438 (95% CI, 188-846). The sensitivity for ultrasound scanning to detect spinal anomalies in this high-risk group was poor at 50% (95% CI, 18.7%-81.3%), with a specificity rate of 77.8% (95% CI, 40%-97.2%).

Conclusions.—Infants and children with midline lumbosacral infantile hemangiomas are at increased risk for spinal anomalies. Screening magnetic resonance imaging is recommended for children with these lesions.

▶ Spinal dysraphism is now categorized into 2 types: obvious and occult. The diagnosis of spinal dysraphism is a broad one encompassing a heterogenous group of congenital spinal anomalies that result from defective closure of the neural tube early in fetal life and anomalous development of the caudal cell mass. Currently 0.5 to 0.8 infants are affected per 1000 live births. Larger defects are readily detected prenatally or at birth. In cases of occult spinal dysraphism (OSD), the delayed presentation of symptoms when the neural tissue is skin covered and not exposed may allow slowly progressive damage to the spinal cord. The diagnosis of OSD is usually suspected because of overlying abnormalities of the skin. Somewhere between 50% and 90% of affected infants and children with OSD have associated skin abnormalities. Unfortunately, there is little in the way of literature telling us about the probability that the presence of a specific skin lesion predicts OSD. This is particularly true with a congenital vascular birthmark in the lumbosacral area. These infantile hemangioma or capillary malformations may fade with maturity (nevus simplexes) and others persist. Currently we lack clear evidence-based guidelines for screening infants with infantile hemangiomas in the lumbosacral region. This report helps to address this issue.

The study of Drolet et al represents a multicenter prospective investigation performed by the Hemangioma Investigator Group. This study looked at infants and children younger than 18 years with an infantile hemangioma, hemangioma precursor, or definitive residual hemangioma greater than 2.5 cm in diameter overlying the midline lumbar spine or sacral spine. Patients with infantile hemangiomas isolated to the skin of the perineum or coccygeal region or with legions not involving the midline were excluded from the study. Subjects underwent ultrasound scanning, MRI, or both of the spine. When the study subject was younger than 4 months, ultrasound scanning was used for screening evaluation at some of the institutions involved with the study. Of 41 study subjects, intraspinal abnormalities were detected in 21 (positive predictive value of infantile hemangioma for spinal dysraphism = 51.2%). The relative risk for all patients with lumbosacral infantile hemangiomas for spinal abnormalities was 640. Unfortunately, the sensitivity for ultrasound scanning to detect spinal abnormalities, particularly in high-risk infants was poor at 50% (specificity, 77.8%). These data suggest that MRI is the preferred screening test for all infants with infantile hemangiomas of the lumbosacral skin. The authors specifically indicate that hemangiomas $\geq$2.5 cm in particular are at high risk for underlying spinal anomalies and should undergo MRI as part of their evaluation. They also say that when no evidence of patent sinus track, ulceration of skin, or neurologic signs or symptoms are evident, MRI can be deferred until 4 to 6 months of age.

This commentary addresses colophonium contact allergy.[1] Recently a doctor presented with a 2-year history of episodes of reddened skin on his cheeks. He was treated with penicillin for presumed streptococcal cellulitis and was then given a prophylactic dose of antibiotics, but despite this treatment, he developed a strip of dusky erythema on his left cheek. Further questioning revealed that he had played the cello the night before the rash appeared and had applied lots of rosin to his bow. It emerged that the rash had also been worse after his wedding, when he had been kissed on the cheek many times by women wearing lipstick. Another case of "cello cheeks" has appeared in the literature.

J. A. Stockman III, MD

Reference

1. Editorial comment. Colophonium contact allergy. *BMJ*. 2010;341:c4860.

LUMBAR: Association between Cutaneous Infantile Hemangiomas of the Lower Body and Regional Congenital Anomalies
Iacobas I, Burrows PE, Frieden IJ, et al (Baylor College of Medicine, Houston, TX; Univ of California San Francisco; et al)
J Pediatr 157:795-801, 2010

Objective.—To define the clinical spectrum of regional congenital anomalies associated with large cutaneous hemangiomas of the lower half of the body, clarify risk for underlying anomalies on the basis of hemangioma location, and provide imaging guidelines for evaluation.

Study Design.—We conducted a multi-institutional, retrospective case analysis of 24 new patients and review of 29 published cases.

Results.—Hemangiomas in our series tended to be "segmental" and often "minimal growth" in morphology. Such lesions were often extensive, covering the entire leg. Extensive limb hemangiomas also showed potential for extracutaneous anomalies, including underlying arterial anomalies, limb underdevelopment, and ulceration. The cutaneous hemangioma and underlying anomalies demonstrated regional correlation. Myelopathies were the most common category of associated anomalies.

Conclusions.—We propose the acronym "LUMBAR" to describe the association of Lower body hemangioma and other cutaneous defects, Urogenital anomalies, Ulceration, Myelopathy, Bony deformities, Anorectal malformations, Arterial anomalies, and Renal anomalies. There are many similarities between LUMBAR and PHACE syndrome, which might be considered regional variations of the same. Although guidelines for imaging are suggested, prospective studies will lead to precise imaging recommendations and help determine true incidence, risk and long-term outcomes.

▶ This is another report providing additional information on the relationship between cutaneous infantile hemangiomas and congenital anomalies. Infantile hemangioma (IH) is in fact the most common childhood tumor, and it is technically a tumor. When IH is located in certain areas of the skin, it can be associated with underlying or related congenital anomalies. The best-known example of this is PHACE syndrome, the association between large characteristically segmental IH on the face and developmental defects of the cerebrovasculature, cardiovascular, eyes, and chest wall. PHACE syndrome is now well understood. What is not as well understood is the occurrence of large IH on the lower half of the body and any potential regional congenital anomalies associated with it. Iacobas et al tell us about the latter in much more detail than has been discussed previously in the literature.

What Iacobas et al have done is to report on a multiinstitutional retrospective analysis of 24 new patients and a review of 29 published cases in the literature. After analyzing all this information, the authors of this article felt like they were able to describe a new syndrome that they call by the acronym LUMBAR, an association of findings including lower body hemangioma and other cutaneous defects: urologic anomalies, ulceration, myelopathy, boney deformities, anorectal malformations, arterial anomalies, and renal anomalies (Fig 3).

Studies of the PHACE syndrome have demonstrated a regional correlation between the cutaneous IH and underlying anomalies present. The findings from the report of Iacobas support a similar observation in LUMBAR. Myelopathies, notably tethered cord or lipomyelocele/lipomyelomeningocele, are the most common categories of anomalies seen in the patients described. A previously undescribed association in LUMBAR syndrome is the potential for underlying arterial anomalies, particularly when the IH extends over the entirety of a lower limb. For example, one child with LUMBAR syndrome has demonstrated a primitive sciatic artery arising from the left common iliac artery, presumably a cause of a deformed and shortened limb. A report of arterial anomalies is not surprising because of their known association and PHACE syndrome. For example, renal artery stenosis has been reported in PHACE syndrome.

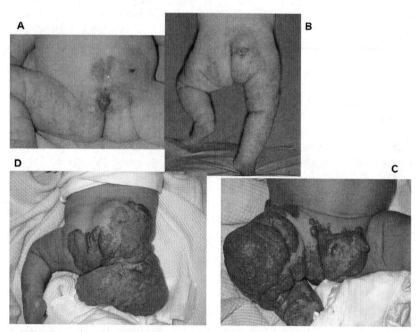

FIGURE 3.—Clinical features of LUMBAR association. A and B, case 19; C and D, case 1. Both cases involve regions ABCD, but case 19 is segmental minimal-growth phenotype and case 1 segmental normal growth. Note the ulceration present in both cases, the lumbar lipoma and urogenital anomalies in case 19, and the pterygium in case 1 (Table I in the original article). (Reprinted from Journal of Pediatrics, Iacobas I, Burrows PE, Frieden IJ, et al. LUMBAR: Association between cutaneous infantile hemangiomas of the lower body and regional congenital anomalies. *J Pediatr.* 2010;157:795-801. Copyright 2010 with permission from Elsevier.)

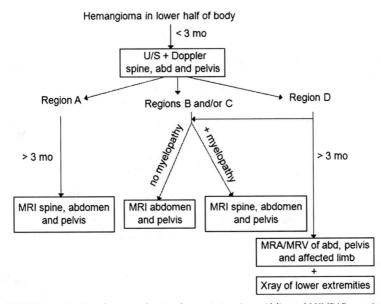

Hemangioma in lower half of body

↓ < 3 mo

U/S + Doppler
spine, abd and pelvis

Region A ← Regions B and/or C → Region D

> 3 mo   > 3 mo

no myelopathy   + myelopathy

MRI spine, abdomen   MRI abdomen   MRI spine, abdomen
and pelvis   and pelvis   and pelvis

MRA/MRV of abd, pelvis
and affected limb
+
Xray of lower extremities

FIGURE 5.—Algorithm for comprehensive diagnostic imaging guidelines of LUMBAR association. (Reprinted from Journal of Pediatrics, Iacobas I, Burrows PE, Frieden IJ, et al. LUMBAR: Association between cutaneous infantile hemangiomas of the lower body and regional congenital anomalies. *J Pediatr.* 2010;157:795-801. Copyright 2010 with permission from Elsevier.)

The pathogenesis of LUMBAR syndrome is unknown. It is also not clear what the thoroughness of a diagnostic evaluation ought to be when skin findings are observed. It certainly should start with a thorough physical examination of the abdomen, pelvis, and lower extremities with emphasis on the genital and paraspinal regions. Judicious use of MRI is of value, presumably after the age of 3 to 4 months (Fig 5). Before that, ultrasound and Doppler studies of the abdomen and pelvis may be useful. Unless there is some urgency in performance of an MRI, it is generally easier to perform in a slightly older infant.

J. A. Stockman III, MD

Efficacy of Propranolol in Hepatic Infantile Hemangiomas with Diffuse Neonatal Hemangiomatosis

Mazereeuw-Hautier J, Hoeger PH, Benlahrech S, et al (Paul Sabatier Univ, Toulouse, France; Catholic Children's Hosp, Hambourg, Germany; René Descartes Paris V Univ, France; et al)
J Pediatr 157:340-342, 2010

We report the rapid and dramatic efficacy of propranolol in 8 infants with infantile hepatic hemangiomas. The degree of response varied from a significant improvement to a complete resolution of hepatic lesions.

Heart failure and hypothyroidism resolved, and hepatomegaly decreased. No side-effects of the drug were noted.

▶ This report teaches us a lot about hemangiomas. One of the more perplexing varieties of hemangiomas is that of the infantile hepatic variety. This report reminds us that there are 3 categories of infantile hepatic hemangiomas (IHH). These include focal, multifocal, or diffuse. Diffuse IHH are life threatening because they may induce congestive heart failure associated with high-volume vascular shunting. A little-known fact is that hypothyroidism may be associated with these hemangiomas and is caused by overproduction of type 3 iodothyronine deiodinase. The traditional management of IHH is similar to the management of hemangiomas elsewhere that need to be treated. Such management usually includes the use of systemic corticosteroids. Embolization is also part of the treatment in cases with severe high output failure as a result of direct shunting. Interferon and chemotherapeutic agents such as vincristine have been used as well, although the outcomes associated with such therapies at best are vagarious.

The report of Mazereeuw-Hautier et al tells us about the management of diffuse neonatal hemangiomatosis associated with IHH in 8 infants who were treated in France and Germany with the β-blocker propranolol. These were patients in whom traditional approaches with steroids and/or embolization had failed. Propranolol was then introduced during the first 4 months of life except in 1 patient, who began the β-blocker at 10 months of age. In each patient, the condition rapidly improved with propranolol dose allowing tapering and discontinuation of other therapies. Two patients had undetectable hepatic lesions after 1 month on the β-blocker. For the other patients, the size of liver hemangiomas decreased an average of 50% or more after 2 to 4 months.

This is not the first report to talk about the efficacy of propranolol as part of the treatment of cutaneous hemangiomas.[1] These earlier reports were based on small numbers of patients. Although 8 patients is not a lot of patients, there are more patients treated with propranolol in this report than in any previous report. Exactly how propranolol would work is not clear, but when it comes to the liver, it is likely that propranolol decreases hepatic blood flow, diminishing the arterial feeders to the hepatic hemangiomas.

Generally speaking, propranolol is a well-tolerated drug, particularly well tolerated in comparison with drugs such as alpha interferon and vincristine. It does not work immediately, and therefore if there is life-threatening high-output cardiac failure associated with direct shunts, one may need to move expeditiously to embolization.

These authors note that propranolol was effective in every patient in whom it was tried, those with diffuse or multifocal hepatic hemangiomas, both in the presence and absence of heart failure, and irrespective of whether propranolol was used as a frontline therapy, alone or in combination with other therapies. Given that it is a quite benign modality of treatment, one may even think about using it in lieu of steroids at the start of initial therapy.

This commentary closes with an unrelated skin observation. Skin lightening (bleaching) cosmetics designed to lighten the color of darker skin may be associated with serious medical consequences. The active ingredients of these products include hydroquinone, mercury, and a highly potent fluorinated corticosteroid ointment or cream. These products are associated with serious and life-threatening complications because their use for long periods on a large body surface are often associated with hot and humid tropical conditions that promote percutaneous absorption. Two well-described complications include exogenous ochronosis and colloid milium, initially reported in people of color more than 30 years ago. Exogenous ochronosis is related to the use of hydroquinone, and it presents with a dirty grayish brown waxy pigmentation on sun-exposed areas of skin. The primary lesion of colloid milium is a translucent flesh or cream colored papule of 1mm to 5mm in diameter on sun-exposed skin. Other complications of topical bleaching agents include impaired wound healing, a fishy odor, nephropathy, steroid addiction syndrome, and suppression of the hypothalamic-pituitary-adrenal axis. The culture of bleaching has become fairly common among black Africans. Outside Africa, these products are not sold in the regular cosmetic sections of department stores or pharmacies. Rather, they are purchased directly from the manufacturers in Africa. To learn more about the consequences of skin lightening creams, see the editorial by Olumide.[2]

J. A. Stockman III, MD

References

1. Sans V, de la Roque ED, Berge J, et al. Propranolol for severe infantile hemangiomas: follow-up report. *Pediatrics.* 2009;31:e423-e431.
2. Olumide YM. Use of skin lightening creams: Lack of recognition and regulations is having serous medical consequences. *BMJ.* 2011;342:345-346.

Mutations in *GNA11* in Uveal Melanoma
Van Raamsdonk CD, Griewank KG, Crosby MB, et al (Univ of British Columbia, Vancouver, Canada; Univ of California San Franciso; et al)
N Engl J Med 363:2191-2199, 2010

Background.—Uveal melanoma is the most common intraocular cancer. There are no effective therapies for metastatic disease. Mutations in *GNAQ*, the gene encoding an alpha subunit of heterotrimeric G proteins, are found in 40% of uveal melanomas.

Methods.—We sequenced exon 5 of *GNAQ* and *GNA11*, a paralogue of *GNAQ*, in 713 melanocytic neoplasms of different types (186 uveal melanomas, 139 blue nevi, 106 other nevi, and 282 other melanomas). We sequenced exon 4 of *GNAQ* and *GNA11* in 453 of these samples and in all coding exons of *GNAQ* and *GNA11* in 97 uveal melanomas and 45 blue nevi.

Results.—We found somatic mutations in exon 5 (affecting Q209) and in exon 4 (affecting R183) in both *GNA11* and *GNAQ*, in a mutually exclusive pattern. Mutations affecting Q209 in *GNA11* were present in 7% of blue nevi, 32% of primary uveal melanomas, and 57% of uveal melanoma metastases. In contrast, we observed Q209 mutations in *GNAQ* in 55% of blue nevi, 45% of uveal melanomas, and 22% of uveal melanoma metastases. Mutations affecting R183 in either *GNAQ* or *GNA11* were less prevalent (2% of blue nevi and 6% of uveal melanomas) than the Q209 mutations. Mutations in *GNA11* induced spontaneously metastasizing tumors in a mouse model and activated the mitogen-activated protein kinase pathway.

Conclusions.—Of the uveal melanomas we analyzed, 83% had somatic mutations in *GNAQ* or *GNA11*. Constitutive activation of the pathway involving these two genes appears to be a major contributor to the development of uveal melanoma. (Funded by the National Institutes of Health and others.)

▶ Before this report appeared, I was not aware that ocular melanoma was the most common intraocular cancer. This form of cancer arises from melanocytes within the choroidal plexus of the eye and metastasizes almost exclusively to the liver. Van Raamsdonk et al report that more than 80% of ocular melanomas carry mutations in either *GNA11* or *GNAQ*. These genes encode members of the q class of G protein alpha subunits, which are involved in mediating signals between G protein–coupled receptors and downstream effectors. Mutations of this nature are emerging as an important source of susceptibility to cancers in humans. Such cancers include ovarian carcinomas and certain forms of breast cancer.

What we also learn from this report of Van Raamsdonk et al is that the presence of *GNAQ* and *GNA11* mutations in blue nevi (benign intradermal melanocytic proliferations affecting the conjunctiva and periorbital skin) also places a patient at risk for ocular melanoma. Epidemiologic studies point to a causative role for ultraviolet irradiation in ocular and cutaneous melanoma, but the types of mutations seen in *GNAQ* and *GNA11* are not typically induced by medium-wave UV-B light (315-280 nm). It is less clear what effects UV-A light (320-400 nm) has on ocular DNA.

Please note that therapy for melanoma is making remarkable progress. After only about 10 years from the initial discovery of mutations in the *BRAF* oncogene, a new small molecule inhibitor specific for these mutations has been found. It induces tumor shrinkage in more than 80% of patients with cutaneous melanoma containing *BRAF* mutations and has extended progression-free survival by an average of 7 months. About 50% of cutaneous melanomas have this *BRAF* mutation, but it is absent from certain other subtypes of the disease such as ocular melanoma, the subject of this report. Ocular melanoma represents about 5% of all melanomas. The more we learn about the management of melanoma in general, the closer we get to a cure.

This commentary closes with a few fast facts having to do with melanoma:

- Eight out of 10 melanomas have been recently described to respond to a new drug called PLX4032, if the melanoma shows a V600E mutation.[1] Other research indicates that treatment with this agent could be actually harmful in people with melanomas that lack this mutation.

- Recently, the governments of England and Wales have banned sun bed use for those under the age of 18. Businesses that break the law can be fined up to £20 000.[2]

- Data from the United Kingdom show that almost half (46%) of 2000 adults taking part in a survey say they had a sunburn during the preceding 12 months. Nearly one-third (32%) of these said their motivation was to get a tan and half of those who experienced a sunburn while attempting to get a tan said they would risk a sunburn again the following year. So much for common sense.[3]

- Finally, please recognize that whales get sunburned too. In the last decade there have been increasing reports about skin lesions on whales and dolphins, thought to be related to ultraviolet radiation exposure. Studies of sperm whales and blue whales have documented this. Just as in humans, lighter-skinned whales seem to suffer more from the sun's rays whereas the darkest whales (fin whales) have the fewest skin abnormalities. Over a recent 3-year study period, the number of blue whales with blisters has increased by some 56%, suggesting that ongoing ozone depletion may be causing more skin damage in this animal species being hammered by ultraviolet rays every day when they surface.[4]

J. A. Stockman III, MD

References

1. Editorial comment. Eight of 10 melanomas with V500E mutation respond to new drug. *BMJ*. 2010;341:c4726.
2. Editorial comment. Sunbed use is made illegal for under 18s in England and Wales. *BMJ*. 2011;342:d2284.
3. Editorial comment. Half of UK adults got sunburnt this summer. *BMJ*. 2010;341: c4850.
4. Morell V. Whales get sunburns too. ScienceNOW. http://news.sciencemag.org/sciencenow/2010/11/whales-get-sunburns-too.html?ref=hp. Published November 9, 2010. Accessed July 25, 2011.

3 Blood

Red Blood Cell Morphology Reporting: How Much is a Waste of Time?
Ford JC, Milner R, Dix DB (BC Children's Hosp, Vancouver, Canada)
J Pediatr Hematol Oncol 33:10-14, 2011

Red blood cell morphology (RBC-M) reporting is a routine requirement for hospital laboratories when reporting complete blood counts. However, there is little evidence that RBC-M reporting is useful to pediatric clinicians. We surveyed pediatric hematology specialists and nonspecialists at the BC Children's Hospital (Vancouver, Canada), to evaluate the perceived clinical utility of this reporting. Although a large majority of pediatric clinicians refer to RBC-M reports in their clinical practice, less than half consider these reports to be clinically useful. Hematology specialists were more likely than nonspecialists to identify individual RBC-M descriptions as clinically useful. Some RBC-M descriptions, such as anisocytosis, were considered not useful by specialists and by nonspecialists. A large proportion of nonspecialist respondents noted that they did not know the clinical significance of some of the RBC-M terms. Educational initiatives to inform nonspecialists about the clinical significance of some RBC-M descriptions should be considered. A few RBC-M descriptions are not clinically useful to either specialists or nonspecialists, and these could be omitted from RBC-M reports as a step toward improved hematology laboratory reporting (Tables 1, 2 and 4).

▶ Most pediatricians rotated onto a hematology service sometime during their training. Many were taught to carefully review a red blood cell smear for abnormalities in red cell size and/or shape (dysmorphology). Hematology laboratories routinely report descriptions of red blood cell morphology as part of a complete blood count (CBC). While some laboratories divide abnormal findings into just a few categories, other laboratories provide a much longer menu of reportable red blood cell morphology findings. Table 1 provides a list of what the literature suggest are clinically significant red blood cell morphologies, while Table 2 shows a full range of potential red cell morphologies.

The authors of this report tell us that giving too much information about red cell morphology actually provides excessive overload to the clinician, specifically, the provision of clinically irrelevant information. Both hematology subspecialists and nonsubspecialists in Vancouver were asked to evaluate the perceived clinical utility of red cell morphology as reported from the clinical laboratory. Table 4 tells us just how important these clinicians find reports of red cell morphology.

TABLE 1.—Clinically Significant Red Blood Cell Morphologies Noted in the Literature

From Williams Hematology[1]	From Nathan and Oski[2]
Acanthocytes	Basophilic stippling
Dacrocytes [teardrops]	Bizarre poikilocytes
Echinocytes	Elliptocytes
Elliptocytes	Intraerythrocytic parasites
Schistocytes	Sickle cells
Spherocytes	Spherocytes
Stomatocytes	Spiculated/crenated cells
Target cells	Stomatocytes
	Target cells

Editor's Note: Please refer to original journal article for full references.

TABLE 2.—RBC Morphologies Reported at BC Children's Hospital

Abnormally constricted cells
Acanthocytes
Anisocytosis
Basophilic stippling
Echinocytes
Elliptocytes
Howell Jolly bodies
Hypochromasia
Macrocytosis
Malaria parasites seen
Microcytosis
Pappenheimer bodies
Poikilocytosis
Polychromasia
RBC agglutination
Rouleaux
Schistocytes
Sickle cells
Spherocytes
Stomatocytes
Target cells
Teardrop forms

RBC indicates red blood cell

I am a pediatric hematologist. I strongly believe that if clinicians are concerned about a hematologic disorder, they should look at a red blood cell smear themselves. All too often laboratory technicians are not well trained in interpreting the red cell smear. The findings as reported by automated equipment are not as good as the trained human eye. The authors of this report are correct that it would be useful for hospitals and laboratories to improve their reporting process by omitting red blood cell descriptions that are clinically useless or irrelevant. This would make for a more streamline reporting system that would be easier for clinicians to use CBC reports and would also have the benefit of saving technologists time.

To conclude, it might be beneficial to learn about the origins of the word "blood." Blood is an English noun, verb, and explicative with many different

TABLE 4.—Proportion of All Respondents Describing Each RBC Morphology as Clinically Useful

RBC Morphology	% Useful
Sickle cells	95.3
Malaria parasites seen	91.4
Howell Jolly bodies	83.5
Microcytosis	82.8
Macrocytosis	82.5
Spherocytes	81.9
Schistocytes	77.8
Target cells	75.6
Hypochromasia	70.5
Basophilic stippling	63
Elliptocytes	48
Acanthocytes	46.8
Rouleaux	46
Teardrop forms	46
Poikilocytosis	44.4
RBC agglutination	42.4
Stomatocytes	42
Polychromasia	41.9
Anisocytosis	40
Echinocytes	30.6
Pappenheimer bodies	25.4
Abnormally constricted cells	21.8

RBC indicates red blood cell.

meanings. The 2 predominant ones—as a bodily humour and kinship—are linked by the assumption that blood is the vital fluid, the bearer of life. The English word is of Teutonic origin. When denoting the fluid (blod, blude, bloud), it can be traced to old English text in the 11th century. When signifying a racial and family connection, it dates from the 14th century. It is impossible to demarcate a strict medical usage in time from the word's usage for other purposes. In 1398, an English translation of a medieval treatise on the properties of things, talks of "foure humours, Blood, Flewme, Colera, and Melencolia," while the *King James Bible* of 1611 states "The life of all flesh is the blood thereof." Figuratively and literally at this period, temperament, feeling, and emotions all lie in the blood. By 1650, ancient ideas of blood had changed with William Harvey's account of the circulation in 1628. In fact, experiments with blood transfusion began as early as 1667. From about 1800 onward, the modern technical language of blood was created. Yet it failed to demystify many things including beliefs in vampires fueled by blood. Modern day blood banking, of course, came with the description of blood groups by Karl Landsteiner in 1900. To read more about the historical origins of the word blood, see the commentary by Lawrence.[1]

J. A. Stockman III, MD

Reference

1. Lawrence C. Blood. *Lancet.* 2011;377:1231.

The Etiology and Treatment Outcome of Iron Deficiency and Iron Deficiency Anemia in Children

Huang S-C, Yang Y-J, Cheng C-N, et al (Natl Cheng Kung Univ and Hosp, Tainan, Taiwan)

J Pediatr Hematol Oncol 32:282-285, 2010

This study aimed to evaluate the frequency of the diverse causes of iron deficiency (ID) and iron deficiency anemia (IDA) and to investigate the treatment outcomes in children. ID was defined as a serum ferritin level < 12 μg/L and a transferrin saturation < 10%. IDA was established as ID combined with a low hemoglobin level judged by age and gender-specific reference intervals. A total of 116 ID patients were categorized into 4 groups: group I: < 2 years old (n = 45), group II: 2 to 10 years old (n = 13), group III: > 10 years old, male (n = 18), and group IV: > 10 years old, female (n = 40). One hundred of them (86.2%) were diagnosed with IDA. The most common causes of ID were inadequate intake in group I (55.6%) and blood loss in groups II (46.1%) and IV (37.5%). *Helicobacter pylori*-associated ID mainly occurred in children more than 10 years old. Forty-five of 57 (78.9%) IDA patients who had underlying diseases treatment and/or iron supplementation for 3 months recovered their hemoglobin levels (followup range: 6−27 mo). In conclusion, the peak incidences of childhood ID were ages under 2 years old and 10−18 years old. Different age groups and sexes showed characteristic etiologies. The outcomes of childhood ID were good (Table 2).

▶ This report emanates from Taiwan, but the information contained in it is still quite useful for those who practice in the United States. The report catalogs the etiology of iron deficiency and iron deficiency anemia by age and also gives some insights into how responsive iron deficiency anemia is to treat, based on age and the etiology of the problem. By way of background, the prevalence of iron deficiency and iron deficiency anemia in Taiwanese school children is running somewhere between 2% and 3%. Table 2 lists the various etiologies of iron deficiency in infants, children, and adolescents based on age and mechanism of the anemia. As one might suspect, the problem breaks down into 1 or 2 causes: inadequate intake/malabsorption or blood loss. There are 2 major deficiencies in the information provided. In the United States, one of the most common causes of iron deficiency does not appear in the table. That is celiac disease. When you are seeing an older toddler, child, or adolescent with iron deficiency for whom no apparent cause is noted, think celiac disease. Perhaps children in Taiwan have such a low prevalence of the latter condition that it does not appear on the list. Also, remember that loss of iron can result from losses other than via shedding blood. Iron can be lost in the urine as hemosiderin, a common problem in those with intravascular hemolysis. Iron can also be lost into joint spaces in hemophiliac children. Bleeding into a joint can result in iron being sequestered within the synovial membrane of a joint, making it unavailable for reuse. Thus there are many other causes of

TABLE 2.—Etiologies of Iron Deficiency in Children and Adolescents by Different Mechanisms Between Different Age and Gender Groups

Groups Etiology	<2 y (n = 45)	2–10 y (n = 13)	10–18 y, Male (n = 18)	10–18 y, Female (n = 40)
Inadequate intake, no. (%)	25 (55.6)	2 (15.4)	7 (38.9)	3 (7.5)
Breastfeeding with inadequate supplementary food	15			
Inadequate calorie intake	4	2	6	2
Preterm with low birth weight	6			
Vegetarian diet			1	1
Malabsorption, no. (%)	0 (0)	0 (0)	5 (27.7)	8 (20)
H. pylori infection with peptic ulcers			5	3
H. pylori gastritis				5
Blood loss, no. (%)	7 (15.5)	6 (46.1)	3 (16.7)	15 (37.5)
Polymenorrhea				12
Ulcerative colitis	1			3
Non-H. Pylori-related peptic ulcers		3		
Eosinophilic gastroenteritis	2	1		
Meckel diverticulum			2	
Gastrointestinal surgery	2			
Portal hypertension, esophageal varices	1	1		
Colonic angiodysplasia	1			
Colonic adenoma		1		
Ileal lymphoma			1	
Unknown etiology, no. (%)	13 (28.9)	5 (38.5)	3 (16.7)	14 (35.0)

iron deficiency, all of them more rare than those that appear in this report, and we should look for these when no obvious cause jumps out.

In 1999, researchers began a trial of micronutrient supplement for pregnant women in rural Nepal. Between 2007 and 2009, the same researchers tested the cognitive function of some of the participants' children, aged 7 to 9 years. Children of women who took iron, folic acid, and vitamin A during pregnancy performed slightly, but significantly, better on tests of general intelligence, executive function, and fine motor ability in comparison with children of control women who took vitamin A alone. The authors have suggested a link between extra iron in utero and better cognitive function in childhood, a biologically plausible relationship, particularly in populations with a high prevalence of iron deficiency.[1]

J. A. Stockman III, MD

Reference

1. Editorial comment. Antenatal iron and folic acid linked to cognitive performance in school age children. *BMJ.* 2011;342:17.

Orange But Not Apple Juice Enhances Ferrous Fumarate Absorption in Small Children

Balay KS, Hawthorne KM, Hicks PD, et al (Baylor College of Medicine and Texas Children's Hosp, Houston; Children's Nutrition Res Ctr, Houston, TX; et al)

J Pediatr Gastroenterol Nutr 50:545-550, 2010

Objective.—Ferrous fumarate is a common, inexpensive iron form increasingly used instead of ferrous sulfate as a food iron supplement. However, few data exist as to whether juices enhance iron absorption from ferrous fumarate.

Subjects and Methods.—We studied 21 children, ages 4.0 to 7.9 years using a randomized crossover design. Subjects consumed a small meal including a muffin containing 4 mg ^{57}Fe as ferrous fumarate and either apple (no ascorbic acid) or orange juice (25 mg ascorbic acid). They were separately given a reference dose of ^{58}Fe (ferrous sulfate) with ascorbic acid.

Results.—Iron absorption increased from 5.5% ± 0.7% to 8.2% ± 1.2%, $P < 0.001$ from the muffins given with orange juice compared with muffins given with apple juice. The absorption of ferrous fumarate given with orange juice and enhancement of absorption by the presence of juice were significantly positively related to height, weight, and age ($P < 0.01$ for each). Although iron absorption from ferrous fumarate given with apple juice was significantly inversely associated with the (log transformed) serum ferritin, the difference in absorption between juice types was not ($P > 0.9$).

Conclusions.—These data demonstrate an overall benefit to iron absorption from ferrous fumarate provided with orange juice. The effect was age related such that in children older than 6 years of age, there was a nearly 2-fold increase in iron absorption from ferrous fumarate given with orange juice.

▶ Despite efforts to eliminate iron deficiency through the provision of adequate iron in fortified foods, this deficiency remains pervasive throughout the world, including being a problem on American shores. Although ferrous sulfate is generally considered to be the optimal source of iron in fortification strategies, it is not practical to add this form of iron to all foods. In some instances, elemental iron is used, but depending on its physical characteristics, it can have poor availability. Elemental iron is nothing more than raw iron that is pulverized into microsized particles rather than being provided as a salt. Increasingly, both in the United States and in the developing world, ferrous fumarate is being selected as an iron fortificant. This form of iron is a compromise between other varieties of iron in terms of cost, bioavailability, and sensory/shelf-life characteristics. The absorption of iron from ferrous fumarate is not quite as good as that from ferrous sulfate. Its absorption is largely dependent on enhancement by other food ingredients, especially ascorbic acid. The data on ascorbic acid enhancing the absorption of ferrous fumarate, however, are quite limited compared with that of ferrous sulfate, thus the value of this report of Balay et al, which looked at the absorption of this salt using a population of well-nourished children aged 4 to 7 years.

What we learn from this report is that ferrous fumarate when added to a diet is absorbed at a rate of about 5.5%. This absorption increases by almost 50% if ferrous fumarate is ingested in the presence of orange juice. On the other hand, while an apple a day may keep the doctor away, apple juice does nothing to enhance the absorption of iron. For whatever reason, we are seeing more and more mothers using apple juice these days and as natural as this product may be, it does have some deficiencies, one of them being its inability to enhance iron absorption.

While on the topic of iron deficiency, another report from Armony Sivan et al tells us how iron deficiency anemia seriously affects the quality of mother-infant interaction.[1] In a report of infants and caregivers being screened at their 9- to 10-month-old health maintenance visit at an inner-city clinic in Detroit, iron-deficient infants were rated significantly lower in interactions with their mothers while observed during periods of feeding. These results and previous studies of mother-infant interactions in iron deficiency anemia confirm that iron deficiency anemia in infancy is associated with less optimal mother-infant interaction during feeding.

J. A. Stockman III, MD

Reference

1. Armony Sivan R, Kaplan-Estrin M, Jacobson SW, Lozoff B. Iron-deficiency anemia in infancy and mother-infant interaction during feeding. *J Dev Behav Pediatr.* 2010;31:326-332.

Prevalence of Iron Deficiency in Children with Down Syndrome

Dixon NE, Crissman BG, Smith PB, et al (Duke Univ Med Ctr, Durham, NC)
J Pediatr 157:967-971, 2010

Objectives.—To determine the prevalence of iron deficiency (ID) and iron deficiency anemia (IDA) in a sample of children with Down syndrome (DS) and to evaluate the effect of macrocytosis on the diagnosis of ID/IDA in these children.

Study Design.—Children with DS ≥12 months of age who were followed at the Duke University Medical Center Comprehensive DS Clinic from December 2004 to March 2007 were screened for ID/IDA with a complete blood count, reticulocyte count, iron panel, and erythrocytic protoporphyrins.

Results.—A total of 114 children were enrolled, with a median age of 4.7 years. ID was identified in 12 subjects (10%), and IDA was identified in 3 subjects (3%). ID/IDA would not have been accurately diagnosed in 13 of 15 subjects (86%) if red blood cell (RBC) indices alone had been used for screening. Abnormal RBC indices with low transferrin saturation were 100% sensitive for ID/ IDA screening.

Conclusions.—Prevalence of ID/IDA in children with DS was comparable with that in the general pediatric population. Macrocytosis had implications for screening of ID/IDA with only RBC indices. We suggest ID/IDA screening in DS children be done with a laboratory panel at least including complete blood count, reticulocyte count, transferrin saturation, and serum ferritin.

▶ It is well known that a large percentage of—in fact most—youngsters with Down syndrome have macrocytosis. The cause of this large red cell volume (mean corpuscular volume [MCV]) remains unknown. It is not because of the usual list of suspects (hypothyroidism, reticulocytosis, folate deficiency, or vitamin B12 deficiency). It is also not because of fetal hematopoiesis. Some believe that the macrocytosis is the result of some primitive form of erythropoiesis that sets some of these children up for stem cell disorders, including some forms of leukemia. Whatever the cause of the macrocytosis, it does potentially confuse clinicians if a patient with Down syndrome were to develop iron deficiency. A patient with Down syndrome may very well have iron deficiency with a normal MCV that is otherwise abnormally low for the macrocytosis that the patient with Down syndrome might normally have.

The authors of this study report the prevalence of iron deficiency and iron deficiency anemia in a population of children and adolescents with Down syndrome. The prevalence of iron deficiency ran 10.5%, and iron deficiency anemia ran 2.6%—figures that are comparable to that found in the general pediatric population. Only 2 of the 114 subjects had an MCV result that was below the reference range for age, and both of these patients did have clear-cut iron deficiency anemia. Aside from these 2 patients, the distribution of MCV values overlaps between the normal, iron deficiency, and iron deficiency anemia groups. Thus, a low MCV and low mean corpuscular hemoglobin individually have poor sensitivity for screening for iron deficiency and iron deficiency anemia. Even when examined with a combination of other red cell indices including red blood cell distribution width, the sensitivity rate is unacceptably low at just 61%. The bottom line is that the data indicate that the macrocytosis of Down syndrome can often mask the diagnosis of iron deficiency and iron deficiency anemia.

So what is a clinician to do? One good piece of information would be to have a baseline MCV in every child with Down syndrome to know if that MCV declines for any reason. The authors of this report recommend obtaining a complete blood count (CBC) and reticulocyte count at diagnosis and subsequent follow-up after iron replacement has been initiated to not only determine response to therapy but also establish the true baseline for these red blood cell indices in the individual patient. Serum ferritin concentration as a sole indicator of iron depletion is not sensitive enough for screening of iron deficiency or iron deficiency anemia in this population. A low serum ferritin, however, is an important diagnostic clinical tool confirming iron depletion when used with other measures of iron status. The final recommendation of these authors is that when a child with Down syndrome is screened for iron deficiency/iron deficiency anemia, an expanded laboratory panel should be used, including a CBC, reticulocyte count, serum iron, total iron binding capacity, and serum ferritin concentration. Ideally, a baseline MCV would be done at 9 to 12 months of age and then annually.

It is critically important not to miss iron deficiency or iron deficiency anemia in a child with Down syndrome. These children are as susceptible as any other child to the nonhematologic manifestations of iron deficiency including alterations in cognitive/behavioral performance, attention-deficit/hyperactivity symptoms, pediatric restless legs syndrome, and sleep disturbances. Iron deficiency has also been suspected to be a significant underlying cause in many children for breath-holding spells. Lastly, iron-deficient red cells are very rigid, and should a child with Down syndrome have cyanotic congenital heart disease and polycythemia, he/she is at much higher risk for developing a stroke.

J. A. Stockman III, MD

Sickle cell disease resulting from uniparental disomy in a child who inherited sickle cell trait
Swensen JJ, Agarwal AM, Esquilin JM, et al (Univ of Utah, Salt Lake City; Columbia Univ Med Ctr, NY; et al)
Blood 116:2822-2825, 2010

Sickle cell disease (SCD) is a classic example of a disorder with recessive Mendelian inheritance, in which each parent contributes one mutant allele to an affected offspring. However, there are exceptions to that rule. We describe here the first reported case of conversion of inherited sickle cell trait to SCD by uniparental disomy (UPD) resulting in mosaicism for SS and AS erythrocytes. A 14-year-old boy presented with splenomegaly and hemolysis. Although his father has sickle cell trait, his mother has no abnormal hemoglobin (Hb). DNA sequencing, performed to rule out Hb S/β-thalassemia, detected homozygous Hb SS. Further studies revealed mosaic UPD of the β-globin locus, more SS erythroid progenitors than AS, but a reverse ratio of erythrocytes resulting from the survival advantage of AS erythrocytes. This report exemplifies non-Mendelian genetics wherein a patient who inherited sickle cell trait has mild SCD resulting from postzygotic mitotic recombination leading to UPD.

▶ It has been just over one century since Dr Herrick first described sickle cell disease as a specific entity, a description that was published based on a patient in Chicago, Illinois. In the interim century, we have learned a lot about the inheritance of sickle cell disease. It is a prototypic autosomal recessive disease with Mendelian inheritance wherein each parent contributes one mutation to an affected offspring. There are, however, rare instances in which a child may develop a recessive disorder when only one parent carries a mutation. Uniparental disomy (UPD) may unmask a recessive mutation or a second mutation may occur de novo in a person who has inherited a single mutation. In UPD, both copies of all or part of a chromosome are received from the same parent. If the copies are from the same chromosome (isodisomy), then any mutation present on that chromosome becomes homozygous and can cause recessive disease. Whole chromosome UPD is most commonly the result of trisomic rescue (exclusion of 1 of 3 chromosome copies from trisomic embryo), whereas segmental UPD results from postzygotic mitotic recombination or gene conversion of a segment of a chromosome.

With this as a background, Swensen et al report a patient with mild sickle cell disease who inherited hemoglobin S (Hb S) from his father and a normal beta-globin gene from his mother. Postzygotic mitotic recombination led to a mosaic segmental paternal isodisomy of chromosome 11, resulting in a subpopulation of erythroid progenitors homozygous for Hb S. The report of Swensen et al is the first one describing sickle cell disease resulting from UPD in a person with the inherited sickle cell trait. This report demonstrates the importance of considering non-Mendelian modes of inheritance when evaluating a patient for possible recessive disorder. Accurate interpretation of genetic testing in such cases requires correlation with results from other family members. When a diagnosis of sickle cell disease is made in such rare circumstances, one will find one parent who appears totally normal and the other as having sickle cell trait. One should not assume erroneous parenting with all of its negative potential implications. The father is the real father, and the mother is the real mother.

While on the topic of sickle cell trait, on April 13, 2010, the legislative council for Division I of the National Collegiate Athletic Association (NCAA) approved mandatory testing for sickle cell carrier status (sickle cell trait) for all student athletes participating in Division I sports. The new rule took effect during the academic year 2010 to 2011. The requirement will ultimately affect about 165 000 student athletes. The screening program resulted from the settlement of a lawsuit brought by the family of Dale Lloyd II against the NCAA and Rice University. Lloyd was a 19-year-old freshman at Rice when he died after a football practice in 2006. His death was attributed to acute exertional rhabdomyolysis associated with the sickle cell trait. Lloyd's family took legal action in the hope of preventing other deaths. Although the NCAA program differs in scope and purpose from earlier sickle cell trait screening programs, it shares the potential for unintended consequences. Will the NCAA assist student athletes and their parents in making informed decisions regarding testing and understanding the implications of the test results? Will the first-line test, hemoglobin solubility, be followed by a second test to eliminate false positives? What role will primary care providers play in screening and counseling? How would the knowledge of carrier status affect student athletes and their families? How will the athletic program and the institution protect the privacy of athletes who test positive? Surveillance and research aimed at understanding the program's effects on universities, athletes, and families will need to be conducted if inadvertent harm is to be avoided.

To read more about screening student athletes for sickle cell trait, see the excellent perspective on this topic by Bonham et al.[1] The screening program may also open the door to additional genetic testing for other entities, such as inherited cardiac arrhythmias and cardiomyopathy syndromes, that have been implicated as the most important nontraumatic cause of death among athletes.

J. A. Stockman III, MD

Reference

1. Bonham VL, Dover GJ, Brody LC. Screening student athletes for sickle cell trait—a social and clinical experiment. *N Engl J Med.* 2010;363:997-999.

Dietary Water and Sodium Intake of Children and Adolescents With Sickle Cell Anemia

Fowler KT, Williams R, Mitchell CO, et al (Univ of Memphis, TN; St Jude Children's Res Hosp, Memphis, TN)
J Pediatr Hematol Oncol 32:350-353, 2010

Dietary fluid and sodium intake may influence the risk for vasoocclusive events in persons with sickle cell anemia (SCA). The objective of this study was to examine the dietary intake of water and sodium in children and adolescents with SCA and identify possible factors influencing intake. We compared water (mL) and sodium (mg) intake in 21 patients with SCA, aged 5 to 18 years, to reported adequate intake for water, daily fluid requirement, upper limit for sodium, and National Health and Nutrition Examination Survey 2005 to 2006 data for sodium, and sociodemographic factors. Dietary intake from 3-day food records was evaluated retrospectively. Median water intake was significantly lower than adequate intake, and median sodium intake was significantly higher than sodium upper limit. Sociodemographic factors were not associated with dietary water or sodium intake. Our results suggest that children and adolescents with SCA would benefit from education regarding increasing fluid intake and limiting high sodium foods.

► It is well known that patients with sickle cell disease need to maintain proper levels of hydration. Such patients are indeed at risk of dehydration as a result of the poor concentrating ability of the kidneys. Indeed, hyposthenuria is the most common abnormality of renal function seen in patients with sickle cell anemia, and this results in increased obligatory urine output, fluid requirement, and susceptibility to dehydration. Currently, the fluid requirement for children with sickle cell anemia is estimated at 150 mL/kg/d, whereas for adults this number increases to 3 to 4 L/d. In children and adolescents, between 1 and 1.5 times of the estimated daily fluid maintenance requirement is recommended during vaso-occlusive pain crises. Extraoral fluid intake in mild cases may shorten an episode in affected individuals. For more severe pain, of course, intravenous hydration is recommended.

Fowler et al assist us in understanding the food requirements of patients with sickle cell anemia by studying dietary water and sodium intake in children and adolescents with the disorder. What was found was that only 80% of daily fluid requirements were observed for patients with sickle cell anemia in comparison to healthy peers. Alarmingly, the median of the percent for water intake was just 34.2%. These results indicate that total dietary water intake for this population is well below current recommendations. Median sodium intake differs significantly (on the high side) compared with recommended amounts of sodium. Mean sodium intakes were found to be above the recommended levels for most children with sickle cell anemia.

Children with sickle cell anemia, their families, and care providers should be made aware of the findings from this report. Specifically, the findings of this study indicate that this population would benefit from education regarding increasing fluid intake and limiting foods that are high in sodium. The authors of this report note that it is unclear what cultural, economic, or knowledge differences or other dietary patterns may be contributing to this population's failure to meet dietary water recommendations or to its exceeding sodium recommendations. To date, no one has looked at thirst studies in this patient population. It could well be that the diet of these patients simply reflects the high-sodium diet of the entire family.

Please note that 2010 marked the 100th anniversary of the initial description of sickle cell disease. Also, just over 60 years ago, sickle cell disease was heralded as the first molecular disease, having then been defined as resulting from a single amino acid substitution in the β-globin chain of hemoglobin A. We have not yet conquered this disease. For example, the World Health Organization estimates that many of the more than 200 000 babies with sickle cell disease born annually in Africa will die before the age of 5 from anemia and infection. In the United States, approximately 50 000 individuals are afflicted with sickle cell disease. Most feel that the ultimate cure for this disorder will come from some unique therapy that reactivates fetal hemoglobin production in sickle cell disease-affected patients, a treatment that would also significantly benefit patients with β-thalassemia.

To read more about sickle cell disease at its 100-year anniversary, see the wonderful summary by Orkin and Higgs.[1] Also, see the excellent review by Ware[2] describing how hydroxyurea can be used to treat patients with sickle cell anemia, as 1 method to increase the production of fetal hemoglobin.

J. A. Stockman III, MD

References

1. Orkin SH, Higgs DR. Sickle cell disease at 100 years. *Science*. 2010;329:291-292.
2. Ware RE. How I use hydroxyurea to treat young patients with sickle cell anemia. *Blood*. 2010;115:5300-5311.

Neuropsychological Dysfunction and Neuroimaging Abnormalities in Neurologically Intact Adults With Sickle Cell Anemia
Vichinsky EP, for the Neuropsychological Dysfunction and Neuroimaging Adult Sickle Cell Anemia Study Group (Children's Hosp & Res Ctr Oakland, CA; et al)
JAMA 303:1823-1831, 2010

Context.—Sickle cell anemia (SCA) is a chronic illness causing progressive deterioration in quality of life. Brain dysfunction may be the most important and least studied problem affecting individuals with this disease.

Objective.—To measure neurocognitive dysfunction in neurologically asymptomatic adults with SCA vs healthy control individuals.

Design, Setting, and Participants.—Cross-sectional study comparing neuropsychological function and neuroimaging findings in neurologically asymptomatic adults with SCA and controls from 12 SCA centers, conducted between December 2004 and May 2008. Participants were patients with SCA (hemoglobin [Hb] SS and hemoglobin level ≤10 mg/dL) aged 19 to 55 years and of African descent (n=149) or community controls (Hb AA and normal hemoglobin level) (n=47). Participants were stratified on age, sex, and education.

Main Outcome Measures.—The primary outcome measure was nonverbal function assessed by the Wechsler Adult Intelligence Scale, third edition (WAIS-III) Performance IQ Index. Secondary exploratory outcomes included performance on neurocognitive tests of executive function, memory, attention, and language and magnetic resonance imaging measurement of total intracranial and hippocampal volume, cortical gray and white matter, and lacunae.

Results.—The mean WAIS-III Performance IQ score of patients with SCA was significantly lower than that of controls (adjusted mean, 86.69 for patients with SCA vs 95.19 for controls [mean difference, −5.50; 95% confidence interval {CI}, −9.55 to −1.44]; P=.008), with 33% performing more than 1 SD (<85) below the population mean. Among secondary measures, differences were observed in adjusted mean values for global cognitive function (full-scale IQ) (90.47 for patients with SCA vs 95.66 for controls [mean difference, −5.19; 95% CI, −9.24 to −1.13]; P=.01), working memory (90.75 vs 95.25 [mean difference, −4.50; 95% CI, −8.55 to −0.45]; P=.03), processing speed (86.50 vs 97.95 [mean difference, −11.46; 95% CI, −15.51 to −7.40]; P<.001), and measures of executive function. Anemia was associated with poorer neurocognitive function in older patients. No differences in total gray matter or hippocampal volume were observed. Lacunae were more frequent in patients with SCA but not independently related to neurocognitive function.

Conclusion.—Compared with healthy controls, adults with SCA had poorer cognitive performance, which was associated with anemia and age.

▶ As management techniques have improved over the years, patients with sickle cell disease are surviving longer and longer. Nonetheless, the Cooperative Study of Sickle Cell Disease has found that 24% of individuals with sickle cell disease have experienced a clinical stroke by the age of 45 years.[1] In addition, prospective pediatric imaging and neurocognitive studies have identified the serious problem of unrecognized brain injury in children with sickle cell disease. Not only do those with a history of overt strokes have problems, but neurologically intact children also may have impaired neurocognitive functioning that worsens with age. Current data suggest declining intelligence quotient (IQ) scores, difficulties with learning, and impairment of executive brain functioning being common in children, even those with normal findings on imaging studies and normal neurologic examinations.

The Neuropsychological Dysfunction and Neuroimaging Adult Sickle Cell Anemia Study Group undertook the study abstracted, which hypothesizes that neurological asymptomatic adult patients with sickle cell anemia and chronic anemia (hemoglobin level 10 g/dL) would score lower on Performance IQ index of the Wechsler Adult Intelligence Scale compared with controls. This measure of nonverbal function was chosen as the primary outcome because of the strong association between nonverbal abilities and central nervous system dysfunction in children with sickle cell anemia. The hypothesis proved to be correct. Adult patients with sickle cell anemia who are neurologically asymptomatic are still at risk for neurocognitive performance deficits because their anemia may be reducing neurocognitive impairment secondary to cerebral hypoxemia undetectable by standard neuroimaging techniques. These are exactly the patients who could theoretically benefit from early identification and enrollment in cognitive rehabilitation programs. This study group presumably will be following up on these patients to determine whether or not there is any progression of the cognitive impairment over time.

Please be aware that these data are derived from patients with sickle cell disease in the United States. More than 80% of all children with sickle cell disease are born in Africa, but there, more than 90% of children with the disease will in fact die before a diagnosis is made. Bacterial infection is a major risk factor for all children with sickle cell disease, but it has been unclear what the main pathogens in Africa are. A recent study at Kilifi District Hospital on the Kenyan coast has shown that the pathogens there are the same as in the United States and Europe.[2] The only way of dealing with this high morbidity problem is early detection and careful management that includes the appropriate vaccines and antibiotic prophylaxis.

J. A. Stockman III, MD

References

1. Ohene-Frempong K, Weiner SJ, Sleeper LA, et al. Cerebrovascular accidents in sickle cell disease: rates and risk factors. *Blood.* 1998;91:288-294.
2. Williams TN, Uyoga S, Macharia A, et al. Bacteraemia in Kenyan children with sickle-cell anaemia: a retrospective cohort and case-control study. *Lancet.* 2009; 374:1364-1370.

Transcranial Doppler Ultrasonography and Prophylactic Transfusion Program Is Effective in Preventing Overt Stroke in Children with Sickle Cell Disease
Enninful-Eghan H, Moore RH, Ichord R, et al (Children's Hosp of Philadelphia, PA; Univ of Pennsylvania, Philadelphia)
J Pediatr 157:479-484, 2010

Objective.—To assess the impact of our transcranial Doppler ultrasonography (TCD) program on the incidence of first stroke and the rate of transfusion for stroke prevention in children with sickle cell disease.

Study Design.—In this single-institution, retrospective study, we compared the incidence of stroke and of transfusion for stroke prevention in 475 patients observed in the 8-year period before instituting TCD screening with the rate in 530 children in the 8-year period after.

Results.—The incidence of overt stroke in the pre-TCD period was 0.67 per 100 patient-years, compared with 0.06 per 100 patient-years in the post-TCD period ($P < .0001$). Of the 2 strokes in the post-TCD period, 1 occurred in a child too young for the screening protocol, and 1 occurred in a child with high velocities solely in the anterior cerebral arteries. The rate of transfusion therapy for stroke prevention increased from 0.67 per 100 patient-years to 1.12 per 100 patient-years since instituting our program ($P = .008$).

Conclusions.—Our program has been successful in reducing the rate of first overt stroke, but with increased use of transfusion. Additional modifications to screening might further reduce the risk of first stroke, and studies of alternative treatments may be beneficial.

▶ Many years ago, it was shown that patients with sickle cell disease frequently develop central nervous system major-vessel occlusive disease leading to stroke. The prevalence of stroke is highest in children under the age of 10 years. Overall, the incidence of overt stroke in persons with homozygous sickle cell disease of all ages runs 0.61 events per 100 patient-years, but this number increases to a rate of 1.02 per 100 patient-years in children aged 2 to 5 years and 0.79 per 100 patient-years in children aged 6 to 9 years.[1] In the last 15 to 20 years, it has been increasingly common to see the use of transcranial Doppler ultrasonography in the detection of children at high risk of stroke. Identified children are best managed with regular transfusions, which, as we see in this report of Enninful-Eghan et al, are an effective mode of therapy.

The object of the study of Enninful-Eghan et al was to assess the impact of transcranial Doppler ultrasonography screening and prophylactic transfusion programs on the incidence of first stroke in children with sickle cell disease followed up in a large comprehensive sickle cell disease center at the Children's Hospital of Philadelphia. It was clear that the incidence of overt stroke in youngsters managed with transfusion therapy is reduced by a magnitude of greater than 10-fold. The screening program failed to detect 2 youngsters. The first was a child who failed to meet the protocol criteria for transfusion because his velocities in the internal carotid and middle cerebral arteries were not significantly elevated prior to the onset of first stroke. The second stroke was not prevented with the transcranial Doppler ultrasonography protocol because the stroke occurred in a 14-month-old child, and the protocol did not begin until children were 2 years of age, suggesting a need to begin such screening at an earlier age.

Needless to say, with the use of transcranial Doppler ultrasonography, more children are being put on hypertransfusion programs. Such regular transfusions have the added benefit of preventing other complications of sickle cells disease such as acute chest syndrome and painful crises but carry the risks of infection, alloimmunization, and iron overload. Some centers are attempting to minimize the amount of iron overload by using exchange transfusion rather than booster transfusion. The authors of this report from Philadelphia suggest that exchange transfusions are of definitive benefit but do involve greater blood donor exposure than simple transfusion and may increase the risk of alloimmunization and transfusion-transmitted infection. Obviously, these children are also managed with iron-chelation agents. Deferasirox, an oral chelator, only became commercially available in early 2006, and thus the impact of this form of iron chelation is not yet well documented.

Given the disastrous consequences of a stroke, transcranial Doppler ultrasonography and prophylactic transfusion are warranted methods to prevent overt stroke. However, more work needs to be done to optimize transfusion protocols and chelation regimens.

J. A. Stockman III, MD

Reference

1. Ohene-Frempong K, Weiner SJ, Sleeper LA, et al. Cardiovascular accidents in sickle cell disease: rates and risk factors. *Blood.* 1998;91:288-294.

White Matter Integrity and Core Cognitive Function in Children Diagnosed With Sickle Cell Disease
Scantlebury N, Mabbott D, Janzen L, et al (Univ of Toronto, Ontario, Canada)
J Pediatr Hematol Oncol 33:163-171, 2011

Children diagnosed with sickle cell disease (SCD) have an increased risk of stroke, often associated with white matter damage and neurocognitive morbidity. Growing evidence suggests that subtle changes in white matter integrity, which do not pass the threshold to be visible on a clinical magnetic resonance image and classified as stroke, may contribute to decreased cognitive performance. We used archived diffusion-weighted imaging and neurocognitive assessment data to identify associations between microstructural changes in normal-appearing white matter and cognitive performance in children with SCD. Study participants included 10 healthy children and 15 pediatric SCD patients (5 with identified lesions and 10 without lesion). After excluding lesioned tissue from analyses, we detected significant increases in apparent diffusion coefficient across the brains of patients in comparison with control children, suggesting compromise to the structure of normal-appearing white matter. Deficits in working memory and processing speed were also apparent in patients. Increased apparent diffusion coefficient and deficiencies in processing speed were again detected in a subanalysis including only the patients without lesion. Correlation analyses evidenced associations between the microstructure of the right frontal lobe and cerebellum, and processing speed. This outcome suggests a relationship between tissue integrity and cognitive morbidity in SCD patients.

▶ It is well known that children with sickle cell disease (SCD) who suffer a stroke may very well have neurocognitive morbidity as a consequence of this problem. The traditional diagnosis of a stroke is made with an MRI. What Scantlebury et al have done is to document that it does not take a stroke to produce neurocognitive morbidity in SCD. These investigators studied patients with SCD using diffusion-weighted imaging (DWI), a specialized MRI sequence that translates the microstructural diffusion properties of water into a measure, known as the apparent diffusion coefficient, that can be used to evaluate white matter integrity. DWI-MRI can detect white matter findings that are not seen normally on MRI. A patient can have brain injury and normal findings on an MRI, but show abnormalities on a DWI-MRI study.

Scantlebury et al report reduced performance on tasks requiring working memory and efficient processing speed in their patient population with abnormal DWI-MRI. While white matter injury caused by overt or even silent strokes will reduce intelligence scores and the gradual accumulation of lesions can result in reduced intellectual quotient, microstructural modifications in normal-appearing white matter can also account for neurocognitive issues in this same patient population. This study also has laid the groundwork for the use of diffusion imaging to assess the relationship between the integrity of normal-appearing white matter and core cognitive function in the SCD population. Needless to say, all this provides more work and full employment for the neuroradiologist.

J. A. Stockman III, MD

Left ventricular hypertrophy and diastolic dysfunction in children with sickle cell disease are related to asleep and waking oxygen desaturation

Johnson MC, Kirkham FJ, Redline S, et al (Washington Univ School of Medicine, St Louis, MO; UCL Inst of Child Health, UK; Case Western Reserve Univ, Cleveland, OH; et al)
Blood 116:16-21, 2010

Premature death and cardiac abnormalities are described in individuals with sickle cell disease (SCD), but the mechanisms are not well characterized. We tested the hypothesis that cardiac abnormalities in children with SCD are related to sleep-disordered breathing. We enrolled 44 children with SCD (mean age, 10.1 years; range, 4-18 years) in an observational study. Standard and tissue Doppler echocardiography, waking oxygen saturation averaged over 5 minutes, and overnight polysomnography were obtained in participants, each within 7 days. Eccentric left ventricular (LV) hypertrophy was present in 46% of our cohort. After multivariable adjustment, LV mass index was inversely related to average asleep and waking oxygen saturation. For every 1% drop in the average asleep oxygen saturation, there was a 2.1 $g/m^{2.7}$ increase in LV mass index. LV diastolic dysfunction, as measured by the E/E' ratio, was present in our subjects and was also associated with low oxygen saturation (sleep or waking). Elevated tricuspid regurgitant velocity ($\geq$ 2.5 m/sec), a measure of pulmonary hypertension, was not predicted by either oxygen saturation or sleep variables with multivariable logistic regression analysis. These data provide evidence that low asleep and waking oxygen saturations are associated with LV abnormalities in children with SCD.

▶ This report by Johnson et al describes echocardiography and polysomnography results from 44 children with sickle cell disease (SCD). The results demonstrate left ventricular hypertrophy and diastolic dysfunction significantly correlating with low oxygen tensions, both asleep and awake, and with systolic blood pressure. The report confirms the association of left ventricular hypertrophy, diastolic dysfunction, and low waking oxygen tensions in patients with SCD previously reported.

The fact that patients with SCD may desaturate during sleep, as seen in otherwise normal patients with obstructive sleep apnea, should be considered very worrisome since in normal individuals, sleep desaturations are associated with markers of activated endothelium, platelets and leukocytes, leukotriene B4, high von Willebrand factor, low hemoglobin count, and high reticulocyte count. This constellation of findings represents ones that are known to correlate with cardiac disease and stroke.

It is also well known in the adult population that left ventricular hypertrophy and diastolic dysfunction are linked to systemic hypertension. Interestingly, the resting blood pressure range in patients with SCD is actually lower than in the general population, but it has been documented that in patients with SCD, relative systemic hypertension that still falls within the normal population norms predicts early mortality. The report of Johnson et al documents that systolic blood pressures even within the upper ranges of normal are independent predictors of left ventricular mass dysfunction in patients with SCD.

The authors of this report are clearly on to something that hopefully we could do something to diminish some of the long-term complications of SCD. If those with SCD desaturate more during sleep, perhaps management in the way we manage sleep apnea would be advisable. Stay tuned.

For more on the topic of SCD and the current role of hydroxyurea, refer to the superb editorial explaining all the excellent evidence for using hydroxyurea to manage patients with sickle cell anemia. This review was prepared by Dr Russell Ware.[1]

J. A. Stockman III, MD

Reference

1. Ware RE. How I use hydroxyurea to treat young patients with sickle cell anemia. *Blood.* 2010;115:5300-5311.

Apparent Desaturation on Pulse Oximetry Because of Hemoglobinopathy
Mounts J, Clingenpeel J, White N, et al (Children's Hosp of The King's Daughters, Norfolk, VA)
Pediatr Emerg Care 26:748-749, 2010

Hemoglobinopathies are an uncommon cause of cyanosis and low oxygen saturation on pulse oximetry. However, when they do occur, they can present a complex clinical scenario for the emergency physician. We report the index case of a previously undescribed hemoglobinopathy that presented to the pediatric emergency department. The evaluation and management of the cyanotic/hypoxic child and review of hemoglobinopathies are presented here.

▶ This report highlights an unusual circumstance in which a patient with a hemoglobinopathy showed apparently abnormally low pulse oximetry results. It highlights not only this unusual circumstance but also other circumstances where similar pulse oximetry findings may be observed. The case was that of a 10-month-old African American infant girl who was transferred to an emergency department in Norfolk, Virginia, for evaluation of hypoxia. She had a 2-day history of cough and congestion and increased work of breathing. On evaluation in a referring facility, a pulse oximetry reading was obtained and revealed oxygen saturations of just 75% on room air. After being placed on oxygen via a nonrebreather face mask, her saturation levels increased only to 85%. She received both albuterol and racemic epinephrine nebulizations without further improvement in her oxygen saturation levels, where upon she was transferred for further evaluation. The medical history was otherwise unremarkable. The physical examination showed an alert, awake, interactive child with only mild respiratory distress. Her lungs were clear to auscultation bilaterally without wheezing or rails. Cardiac examination was normal. The rest of the examination was unremarkable. There was no evidence of cyanosis. An arterial blood gas obtained on 15 L/min via a nonrebreathing face mask showed a pH of 7.41, a Pco_2 of 34 mm Hg, Pao_2 of 300 mm Hg, bicarbonate of 21 mmol/L, and oxygen saturations of 100%. Methemoglobin levels were unremarkable, and the oxygen dissociation curve was unremarkable with a normal P50. An echocardiogram was normal. DNA sequencing analysis of the α-globin gene identified a previously unreported substitution.

So what was occurring with this youngster? Unfortunately, for many of us, pulse oximetry is used as a gold standard for oxygen status in a patient when, in fact, most of us do not understand the nuances of pulse oximeters. The most common causes of abnormal pulse oximetry findings are cyanotic congenital heart disease and methemoglobinemia. The child had neither of these, leaving the attending physician to wonder about the possibility of a hemoglobinopathy, which was confirmed. There are 2 main reasons why certain hemoglobinopathies are thought to cause low pulse oximetry readings. One postulation is that there is variance in light absorption by the hemoglobin at the 2 wavelengths measured by the pulse oximeter, causing one to believe that there is more deoxygenated hemoglobin than is truly present. Another theory is that the enhanced peripheral unloading of oxygen of low—oxygen affinity hemoglobin results in a lowered ratio of oxygenated hemoglobin to deoxygenated hemoglobin, therefore affecting the pulse oximetry calculations of oxygen saturation. This patient did not have an abnormal hemoglobin oxygen saturation curve, leading one to therefore suspect that altered light absorption caused the apparent hypoxemia.

Please be aware that pulse oximetry measures the absorption of 2 wavelengths of light (red and infrared) by oxygenated and deoxygenated hemoglobin. It uses the ratio of these absorptions and compares it with a standardized ratio to determine the percentage of oxygenated and deoxygenated hemoglobin present. Abnormal hemoglobin such as found in this youngster will show varying patterns of absorption leading to erroneously low pulse oximetry readings.

If there is a teachable moment in all this, it is that if you find an abnormally low pulse oximetry reading and there is no obvious explanation for it, think about the possibility of a hemoglobinopathy. Although it is rare to see a hemoglobinopathy presenting in such a way, the possibility does need to be considered.

J. A. Stockman III, MD

Nucleic Acid Testing to Detect HBV Infection in Blood Donors

Stramer SL, Wend U, Candotti D, et al (American Red Cross, Gaithersburg, MD; Univ of Giessen, Germany; Natl Health Service Blood and Transplant, Cambridge, UK; et al)
N Engl J Med 364:236-247, 2011

Background.—The detection of hepatitis B virus (HBV) in blood donors is achieved by screening for hepatitis B surface antigen (HBsAg) and for antibodies against hepatitis B core antigen (anti-HBc). However, donors who are positive for HBV DNA are currently not identified during the window period before seroconversion. The current use of nucleic acid testing for detection of the human immunodeficiency virus (HIV) and hepatitis C virus (HCV) RNA and HBV DNA in a single triplex assay may provide additional safety.

Methods.—We performed nucleic acid testing on 3.7 million blood donations and further evaluated those that were HBV DNA−positive but negative for HBsAg and anti-HBc. We determined the serologic, biochemical, and molecular features of samples that were found to contain only HBV DNA and performed similar analyses of follow-up samples and samples from sexual partners of infected donors. Seronegative HIV and HCV-positive donors were also studied.

Results.—We identified 9 donors who were positive for HBV DNA (1 in 410,540 donations), including 6 samples from donors who had received the HBV vaccine, in whom subclinical infection had developed and resolved. Of the HBV DNA−positive donors, 4 probably acquired HBV infection from a chronically infected sexual partner. Clinically significant liver injury developed in 2 unvaccinated donors. In 5 of the 6 vaccinated donors, a non-A genotype was identified as the dominant strain, whereas subgenotype A2 (represented in the HBV vaccine) was the dominant strain in unvaccinated donors. Of 75 reactive nucleic acid test results identified in seronegative blood donations, 26 (9 HBV, 15 HCV, and 2 HIV) were confirmed as positive.

Conclusions.—Triplex nucleic acid testing detected potentially infectious HBV, along with HIV and HCV, during the window period before seroconversion. HBV vaccination appeared to be protective, with a breakthrough subclinical infection occurring with non-A2 HBV subgenotypes and causing clinically inconsequential outcomes.

▶ Currently, blood is screened for hepatitis B by testing for hepatitis B surface antigen and for antibodies against hepatitis B core antigen. Blood that is free of hepatitis B surface antigen but has high-titer antibodies against hepatitis core antigen in the absence of antibodies against hepatitis B surface antigen can also transmit hepatitis B virus (HBV). Blood that is collected during the early window period of HBV infection is highly infectious, but this risk declines as antihepatitis B surface antigen develops. The estimated residual risk of HBV infection from donations to the American Red Cross ranges from 1 in 280 000 to 1 in 357 000 donations. After the introduction of nucleic acid testing for screening of mini pools (pools of 6-16 donors), the estimated yield of HBV infection now ranges from 1 in 830 000 to 1 in 2 000 000 donations. These estimates, however, do not capture the possibility of HPV infection in vaccinated donors who have acute infection with low or no expression of hepatitis B surface antigen. HBV-seronegative but infected donors have been identified by means of nucleic acid testing at a rate of approximately 1 in 600 000 donations screened. Although the risk of transmission of HBV by transfusion has decreased progressively over the years, it remains higher than the estimated risk for human immunodeficiency virus and hepatitis C virus. The latter risks are 1 in 1 467 000 donations and 1 in 1 449 000 donations, respectively.

Stramer et al conducted a study to evaluate the use of nucleic acid testing in determining the number of seronegative donors who have HBV DNA in their circulation. They also characterized these donors according to their risk factors. The investigators observed some unexpected patterns of early HBV infection as a result of evaluating HBV nucleic acid testing in some 3.7 million blood donors. In this large population, they expected to see 2 to 4 seronegative, HBV DNA—positive samples from mini pool nucleic acid testing and 1 seronegative, HBV DNA—positive sample from single-donation testing. In fact, they found 9 seronegative HBV DNA—positive samples, and all but one were detected on mini pool nucleic acid testing for a total rate of 1 per 410 540 donations. Three of the infected donors appear to have had conventional window-period infection, which is consistent with expected findings. Unexpectedly, 5 of the other 6 infected donors had low-level antihepatitis B surface antigen or a rapid anamnestic response, presumably attributable to the receipt of HBV vaccine some 7 to 27 years earlier. The 5 vaccinated donors had a brief transient course of infection with no evidence of disease and very low or absent expression of hepatitis B surface antigen. Their level of viremia was very low. Thus, even those who have been vaccinated against hepatitis B may for a short period of time after exposure to HBV become transiently infectious as blood donors, although they themselves will not suffer any consequence of having been exposed to HBV because they were vaccinated.

In summary, this study showed a higher than expected rate of HBV infection with the use of nucleic acid testing, mainly in donors who had been vaccinated some years earlier against HBV and who would not have been identified by routine screening for hepatitis B surface antigen or antihepatitis B core. These HBV infections are of no consequence whatsoever to vaccinated donors, but the potential for transmission to a recipient of infected blood remains to be seen. The study is important because it shows the efficacy of hepatitis B vaccine for the prevention of clinical disease in those who are vaccinated but not necessarily prevention of transmissible infection.

J. A. Stockman III, MD

Romiplostim or Standard of Care in Patients with Immune Thrombocytopenia

Kuter DJ, Rummel M, Boccia R, et al (Massachusetts General Hosp, Boston; Klinikum der Justus-Liebig-Universität, Giessen, Germany; Ctr for Cancer and Blood Disorders, Bethesda, MD; et al)
N Engl J Med 363:1889-1899, 2010

Background.—Romiplostim, a thrombopoietin mimetic, increases platelet counts in patients with immune thrombocytopenia, with few adverse effects.

Methods.—In this open-label, 52-week study, we randomly assigned 234 adult patients with immune thrombocytopenia, who had not undergone splenectomy, to receive the standard of care (77 patients) or weekly subcutaneous injections of romiplostim (157 patients). Primary end points were incidences of treatment failure and splenectomy. Secondary end points included the rate of a platelet response (a platelet count $>50\times10^9$ per liter at any scheduled visit), safety outcomes, and the quality of life.

Results.—The rate of a platelet response in the romiplostim group was 2.3 times that in the standard-of-care group (95% confidence interval [CI], 2.0 to 2.6; P<0.001). Patients receiving romiplostim had a significantly lower incidence of treatment failure (18 of 157 patients [11%]) than those receiving the standard of care (23 of 77 patients [30%], P<0.001) (odds ratio with romiplostim, 0.31; 95% CI, 0.15 to 0.61). Splenectomy also was performed less frequently in patients receiving romiplostim (14 of 157 patients [9%]) than in those receiving the standard of care (28 of 77 patients [36%], P<0.001) (odds ratio, 0.17; 95% CI, 0.08 to 0.35). The romiplostim group had a lower rate of bleeding events, fewer blood transfusions, and greater improvements in the quality of life than the standard-of-care group. Serious adverse events occurred in 23% of patients (35 of 154) receiving romiplostim and 37% of patients (28 of 75) receiving the standard of care.

Conclusions.—Patients treated with romiplostim had a higher rate of a platelet response, lower incidence of treatment failure and splenectomy, less bleeding and fewer blood transfusions, and a higher quality of life than patients treated with the standard of care. (Funded by Amgen; ClinicalTrials.gov number, NCT00415532.)

▶ I selected this report to demonstrate how rapidly the world is changing when it comes to the management of patients with immune thrombocytopenia. The report of Kuter et al does include teenagers with immune thrombocytopenia, an age group in the pediatric population more likely to develop chronic immune thrombocytopenia. The information provided by this report therefore may not apply to all of the pediatric population, but the data from the study yield valuable information for all of us who care for children.

It was back in 2004 that reports first appeared showing that 2 biotechnology products, romiplostim and eltrombopag, mimicked the biologic effects of thrombopoietin, the physiologic regulator of platelet production. These novel thrombopoietic agonists promoted megakaryocyte growth and maturation by binding to the thrombopoietin receptor, c-mpl. The primary disease target of thrombopoietin mimetics is chronic immune thrombocytopenia (also known as immune thrombocytopenic purpura [ITP]) in which autoantibodies accelerate platelet destruction and block platelet production, leading to low and sometimes dangerous decreases in platelet counts. Romiplostim and eltrombopag were shown to restore platelet counts in most patients with chronic ITP who were resistant to standard therapy (steroids, immunoglobulins, and splenectomy). The success of these 2 agents led the US Food and Drug Administration to quickly approve their use as second-line treatment for chronic ITP. Unlike romiplostim, which is given weekly by injection, eltrombopag is a once-daily oral nonpeptide agonist functioning at the thrombopoietin receptor.

The study by Kuter et al is an example of the enormous energy required to study an uncommon disorder such as ITP. In this randomized study, 85 investigational sites and 14 countries enrolled 234 patients, including teenagers, comparing romiplostim with standard care in patients who had not undergone splenectomy and in whom at least 1 previous treatment for immune thrombocytopenia had failed. The conclusions are quite clear. Outcomes were better in patients receiving romiplostim than in patients receiving standard care (short of splenectomy). Romiplostim was associated with a greater incidence of sustained platelet response, less bleeding, and fewer transfusions, a decreased requirement for other treatments (including splenectomy), and a greater improvement in quality of life. The side effects of this therapy were minimal.

The standard first treatment for immune thrombocytopenia continues to be the use of glucocorticoids, which are well known to care providers, inexpensive, and usually effective in those in whom the natural history of ITP does not allow resolution on its own. Unfortunately, durable remission with steroids in those with chronic ITP is uncommon. Historically, splenectomy was the first and is still the most effective treatment for persistent immune thrombocytopenia. The risks of splenectomy, however, are well known. In view of this, George, in a commentary that accompanied the report of Kuter et al, asked the question whether the new standard of care for management of chronic ITP ought to be the use of romiplostim.[1]

There is no question that the availability of thrombopoietin mimetic agents that stimulate platelet production has been an enormous advance for patients with immune thrombocytopenia. These agents can be effective in inducing safe platelet counts when all other treatments, including splenectomy and rituximab, have failed and therefore provide hope for patients with the most severe thrombocytopenia. It will be interesting to see whether the issues raised by Dr George will translate into high-quality studies that could lead us toward the more routine use of thrombopoietin mimetic agents.[1]

J. A. Stockman III, MD

Reference

1. George JN. Management of immune thrombocytopenia—something old, something new. *N Engl J Med.* 2010;363:1959-1961.

Neoangiogenesis contributes to the development of hemophilic synovitis
Acharya SS, Kaplan RN, Macdonald D, et al (Natl Insts of Health, Bethesda, MD; et al)
Blood 117:2484-2493, 2011

Joint arthropathy secondary to recurrent hemarthroses remains a debilitating complication of hemophilia despite the use of prophylactic factor concentrates. Increased vascularity and neoangiogenesis have been implicated in the progression of musculoskeletal disorders and tumor growth. We hypothesized that de novo blood vessel formation could play a major role in the pathogenesis of hemophilic joint disease (HJD). We observed a 4-fold elevation in proangiogenic factors (vascular endothelial growth factor-A [VEGF-A], stromal cell–derived factor-1, and matrix metalloprotease-9) and proangiogenic macrophage/monocyte cells (VEGF$^+$/CD68$^+$ and VEGFR1$^+$/CD11b$^+$) in the synovium and peripheral blood of HJD subjects along with significantly increased numbers of VEGFR2$^+$/AC133$^+$ endothelial progenitor cells and CD34$^+$/VEGFR1$^+$ hematopoietic progenitor cells. Sera from HJD subjects induced an angiogenic response in endothelial cells that was abrogated by blocking VEGF, whereas peripheral blood mononuclear cells from HJD subjects stimulated synovial cell proliferation, which was blocked by a humanized anti-VEGF antibody (bevacizumab). Human synovial cells, when incubated with HJD sera, could elicit up-regulation of HIF-1α mRNA with HIF-1α expression in the synovium of HJD subjects, implicating hypoxia in the neoangiogenesis process. Our results provide evidence of local and systemic angiogenic response in hemophilic subjects with recurrent hemarthroses suggesting a potential to develop surrogate biologic markers to identify the onset and progression of hemophilic synovitis.

▶ Sood et al[1] reported about the use of an anti–vascular endothelial growth factor (anti-VEGF) monoclonal antibody that appears to have terrific promise in the management of retinopathy of prematurity, a disease characterized in many instances by the proliferation of small blood vessels in the retina of newborns. Now we see in this report of Acharya et al evidence for the role of angiogenesis in the pathophysiology of hemophiliac joint disease.

Joint disease has always been the hallmark of severe hemophilia, but the introduction of regular infusions of intravenous factor VIII or IX (prophylaxis) from an early age has lessened its impact. Prophylaxis is of course now the standard of care for children with hemophilia, but for those born in the preprophylaxis era or who demonstrate bleeding despite the regular infusion of factor concentrate, the treatment of established joint disease must include (alone or in combination) ongoing infusions of factor concentrate, or surgical synovectomy, or for those with end-stage arthropathy, chronic anti-inflammatory and pain management or joint replacement.

The hallmarks of hemophiliac arthropathy involve joint bleeding, inflammation, synovial hypertrophy/villous formation, and cartilage/bony destruction, in essence, inflammation and cellular proliferation (angiogenesis). Some of this inflammation is the consequence of iron deposition from blood in the joint that stimulates inflammation through increased c-myc expression. Now we see in this report of Acharya et al evidence for the role of key angiogenic factors (VEGF) in cellular proliferation. The authors of this report suggest that the use of an angiogenic profile that might include VEGF might help better delineate the temporal and etiologic role of angiogenesis in hemophilic synovitis. Perhaps we will soon see reports of the use of anti-VEGF intra-articular injections as part of the successful management of hemophilia-related hemarthroses.

J. A. Stockman III, MD

Reference

1. Sood BG, Madan A, Saha S, et al. Perinatal systemic inflammatory response syndrome and retinopathy of prematurity. *Pediatr Res.* 2010;67:394-400.

Rational design of a fully active, long-acting PEGylated factor VIII for hemophilia A treatment

Mei B, Pan C, Jiang H, et al (Bayer HealthCare LLC, Berkeley, CA; Bayer HealthCare LLC, Richmond, CA)
Blood 116:270-279, 2010

A long-acting factor VIII (FVIII) as a replacement therapy for hemophilia A would significantly improve treatment options for patients with hemophilia A. To develop a FVIII with an extended circulating half-life, but without a reduction in activity, we have engineered 23 FVIII variants with introduced surface-exposed cysteines to which a polyethylene glycol (PEG) polymer was specifically conjugated. Screening of variant expression level, PEGylation yield, and functional assay identified several conjugates retaining full in vitro coagulation activity and von Willebrand factor

(VWF) binding. PEGylated FVIII variants exhibited improved pharmaco-kinetics in hemophilic mice and rabbits. In addition, pharmacokinetic studies in VWF knockout mice indicated that larger molecular weight PEG may substitute for VWF in protecting PEGylated FVIII from clear-ance in vivo. In bleeding models of hemophilic mice, PEGylated FVIII not only exhibited prolonged efficacy that is consistent with the improved pharmacokinetics but also showed efficacy in stopping acute bleeds comparable with that of unmodified rFVIII. In summary site-specifically PEGylated FVIII has the potential to be a long-acting prophylactic treat-ment while being fully efficacious for on-demand treatment for patients with hemophilia A.

▶ Most of us are familiar with the fact that hemophilia A is caused by defi-ciencies in coagulation factor VIII (FVIII) and is the most common hereditary coagulation disorder, affecting about 1 in 5000 boys. The current treatment for hemophilia A involves intravenous injection of recombinant human FVIII (rFVIII) or plasma-derived human FVIII. Injections of FVIII are either given on demand in response to a bleeding episode or as prophylactic therapy adminis-tered 2 to 4 times a week. Quality of life measures now track similar to un-affected peers, and patients engage regularly in sporting activities unimagined in previous generations. Prophylaxis for severe hemophilia is now recognized as the standard of care with optimal initiation early in life before the onset of repeated hemarthrosis, typically between 1 and 3 years of age.

Despite all the successes in managing patients with hemophilia A, barriers still remain to accomplish the goals of universal prophylaxis. Generally speaking, the cost for prophylactic replacement therapy runs in excess of $100 000 per patient per year. Accessing a vein several times a week also produces its own set of problems with the frequent need for central venous access devices to be placed in the youngest of patients. As time passes, suboptimal adherence to a prophylactic regimen commonly occurs. While plasma-derived products can be effective, one interesting aspect of rFVIII is the ability in the laboratory to tinker with such products to slightly modify their structure or function by engineering modifications to enhance functional properties. A number of bioengineering strategies have led to rFVIII variants with improved efficiency of expression, increased potency and resistance to inactivation, as well as resistance to inhibitors. A great deal of emphasis is being placed these days on trying to bioengineer rFVIII to increase its half-life. A longer-acting FVIII would hold promise in overcoming some of the barriers to the adoption of and adherence to long-term prophylaxis.

It is well known that FVIII is too large a molecule to be cleared by the kidney. Cellular clearance occurs primarily in the liver through the interaction with a family of low-density lipoprotein receptor-related proteins and heparin sulfate proteoglycan receptors, among others. One of the bioengineering techniques that is currently being looked at is creating an association of rFVIII with PEGy-lated liposomes as well as chemical modifications (eg, direct PEGylation) and bioengineering rFVIII through mutagenesis or the generation of fusion proteins (eg, with an Fc antibody fragment). For most other products, PEGylation results in a larger product that cannot be filtered through the kidney, enhancing half-life. This is of no particular advantage for FVIII since it is already too large to be filtered by the kidney but somehow or other PEGylation does significantly increase the half-life of FVIII as demonstrated by Mei et al, who used a unique bioengineering approach to identify promising PEGylated FVIII molecules with extended half-life.

Needless to say, the data from the study abstracted need to be replicated in clinical trials. The data suggest that FVIII half-life may be doubled with PEGylation. This could mean the possibility of once-a-week injections of FVIII, maintaining trough FVIII levels in plasma above critical thresholds for the prevention of spontaneous bleeding (typically 1%). This truly would be a welcome innovation for parents and children struggling to find venous access every other day, such as in an infant or toddler or for the busy adolescent striving to adhere to a regular prophylactic regimen.

It is difficult to tell whether the half-life extension of biological FVIII through bioengineering will pan out as a major therapeutic step in the evolution of the management of patients with hemophilia A. To read more about this topic, including some of the cautions about the use of PEG polymers, see the excellent commentary by Pipe.[1]

J. A. Stockman III, MD

Reference

1. Pipe SW. Go long! A touchdown for factor VIII? *Blood.* 2010;116:153-154.

Cost-utility analysis of von Willebrand disease screening in adolescents with menorrhagia
Sidonio RF Jr, Smith KJ, Ragni MV (Children's Hosp of Pittsburgh/Univ of Pittsburgh Med Ctr, PA; Univ of Pittsburgh School of Medicine, PA; Univ of Pittsburgh Med Ctr and Hemophilia Ctr of Western Pennsylvania)
J Pediatr 157:456-460, 2010

Objective.—To construct a decision analysis model to evaluate the cost utility of von Willebrand disease (VWD) testing in adolescents with menorrhagia.

Study Design.—A 20-year Markov decision analytic model was constructed to evaluate the cost utility of two strategies: testing or not testing for VWD. The model includes probabilities of remaining well, suffering an acute menorrhagia bleeding event, surgical complications, oral contraceptive pill complications, or dying. Probabilities, costs, and utilities were estimated from published literature. The prevalence of type 1 VWD in adolescent females with menorrhagia was estimated at 13%.

Results.—The cost of testing adolescents with menorrhagia for VWD was $1790, versus $1251 for not testing for VWD. The effectiveness of not testing in quality-adjusted life-years (QALYs) gained (14.237 QALYs) was similar to the VWD testing strategy (14.246 QALYs). Compared with not testing for VWD, screening for VWD had an incremental cost-effectiveness ratio of $62 791 per QALY, a value typically considered economically reasonable.

Conclusions.—In adolescents with menorrhagia, testing for VWD before the initiation of oral contraceptives is cost-effective.

▶ One of the difficult decisions pediatricians and obstetricians/gynecologists face is whether to evaluate adolescents with menorrhagia for an inherited bleeding disorder, specifically von Willebrand disease (VWD), the most common bleeding disorder in humans, found in 1% of the general population. About 1 in 7 adolescents with menorrhagia will be found to have VWD. Menorrhagia alone, therefore, places one at a higher risk for having VWD but is certainly not fully predictive of the disorder. In 2001, the American College of Obstetricians and Gynecologists recommended screening all adolescent women with menorrhagia for VWD, but this recommendation was not based on firm data.

One should not undertake a VWD evaluation in an adolescent with VWD without knowing some of the pitfalls that one may encounter. VWD involves testing that is quite complex and can be affected by blood type, stress, and exogenous estrogen. For example, the estrogen in oral contraceptives pills can increase coagulation factor levels masking a diagnosis of VWD, the effect lasting up to 8 weeks after cessation of the pill. Thus, the timing of any bleeding evaluation is extremely important.

What Sidonio et al have done is to examine whether screening for VWD in adolescents who have menorrhagia before the start of standard treatment, oral contraceptives, is cost-effective as opposed to waiting out the problem to see if it resolves. The data are fairly clear. Compared with not testing for VWD, screening for VWD before administration of oral contraceptives has an incremental cost-effective ratio of $62 791 per quality year of life, value typically considered to be economically reasonable.

The cost of screening for VWD is not cheap. In this report, we saw it ran about $1790. The suggestion is, however, that in the long run, the expenditure of such sums will pay off. The data from this report should keep a lot of laboratories busy if the recommendations are followed.

J. A. Stockman III, MD

Safety of Recombinant Activated Factor VII in Randomized Clinical Trials
Levi M, Levy JH, Andersen HF, et al (Univ of Amsterdam, the Netherlands; Emory Univ School of Medicine, Atlanta, GA; Novo Nordisk, Bagsværd, Denmark)
N Engl J Med 363:1791-1800, 2010

Background.—The use of recombinant activated factor VII (rFVIIa) on an off-label basis to treat life-threatening bleeding has been associated with a perceived increased risk of thromboembolic complications. However, data from placebo-controlled trials are needed to properly assess the thromboembolic risk. To address this issue, we evaluated the rate of thromboembolic events in all published randomized, placebo-controlled trials of rFVIIa used on an off-label basis.

Methods.—We analyzed data from 35 randomized clinical trials (26 studies involving patients and 9 studies involving healthy volunteers) to determine the frequency of thromboembolic events. The data were pooled with the use of random-effects models to calculate the odds ratios and 95% confidence intervals.

Results.—Among 4468 subjects (4119 patients and 349 healthy volunteers), 498 had thromboembolic events (11.1%). Rates of arterial thromboembolic events among all 4468 subjects were higher among those who received rFVIIa than among those who received placebo (5.5% vs. 3.2%, P = 0.003). Rates of venous thromboembolic events were similar among subjects who received rFVIIa and those who received placebo (5.3% vs. 5.7%). Among subjects who received rFVIIa, 2.9% had coronary arterial thromboembolic events, as compared with 1.1% of those who received placebo (P = 0.002). Rates of arterial thromboembolic events were higher among subjects who received rFVIIa than among subjects who received placebo, particularly among those who were 65 years of age or older (9.0% vs. 3.8%, P = 0.003); the rates were especially high among subjects 75 years of age or older (10.8% vs. 4.1%, P = 0.02).

Conclusions.—In a large and comprehensive cohort of persons in placebo-controlled trials of rFVIIa, treatment with high doses of rFVIIa on an off-label basis significantly increased the risk of arterial but not venous thromboembolic events, especially among the elderly. (Funded by Novo Nordisk.)

▶ Recombinant activated coagulation factor VII (rFVIIa) has been approved for the treatment of bleeding in patients with hemophilia A and B who have inhibiting antibodies to coagulation factor VIII or IX and who therefore are not easily managed with simple factor replacement. In patients in whom inhibitors develop, either as a result of hemophilia therapy or through an autoimmune mechanism, the use of rFVIIa has become an important addition to management. The mechanism of action of rFVIIa is the activation of coagulation by 2 mechanisms: platelets and tissue factors. The use of rFVIIa is associated with the potential for thrombosis since this recombinant product activates coagulation by bypassing normal mechanisms of coagulation.

Once rFVIIa was introduced, there was an enormous potential temptation to use it more widely other than as part of the management of hemophilia A or B. Off-label indications have been broadened to include the treatment of episodes of bleeding and the prevention of bleeding episodes related to surgical or invasive procedures in patients with congenital and acquired other—coagulation factor deficiencies, including factor VII deficiency or Glanzmann thrombasthenia. A growing number of case reports in small controlled or uncontrolled studies have shown the successful use of rFVIIa for various clinical indications other than the management of hemophilia including the treatment of severe traumatic injury, control of bleeding during surgery and transplantation, treatment of intra-cerebral hemorrhage, and the management of bleeding due to anticoagulation therapy. The concern about thrombosis is related to the fact that when rFVIIa is administered, it is given in doses up to 1000 times the physiological level. This activated factor also has a relatively long half-life of 2.5 hours. Once thrombosis is induced by generation of thrombin by rFVIIa, the thrombus formation may be difficult to control. The report of Levi et al is helpful in that it reports on data obtained from all published studies of off-label clinical trials of rFVIIa. Some 26 trials involving 4119 patients were included in this report because they were placebo-controlled and randomized. Nine other trials were looked at that involved 349 healthy volunteers. The authors reviewed 483 anecdotal reports of both the on-label and off-label use of rFVIIa. The conclusion was that the incidence of thromboembolic complications was just 1% to 2%. Thromboembolic events included coronary and cerebrovascular clotting as well as events involving the limbs and organs such as liver as well as venous occlusions such as deep-vein thrombosis, pulmonary embolism, and events involving the liver (eg, Budd-Chiari syndrome).

Recombinant factor VIII is used in pediatrics. The authors of this report appropriately warn us that the data from their review warrant scrutiny when rFVIIa is used on an off-label basis. The thrombotic sequelae, although infre-quent, are hardly inconsequential. The young and the old are those who are most seriously affected. As in any other management situation, the decision to use a risky agent is always based on whether the benefit is likely to outweigh the perceived/real risk.

Finally, there is a new substance that causes bleeding to cease. A novel gel may provide a cheap means of staunching blood flow on the battlefield or in any other situation where there is not time for sutures. Estimates suggest that the gel would cost less than $10 per application, a fraction of the cost of other gels in use today. The new blood-clotting material is a hydrogel, a jelly-like mixture of water and a fibrous polymer, in this case acrylamide deco-rated with positively charged nitrogen-containing groups. Experiments with blood plasma revealed that the gel activates factor VIII. You just slap it on the wound, the investigators say. In experiments on incisions made into sheep lung and liver tissue, clotting took place within a matter of minutes. Johnson and Johnson Pharmaceutical is the manufacturer of this substance.[1]

J. A. Stockman III, MD

Reference

1. Ehrenberg R. New gel can seal wounds quickly: low-cost synthetic material speeds up blood clotting. *Science News*. September 25, 2010:8.

Difficulties in Diagnosing Congenital Thrombotic Thrombocytopenic Purpura

Klukowska A, Niewiadomska E, Budde U, et al (Warsaw Med Univ, Poland; Univ Med Ctr Hamburg-Eppendorf, Germany)
J Pediatr Hematol Oncol 32:103-107, 2010

Thrombotic thrombocytopenic purpura is a very rare condition, espe-cially its familial, genetically determined type called Upshaw Schulman Syndrome (OMIM #274150). The study presents 2 families of patients in which congenital thrombotic thrombocytopenic purpura were diag-nosed. Symptoms of the disease, such as thrombocytopenia, microangio-pathic hemolytic anemia, and kidney disorders were pronounced with varying degrees of severity in 5 children of various ages from these fami-lies. Before the final diagnosis, patients were treated for idiopathic throm-bocytopenia, hemolytic anemia, and hemolytic-uremic syndrome, respectively. The study was focused on finding the factors responsible for hemolytic anemia. The activity of a disintegrin and metalloprotease with thrombospondin type 1 motif, 13 (ADAMTS13) and ADAMTS13 antibodies were evaluated and genetic tests were performed. Severe ADAMTS13 deficiency was detected in all affected siblings. The diagnosis of Upshaw Schulman Syndrome was confirmed by molecular testing of the gene encoding the von Willebrand factor cleaving protease ADAMTS13 which revealed compound heterozygosity for 1045C > T (R349C) and 3107C > A (S1036X) in the patients of family 1 and homozygosity for the common mutation 4143insA in the patients of family 2. Regular fresh-frozen plasma transfusions were sufficient to control the disease.

▶ In recent years, there has been a lot learned about a relatively rare blood condition known as thrombotic thrombocytopenic purpura (TTP). TTP occurs considerably less frequently in children than in adults and our level of knowl-edge as pediatricians about this disease clearly is lower in comparison with our adult colleagues in internal medicine. TTP often begins with jaundice in the newborn period, but its symptoms and signs are different than those of physiologic jaundice. Sometimes, the only sign is thrombocytopenia, which may later occur together with hemolytic anemia and be initially misdiagnosed as an autoimmunologic thrombocytopenia or Evans syndrome. The fully symp-tomatic disease frequently develops later in childhood, with periods of relapse. Episodes are triggered by inflammation, stress, pregnancy, or by unknown factors. Historically, 4 out of 5 patients with TTP have a history of requiring exchange transfusion during the neonatal period because of hyperbilirubinemia. Episodes of thrombocytopenia and hemolytic anemia can occur in early infancy but frequently occur in later childhood. Many have relapsing proteinuria and hematuria of varying severity. Renal failure is a common complication of the disorder. The diagnosis is frequently thought of when the peripheral blood smear shows characteristic damaged red blood cells, which are fragmented, helmet-shaped, or frank schistocytes. Such red blood cells, however, appear also in the hemolytic-uremic syndrome (HUS), Kasabach-Merritt syndrome, and other forms of microangiopathic hemolytic anemia.

What is new about TTP is our understanding of its genetic/congenital causes. TTP is associated with a deficiency of a disintegrin and metalloprotease with the thrombospondin type 1 motif 13 (ADAMTS13). This metalloprotease is responsible for cleaving very large multimers of the von Willebrand factor. Adults are most frequently diagnosed with the acquired type of disease caused by the production of ADAMTS13 antibodies. There is a recessively inherited form of the disease characterized by life-threatening episodes of microangiopathic hemolytic anemia, thrombocytopenia, fever, kidney disease, and neurologic disorders. These symptoms are caused by microthrombi precipitating in capillary vessels. These microthrombi are not broken down because of the absence of the metalloprotease. Virtually identical clinical findings are seen in HUS. However, severe deficiency of ADAMTS13 characteristic of TTP is found in normal levels in classical HUS, allowing a distinction between these 2 diseases.

One should be aware that TTP was once considered a fatal disease prior to the institution of plasma exchange treatment. Plasma exchange removes antibodies from the circulation system in patients with acquired TTP and also allows the substitution of ADAMTS13.

The bottom line is that although TTP is a rare disease, it does occur in pediatrics, and its diagnosis may be considerably delayed because of the general lack of knowledge of this entity. The authors of this report remind us that in patients with an atypical presentation or familial occurrence of immune thrombocytopenia or Evans syndrome, one should test for ADAMTS13 activity to rule out congenital TTP. Early commencement of regular prophylactic plasma transfusions is the treatment of choice in congenital TTP.

J. A. Stockman III, MD

High Prevalence of Thrombophilic Traits in Children with Family History of Thromboembolism

Calhoon MJ, Ross CN, Pounder E, et al (Univ of Colorado Denver and The Children's Hosp, Aurora)
J Pediatr 157:485-489, 2010

Objectives.—To determine a proximate family history of venous thromboembolism (VTE) in (1) the prevalence of thrombophilia; (2) the frequency of recommended changes in management resulting from thrombophilia evaluation; and (3) outcomes in longitudinal follow-up.

Study Design.—Laboratory thrombophilia investigation was performed in 56 children with first- or second-degree family history of thromboembolism before age 55 years, but without personal history of thromboembolism, who were enrolled in a prospective inception cohort. VTE risk factors, family history, thrombophilia findings, and management recommendations were systematically collected, along with thromboembolism risk episodes/exposures, prophylactic anticoagulation, major bleeds, and thromboembolism events during follow-up.

Results.—The frequencies of all thrombophilia traits were higher than the general population. Among 32 children who underwent complete laboratory evaluation, 34% had ≥2 traits. Thrombophilia testing led to recommendations for risk-based transient antithrombotic prophylaxis in 71% of subjects. No thromboembolism episodes developed during more than 900 patient-months of follow-up, although at-risk exposures were infrequent.

Conclusion.—Risk-stratified approaches to primary prevention of pediatric VTE should be further evaluated in cooperative prospective studies (Table 1).

▶ This report teaches us a classical piece of medical dictum that the history is always important. This is especially true when there is a family history of thromboembolism. While children very infrequently have evidence of venous thromboembolism, the risk of this is increased by orders of magnitude if there is family history of the problem. The investigators from the University of Colorado add to our body of knowledge by designing a study to determine thrombophilia findings, recommendations for targeted antithrombotic primary prevention, and outcomes in longitudinal follow-up of symptom-free children with a close family history of early thromboembolism. The premise of the study was that, among such children, comprehensive thrombophilia testing would frequently reveal underlying thrombophilia and would lead to a recommendation for the use of

TABLE 1.—Prevalence of Thrombophilia Traits, by Type, in the Study Population of Symptom-Free Children with a Proximate Family History of Early Thromboembolism

Factor V Leiden	
Heterozygous	34% (17/50)
Homozygous	0% (0/50)
FII G20210A	
Heterozygous	17% (8/47)
Homozygous	0% (0/47)
Protein C deficiency	
Mild	7% (3/46)
Severe	0% (0/46)
Protein S deficiency	
Mild	0% (0/45)
evere	0% (0/45)
Antithrombin deficiency	
Mild	2% (1/47)
Severe	0% (0/47)
Elevated lipoprotein(a)	28% (13/46)
Elevated homocysteine	0% (0/49)
Elevated factor VIII	17% (7/41)
Antiphospholipid antibody	
Lupus anticoagulant	8% (4/48)
Anticardiolipin IgG, IgM	7% (3/46), 0% (0/46)
Beta-2-glycoprotein-I IgG, IgM	4% (2/45), 0% (0/45)
Any	20% (9/45)

For definitions and thresholds used, see Methods.

at least temporary anticoagulation as a primary prophylaxis during periods of heightened clinical thrombotic risk. The authors investigated children with a close family history (ie, first- or second-degree relative) of a venous or arterial thromboembolism that occurred before the age of 55 years. These youngsters were enrolled in an institutional-based prospective study. Comprehensive testing included the following panel: plasma protein C and antithrombin activities, plasma-free protein S antigen concentration, plasma homocysteine concentration, factor V Leiden polymorphism, factor II G20210A polymorphism, lupus anticoagulant concentration in plasma, serum immunoglobulin G and M levels of anticardiolipin, plasma factor VIII activity, and serum lipoprotein concentration.

Table 1 shows the prevalence of thrombophilia traits, by type, in the study population. Factor V Leiden polymorphism, elevated factor VIII activity, elevated lipoprotein(a) concentration, and antiphospholipid antibody positivity were the most common findings. Thrombophilia testing led to a change in recommended management in 70% of subjects, consisting principally of transient anticoagulation prophylaxis during periods of heightened risk for venous thromboembolism. The latter included such events as undergoing surgical procedures that would reduce postoperative mobility for a period of at least 48 hours. Additionally, restricting the use of estrogen-containing oral contraceptive pills was advised in a significant proportion of women on the basis of factor V Leiden testing. The children were followed up for a total of 923 patient-months (over an actual period of 22 months). There were 6 episodes involving a heightened risk of thromboembolism. No thromboembolism events occurred.

It has been several years now since the US Surgeon General issued a call to action aimed at increasing our awareness of venous thromboembolism risks to reduce the incidence, morbidity, and mortality rates of this problem. In children, given the low incidence of venous thromboembolism in the general pediatric population, widespread unselected thrombophilia screening would be neither ethical nor cost effective. The authors of this report from Colorado advocate a risk-stratified approach to thrombophilia evaluation in asymptomatic children, targeting individuals with a family history of early thromboembolism. The findings from the report have important potential implications for the evaluation and management of symptom-free children with a close family history of early thromboembolism. At highest risk are children who on testing are found to have multitrait thrombophilia, that is, an aggregate of more than 1 risk factor for thrombosis. Needless to say, this study was not sufficiently large to give clear-cut indications as to the best way to prevent thromboembolism. A long overdue collaborative is necessary to address the many unknowns that exist in the area of coagulation disorders.

It has been recently noted that sitting at a computer all day, while unhealthy for lots of reasons, creates a risk of venous thromboembolism. A case control study found that 33 of 197 (17%) people admitted for venous thromboembolism had been exposed to prolonged work and computer-related immobility in the previous 4 weeks, compared with 19 of 197 (10%) matched controls. This basically means that those sitting on their bottoms in front of computers have a 2.8-fold increased risk of developing a venous thrombosis. The acronym for all this, by the way, is "SIT": Seated Immobility Thromboembolism.[1]

J. A. Stockman III, MD

Reference

1. Healy B, Levin E, Perrin K, Weatherall M, Beasley R. Prolonged work- and computer-related seated immobility and risk of venous thromboembolism. *J R Soc Med.* 2010;103:447-454.

4 Child Development/ Behavior

Effects of a restricted elimination diet on the behaviour of children with attention-deficit hyperactivity disorder (INCA study): a randomised controlled trial
Pelsser LM, Frankena K, Toorman J, et al (ADHD Res Centre, Eindhoven, Netherlands; Wageningen Univ, Netherlands; Catharina Hosp, Eindhoven, Netherlands; et al)
Lancet 377:494-503, 2011

Background.—The effects of a restricted elimination diet in children with attention-deficit hyperactivity disorder (ADHD) have mainly been investigated in selected subgroups of patients. We aimed to investigate whether there is a connection between diet and behaviour in an unselected group of children.

Methods.—The Impact of Nutrition on Children with ADHD (INCA) study was a randomised controlled trial that consisted of an open-label phase with masked measurements followed by a double-blind crossover phase. Patients in the Netherlands and Belgium were enrolled via announcements in medical health centres and through media announcements. Randomisation in both phases was individually done by random sampling. In the open-label phase (first phase), children aged 4–8 years who were diagnosed with ADHD were randomly assigned to 5 weeks of a restricted elimination diet (diet group) or to instructions for a healthy diet (control group). Thereafter, the clinical responders (those with an improvement of at least 40% on the ADHD rating scale [ARS]) from the diet group proceeded with a 4-week double-blind crossover food challenge phase (second phase), in which high-IgG or low-IgG foods (classified on the basis of every child's individual IgG blood test results) were added to the diet. During the first phase, only the assessing paediatrician was masked to group allocation. During the second phase (challenge phase), all persons involved were masked to challenge allocation. Primary endpoints were the change in ARS score between baseline and the end of the first phase (masked paediatrician) and between the end of the first phase and the second phase (double-blind), and the abbreviated Conners' scale (ACS) score (unmasked) between the same timepoints. Secondary endpoints included food-specific IgG levels at baseline related to the behaviour of the diet group responders after IgG-based food challenges.

The primary analyses were intention to treat for the first phase and per protocol for the second phase. INCA is registered as an International Standard Randomised Controlled Trial, number ISRCTN 76063113.

Findings.—Between Nov 4, 2008, and Sept 29, 2009, 100 children were enrolled and randomly assigned to the control group (n=50) or the diet group (n=50). Between baseline and the end of the first phase, the difference between the diet group and the control group in the mean ARS total score was $23 \cdot 7$ (95% CI $18 \cdot 6-28 \cdot 8$; p<0·0001) according to the masked ratings. The difference between groups in the mean ACS score between the same timepoints was $11 \cdot 8$ (95% CI $9 \cdot 2-14 \cdot 5$; p<0·0001). The ARS total score increased in clinical responders after the challenge by $20 \cdot 8$ (95% CI $14 \cdot 3-27 \cdot 3$; p<0·0001) and the ACS score increased by $11 \cdot 6$ ($7 \cdot 7-15 \cdot 4$; p<0·0001). In the challenge phase, after challenges with either high-IgG or low-IgG foods, relapse of ADHD symptoms occurred in 19 of 30 (63%) children, independent of the IgG blood levels. There were no harms or adverse events reported in both phases.

Interpretation.—A strictly supervised restricted elimination diet is a valuable instrument to assess whether ADHD is induced by food. The prescription of diets on the basis of IgG blood tests should be discouraged.

▶ Disorders such as attention-deficit hyperactivity disorder (ADHD) are ripe for good and not-so-good studies of psychopharmacological and psychosocial treatments. Concerns about the side effects of psychoactive drugs and the many barriers to ready access to psychosocial treatments have led to alternative methods to manage ADHD, including restrictive diets. Unfortunately, there have been few quality studies about the successful use of the latter. This is the importance of the report by Pelsser et al.

Pelsser et al report a 2-phase randomized trial using a control and diet group in 100 children diagnosed with ADHD who were aged 4 to 8 years and were unselected for any food sensitivity. After a 2-week baseline period, controls were placed on a waiting list and continued normal eating. Their parents received healthy food advice and kept a diary of their child's behavior. The diet group received a 5-week open trial with a restricted eliminated diet of oligoantigenic few foods (rice, meat, vegetables, pears, water) complemented with specific foods such as potatoes, fruit, and wheat. Of the 41 diet-group children who completed first phase, 41.5% had no behavioral response to the diet by the end of week 2, and their diet was further restricted to a few foods. At the end of the first phase, symptoms of ADHD in oppositional defiant disorder significantly improved in 64% of children in the diet group compared with no improvement in the controls. The first phase clinical responders then had a double-blind crossover food challenge in random order with 2 weeks each of 3 high immunoglobulin G (IgG) and 3 low IgG foods added to the elimination diet. Relapse of ADHD symptoms occurred with the first, second, or both food challenges in 19 of the 30 children entering the crossover phase. IgG levels against foods did not predict which foods might lead to a negative effect on behavior because an equal amount of low and high IgG food challenges resulted in relapse of ADHD symptoms.

Needless to say, studies using restricted elimination diets are complex and quite challenging. This report of Pelsser et al was well designed and carefully done and did appear to show benefit with a very strict supervised elimination diet. The study provides additional treatment options for some young children with ADHD, although the options require some significant rigor. It is important to note, however, that 36% of children either did not respond to the elimination diet or were noncompliant.

Needless to say there has been much written recently about elimination diets, artificial food colorings, etc. The report of Pelsser et al will only add fuel to the fire of the debate around elimination diets. Diagnosing food sensitivity is a complex affair, can take several weeks, and is quite burdensome for families to implement. To read more about elimination diets and ADHD, see the excellent editorial that accompanied the report abstracted.[1] Despite the rigor of the Impact of Nutrition on Children with ADHD study, we should all be very cautious about where the real evidence lies for using elimination diets.

To close, we have an observation having to do with one aspect of child development: how children learn words. Toddlers certainly get a kick out of giving adults a hard time. True to form, these creatures who seem to absorb new knowledge like sponges actually learn virtually nothing from best-selling DVDs that parents might think boost vocabulary and trigger academic superstardom, at least with respect to the acquisition of words. Children who viewed a popular educational DVD regularly for one month, either with or without their parents, showed no greater understanding of words from the program than did kids who never saw it. In this study, youngsters displayed word-learning advantages if their moms and dads spent a month trying to teach words from the DVD whenever the parents had time. This indicates the importance of having a social partner in the learning process. Nonetheless, toddlers can become addicted to looking at the boob-tube while such DVDs are playing, which most likely erroneously leads parents to believe that they are of more educational value than they are.[2]

J. A. Stockman III, MD

References

1. Ghuman JK. Restricted elimination diet for ADHD: the INCA study. *Lancet.* 2011;377:446-448.
2. Bower B. DVDs don't turn toddlers into vocabulary Einsteins. *Science News.* September 25, 2010:15.

Food Selectivity in Children with Autism Spectrum Disorders and Typically Developing Children
Bandini LG, Anderson SE, Curtin C, et al (Univ of Massachusetts Med School, Waltham; Ohio State Univ, Columbus; et al)
J Pediatr 157:259-264, 2010

Objectives.—To define food selectivity and compare indices of food selectivity among children with autism spectrum disorders (ASDs) and typically developing children, and to assess the impact of food selectivity on nutrient adequacy.

Study Design.—Food selectivity was operationalized to include food refusal, limited food repertoire, and high-frequency single food intake using a modified food frequency questionnaire and a 3-day food record. Food selectivity was compared between 53 children with ASDs and 58 typically developing children age 3-11 years. Nutrient adequacy was assessed relative to the dietary reference intakes.

Results.—The children with ASDs exhibited more food refusal than typically developing children (41.7% of foods offered vs 18.9% of foods offered; *P* <.0001). They also had a more limited food repertoire (19.0 foods vs 22.5 foods; *P* <.001). Only 4 children with ASDs and 1 typically developing child demonstrated high-frequency single food intake. Children with a more limited food repertoire had inadequate intake of a greater number of nutrients.

Conclusions.—Our findings suggest that food selectivity is more common in children with ASDs than in typically developing children, and that a limited food repertoire may be associated with nutrient inadequacies.

▶ What parent from time to time does not worry about his/her offspring being a picky eater? As we see in this report from Boston, youngsters with autism spectrum disorder can be really picky eaters. Unfortunately, despite numerous reports focusing on pickiness, rigidity, selective eating, and mealtime food refusal in children with autism spectrum disorders, a standardized definition of food selectivity has been lacking. To address the gaps in our knowledge, Bandini et al developed a definition of food selectivity based on clinical experience and pilot studies describing eating patterns of children with autism spectrum disorders focusing on 3 areas: food refusal, limited food repertoire, and high frequency of single food intake. With these definitions, the authors of this report hypothesized that children with autism spectrum disorders would exhibit more food selectivity than typically developing children and that food selectivity would decline with age in typically developing children but would not be associated with age in children with autism spectrum disorders. They also explored whether food selectivity is associated with inadequate nutritional intake, which could of course have important implications for nutritional management. In a study including a total of 53 children with autism spectrum disorders and 58 typically developing children, they were able to carry out an investigation that yielded valuable new information.

So what did these investigators find? They observed food refusal in both typically developing children and children with autism spectrum disorders. On average, children with autism spectrum disorders refused more foods and refused more foods as a percentage of those offered compared with typically developing children, doing so with a frequency at least twice than that in normal children. Vegetables were typically refused by youngsters with autism spectrum disorders. Interestingly, contrary to expectations, high-frequency single-food intake was rarely seen in either normal children or children with autism spectrum disorders. When it came to limited food repertoire, on average, parents of children with autism spectrum disorders recorded that their children ate significantly fewer types of food over a several-day period in comparison with typically developing children. The commonly held belief that dietary pickiness is outgrown with age was not supported by the findings of this report.

The association between limited food repertoire and nutrient inadequacy in children with autism spectrum disorder suggests that a very limited diet may put a youngster at risk for nutritional deficiencies. Some of the children with autism spectrum disorders have been put on special diets, including gluten-free diets and lactose-free diets, which can add to the risk of nutritional deficiency.

This report is useful in that it operationalizes the definitions of food selectivity and provides data from a reasonable size sample from which firm conclusions can be made about the eating habits of children with autism spectrum disorder. Unfortunately, the report does nothing to help parents or care providers to figure out how to address the eating habits of these youngsters. Longitudinal studies examining food selectivity are badly needed to explore whether food selectivity persists well into adolescence and adulthood.

It should be noted that there has been an explosion in the number of cases diagnosed under the category of autism spectrum disorders in recent years, in part related to the addition of Asperger disorder to the *Diagnostic and Statistical Manual of Mental Health Disorders* (*Fourth Edition*) manual. Autistic disorder, Asperger disorder, and pervasive developmental disorders not otherwise specified are expected to be combined in the 2013 DSM-V into 1 label: autism spectrum disorder. For one of the best and certainly easy-to-read reviews of the clinical spectrum of autism, refer to the excellent article by Golnik and Maccabee-Ryaboy.[1]

J. A. Stockman III, MD

Reference

1. Golnik A, Maccabee-Ryaboy N. Autism: clinical pearls for primary care. *Contemp Pediatr.* 2010:42-60.

Mitochondrial Dysfunction in Autism

Giulivi C, Zhang Y-F, Omanska-Klusek A, et al (Univ of California, Davis)
JAMA 304:2389-2396, 2010

Context.—Impaired mitochondrial function may influence processes highly dependent on energy, such as neurodevelopment, and contribute to autism. No studies have evaluated mitochondrial dysfunction and mitochondrial DNA (mtDNA) abnormalities in a well-defined population of children with autism.

Objective.—To evaluate mitochondrial defects in children with autism.

Design, Setting, and Patients.—Observational study using data collected from patients aged 2 to 5 years who were a subset of children participating in the Childhood Autism Risk From Genes and Environment study in California, which is a population-based, case-control investigation with confirmed autism cases and age-matched, genetically unrelated, typically developing controls, that was launched in 2003 and is still ongoing. Mitochondrial dysfunction and mtDNA abnormalities were evaluated in lymphocytes from 10 children with autism and 10 controls.

Main Outcome Measures.—Oxidative phosphorylation capacity, mt-DNA copy number and deletions, mitochondrial rate of hydrogen peroxide production, and plasma lactate and pyruvate.

Results.—The reduced nicotinamide adenine dinucleotide (NADH) oxidase activity (normalized to citrate synthase activity) in lymphocytic mitochondria from children with autism was significantly lower compared with controls (mean, 4.4 [95% confidence interval {CI}, 2.8-6.0] vs 12 [95% CI, 8-16], respectively; $P = .001$). The majority of children with autism (6 of 10) had complex I activity below control range values. Higher plasma pyruvate levels were found in children with autism compared with controls (0.23 mM [95% CI, 0.15-0.31 mM] vs 0.08 mM [95% CI, 0.04-0.12 mM], respectively; $P = .02$). Eight of 10 cases had higher pyruvate levels but only 2 cases had higher lactate levels compared with controls. These results were consistent with the lower pyruvate dehydrogenase activity observed in children with autism compared with controls (1.0 [95% CI, 0.6-1.4] nmol × [min × mg protein]$^{-1}$ vs 2.3 [95% CI, 1.7-2.9] nmol × [min × mg protein]$^{-1}$, respectively; $P = .01$). Children with autism had higher mitochondrial rates of hydrogen peroxide production compared with controls (0.34 [95% CI, 0.26-0.42] nmol × [min × mg of protein]$^{-1}$ vs 0.16 [95% CI, 0.12-0.20] nmol × [min × mg protein]$^{-1}$ by complex III; $P = .02$). Mitochondrial DNA overreplication was found in 5 cases (mean ratio of mtDNA to nuclear DNA: 239 [95% CI, 217-239] vs 179 [95% CI, 165-193] in controls; $P = 10^{-4}$). Deletions at the segment of cytochrome *b* were observed in 2 cases (ratio of cytochrome *b* to *ND1*: 0.80 [95% CI, 0.68-0.92] vs 0.99 [95% CI, 0.93-1.05] for controls; $P = .01$).

Conclusion.—In this exploratory study, children with autism were more likely to have mitochondrial dysfunction, mtDNA overreplication, and mtDNA deletions than typically developing children.

▶ This is an intriguing report. Some studies have already suggested that mitochondrial dysfunction and altered energy metabolism may influence the social and cognitive defects in subjects with autism. Unfortunately, the suspicions in this regard are based on only a handful of isolated cases. A significantly larger study of school-aged children with confirmed autism between the ages of 10 and 14 years found mitochondrial respiratory chain dysfunction in 7.2% of those with autism or autism spectrum disorders.[1] Giulivi et al note that there are no systematic studies aimed at investigating changes in mitochondrial function, mitochondrial DNA copy number, mitochondrial DNA deletions, and oxidative stress in well-characterized children with autism. Taking off on the challenge of pursuing this, these investigators undertook a study to look at whether youngsters with autism or autism spectrum disorders have dysfunctional mitochondria using the data provided by peripheral blood lymphocytes. You will need to read this article in some detail (it will require a fair amount of concentration), but the bottom line is that children with autism are remarkably more likely to have evidence of mitochondrial dysfunction compared with their normal peers.

So what does all this mean? The high prevalence of mitochondrial dysfunction observed in this preliminary study performed in children with full syndrome autism may or may not indicate an etiological role. Whether the mitochondrial dysfunction in children with autism is primary or secondary to an as yet unknown event remains the subject of future work. Mitochondrial dysfunction could greatly amplify and propagate brain dysfunction, such as that found in autism, given that the highest levels of mitochondrial DNA abnormalities are observed in postmitotic tissues with high energy demands, such as the human brain. While this study does find evidence of mitochondrial dysfunction in children presenting with full syndrome autism, more research is needed to understand the molecular causes of the mitochondrial dysfunction and how this and other metabolic defects may contribute to the disorder. Despite this disclaimer, this report does provide us with some badly needed insights into the possible pathophysiology of autism in children.

This commentary closes with an unrelated observation about music as a learning experience. Nearly 20 years ago, a small study advanced the notion that listening to Mozart's *Sonata for Two Pianos in D Major* could boost mental functioning. It was not long before trademark "Mozart Effect" products appealed to many parents aiming to put toddlers on the fast track to the Ivy League. Georgia's governor at the time even proposed giving every newborn there a classical CD (or actually a cassette), a sign of the time. The evidence for Mozart therapy turned out to be somewhat flimsy, and perhaps nonexistent, although the original study never claimed anything more than a temporary and limited effect. In recent years, however, neuroscientists have examined the benefits of a concerted effort to study and practice music, as opposed to playing a Mozart CD or a computerized "brain fitness" game once in a while. It has now been found that music lessons can produce profound and lasting changes that enhance the general ability to learn. These results should disabuse public officials of the idea that music classes are a mere frill, ripe for discarding during periods of budget crises. Studies have clearly shown that assiduous instrument playing from an early age can help the brain to process sounds better, making it easier to stay focused when absorbing other subjects, from literature to high-level calculus. To learn more about honing the mind with music, see the excellent editorial that appeared on this topic in *Scientific American*.[2]

J. A. Stockman III, MD

References

1. Oliveira G, Diogo L, Grazina M, et al. Mitochondrial dysfunction in autism spectrum disorders: a population-based study. *Dev Med Child Neurol.* 2005;47: 185-189.
2. McMurdo W. Hearing the music, honing the mind: Music produces profound and lasting changes in the brain. Schools should add classes not cut them. *Scientific American.* November 2010:16.

Lack of Association Between Measles-Mumps-Rubella Vaccination and Autism in Children: A Case-Control Study

Mrożek-Budzyn D, Kiełtyka A, Majewska R (Jagiellonian Univ, Krakow, Poland)
Pediatr Infect Dis J 29:397-400, 2010

Objective.—The first objective of the study was to determine whether there is a relationship between the measles-mumps-rubella (MMR) vaccination and autism in children. The second objective was to examine whether the risk of autism differs between use of MMR and the single measles vaccine.

Design.—Case-control study.

Study Population.—The 96 cases with childhood or atypical autism, aged 2 to 15, were included into the study group. Controls consisted of 192 children individually matched to cases by year of birth, sex, and general practitioners.

Methods.—Data on autism diagnosis and vaccination history were from physicians. Data on the other probable autism risk factors were collected from mothers. Logistic conditional regression was used to assess the risk of autism resulting from vaccination. Assessment was made for children vaccinated (1) Before diagnosis of autism, and (2) Before first symptoms of autism onset. Odds ratios were adjusted to mother's age, medication during pregnancy, gestation time, perinatal injury and Apgar score.

Results.—For children vaccinated before diagnosis, autism risk was lower in children vaccinated with MMR than in the nonvaccinated (OR: 0.17, 95% CI: 0.06−0.52) as well as to vaccinated with single measles vaccine (OR: 0.44, 95% CI: 0.22−0.91). The risk for vaccinated versus nonvaccinated (independent of vaccine type) was 0.28 (95% CI: 0.10−0.76). The risk connected with being vaccinated before onset of first symptoms was significantly lower only for MMR versus single vaccine (OR: 0.47, 95% CI: 0.22−0.99).

Conclusions.—The study provides evidence against the association of autism with either MMR or a single measles vaccine.

▶ It seems a bit late in the now apparently resolved controversy about the relationship between measles-mumps-rubella (MMR) vaccination and autism to still be reporting on this topic, but it is a topic that does not seem to have any real end. Wakefield et al were the first to propose that the MMR vaccine might be causally linked to autism. It was also suggested that gastrointestinal and developmental symptoms constituted an actual syndrome that might be triggered by this vaccine. Their study was widely criticized, but generated immense media attention, leading to a fall in MMR coverage in some European countries, much to the detriment of children. Since that report, a number of other studies have found no evidence to support a link between MMR vaccination and autism. The controversy ultimately culminated in a retraction of the original article.[1] The report of Mrożek-Budzyn et al tells a bit about the experience in Poland where MMR vaccination coverage continued throughout all this, but questions about the safety of this vaccine boosted by periodic antivaccination campaigns has persisted. When first introduced in Poland, MMR was not covered by the National Health Services of Poland, and parents who wished to vaccinate their children with MMR, as opposed to the single mandatory measles vaccine, had to pay extra. For this reason, few children were immunized with MMR. The Polish mandatory vaccination schedules did not include MMR for all children until 2004. Since then, already high levels of immunization against measles have slightly grown. Interestingly, Poland's heterogeneous population (ie, vaccinated with MMR, vaccinated against measles only, and nonvaccinated) now serves as a unique group for studying the debated association of these vaccines with autism in children. That is why the report of Mrożek-Budzyn et al is so important, because it is one of the purest studies available that looks at the specific conse-quences of MMR on the possibility of it triggering autism. The study is the first objective report to determine whether a relationship exists between MMR vacci-nation and autism in children and clearly documents that the autism risk is actu-ally lower in children vaccinated with MMR than in the nonvaccinated group as well as in those infants/children vaccinated with the single measles vaccine (odds ratio 0.44). The study therefore provides unequivocal evidence against the association of autism with either MMR or the single measles vaccine.

Please note that this report from Poland only deals with the relationship between MMR vaccination and autism, not with the issue of a potential link between MMR and autistic enterocolitis, a term introduced by Andrew Wakefield in his original *Lancet* article in which the authors believed they were describing a new form of inflammatory bowel disease linked to autism. Not a lot has been said in Great Britain where all this started about retracting autistic colitis, but apparently an association with MMR is now also being debunked.[2] Little survives of autistic enterocolitis after the retraction of Wakefield's article and his subsequent disgrace in Great Britain. Dr Wakefield had been hired by a solic-itor to help launch a speculative lawsuit against drug companies that manufac-tured the MMR vaccine. The instrument of their attack was to find what he called at the time a new syndrome of bowel and brain disease caused by the vaccine. Even the pathologist who described the findings in blind reviews of colon biopsies has added his retraction to the original article. Unfortunately, the original biopsy specimens can no longer be located for a formal review.

J. A. Stockman III, MD

References

1. Wakefield AJ, Murch SH, Anthony A, et al. Ileal-lymphoid-nodular hyperplasia, non-specific colitis, and pervasive developmental disorder in children. *Lancet*. 1998;351:637-641.
2. Deer B. Wakefield's "autistic enterocolitis" under the microscope. *BMJ*. 2010;340: c1127.

Predicting Persistence of and Recovery from Stuttering by the Teenage Years Based on Information Gathered at Age 8 Years
Howell P, Davis S (Univ College London, UK)
J Dev Behav Pediatr 32:196-205, 2011

Objectives.—Information obtained at around age 8 years was used to construct a model that predicted persistence of, and recovery from, stuttering several years later. A logistic regression model that classified children as persistent or recovered at the teenage years using stuttering history and symptom information obtained at around age 8 years was constructed and validated.

Methods.—A longitudinal study of 222 children who stuttered was conducted. The children were followed up from around age 8 until the teenage years. Persistence and recovery outcomes were established at the teenage years for 206 of the children, based on agreement across 3 standardized instruments. The data from 132 children were used to develop the model, and the data from the remaining 74 children were used to validate the model. Risk factors assessed at the beginning of the study were head injury, age at stuttering onset, family history of stuttering, handedness, whether a second language was spoken in the home, gender, and scores from the Stuttering Severity Instrument Version 3. The information about risk factors was obtained at around age 8 years by interview, except for the severity estimate, which was obtained by analysis of recordings and observations of physical concomitants associated with stuttering. The model was developed using logistic regression procedures.

Results.—The only factor to predict the persistence of, and recovery from, stuttering at the teenage years was stuttering severity at around age 8 years (none of the other factors being significant). For the initial model, the sensitivity (percentage of the group that was classified as persistent) was 84.1% and specificity (the percentage of the group that was classified as recovered) was 78.3%. For the validation, sensitivity was 76.3% and specificity was 72.2%.

Conclusions.—Persistence and recovery at teenage can be predicted from information that can be collected at around age 8 years with sensitivity and specificity of ~80%.

▶ This report contains an enormous amount of data on children who stutter. In children with developmental stuttering evaluated by 8 years, about 60% of cases started before 3 years and 85% had started by 3.5 years. Many of these children will recover relatively soon after the problem begins. Recovery rates of 65% to 80% have been reported 3 to 5 years after the onset of stuttering. It should be noted, however, that developmental stuttering can start after 8 years of age, and recovery can occur at any age up to the teenage years. Approximately 50% of children still stuttering at 8 years of age will recover by their teenage years. It has not been clear what the prognostic factors are for the likely persistence or recovery for these older stutterers. A large-scale retrospective study of more than 14 000 adult Swiss Army conscripts identified 6 factors that were significant predictors of stuttering.[1] These included obsessive-compulsive disorder in a family member, an alcoholic mother, an alcoholic father, a foreign parent (a proxy for a second language being spoken in the home), prematurity, and being restless and fidgety at school.

Howell and Davis looked for predictive factors for recovery of stuttering among a total of 222 children with stuttering in London who were referred to specialist clinics. The authors of the report looked at a number of different potential predictors of persistence/recovery by the teenage years. Only symptom severity, measured by Stuttering Severity Instrument Version 3, was a significant predictor for risk of persistence. A logistic regression model that included symptom severity at first assessment was able to correctly predict 80% of the outcomes by teenage years with a high degree of sensitivity and specificity.

The authors of this report suggest that consultation needs to take place between clinicians and patients and their families to establish the best way of using the information derived from this study. Care providers may not want to know the likelihood that a child will persist or recover, as this may affect their approach to the child's treatment. Parents and children might not want to know that they are likely to have ongoing fluency problems. That said, surveys done by the authors of this report suggest that clinicians seem to show a clear preference toward having the information.

A great deal of attention has been paid in recent years to stuttering as a developmental problem. This was true even before the first showing of the King's Speech. The latter film was a boost to many families of children with stuttering. It provided a ray of hope for those with even the most severe forms of the problem.

This commentary concludes with a couple of observations having to do with multilingual families and the development of speech in the offspring. Babies living in bilingual homes do get a perceptual boost by 8 months of age that may set the stage for more resilient thinking later on, or so say scientists.[2] Infants raised bilingual from birth can distinguish not only their native tongues, but between languages they have never encountered, even when they see adults speak without hearing what they say. It appears that babies in monolingual households lack these discrimination skills. Given exposure to 2 tongues, infants develop an ability to track closely what they hear to decode languages. Early perceptual strides by infants in bilingual homes may mark the beginnings of an increased ability to focus attention and think in complex ways later in life. Interestingly, in an unrelated report, data suggest that lifelong bilingualism is a form of "cognitive reserve." A study of 102 bilingual patients and 109 monolingual patients with Alzheimer disease reports that bilingual patients had been diagnosed 4.3 years later and had reported the onset of symptoms 5.1 years later than monolingual patients. The groups were equivalent on measures of cognitive and occupational level and immigration status. The monolingualist had actually received more formal education than the bilingualist.[3] Thus it is that those who are capable with speaking with "forked tongue" are not crazy. They are probably smarter than the rest of us who are lingo-deprived.

J. A. Stockman III, MD

References

1. Ajdacic-Gross V, Vetter S, Müller M, et al. Risk factors for stuttering: a secondary analysis of a large data base. *Eur Arch Psychiatry Clin Neurosci.* 2010;260:279-286.
2. Bower B. Bilingual babies discern languages: Early challenge of learning two tongues may hone thinking. *Science News.* March 12, 2011:16.
3. Craik FIM, Bialystok E, Freedman M. Delaying the onset of Alzheimer disease: Bilingualism as a form of cognitive reserve. *Neurology.* 2010;75:1726-1729.

Transient idiopathic dystonia in infancy
Calado R, Monteiro JP, Fonseca MJ (Hospital do Espírito Santo, Évora – EPE, Portugal; Hospital Garcia de Orta, Almada, Portugal)
Acta Paediatr 100:624-627, 2011

Aim.—Review of transient idiopathic dystonia cases to improve knowledge on this entity, in relation to frequency, characterization and evolution.

Methods.—Retrospective review and characterization of clinical cases seen in paediatric neurology consultation, diagnosed with transient idiopathic dystonia, between February 2001 and June 2009, using clinical files complemented with photographic records and updated information through the physician.

Results.—Thirteen infants were referred to the paediatric neurology consultation over a period of 8 years, for asymmetric tone, posture and movements of the upper limb with onset before 6 months, with spontaneous favourable evolution and disappearance without sequelae, although the reason for referral was, in most cases, the suspicion of a hemiplegic cerebral palsy.

Conclusion.—Transient changes of tone, posture and movement can be observed during the first months of life. Differential diagnosis is extensive and complex, based on a careful history and neurological examination. Distinction between neurological, neuromuscular and orthopaedic pathology is difficult, particularly at the onset of clinical manifestations. The cases presented are similar to those previously reported by Willemse and Deonna, classified as transient idiopathic dystonia of childhood. Pathophysiology is unknown; some findings support a genetic susceptibility to functional imbalance in brain neurotransmitters and synaptogenesis.

▶ This report is included to make all of us aware of a disorder that many of us may not be very familiar with, if at all. That disorder is transient idiopathic dystonia in infancy. The disorder was in fact first described almost 20 years ago by Willemse[1] who reported the presence of segmental dystonia that was self-limiting and not associated with the appearance of sequelae. The initial report involved 4 infants aged 5 months to 1 year. Willemse termed the disorder benign idiopathic dystonia.

Since the initial description back in the mid-1980s of transient idiopathic dystonia of infancy, additional cases have been described, including ones that are familial. Few centers get to see many of these patients, thus the importance of this report from Portugal describing 13 infants referred for pediatric neurology consultation over a period of 8 years. The infants described did in fact have a benign transitory neurological presentation consisting of a change in tone, posture, or movement, appearing in early development, usually up to age 1 year and most often in the first 6 months of life. The neurologic findings affect mostly 1 upper limb, occasionally both, and rarely the lower limbs, trunk, or cervical region. The most commonly found sign is forearm hyperpronation with palmar flexion of the wrist. Dystonic posture is usually intermittent and triggered by movements, positions, or specific situations such as being placed prone, crawling, and bathing, among others. The findings persist for seconds to hours and usually disappear during voluntary movements. The latter helps define the diagnosis. The association of fine tremor with dystonia may also be seen. This presents as a slight tremor of the head, trunk, and/or upper limbs. There are no other neurologic findings, and there is no psychomotor developmental delay.

If you ever see an infant with the findings noted above that disappear when the infant is repositioned, think benign idiopathic dystonia and assure the parents that in the absence of any other abnormalities, their baby will get over this. The findings are specific enough that unnecessary diagnostic procedures should be able to be avoided.

J. A. Stockman III, MD

Reference

1. Willemse J. Benign idiopathic dystonia with onset in the first year of life. *Dev Med Child Neurol.* 1986;28:355-360.

Physician "Costs" in Providing Behavioral Health in Primary Care
Meadows T, Valleley R, Haack MK, et al (Univ of Nebraska Med Ctr, Omaha, NE; Mendota Heights, MN)
Clin Pediatr 50:447-455, 2011

Objective.—To examine pediatricians time spent, and resulting reimbursement payments for, addressing behavioral health concerns in a rural primary care pediatric practice.

Methods.—Research assistants observed 228 patient visits in a rural pediatric primary care office. The length of the visit (in minutes), content of visit, number and type of codes billed, and related insurance reimbursement amounts were recorded. Interrater reliability, scored for 22% of patient visits, was ≥90%.

Results.—Medical only visits lasted, on average, 8 minutes as compared with behavioral only visits that required nearly 20 minutes of physician time. Pediatricians billed up to 10 different billing codes for medical only visits but only billed 1 code for behavioral only visits. Consequently, pediatricians were reimbursed significantly less, per minute, for behavioral only visits as compared with those sessions addressing medical only or a combination of medical and behavior concerns.

Conclusion.—Findings converge with previous research, demonstrating that behavioral health concerns dramatically affect the length of visit for primary care physicians. Moreover, this study is the first to document the specific impact of such concerns on pediatrician reimbursement for providing behavioral services. These results provide further support for integrating behavioral health services into pediatric primary care settings, thus allowing physicians to refer more difficult patients with behavioral issues to in-house collaborating behavioral health providers who can spend additional time necessary to address the behavioral health issue and who are licensed to receive mental health reimbursement.

▶ Most pediatricians are very familiar with the fact that pediatric visits for behavioral disorders are not well reimbursed. Behavioral health concerns are the primary reason for visits to the pediatrician's office in as many as 15% of cases.[1] Parents or physicians raise behavioral or psychosocial concerns during 50% to 80% of all child health care visits. The question that remains, however, is whether or not pediatricians can cost-effectively diagnose and provide ongoing treatment services for behavioral health problems within the parameters of the typical 12- to 15-minute patient sessions in the primary care setting.

Meadows et al looked at the typical time to see children in a rural free-standing physician clinic in the Midwest. Pediatric patients being seen for medical visits only required a visit lasting just 8 minutes as compared with behavioral visits only that required nearly 20 minutes of physician time. The reimbursement rate per minute when calculated was $18.12 for purely medical visits and $4.36 per minute for behavioral visits. If issues were raised at the time of a scheduled medical visit, the visit time extended to 17 minutes and resulted in a reimbursement rate per minute of $5.86.

This study is one of the very first to begin to document the financial cost to pediatricians in providing behavioral diagnostic and treatment services by examining reimbursement rates. The findings support the need for alternative models of care, such as the integrated behavioral health specialist in primary care setting as a way to ensure more cost-effective use of pediatrician time and maximization of reimbursement. This recommendation by the authors is based on the assumption that primary care pediatricians will be unlikely to see better reimbursement rates for the management of behavioral disorders in their routine office setting.

Clearly behavioral issues are a part of normal child development and we conclude with an observation having to do with how interactive games relate to behavior. Games are now a dominant form of entertainment at all ages. Zynga Inc., a Facebook game developer, claims 215 million players worldwide use that social website's online gaming programs. Games targeting healthy behaviors are also proliferating. For example, web-based games offered by Humana, the large insurance company, are based on conventional objectives for diet and exercise. *Packy & Marlon*, a Nintendo game published first in 1994 that allowed children and adolescents to play the role of a character with type 1 diabetes mellitus, monitoring glucose levels, using insulin and selective foods, has shown a high degree of educational value. In a 6-month placebo-controlled study, study participants who played the *Packy & Marlon* game had a 77% reduction in diabetes-related emergency department visits and urgent care visits.[2] More recently, *Re-Mission*, a game for adolescent and young-adult patients with cancer, has been shown in a randomized trial to improve adherence to chemotherapy and treatment plans.[3]

The substantial growth of new interactive game technologies and genres raises great opportunities for high quality learning, including health learning for children. The size and level of engagement of the audience means that health games can affect a wide range of individuals, including those who are difficult to reach with traditional messaging. To learn more about interactive games to promote health behavior, see the commentary by Read and Shortell.[4]

J. A. Stockman III, MD

References

1. Williams J, Klinepeter K, Palmes G, Pulley A, Foy JM. Diagnosis and treatment of behavioral health disorders in pediatric practice. *Pediatrics.* 2004;114:601-606.
2. Brown SJ, Lieberman DA, Germeny BA, Fan YC, Wilson DM, Pasta DJ. Educational video game for juvenile diabetes: Results of a controlled trial. *Med Inform (Lond).* 1997;22:77-89.
3. Kato PM, Cole SW, Bradlyn AS, Pollock BH. A video game improves behavioral outcomes in adolescents and young adults with cancer: a randomized trial. *Pediatr.* 2008;122:e305-e317.
4. Read JL, Shortell SM. Interactive games to promote behavior change in prevention and treatment. *JAMA.* 2011;305:1704-1705.

5 Dentistry and Otolaryngology (ENT)

Toothache in US Children
Lewis C, Stout J (Univ of Washington School of Medicine, Seattle)
Arch Pediatr Adolesc Med 164:1059-1063, 2010

Objectives.—To describe the prevalence of and risk factors for recent toothache among US children and to estimate frequency of contact between children with toothache and their pediatric primary care providers (PPCP).

Design.—Cross-sectional analysis of nationally representative data.

Setting.—The 2007 National Survey of Children's Health.

Participants.—Population-based sample of parents/guardians of 86 730 children aged 1 through 17 years from 50 states and the District of Columbia.

Outcome Measure.—Parent-reported toothache in the last 6 months.

Results.—A total of 10.7% of US children and 14% of children aged 6 to 12 years experienced toothache in the last 6 months. Poor and low-income minority children and those with special needs were significantly more likely to have had a toothache on multivariable analysis. Most children with toothache in the last 6 months had their own physician (88.9%) and had a preventive medical visit in the last year (88.1%), pointing to opportunities for PPCP to identify and intervene with children who have untreated dental decay and toothache.

Conclusions.—Toothache is not the universal experience it was before the advent of modern dentistry. Nevertheless, a substantial number of US children recently had a toothache, with noteworthy variability between states. There are opportunities for PPCP to address oral health prevention, assess for dental decay and toothache, and treat complications. We propose toothache as a potential quality indicator reflecting disparities in oral health for a population.

▶ When was the last time you saw an article on toothache? Well, now you have. This report emanates from the Department of Pediatrics at the University of Washington, School of Medicine, Seattle, and describes a cross-sectional analysis of nationally representative data on the prevalence of and risk factors for toothache in children in our country. Every primary care provider should become familiar with the information in this report since it is not likely that you will see another comprehensive analysis anytime soon.

This report begins with a basic description of what a toothache is. Destruction of the tooth's structure in the form of a cavity results from acidic byproducts of bacterial carbohydrate metabolism that erode through the enamel and dentin and then into the pulp. Within the pulp lies the nerve that when inflamed will result in pain, often excruciating pain. Recent data suggest that about one-third of youngsters of school age living at or below 200% of the federal poverty level have untreated tooth decay, twice the rate than among children with families above 200% of the federal poverty level.[1]

The 2007 National Survey of Children's Health provides a wealth of information about a number of subject areas, including information on children with toothaches. Lewis and Stout have taken a deep dive into the data from the survey to better define the scope of dental issues in children aged 1 through 17 years. They observed that about 7.5 million US children had experienced a toothache in the previous 6 months. Approximately, 1 in 7 youngsters aged 6 to 12 years experienced a toothache in the preceding 6 months. If there was a current history of dental cavities, the prevalence of toothache rose to 32%. Even controlling for financial status, black and multiracial children had significantly higher odds of toothache than white children. Toothache also inversely correlates with per capita dentist supply. If one looks carefully, for example, Massachusetts has twice the per capita dentist supply (1.1 dentists per 1000 persons) than that of Mississippi (0.5 dentists per 1000 persons). In fact, Mississippi is tied for last, while the District of Columbia has the highest per capita number of dentists. If one translates the data from this report to the real world, one can estimate that in an elementary school class of 20, on average, 4 children in the classroom have or recently have had a toothache.

Needless to say, we are not doing a very good job in caring for our offsprings' teeth. We should not be trivializing the problem. At the far end of the spectrum of complications, a simple toothache can have disastrous consequences. In 2007, there was reported a well-publicized case of a 12-year-old African American boy from Maryland who actually died as the result of an infection in an abscessed tooth that spread to his brain.[2]

Add to this the long-term consequences of tooth loss. In a large study of 80-year-old Japanese people living in their own community, it appears that tooth loss is a strong predictor of death—independent of other health factors and also independent of socioeconomic status and lifestyle in octogenarians. The relationship is stronger in women than in men. The bottom line is that when push comes to shove, it is better to have your own "choppers" than manufactured ones![3]

J. A. Stockman III, MD

References

1. Gehshan S, Snyder A, Paradise J. *Filing an Urgent Need: Improving Children's Access to Dental Care in Medicaid and SCHIP.* Menlow Park, CA: Keiser Commission on Medicaid and the Uninsured; 2008.

2. Otto M. For Want of a Dentist: Boy Dies After Bacteria From Tooth Spread to Brain. *Washington Post;* February 28, 2007.
3. Ansai T, Takata Y, Soh I. Relationship between tooth loss and mortality in 80-year-old Japanese community-dwelling subjects. *BMC Public Health.* 2010;10:386.

Preventive Oral Health Care in Early Childhood: Knowledge, Confidence, and Practices of Pediatricians and Family Physicians in Florida

Herndon JB, Tomar SL, Lossius MN, et al (Univ of Florida College of Medicine, Gainesville; Univ of Florida College of Dentistry, Gainesville)

J Pediatr 157:1018-1024, 2010

Objective.—To examine the relationships among pediatricians' and family physicians' oral health training, knowledge, confidence, and practice patterns.

Study Design.—A survey of physicians identified through the membership databases of the Florida Academy of Family Physicians and the Florida Pediatric Society was conducted in 2008. Responses of pediatricians and family physicians were compared through bivariate and multivariate analyses.

Results.—Although training was not directly associated with performing recommended practices, there were positive associations between training and confidence and between confidence and performing recommended practices ($P < .05$). Pediatricians were more likely than family physicians to answer fluoride-related knowledge questions correctly and reported greater confidence ($P < .05$). Less than 20% of the respondents reported counseling parents about bringing their child to the dentist before age 1 year or inquiring about the parents' dental health.

Conclusions.—Oral health training appears to promote confidence in performing recommended oral health practices. Differences in fluoride knowledge by provider type suggest that fluoride guidance has been disseminated more effectively among pediatricians than among family physicians. Educational content of oral health training programs should place increased emphasis on current fluoride guidance, early dental visits, and assessing parents' oral health. Instructional methods should address physicians' confidence, particularly among family physicians.

▶ This report is full of extremely useful information for the pediatric practitioner when it comes to important strategies to reduce early childhood caries. It has only been for this generation of pediatricians that we have recognized the key role that we play in this regard. This is especially true for preschool-aged children. Because preschool-aged children are significantly more likely to visit a physician's office than a dentist's office, the American Academy of Pediatric Dentistry and the American Academy of Pediatrics both recommend that medical care providers adopt several oral health prevention strategies. These include the performance of periodic risk assessments to determine a child's relative likelihood of developing dental caries; the provision of anticipatory guidance to parents about oral hygiene, diet, and fluoride exposure; the application of appropriate preventive therapies including fluoride varnish; and assistance to parents in establishing a dental home for their children by no later than 12 months of age.[1] No policy is very good unless the policy is embraced by those to whom the policies are targeted. The report of Herndon et al is useful in that it tells us what family physicians and pediatricians (in this case in Florida) know about these preventive measures.

We learn from this report that there is no direct effective training related to either a family physician's or pediatrician's oral health practices. What appears to be needed is what is known as applied training. This might include interactive training sessions actually carried out in a physician's office, which are shown to be more efficacious than more passive educational formats such as didactic presentations either in residency training or as part of continuing medical education. Hands-on experience may actually increase physicians' confidence in their ability to competently perform recommended practices and thereby increase the likelihood that they will incorporate those practices into patient care. The report also found that pediatricians were more likely than family physicians to answer fluoride-related knowledge questions correctly, even after controlling for oral health training. However, the finding that almost one-half of pediatricians incorrectly responded to fluoride supplementation questions suggests that they too can benefit from additional training. Despite recommendations emanating from the American Academy of Pediatrics, less than 20% of pediatricians reported counseling parents on bringing their child for a dental visit before 1 year of age or inquiring about parent's dental health. These statistics apply equally to family physicians.

It is hard to say if some of the recommendations emanating from the American Academy of Pediatric Dentistry or from the American Academy of Pediatrics can actually be carried out. There is some suspicion that if every child by 1 year of age was to be seen by a dentist (much less a pediatric dentist), there would not be the capacity in the provider arena, workforce-wise, to carry out the mandate. In fact, a decision-tree analysis has suggested that under a fixed dental care capacity for Medicaid-insured children, such a policy would crowd out those children at greatest risk for oral disease and that without an increase in dental capacity for Medicaid-insured children, universal dental visits by every child by 1 year of age would actually increase the prevalence of untreated dental caries overall because those at highest risk would simply be in a queue with everyone else.[2]

Given the fact that there appears to be no significant shortage of primary care provider physicians for the care of children, while there are significant shortages of trained dentists to care for very young children, it is incumbent on us as pediatricians to figure out how to fill the gap in our own offices. We can go a long way with our own skills in supporting the oral health of young ones, including providing expert fluoride guidance and fluoride varnishes. Similar approaches by family physicians are also critical, given the significant proportion of children cared for in family practice offices.

Read this report of Herndon et al to learn more about the issue of preventive oral care for young children.

Also, if you want to read more about how teeth have evolved over time, see the interesting story of when large animals eventually developed the ability to have proper dental occlusion.[3] It appears that mammals evolved within a group of tetrapods, the therapsids, which arose during the lower Permian period about 270 million years ago. After the end of the Permian Age, a group of therapsids evolved as mammal-like reptiles that differentiated into an extremely diverse group of herbivores—from small burrowing animals to large browsers. From these a new anomodont, *Tiarajudens*, emerged with the ability to occlude their teeth. Dental occlusion is a key component of successful herbivory that facilitates efficient processing of tough cellulosic plant materials through thorough grinding between hard teeth. The evolution of *Tiarajudens* pushes the date of dental occlusion in this group back to 260 million years ago. To put this into perspective, the behavioral dysfunction occasionally seen in some children of tooth grinding really is a throwback to over a quarter of a billion years ago!

J. A. Stockman III, MD

References

1. American Academy of Pediatric Dentistry. Definition of dental home. 2009-2010 definitions, oral health policies and clinical guidelines. http://www.aapd.org/media/policies.asp. Accessed December 27, 2010.
2. Jones K, Tomar SL. Estimated impact of competing policy recommendations for age of first dental visit. *Pediatrics*. 2005;115:906-914.
3. Editorial comment. My, what new teeth you have. *Science*. 2011;331:1487.

Fluoride Content of Water Used to Reconstitute Infant Formula
Steinmetz JEA, Martinez-Mier EA, Jones JE, et al (Indiana Univ, Indianapolis)
Clin Pediatr 50:100-105, 2011

Objective.—To assess the fluoride content of water used to reconstitute infant formula by a Latino population living in the Indianapolis, Indiana, area.

Background.—Negligible as well as excessive fluoride can be detrimental to oral health. Estimates of fluoride intake and exposure for individuals may aid in the determination of their risk for developing dental fluorosis or caries.

Methods.—Interviews were conducted to determine brands of bottled water used to reconstitute infant formula. Identified brands were analyzed for fluoride concentration.

Results.—Of the 458 samples tested (from 20 brands), fluoride concentration ranged from 0.006 to 0.740 μg/mL. All brands but one had fluoride concentration less than 0.7 μg/mL, with 16 brands having less than 0.22 μg/mL. Most bottled waters analyzed in the study comply with the American Dental Association recommendation to prevent fluorosis. Comparisons made demonstrated that only waters targeted for infants and that are fluoridated do not comply with recent American Dental Association recommendations.

▶ This report is an interesting one because it gives us not only information about the fluoride concentration and content of water used to reconstitute infant formulas, but also some insights into the cultural variations that exist in the United States that increase the likelihood that bottled water will be used to reconstitute concentrated or powdered infant formulas. Infant formulas, of course, come in 3 variations: powdered formula, concentrated liquid formula, and ready-to-use formula. Both the powdered and concentrated liquid forms of formula must be mixed with water. Since the formula itself in such circumstances contains negligible amounts of fluoride, the fluoride that an infant will receive will be based on the concentration and amount of fluoride in the water used to reconstitute the formulas. Too little fluoride and the infant will be at greater risk subsequently for the development of caries. If there is too much fluoride in the water used to mix the formula, then the risk will be the development of fluorosis. Certain segments of the population may be particularly affected by the variations in fluoride concentration in tap or bottled water. It has been demonstrated that infant feeding habits are influenced by both cultural and ethnic factors. A study undertaken about 15 years ago by Weinstein et al showed that Latinos have the highest rate of infant bottle feeding (76%), as compared with other ethnicities.[1] In addition, Latino parents are more likely to give bottled water to their children. Many Latino families avoid drinking tap water because they fear it causes illness. Studies done over the years on bottled water imported from Australia, Brazil, England, Greece, Mexico, and bottled water from the United States have shown significant variations in fluoride content, some with less and some with greater than the optimal recommended range for the populations that consume the water.

What Steinmetz et al have done is to assess the fluoride concentration of water used to reconstitute infant formula by a Latino population living in the Indianapolis, Indiana, area. Of the 18 different bottled waters sampled and tested, fluoride concentration varied from nearly 0 to 0.740 µg/mL. All brands but one had less than 0.7 µg/mL, with 16 brands having less than 0.22 µg/mL. Most bottled waters reported in this study used to reconstitute formula comply with the American Dental Association (ADA) recommendations to prevent fluorosis. Comparisons between bottled water from spring and nonspring sources did not reveal any significant difference. It should be noted that some bottled waters do have added fluoride and in such circumstances do not comply with recent ADA recommendations and may be placing infants at risk for developing dental fluorosis. Currently the ADA recommendations state that fluoridated water should be avoided when reconstituting infant formulas to prevent fluorosis. It should also be noted that the ADA recommends that parents not use fluoride toothpaste for children less than 2 years of age. However, if fluoride-free water is used to reconstitute infant formula in children who already have teeth and who have been determined to be at high risk for caries, not using a fluoride toothpaste may further increase their risk for developing caries. Therefore, in these cases, parents should follow the recommendations of the American Academy of Pediatric Dentistry, which include using a smear of toothpaste for children less than 2 years of age while a pea-size amount of paste is recommended for children 2 to 5 years of age. By following these recommendations, children in high risk for caries would be exposed to fluoride in a topical manner, which has been shown to be most appropriate for caries prevention.[2]

This commentary concludes with a comment for all ye who are pregnant. Make sure you maintain good oral hygiene during your pregnancy. Epidemiologic studies have shown that clinical and subclinical periodontal infections during pregnancy are associated with preterm birth.[3] Infection is thought to result in the release of proinflammatory cytokines, which can have downstream effects on other biological pathways and tissues. This association with preterm delivery was first noted in an association between bacterial vaginosis in the 1980s and 1990s. Polyzos et al have documented that scaling and root planing during pregnancy are associated with a reduced rate of preterm birth.[4] Only 8% of women who have been successfully treated for gum disease had a preterm baby compared with 63% of those whose gum disease treatment was not undertaken or failed. It is hard to believe, but it is true that something as simple as having bad teeth and gums can have monumental effects on a pregnancy!

J. A. Stockman III, MD

References

1. Weinstein P, Oberg D, Domoto PK, et al. A prospective study of the infant and brushing practices of WIC mothers: 6- and 12-month data and ethnicity and family variables. *ASDC J Dent Child.* 1996;63:113-116.
2. American Academy of Pediatric Dentistry. *Guideline on infant oral healthcare.* Chicago, IL: American Academy of Pediatric Dentistry (AAPD); 2009. 5.
3. Macones G. Treatment of periodontal disease in pregnancy. *BMJ.* 2010;342: c7090.
4. Polyzos NP, Polyzos IP, Zavos A, et al. Obstetric outcomes after treatment of periodontal disease during pregnancy: Systematic review and metaanalysis. *BMJ.* 2010;341:c7017.

Familial Cases of Periodic Fever with Aphthous Stomatitis, Pharyngitis, and Cervical Adenitis Syndrome

Adachi M, Watanabe A, Nishiyama A, et al (Kakogawa Municipal Hosp, Japan; et al)
J Pediatr 158:155-159, 2011

We report three familial cases of periodic fever with aphthous stomatitis, pharyngitis, and cervical adenitis syndrome, including a pair of monozygotic twins and their mother. It suggests that periodic fever with aphthous stomatitis, pharyngitis, and cervical adenitis syndrome may have a certain monogenetic background.

▶ We are now 25 years out from the first descriptions appearing in the literature of periodic fever with aphthous stomatitis, pharyngitis, and cervical adenitis (PFAPA) syndrome.[1] Virtually everyone now agrees that this is a distinct clinical entity that presents with periodic fever occurring at intervals, fever that is associated with aphthous stomatitis, pharyngitis, and cervical adenitis. The syndrome usually begins before the age of 5 years. Very specific diagnostic criteria for PFAPA are established now. All agree that PFAPA syndrome is a noninfectious, nonautoimmune, autoinflammatory disease. It shows dramatic responses to steroid therapy.

The etiology of PFAPA syndrome remains unknown. Most cases are sporadic. There have been some reported cases of nontwin siblings being affected and of siblings and their mother, suggesting that the syndrome may be induced by environmental or genetic factors. Adachi et al report 3 familial cases of PFAPA syndrome, namely, a mother and her monozygotic twins.

In cases described by Adachi et al, the mother of biological twins who was aged 29 years when the first of her twins was diagnosed with PFAPA noted that between the ages of 2 and 10 years, she frequently had episodes of acute pharyngitis and aphthous stomatitis. Every time she was seen with this problem, she was given oral antibiotics, but her fevers failed to respond. The fevers lasted between 3 and 5 days and resolved spontaneously and were associated with symptom-free nonfebrile interval periods. After her first pregnancy and delivery, abrupt periodic febrile episodes again started in this woman and were repeated at approximately 30-day intervals. She was eventually diagnosed as having PFAPA. Both her twins had similar clinical courses and were also diagnosed with PFAPA. Although no specific genetic test identified an abnormality in family members, it was strongly speculated that this family did in fact document the existence of a familial variant of PFAPA.

There are a number of periodic illnesses that can present in childhood. Among the various autoinflammatory diseases that can present this way are cyclic neutropenia, hyperimmunoglobulinemia D syndrome, familial Mediterranean fever, and tumor necrosis factor—associated periodic syndrome. Of the periodic syndromes, only PFAPA syndrome still has an unknown genetic background and pathogenesis. Of the autoinflammatory diseases, only PFAPA has been described as a noninherited syndrome. Despite this, a number of cases of PFAPA have been documented to be associated with defective gene regulation of mevalonate kinase. The bottom line, however, is that if you do want to diagnose a patient with PFAPA, take a careful history of related illness in other family members. You may also have a report on your hands.

This commentary closes with a quiz question having to do with the oropharyngeal part of our body. What is the gene that encodes for the ability to experience the fizziness of carbonated drinks? Obviously this is a carbonated drinker aficionado's question. It appears that the fizz of carbonated drinks is picked up by the same tongue cells that register sour taste.[2] The experience of fizziness involves the detection of a physical sensation and the taste of carbon dioxide. Studies have now shown that mice lacking sour sensing cells also fail to taste carbon dioxide. A genetic analysis of these cells revealed the gene that encodes the enzyme carbonic anhydrase 4, which turns carbon dioxide and water into bicarbonate and free protons. It is the latter protons that trigger the sour sensitivity of the cells and gives the sensation of both sourness and fizz. With this new knowledge, the next time you are in a restaurant and ask for water "with gas," you will know why you get that little sparkle in your mouth.

J. A. Stockman III, MD

References

1. Marshall GS, Edwards KM, Butler J, Lawton AR. Syndrome of periodic fever, pharyngitis and aphthous stomatitis. *J Pediatr.* 1987;110:43-46.
2. Chandrashekar J, Yarmolinsky D, von Buchholtz L, et al. The taste of carbonation. *Science.* 2009;326:443-445.

Intraorbital and Intracranial Extension of Sinusitis: Comparative Morbidity
Goytia VK, Giannoni CM, Edwards MS (Baylor College of Medicine, Houston, TX)
J Pediatr 158:486-491, 2011

Objectives.—We hypothesized that intracranial extension of sinusitis carries greater morbidity than extension confined to the orbit and that presenting features can raise suspicion for intracranial extension.

Study Design.—A retrospective review (1997 to 2006) identified 118 children with sinusitis complicated by intracranial extension or intraorbital extension. Presenting features and infecting organisms were compared using χ^2 or Fisher exact tests. Outcomes included duration of hospitalization, length of therapy and sequelae.

Results.—Thirty-three children had intracranial extension and 85 had intraorbital extension. Children with intracranial extension were older (11.4 versus 7.6 years; $P \leq .001$), had more preadmission encounters (1.9 versus 1.3; $P = .012$), longer headache duration (9.5 versus 2.8 days; $P = .009$), and presented more often with vomiting (73% versus 28%; $P < .001$) than those with intraorbital extension. Children with intracranial extension also were hospitalized (26 versus 10 days; $P < .001$) and treated (36 versus 24 days; $P = .001$) longer. Four children (3%) had persistent sequelae.

Conclusions.—Children with intracranial extension are hospitalized and treated longer than those with intraorbital extension of sinusitis but persistent sequelae are uncommon. Prolonged headache and protracted vomiting at presentation should alert caregivers to consider intracranial extension.

▶ Sinusitis is a common problem in both children and adults. One of the serious consequences of sinusitis is extension of the infection beyond the sinuses. The most worrisome areas of extension involve the intraorbital and intracranial areas. Intracranial extension more often occurs in children older than 7 to 8 years than in younger children and also is more common in African American children than in other ethnicities. Goytia et al undertook a study to determine whether the clinical features at presentation could give us a heads up into those youngsters who are more likely to either have or develop intracranial extension of sinusitis. The authors also attempted to determine whether intracranial extension is associated with greater morbidity and a higher risk for sequelae than is intraorbital extension of sinusitis.

The authors were able to mine data from the charts of 33 children with sinusitis who had intracranial extension and 85 who had intraorbital extension. The diagnoses were made between early 1997 and late 2006. Children with intraorbital extension or intracranial extension were equally likely to present with fever, headache, and vomiting. However, prolonged duration of headache (often for more than a week) and persistent emesis were presenting features heightening suspicion for intracranial extension. Although ethmoid involvement was associated with intraorbital extension and frontal sinusitis with intracranial extension of sinusitis, 90% of the children evaluated had opacification of multiple sinuses. Approximately one-half of those with intraorbital extension and all except one child with intracranial extension ultimately underwent drainage of purulent material. About one-half of those with intracranial extension had neurosurgical drainage and one-third required multiple drainage procedures. One in 4 patients had sterile fluid obtained at the time of drainage. These youngsters had preadmission antibiotics. Most positive cultures were polymicrobial. For this reason, it seems reasonable that one starts with broad-spectrum antibiotics until one has culture results in hand.

If there is any lesson from this report, it is that eye swelling, combined with persistent headache and vomiting, is the most helpful finding in identifying children with intracranial extension in routine practice. These youngsters need to be admitted to institutions that have a wide range of subspecialty services including those of pediatric otolaryngologists, neurosurgeons, ophthalmologists, and infectious disease experts.

This commentary closes with an observation from the recent literature that documents how "snot" has the power to alter how things smell. A rose sniffed through a snotty nose may not smell so sweet. It has now been documented that enzymes in a mouse's nasal mucosa transform certain scents before the nose can actually detect them.[1] It appears that the thick goo that serves to lubricate the nose is teaming with proteins and protein-chopping enzymes. Investigators have added odorants to tiny amounts of mucous sucked out of the nose of a mouse and tested the resulting chemical composition of the mix. After 5 minutes of sitting in mucous, about 80% of almond-smelling benzaldehyde was converted to benzyl alcohol (a scent found in some teas and plants) and odorless benzoic acid. Inactivation of enzymes in nasal mucous from boiling did not result in odor conversion. There is much to be said of mice and men being alike. If alike with regard to their noses, the latter having a snotty nose is not particularly good around mealtime if you want to enjoy the aroma of the food you are about to eat.

J. A. Stockman III, MD

Reference

1. Sanders L. Snot has the power to alter scents: Mice studies show sense of smell is modified by mucous. *Science News.* January 1, 2011:12.

Diagnosis, Microbial Epidemiology, and Antibiotic Treatment of Acute Otitis Media in Children: A Systematic Review

Coker TR, Chan LS, Newberry SJ, et al (Mattel Children's Hosp, Los Angeles, CA; Los Angeles County-USC Med Ctr, CA; Southern California Evidence-based Practice Ctr, Santa Monica, CA; et al)

JAMA 304:2161-2169, 2010

Context.—Acute otitis media (AOM) is the most common condition for which antibiotics are prescribed for US children; however, wide variation exists in diagnosis and treatment.

Objectives.—To perform a systematic review on AOM diagnosis, treatment, and the association of heptavalent pneumococcal conjugate vaccine (PCV7) use with AOM microbiology.

Data Sources.—PubMed, Cochrane Databases, and Web of Science, searched to identify articles published from January 1999 through July 2010.

Study Selection.—Diagnostic studies with a criterion standard, observational studies and randomized controlled trials comparing AOM microbiology with and without PCV7, and randomized controlled trials assessing antibiotic treatment.

Data Extraction.—Independent article review and study quality assessment by 2 investigators with consensus resolution of discrepancies.

Results.—Of 8945 citations screened, 135 were included. Meta-analysis was performed for comparisons with 3 or more trials. Few studies examined diagnosis; otoscopic findings of tympanic membrane bulging (positive likelihood ratio, 51 [95% confidence interval {CI}, 36-73]) and redness (positive likelihood ratio, 8.4 [95% CI, 7-11]) were associated with accurate diagnosis. In the few available studies, prevalence of *Streptococcus pneumoniae* decreased (eg, 33%-48% vs 23%-31% of AOM isolates), while that of *Haemophilus influenzae* increased (41%-43% vs 56%-57%) pre- vs post-PCV7. Short-term clinical success was higher for immediate use of ampicillin or amoxicillin vs placebo (73% vs 60%; pooled rate difference, 12% [95% CI, 5%-18%]; number needed to treat, 9 [95% CI, 6-20]), while increasing the rate of rash or diarrhea by 3% to 5%. Two of 4 studies showed greater clinical success for immediate vs delayed antibiotics (95% vs 80%; rate difference, 15% [95% CI, 6%-24%] and 86% vs 70%; rate difference, 16% [95% CI, 6%-26%]). Data are absent on long-term effects on antimicrobial resistance. Meta-analyses in general showed no significant differences in antibiotic comparative effectiveness.

Conclusions.—Otoscopic findings are critical to accurate AOM diagnosis. AOM microbiology has changed with use of PCV7. Antibiotics are modestly more effective than no treatment but cause adverse effects in 4% to 10% of children. Most antibiotics have comparable clinical success.

▶ This report represents one of the most updated surveys providing an overview of the current status of both the diagnosis and management of acute otitis media (AOM). Obviously, AOM remains one of the most prevalent diagnoses seen in the pediatric care provider's office. It is also, in the aggregate, an expensive diagnosis. A study using 2006 Medical Expenditure Panel Survey data documented that an average expenditure per episode of AOM ran about $350 per child. If one runs the math, this totals to an amount of approximately $2.8 billion annually.[1] Needless to say, the more we can continue to learn about the current trends in the diagnosis and management of AOM the better off we and our country will be.

A lot has changed in the last decade or so when it comes to AOM. For one, the use of the heptavalent pneumococcal conjugate vaccine (PCV7) has become widely established as have the clinical guidelines for antibiotic use. What Coker et al have done is to search PubMed, the Cochrane Control Clinical Trials Register Database, the Cochrane Database of Reviews of Effectiveness, and the Web of Science for articles published January 1999 through July 2010 on AOM diagnosis, treatment outcomes, and association of PCV7 use with changes in AOM microbiology using Medical Subject Headings terms related to AOM. The literature searches and reference mining yielded almost 9000 titles. When distilling this list down to ones that were truly systematic reviews and highly relevant research articles, 80 articles were left. Consensus on the clinical diagnosis of AOM includes 3 components: acute signs of infection, evidence of middle ear inflammation, and effusion. Unfortunately, a major limitation to the evidence regarding a precise diagnosis is the lack of a gold standard. The diagnostic tools studied (eg, otoscopy) are often part of the only available gold standard, a clinical diagnosis.

The report of Coker et al also shows that there have been significant shifts in AOM microbiology with the introduction of PCV7. *Streptococcus pneumoniae* has become significantly less prevalent, and *Haemophilus influenzae* has become more prevalent. We are also seeing a shift toward an increase in the proportion of AOM because of nonvaccine *S pneumoniae* serotypes.

When it comes to the information provided from this report on antibiotic treatment, it appears that immediate ampicillin/amoxicillin treatment has only a modest benefit compared with placebo or delayed antibiotic but may also be associated with more secondary side effects such as diarrhea and rash. The data from the literature show that of 100 average-risk children with AOM, approximately 80 would likely get better within about 3 days without antibiotics. If all were treated with immediate ampicillin/amoxicillin, an additional 12 would likely improve but 3 to 10 would develop rash and 5 to 10 would develop diarrhea. Obviously we need to weigh these risks (including the possible long-term effects on antibiotic resistance) against the benefits before prescribing immediate antibiotics for uncomplicated AOM. The tide is gradually changing toward conservative nonantibiotic treatment wherever possible. This major review also concluded that there was no evidence to support the use of one antibiotic over another, including the cheapest, amoxicillin. There was no evidence at all for the first-line use of higher-cost antibiotics (eg, cefdinir, cefixime). In this study, it appeared that amoxicillin was prescribed in 49% of diagnoses of AOM, amoxicillin-clavulanate in 16%, cefdinir in 14%, and other cephalosporins in 6%. Coker et al ran the math and showed that if just half of the estimated 8 million children who received cefdinir were to receive amoxicillin (assuming that half were receiving cefdinir correctly for penicillin allergy etc), the estimated annual savings would exceed $34 million. This report reminds us in its conclusions that clinical trials showing the superiority of one antibiotic over another will be difficult to come by. The authors note that with an 80% spontaneous resolution rate, differences in antibiotic success can only be examined in the remaining 20%. For example, if the success rate is 88% for a particular treatment group and 80% for a control group, a sample size of 1150 per cohort is needed to provide a 95% confidence interval if the difference is 5% to 11%. This sample size is much larger than that of any published AOM comparative effectiveness studies to date.

J. A. Stockman III, MD

Reference

1. Soni A. *Ear Infections (Otitis Media) in Children 0–17): Use and Expeditures, 2006. Statistical Brief No.* Agency for Healthcare Research and Quality Web site. http://www.mep.ahrq.gov/mepsweb/data_files/publications/st228/stat228.pdf. December 2008. Accessed September 20, 2010.

A Placebo-Controlled Trial of Antimicrobial Treatment for Acute Otitis Media

Tähtinen PA, Laine MK, Huovinen P, et al (Turku Univ Hosp, Finland; Natl Inst for Health and Welfare, Turku, Finland)
N Engl J Med 364:116-126, 2011

Background.—The efficacy of antimicrobial treatment in children with acute otitis media remains controversial.

Methods.—In this randomized, double-blind trial, children 6 to 35 months of age with acute otitis media, diagnosed with the use of strict criteria, received amoxicillin—clavulanate (161 children) or placebo (158 children) for 7 days. The primary outcome was the time to treatment failure from the first dose until the end-of-treatment visit on day 8. The definition of treatment failure was based on the overall condition of the child (including adverse events) and otoscopic signs of acute otitis media.

Results.—Treatment failure occurred in 18.6% of the children who received amoxicillin-clavulanate, as compared with 44.9% of the children who received placebo (P<0.001). The difference between the groups was already apparent at the first scheduled visit (day 3), at which time 13.7% of the children who received amoxicillin—clavulanate, as compared with 25.3% of those who received placebo, had treatment failure. Overall, amoxicillin—clavulanate reduced the progression to treatment failure by 62% (hazard ratio, 0.38; 95% confidence interval [CI], 0.25 to 0.59; P<0.001) and the need for rescue treatment by 81% (6.8% vs. 33.5%; hazard ratio, 0.19; 95% CI, 0.10 to 0.36; P<0.001). Analgesic or antipyretic agents were given to 84.2% and 85.9% of the children in the amoxicillin—clavulanate and placebo groups, respectively. Adverse events were significantly more common in the amoxicillin—clavulanate group than in the placebo group.

A total of 47.8% of the children in the amoxicillin–clavulanate group had diarrhea, as compared with 26.6% in the placebo group (P<0.001); 8.7% and 3.2% of the children in the respective groups had eczema (P=0.04).

Conclusions.—Children with acute otitis media benefit from antimicrobial treatment as compared with placebo, although they have more side effects. Future studies should identify patients who may derive the greatest benefit, in order to minimize unnecessary antimicrobial treatment and the development of bacterial resistance. (Funded by the Foundation for Paediatric Research and others; ClinicalTrials.gov number, NCT00299455.)

► Anyone practicing pediatrics in the United States 20 years ago would have found it unimaginable that an article such as this and the one by Hoberman et al would appear in the mainstream literature.[1] Interestingly, 80 years ago, acute otitis media and its suppurative complications accounted for 27% of all pediatric admissions to Bellevue Hospital in New York City.[2] Mastoiditis and suppurative intracranial complications were quite common in those days. Today, severe acute otitis media and related complications still occur but generally in those parts of the world with limited access to medical care. Data began to appear in the literature, however, beginning in the 1980s that the use of antimicrobials may not be absolutely necessary or indicated in all children with acute otitis media. These data first appeared in literature from Western Europe. The suggestion was that antibiotic agents be administered only if the illness persisted for 3 days or longer. Other studies from centers in Western Europe, Britain, and the United States subsequently began to corroborate these earlier observations. Unfortunately, most of the early studies had study design flaws, including the lack of precise criteria for the diagnosis of acute otitis media, participation of physicians who were not validated in their ability to look at the eardrum, inadequate sample size, inclusion of older children, inclusion of children who had minimal or uncertain signs of disease, and ambiguous end points for cure or failure. When the topic of the appropriateness of antibiotic therapy for acute otitis media was reviewed by Wald back in 2003, Dr Wald concluded that evidence from studies to date were insufficient to conclude that acute otitis media in children could be safely managed without antibiotics.[3] Nevertheless, in 2004, the American Academy of Pediatrics and the American Academy of Family Physicians endorsed a guideline that recommended initial observation rather than immediate antibiotic therapy for the management of acute otitis media.

Tähtinen et al have undertaken a very well-designed, randomized, double-blind trial in children aged 6 to 35 months with acute otitis media in which children received either amoxicillin-clavulanate or placebo. The results of the study provide evidence that in children of this age, the treatment of acute otitis media with an antibiotic that gives adequate coverage, such as amoxicillin-clavulanate, is beneficial (Fig 2 in the original article).

To better understand the results of this report, see the one by Hoberman et al, which looks at the treatment of acute otitis media in children younger than 2 years.[1]

J. A. Stockman III, MD

References

1. Hoberman A, Paradise JL, Rockette HE, et al. Treatment of acute otitis media in children under 2 years of age. *N Engl J Med.* 2011;364:105-115.
2. Bakwin H, Jacobinzer H. Prevention of purulent otitis media in infants. *J Pediatr.* 1939;14:730-736.
3. Wald ER. Acute otitis media: more trouble with the evidence. *Pediatr Infect Dis J.* 2003;22:103-104.

Treatment of Acute Otitis Media in Children under 2 Years of Age

Hoberman A, Paradise JL, Rockette HE, et al (Children's Hosp of Pittsburgh of the Univ of Pittsburgh Med Ctr, PA; Univ of Pittsburgh, PA)
N Engl J Med 364:105-115, 2011

Background.—Recommendations vary regarding immediate antimicrobial treatment versus watchful waiting for children younger than 2 years of age with acute otitis media.

Methods.—We randomly assigned 291 children 6 to 23 months of age, with acute otitis media diagnosed with the use of stringent criteria, to receive amoxicillin—clavulanate or placebo for 10 days. We measured symptomatic response and rates of clinical failure.

Results.—Among the children who received amoxicillin—clavulanate, 35% had initial resolution of symptoms by day 2, 61% by day 4, and 80% by day 7; among children who received placebo, 28% had initial resolution of symptoms by day 2, 54% by day 4, and 74% by day 7 (P=0.14 for the overall comparison). For sustained resolution of symptoms, the corresponding values were 20%, 41%, and 67% with amoxicillin—clavulanate, as compared with 14%, 36%, and 53% with placebo (P=0.04 for the overall comparison). Mean symptom scores over the first 7 days were lower for the children treated with amoxicillin—clavulanate than for those who received placebo (P=0.02). The rate of clinical failure—defined as the persistence of signs of acute infection on otoscopic examination—was also lower among the children treated with amoxicillin—clavulanate than among those who received placebo: 4% versus 23% at or before the visit on day 4 or 5 (P<0.001) and 16% versus 51% at or before the visit on day 10 to 12 (P<0.001). Mastoiditis developed in one child who received placebo. Diarrhea and diaper-area dermatitis were more common among children who received amoxicillin—clavulanate. There were no significant changes in either group in the rates of nasopharyngeal colonization with nonsusceptible *Streptococcus pneumoniae.*

Conclusions.—Among children 6 to 23 months of age with acute otitis media, treatment with amoxicillin—clavulanate for 10 days tended to reduce the time to resolution of symptoms and reduced the overall symptom burden and the rate of persistent signs of acute infection on otoscopic examination. (Funded by the National Institute of Allergy and Infectious Diseases; ClinicalTrials.gov number, NCT00377260.)

▶ A study with an adequate design addressing the controversy regarding antibiotic therapy in children with a diagnosis of acute otitis media has been a long time coming. Investigators in both Finland (see the commentary by Tähtinen et al) and Pittsburgh now provide us such studies. The report from Finland suggests that children with acute otitis media benefit from antimicrobial treatment as compared with placebo, although they will have more side effects.[1] The report of Hoberman et al from Pittsburgh sheds more light on this topic. Both the Pittsburgh and Finland studies represent randomized blinded trials of the use of amoxicillin-clavulanate as compared with placebo in age groups at greatest risk for acute otitis media and its complications. Acute otitis media in these children was defined by the acute onset of the condition and the presence of middle-ear effusion, a bulging tympanic membrane, and otalgia or erythema of the tympanic membrane. Acute otitis media was meticulously assessed by experienced otoscopists, and only children with a clear certain diagnosis were enrolled. Both studies showed benefit among children who received the drug with respect to the duration of acute signs of illness. Among children with moderate or severe disease, the rates of clinical failure were higher in the placebo group than in the amoxicillin-clavulanate group. As expected, the condition of many children in the placebo group improved without antibiotics, and more children in the antibiotic groups had associated side effects. Since the physician cannot determine at the onset of the illness which child is likely to benefit from antibiotic therapy, one would need to consider these data as applicable to all young children in whom a certain diagnosis of acute otitis media has been made.

So the question is, is acute otitis media a treatable disease? The bottom line is that acute otitis media—affected children will recover more quickly when they are treated with an appropriate antibiotic. I have been on the fence about this topic and have even favored watchful waiting. I am prepared to eat crow. It is my understanding that chewing on anything, such as bubble gum (and in this instance, crow), may in fact reduce the prevalence of middle-ear effusion, but more on that topic at some other time. This is not to say that most children with acute otitis media will not get better without antibiotics. They indeed will. Resolution, however, is enhanced with the use of an appropriate antibiotic. All this reminds me of the teaching of one of my mentors, Dr Lewis Barness, who once taught the group of residents at the Children' Hospital of Philadelphia that it is critically important to treat disease early; otherwise, the patient may get better on their own.

J. A. Stockman III, MD

Reference

1. Tähtinen PA, Laine MK, Huovinen P, Jalava J, Ruuskanen O, Ruohola A. A placebo-controlled trial of antimicrobial treatment for acute otitis media. *N Engl J Med.* 2011;364:116-126.

Newborn Hearing Screening vs Later Hearing Screening and Developmental Outcomes in Children With Permanent Childhood Hearing Impairment
Korver AMH, for the DECIBEL Collaborative Study Group (Leiden Univ Med Ctr, The Netherlands)
JAMA 304:1701-1708, 2010

Context.—Newborn hearing screening programs have been implemented in many countries because it was thought that the earlier permanent childhood hearing impairment is detected, the less developmentally disadvantaged children would become. To date, however, no strong evidence exists for universal introduction of newborn hearing screening.

Objective.—To study the effect of newborn hearing screening vs distraction hearing screening, conducted at 9 months of age, on development, spoken communication, and quality of life.

Design, Setting, and Participants.—Between 2002 and 2006, all 65 regions in the Netherlands replaced distraction hearing screening with newborn hearing screening. Consequently, the type of hearing screening offered was based on availability at the place and date of birth and was independent of developmental prognoses of individual children. All children born in the Netherlands between 2003 and 2005 were included. At the age of 3 to 5 years, all children with permanent childhood hearing impairment were identified. Evaluation ended December 2009.

Main Outcome Measures.—Performance (education and spoken and signed communication), development (general and language), and quality of life.

Results.—During the study period, 335 560 children were born in a newborn hearing screening region and 234 826 children in a distraction hearing screening region. At follow-up, 263 children in newborn hearing screening regions (0.78 per 1000 children) and 171 children in distraction hearing screening regions (0.73 per 1000 children) had been diagnosed with permanent childhood hearing impairment. Three hundred one children (69.4%) participated in analysis of general performance measures. There was no difference between groups in the primary mode of communication or type of education. Analysis of extensive developmental outcomes included 80 children born in newborn hearing screening regions and 70 in distraction hearing screening regions. Multivariate analysis of variance showed that overall, children in newborn hearing screening regions had higher developmental outcome scores compared with children in distraction hearing screening regions (Wilks $\lambda=0.79$; $F_{12}=2.705$; $P=.003$). For social development, the mean between-group difference in quotient points was 8.8 (95%CI, 0.8 to 16.7) and for gross motor development, 9.1 (95%CI, 1.1 to 17.1). For quality of life, the mean between-group difference was 5.3 (95% CI, 1.7 to 8.9), also in favor of children in newborn hearing screening regions.

Conclusion.—Compared with distraction hearing screening, a newborn hearing screening program was associated with better developmental outcomes at age 3 to 5 years among children with permanent childhood hearing impairment.

▶ It was not long ago that screening for hearing loss was recommended to be done at about 9 months of age. The technique used was known as distraction hearing testing using behavioral detection methods. The latter has been largely replaced by newborn hearing screening in the first few days of life. The basis of screening in the newborn period is that if permanent hearing is diagnosed early, there will be less developmental sequelae. Unfortunately, there have been little data to date to tell us for sure whether the universal implementation of newborn hearing screening has had a major positive impact on developmental outcomes. This is the subject of the report of Korver et al. The report emanates from the Netherlands where newborn hearing screening replaced distraction screening in the early part of the last decade. The experience in the Netherlands permits an analysis of children with prominent hearing impairment diagnosed with either the distraction hearing screening techniques or newborn hearing screening.

The information provided by this report gives us firm data convincingly documenting that early detection of hearing loss permits the best developmental outcomes. Specifically, newborn hearing screening, compared with distraction hearing screening, is associated with statistically significantly fewer words signed and better overall, social, and gross motor development and quality of life at 3 to 5 years of age among children with hearing impairment. Children who have hearing loss as a result of congenital cytomegalovirus infection in particular have more problems that are best detected as early as possible. It is important to realize that despite early hearing screening, the development of children with permanent childhood hearing impairment at 3 to 5 years following newborn hearing screening is still not comparable with that of normally developing children with normal hearing. This is particularly highlighted when it comes to language comprehension, which at best is within the borderline range.

While on the topic of hearing loss, please be aware that the prevalence of hearing loss in teenagers rose by nearly one-third in recent years compared with the late 1980s and early 1990s.[1] Data show that the proportion of US adolescents aged 12 to 19 years with any degree of hearing loss rose from 14.9% during 1988 to 1994 to 19.5% in 2005 to 2006. Extrapolated to the United States as a whole, it is estimated that as many as 6.5 million teens will have some degree of hearing impairment. "Any degree of hearing impairment" is defined as a loss of 15 dB in at least 1 ear. Hearing loss of 25 dB or greater is less common, particularly in children; however, it did rise from 3.5% to 5.3% in the study period time frames. The rate of hearing loss increased in high frequencies but not low frequencies. The study did not look at the cause of this hearing loss. To read more about deafness in children, see the superb medical progress review article on this topic by Kral and O'Donoghue.[2]

Also, to learn more about another form of interesting deafness, beat deafness, see the commentary by Bower.[3] "Beat deafness" is a form of selective deafness. The Go-Go's had a 1982 hit record with "We got the beat," but a 23-year-old man named Mathieu never got the message. Researchers have identified this individual as having the first documented case of beat deafness, a condition in which a person cannot feel music's beat or move in time to it. The study subject, Mathieu flails in a time zone of his own when bouncing up and down to a melody, unlike people who do not dance particularly well, but who generally move in synchrony with a musical beat. Interestingly, this individual fails to recognize when someone else dances out of synchrony to a tune. The subject is felt to have a unique form of deafness isolated to inability to follow the beat of music, a rare phenomenon indeed. This individual can sing in tune and recognizes familiar melodies, so musical pitch is apparently normal. Hearing in motor areas of the individual's brain appeared to be also normal. Remember the phenomenon of "beat deafness." This is not just a bad form of dancing. It is a true medical condition.

J. A. Stockman III, MD

References

1. Seppa N. Teens show rise in hearing loss. *Science News*. September 11, 2010:14.
2. Kral A, O'Donoghue GM. Profound deafness in childhood. *N Engl J Med*. 2010; 363:1438-1450.
3. Bower B. A man oblivious to music's tempo. *Science News*. March 26, 2011:9.

Change in Prevalence of Hearing Loss in US Adolescents
Shargorodsky J, Curhan SG, Curhan GC, et al (Brigham and Women's Hosp, Boston, MA; et al)
JAMA 304:772-778, 2010

Context.—Hearing loss is common and, in young persons, can compromise social development, communication skills, and educational achievement.

Objective.—To examine the current prevalence of hearing loss in US adolescents and determine whether it has changed over time.

Design.—Cross-sectional analyses of US representative demographic and audiometric data from the 1988 through 1994 and 2005 through 2006 time periods.

Setting.—The Third National Health and Nutrition Examination Survey (NHANES III), 1988-1994, and NHANES 2005-2006.

Participants.—NHANES III examined 2928 participants and NHANES 2005-2006 examined 1771 participants, aged 12 to 19 years.

Main Outcome Measures.—We calculated the prevalence of hearing loss in participants aged 12 to 19 years after accounting for the complex survey design. Audiometrically determined hearing loss was categorized as either unilateral or bilateral for low frequency (0.5, 1, and 2 kHz) or high frequency (3, 4, 6, and 8 kHz), and as slight loss (>15 to <25 dB) or mild or greater loss (≥25 dB) according to hearing sensitivity in the worse ear. The prevalence of hearing loss from NHANES 2005-2006 was compared with the prevalence from NHANES III (1988-1994). We also examined the cross-sectional relations between several potential risk factors and hearing loss. Logistic regression was used to calculate multivariate adjusted odds ratios (ORs) and 95% confidence intervals (CIs).

Results.—The prevalence of any hearing loss increased significantly from 14.9% (95% CI, 13.0%-16.9%) in 1988-1994 to 19.5% (95% CI, 15.2%-23.8%) in 2005-2006 (*P*= .02). In 2005-2006, hearing loss was more commonly unilateral (prevalence, 14.0%; 95% CI, 10.4%-17.6%, vs 11.1%; 95% CI, 9.5%-12.8% in 1988-1994; *P*= .005) and involved the high frequencies (prevalence, 16.4%; 95% CI, 13.2%-19.7%, vs 12.8%; 95% CI, 11.1%-14.5% in 1988-1994; *P*= .02). Individuals from families below the federal poverty threshold (prevalence, 23.6%; 95% CI, 18.5%-28.7%) had significantly higher odds of hearing loss (multivariate adjusted OR, 1.60; 95% CI, 1.10-2.32) than those above the threshold (prevalence, 18.4%; 95% CI, 13.6%-23.2%).

Conclusion.—The prevalence of hearing loss among a sample of US adolescents aged 12 to 19 years was greater in 2005-2006 compared with 1988-1994.

▶ Can you hear me now? This is not just a popular slogan appearing on advertisements for cellular phone carriers. Such a phrase may very well apply to the teenage population these days. We see from this report by Shargorodsky that the prevalence of hearing loss in teens has increased from about 15% to almost 20%, if one defines hearing loss as any degree of unilateral or bilateral hearing loss for low frequency or high frequency affecting the ability to hear. In particular, high-frequency unilateral hearing loss is becoming more and more prevalent among teens. In fact, when comparing the period 2005 to 2006 with 1988 to 1994, there was a one-third increase in the prevalence of hearing loss. Fortunately, most of the hearing loss was slight, but it was present nonetheless. The prevalence of hearing loss of significance (25 dB or greater) increased from 3.5% to 5.3% indicating that 1 in 20 children in the teen population have mild or worse hearing loss.

The reasons for the demonstrated hearing loss in teens remain elusive. One would have thought that with the introduction of the now commonly administered bacterial vaccines, the prevalence of otitis media would have diminished as a potential cause of hearing loss. The finding of a significant increase in high-frequency hearing loss over the last 20 years may relate to an increase in noise-induced hearing problems.

Most do believe that the leading preventable cause of acquired sensorineural hearing loss is exposure to excessive levels of noise, leading to irreversible loss of cochlear hair cells. When it comes to children and teens, environmental overexposure usually relates to exposure to amplified music, especially through the use of personal music devices such as MP3 players. More than 90% of youngsters use MP3 players. Increasingly, the devices have used earphones that insert into the ear canal, which can produce higher sound levels in the ear than over the earphones used at the same volume, and these sounds can exceed 120 dB, similar in intensity to the noise of a jet engine. Several small studies have found that reported use of personal music players is associated with worse hearing function in adolescents and young adults. Needless to say, we should be advising current users of MP3 players or similar devices to avoid listening to personal music players at maximum volume. We also need to wish ourselves good luck with any success in this regard.

To read more about hearing loss and personal music players, see the excellent commentary on this topic by Rabinowitz.[1]

J. A. Stockman III, MD

Reference

1. Rabinowitz PM. Hearing loss and personal music players. Reducing exposure is prudent. *BMJ.* 2010;341:57-58.

Spoken Language Development in Children Following Cochlear Implantation
Niparko JK, for the CDaCI Investigative Team (Johns Hopkins Univ School of Medicine, Baltimore, MD; et al)
JAMA 303:1498-1506, 2010

Context.—Cochlear implantation is a surgical alternative to traditional amplification (hearing aids) that can facilitate spoken language development in young children with severe to profound sensorineural hearing loss (SNHL).

Objective.—To prospectively assess spoken language acquisition following cochlear implantation in young children.

Design, Setting, and Participants.—Prospective, longitudinal, and multidimensional assessment of spoken language development over a 3-year period in children who underwent cochlear implantation before 5 years of age (n = 188) from 6 US centers and hearing children of similar ages (n = 97) from 2 preschools recruited between November 2002 and December 2004. Follow-up completed between November 2005 and May 2008.

Main Outcome Measures.—Performance on measures of spoken language comprehension and expression (Reynell Developmental Language Scales).

Results.—Children undergoing cochlear implantation showed greater improvement in spoken language performance (10.4; 95% confidence interval [CI], 9.6-11.2 points per year in comprehension; 8.4; 95% CI, 7.8-9.0 in expression) than would be predicted by their preimplantation baseline scores (5.4; 95% CI, 4.1-6.7, comprehension; 5.8; 95% CI, 4.6-7.0, expression), although mean scores were not restored to age-appropriate levels after 3 years. Younger age at cochlear implantation was associated with significantly steeper rate increases in comprehension (1.1; 95% CI, 0.5-1.7 points per year younger) and expression (1.0; 95% CI, 0.6-1.5 points per year younger). Similarly, each 1-year shorter history of hearing deficit was associated with steeper rate increases in comprehension (0.8; 95% CI, 0.2-1.2 points per year shorter) and expression (0.6; 95% CI, 0.2-1.0 points per year shorter). In multivariable analyses, greater residual hearing prior to cochlear implantation, higher ratings of parent-child interactions, and higher socioeconomic status were associated with greater rates of improvement in comprehension and expression.

Conclusion.—The use of cochlear implants in young children was associated with better spoken language learning than would be predicted from their preimplantation scores.

▶ This important report details for us how spoken language is acquired following cochlear transplantation in young children. The report demonstrates findings consistent with the critical period concept for language learning in that early transplantation in infants and toddlers is associated with significantly accelerated spoken language learning. Specifically, performance scores in children who receive implants earlier are closer to scores of normal-hearing controls. Older age at transplantation is associated with greater gaps between chronological and language ages. The rate of improvement in performance on spoken language measures is less steep in children undergoing cochlear implantation at later ages.

The decision of whether to pursue cochlear implantation is not an easy one for some families and care providers. One must weigh the potential benefit of implantation versus the continued amplification of residual hearing using hearing aids. The findings from this report suggest that delaying implantation to extend hearing aid use for children with severe to profound hearing loss may be detrimental to language development following cochlear implantation. Spoken language learning relies on effective hearing. Close monitoring of performance with hearing aids can help determine whether speech is effectively amplified to allow spoken language acquisition to progress. If there is a lesson to be learned from this report, it is that if you are fairly well assured that even with assisted hearing devices (such as hearing aids) a child has or will have significant problems with delayed speech, one might seriously consider moving to cochlear implantation sooner than later.

If you are not aware of how these implant systems work, cochlear implant systems consist of an externally worn microphone and a microprocessor program to extract intensity, frequency, and timing clues from acoustic signals. The system transforms these acoustic clues into an electrical code. Internally, a surgically placed receiver relays the transmitted code to an implanted array of contacts in the cochlea to stimulate surviving auditory neurons. With experience, children understand speech, environmental sounds, and music with varying degrees of success.

This commentary closes with an observation having to do with whales and what they perceive in terms of sound at both audible and subaudible levels. It is well known that sonar unquestionably disturbs beaked whales. During sonar exercises at the US Navy's underwater test range in the Bahamas, beaked whales stopped their chirpy echolocations and fled the area. These findings are very similar to those observed previously in harbor porpoises, which are known to be extraordinarily sensitive to sound. The consequence of such sound exposure can cause whales to beach themselves. Until beaked whales started showing up in unusual mass strandings, the elusive animals were rarely seen. Because these strandings often coincided with nearby Naval sonar exercises, it seems clear that noise is somehow driving these whales to the beach.[1]

J. A. Stockman III, MD

Reference

1. Ehrenberg R. Beaked whales can't stand sonar. New study suggests species are highly sensitive to noise. *Science News.* April 23, 2011:16.

6 Endocrinology

A Genetic Basis for Functional Hypothalamic Amenorrhea

Caronia LM, Martin C, Welt CK, et al (Massachusetts General Hosp, Boston; et al)
N Engl J Med 364:215-225, 2011

Background.—Functional hypothalamic amenorrhea is a reversible form of gonadotropin-releasing hormone (GnRH) deficiency commonly triggered by stressors such as excessive exercise, nutritional deficits, or psychological distress. Women vary in their susceptibility to inhibition of the reproductive axis by such stressors, but it is unknown whether this variability reflects a genetic predisposition to hypothalamic amenorrhea. We hypothesized that mutations in genes involved in idiopathic hypogonadotropic hypogonadism, a congenital form of GnRH deficiency, are associated with hypothalamic amenorrhea.

Methods.—We analyzed the coding sequence of genes associated with idiopathic hypogonadotropic hypogonadism in 55 women with hypothalamic amenorrhea and performed in vitro studies of the identified mutations.

Results.—Six heterozygous mutations were identified in 7 of the 55 patients with hypothalamic amenorrhea: two variants in the fibroblast growth factor receptor 1 gene *FGFR1* (G260E and R756H), two in the prokineticin receptor 2 gene *PROKR2* (R85H and L173R), one in the GnRH receptor gene *GNRHR* (R262Q), and one in the Kallmann syndrome 1 sequence gene *KAL1* (V371I). No mutations were found in a cohort of 422 controls with normal menstrual cycles. In vitro studies showed that *FGFR1* G260E, *FGFR1* R756H, and *PROKR2* R85H are loss-of-function mutations, as has been previously shown for *PROKR2* L173R and *GNRHR* R262Q.

Conclusions.—Rare variants in genes associated with idiopathic hypogonadotropic hypogonadism are found in women with hypothalamic amenorrhea, suggesting that these mutations may contribute to the variable susceptibility of women to the functional changes in GnRH secretion that characterize hypothalamic amenorrhea. Our observations provide evidence for the role of rare variants in common multifactorial disease. (Funded by the Eunice Kennedy Shriver National Institute of Child Health and Human Development and others; ClinicalTrials.gov number, NCT00494169.)

▶ Teens as well as young and older adults can suffer from functional hypothalamic amenorrhea. Cessation of menses can occur in response to a variety of circumstances, particularly life stressors. The latter often include weight loss, excessive exercise, eating disorders, and psychological distress. These stressors through complicated mechanisms suppress the hypothalamic-pituitary-gonadal axis by inhibiting hypothalamic pulsatile secretion of gonadotropin-releasing hormone (GnRH). For those wishing to have children, this is a frequent cause of female infertility. The specific diagnosis of the problem is termed functional hypothalamic amenorrhea. This is defined as the absence of menses, low or normal gonadotropin levels, and hypoestrogenemia without organic abnormality. In affected teens and adults, after the underlying stressors have been eliminated, normal reproductive function generally resumes in most cases.

It is unknown whether the susceptibility of individuals to suppression of menses by stressors is based on a genetic predisposition since there is wide variation between women in this response to stress. Much is known about the genetics of congenital GnRH deficiency (idiopathic hypogonadotropic hypogonadism) in contrast to hypothalamic amenorrhea. The former is characterized by an absence of puberty and by infertility caused by defects in the secretion of GnRH from the hypothalamus or defects in the action of GnRH on the pituitary. The disease is genetically heterogeneous, with several associated loci that account for approximately 40% of cases. There are likely to be multiple gene defects causing the problem.

Caronia et al have hypothesized that mutations in genes involved in idiopathic hypogonadism confer susceptibility to the functional deficiency in GnRH secretion that characterizes the much more common stress-induced hypothalamic amenorrhea. These investigators analyzed the sequences of genes associated with idiopathic hypogonadotropic hypogonadism in individuals with hypothalamic amenorrhea. They did observe that the rare gene variance associated with idiopathic hypogonadotropic hypogonadism is found in women with hypothalamic amenorrhea, suggesting that these mutations may, at least in part, contribute to the susceptibility of some women to the problem of stress-induced hypothalamic amenorrhea. The authors do not necessarily suggest that women affected with stress-induced hypothalamic amenorrhea be routinely screened for gene mutations known to underlie idiopathic hypogonadotropic hypogonadism except in cases of clear familial inheritance of stress-induced hypothalamic amenorrhea or of idiopathic hypogonadotropic hypogonadism. Even though the data from this report do not immediately translate into any effective new understandings of different ways to manage this problem in teens and adults, it is nice to know that in many instances there is a genetic underpinning for the problem and that it does not necessarily just occur out of the blue.

In conclusion, we will close with a brief historical note having to do with an endocrinologic problem, this being pituitary adenomas. Recently, investigators identified a common gene haplotype mutation in 4 family members with familial isolated pituitary adenoma including a family member who was a "giant" from 18th century Northern Ireland.[1] It appears that gigantism and acromegaly have been described since ancient times. Indeed, Wier provided the first accurate medical description of acromegaly in the 16th century.[2] The link between pituitary adenoma and clinical acromegaly and gigantism was not recognized until the second part of the 19th century. Acromegaly was initially considered to be an acquired disease, whereas gigantism was considered to be a congenital disorder. With the data emerging on the *AIP* mutations in patients with familial acromegaly, it appears that this old dogma might ultimately have some truth, since it has now been shown that one of the most famous giants in medical literature, the Irishman, did in fact harbor an inherited predisposition to the disease and that the mutation responsible for this predisposition persists in contemporary society within Ireland. The bottom line is that you can never fool a geneticist these days. They have the tools to prove virtually anything.

J. A. Stockman III, MD

References

1. Chahal HS, Stals K, Unterländer PK, et al. AIP mutation in primary adenomas in the 18ᵗʰ century and today. *N Engl J Med.* 2011;364:43-50.
2. Wier J. Medicarum observationum. In: *Virgo Gygantea Ex Quartana Reddita.* Basel, Switzerland: Oporinus; 1567:7-10.

A National Study of Physician Recommendations to Initiate and Discontinue Growth Hormone for Short Stature

Silvers JB, Marinova D, Mercer MB, et al (Case Western Reserve Univ, Cleveland, OH; Univ of Missouri, Columbia)
Pediatrics 126:468-476, 2010

Objectives.—Overall growth hormone (GH) use depends on decisions to both initiate treatment and continue treatment. The determinants of both are unclear. We studied how physicians decided to begin GH in idiopathic short stature and how, after an initial course of treatment, they decided to continue, intensify (increase the dose), or terminate treatment.

Methods.—We used a national census study of 727 pediatric endocrinologists involving a structured questionnaire with a factorial experimental design. Main outcome measures were GH recommendations for previously untreated children and those children who were treated with GH for 1 year.

Results.—The response rate was 90%. In previously untreated children, recommendations to initiate GH were consistent with guidelines and also influenced by family preferences and physician attitudes ($P < .001$). In children treated with GH, recommendations on whether to continue GH were influenced by the growth response to therapy ($P < .01$) but were divided regarding course of action. With identical growth responses to treatment, physician decisions diverged (intensify versus discontinue GH) and were driven by independent, nonphysiologic, and contextual factors (eg, physician attitudes, family preferences, and GH-initiation recommendation; each $P < .001$). Together, attitudinal and contextual factors exerted more influence on continuation decisions than did the growth response to therapy.

Conclusions.—Physician decisions to initiate GH are largely consistent with evidence-based medicine. However, decisions about continuing GH vary and are strongly influenced by factors other than response to treatment. With a potential market of 500 000 US children and costs exceeding

$10 billion per year, changes in GH use may depend on potentially modifiable physician attitudes and family preferences as much as physiologic evidence.

▶ Until this report appeared, I was not familiar with the statistic that there are more than half a million potential children in our country with idiopathic short stature (ISS). Every one of these youngsters is a potential candidate for making a decision about whether growth hormone (GH) should or should not be administered. The US Food and Drug Administration has provided guidelines for GH treatment initiation.[1] There are a few clear guidelines regarding how and when to discontinue GH administration. Given that GH is an example of one of the fastest growing classes of pharmaceuticals and the fact that it is expensive, it is clear that we need a better understanding about when to discontinue its use.

The report of Silvers et al sheds light on this issue by looking at when pediatric endocrinologists decide to discontinue GH treatment. The study itself is the first to examine physician recommendations for the continuation of GH as part of the management of ISS. The study was based on a survey of 727 pediatric endocrinologists. The results are valuable in that virtually all children with ISS are managed by pediatric endocrinologists. Ninety percent of those surveyed responded. Some three-fourths of pediatric endocrinologists indicated that they continue or increase GH in the face of poor growth responses to standard doses, yet the stated purpose of therapeutic trials of GH by 88% of those responding to the survey was to determine the need for such long-term treatment. Endocrinologists were as likely to continue as to discontinue GH treatment when it is quite clear that the patient in fact is not responding. Decisions for continuing/intensifying GH therapy are tempered by a variety of other factors. Parent influence is one of these factors.

If there is anything one can learn from this report, it is that many endocrinologists are flying by the seat of their pants when they make decisions about discontinuing GH therapy. The implications of the findings from this report are quite substantial and underscore the need for undertaking carefully designed trials of high-dose GH when patients have failed initial treatment. Given the fact that over $10 billion is expended annually on GH therapy, there should be enough money in the pot to fund long-term studies designed to determine what is in the best interest of these youngsters.

To read more about growth and the timing of puberty, including whether it is changing to younger and younger ages, see the excellent review article by Walvoord.[2]

J. A. Stockman III, MD

References

1. US Food and Drug Administration. *Approval Letter for Application Number NDA19–640/S-033: Humatrope.* http:/www.fda.gov/drugsatfda_docs/appletter/003/19640se1-033ltr.pdf. July 25, 2003. Accessed November 25, 2010.
2. Walvoord EC. The timing of puberty: Is it changing? Does it matter? *J Adolesc Health.* 2010;47:433-439.

Variation in Methods of Predicting Adult Height for Children with Idiopathic Short Stature

Topor LS, Feldman HA, Bauchner H, et al (Children's Hosp Boston, MA; et al)
Pediatrics 126:938-944, 2010

Objective.—Recombinant human growth hormone (GH) is approved for treatment of children with idiopathic short stature, and endocrinologists often depend on algorithms to predict adult height. Because algorithm performance often is included in treatment decisions, we sought to evaluate agreement among height prediction formulas.

Methods.—We identified 3 commonly used algorithms for height prediction, the Bayley-Pinneau, Roche-Wainer-Thissen, and Khamis-Roche methods. We constructed simulated samples of children with typical distributions of ages, heights, weights, bone ages, and parental heights seen in patients with idiopathic short stature, and we applied the algorithms to the simulated sample to determine whether predicted adult height was <160 cm for boys or <150 cm for girls (<1.2nd height percentiles for adults).

Results.—We found substantial disagreement among algorithms in the proportions of simulated cases with predicted adult heights of <1.2nd percentile, a cutoff value that may influence GH treatment decisions. With the Bayley-Pinneau formula, 43% of boys and 81% of girls had predicted adult heights below this threshold; with the Khamis-Roche method, only 3% of boys and 0.2% of girls had predicted heights of <1.2nd percentile. Roche-Wainer-Thissen predictions were between those values. Overall agreement of the methods was poor ($\kappa = 0.21$) for boys and negative for girls.

Conclusions.—Wide variation exists among formulas used to predict adult heights. Because these algorithms may be used in decisions regarding whether to initiate GH treatment and assessment of the efficacy of GH in research trials, it is important for parents, pediatricians, and investigators to recognize the considerable variation involved in height predictions.

▶ It has been almost 10 years since the US Food and Drug Administration (FDA) approved the use of recombinant human growth hormone (GH) for the treatment of children with idiopathic short stature, defined by the FDA as height before treatment 2.25 standard deviations (SDs) below the mean for age (1.2nd percentile) without evidence of underlying disease or GH deficiency. Obviously, prior to 2003 many endocrinologists were already using GH for this purpose. Although predicted adult height is not part of the FDA criteria for using GH to treat children with idiopathic short stature, the FDA criteria do include a statement regarding "a growth rate that is unlikely to attain an adult height within the normal range." The FDA criteria identify the 1.2nd percentile cutoff for values in height in adults as 63 in (160 cm) for men and 59 in (150 cm) for women. Straightforward math shows that about 400 000 children in the United States would qualify for GH therapy. Various studies performed over the years have shown height increases with the use of GH ranging from 0 to 0.7 SD, but there is little information comparing near-adult heights with predicted adult heights based on formulas such as the Bayley-Pinneau (BP) method of height prediction.

Needless to say, it is important to be able to predict what a short child's likely adult height would be sans GH administration. The approval of GH treatment for children with idiopathic short stature has substantial cost for the US health care system. Data suggest that the cost-effectiveness of GH is estimated at about $15 000 per year for each inch attained, and given an average incremental height of 1.9 in over 5 years, the incremental cost per child runs almost $100 000. At this average cost per child, the potential cost of treating all eligible children would be expected to be approximately $40 billion. Needless to say, many, if not most, insurers deny coverage for GH for the treatment of idiopathic short stature.

To assess the appropriateness of treatment with GH for children with idiopathic short stature, endocrinologists usually use an algorithm to predict whether a child's predicted adult height will be less than 1.2nd percentile, corresponding to < 160 cm (< 63 in) for adult men and < 150 cm (< 59 in) for adult women. Because the performance of such algorithms often is crucial for decision making regarding treatment with GH, what Topor et al have done is to evaluate the potential agreement between the various formulas used to predict adult height. Using complicated SAS software, the investigators assessed the variation of 3 height prediction algorithms commonly used for children with short stature. They found wide differences in height predictions among the commonly used formulas but showed that on average, the BP method predicted lower adult heights than did the other methods. This is the first study to compare height prediction algorithms using large-scale models to represent typical short children presenting for endocrinologic evaluation.

Future studies are indeed necessary to determine which is the most accurate height algorithm for children with short stature. It is entirely possible that automated bone age measurements will be found to be more precise than measurements by human readers, and the use of such technology might help reduce errors in height prediction allowing more accurate comparisons of the different algorithms. The authors of this report note that given the substantial medical, psychosocial, and financial implications of using GH for children with idiopathic short stature, it is important that parents, clinicians, and investigators understand the considerable uncertainty of height prediction with the currently available mathematical tools.

J. A. Stockman III, MD

Impact of growth hormone therapy on adult height of children with idiopathic short stature: systematic review
Deodati A, Cianfarani S (Tor Vergata Univ, Rome, Italy)
BMJ 342:c7157, 2011

Objective.—To systematically determine the impact of growth hormone therapy on adult height of children with idiopathic short stature.
Design.—Systematic review.

Data Sources.—Cochrane Central Register of Controlled Trials, Medline, and the bibliographic references from retrieved articles of randomised and non-randomised controlled trials from 1985 to April 2010.

Data Extraction.—Height in adulthood (standard deviation score) and overall gain in height (SD score) from baseline measurement in childhood.

Study Selection.—Randomised and non-randomised controlled trials with height measurements for adults. Inclusion criteria were initial short stature (defined as height >2 SD score below the mean), peak growth hormone responses >10 μg/L, prepubertal stage, no previous growth hormone therapy, and no comorbid conditions that would impair growth. Adult height was considered achieved when growth rate was <1.5 cm/year or bone age was 15 years in females and 16 years in males.

Results.—Three randomised controlled trials (115 children) met the inclusion criteria. The adult height of the growth hormone treated children exceeded that of the controls by 0.65 SD score (about 4 cm). The mean height gain in treated children was 1.2 SD score compared with 0.34 SD score in untreated children. A slight difference of about 1.2 cm in adult height was observed between the two growth hormone dose regimens. In the seven nonrandomised controlled trials the adult height of the growth hormone treated group exceeded that of the controls by 0.45 SD score (about 3 cm).

Conclusions.—Growth hormone therapy in children with idiopathic short stature seems to be effective in partially reducing the deficit in height as adults, although the magnitude of effectiveness is on average less than that achieved in other conditions for which growth hormone is licensed. The individual response to therapy is highly variable, and additional studies are needed to identify the responders.

▶ This report of Deodati and Cianfarani tells us about the management of otherwise normal children with idiopathic short stature and the use of recombinant growth hormone. Idiopathic short stature in studies performed to date is defined as prepubertal short stature in children born at appropriate size for gestational age. This review found that the overall adult height of children treated with growth hormone was 0.65 standard deviation (SD) score higher than that of controls (about 4 cm), and they became 0.94 SD score taller than their parents. The overall height gain was 1.2 SD score in children treated with growth hormone versus 0.34 SD score in children not treated with growth hormone (difference 0.8 SD score), with a large interindividual variation in growth response, ranging from 0 to 3 SD score.

It should be noted that growth hormone affects more than just height. It is a major anabolic hormone with effects on most human tissues. Responsiveness to growth hormone varies not only between individuals but also between tissues: brain, fat, and muscle may be more sensitive than bone. The interindividual variation in nongrowth effects of growth hormone can be reduced somewhat by using tailored dose, selected on the basis of mathematical models of responsiveness. Such modeling can reduce the risk of overtreatment or undertreatment with consequent hormone imbalances.

The editors of the *British Medical Journal* that accepted this report on growth hormone in the management of idiopathic short stature noted that the reviewers of the article thought that the study provided the ending of the story since further funding of clinical trials in this regard is highly unlikely at this point. The authors of the report suggest that the debate about the use of growth hormone should now focus on whether the gains seen, around 4 cm, are truly of value. In an editorial that accompanied this report, Albertsson-Wikland emphasizes that the response to growth hormone treatment can vary substantially between individuals and also at different stages of growth. The editorial comments that it would be safer and more efficient to tailor doses to the individual, rather than using a standard dose based on a child's size, the approach that is currently recommended by drug agencies and that was used in the report of Deodati and Cianfarani.

As a segue to the commentary on the growth and development of male external genitalia, it should be noted that at least in the duck population, the length of a duck's penis depends on the companion that duck keeps. And in this case, it is the female who makes all the difference.[1] It appears, for example, that a drake's penis substantially wastes at the end of one breeding season and then regrows as the next season begins. Among lesser ruddy ducks, the regrowth varies in length depending on whether males have to compete with a bunch of others for the females. The study from Yale University is the first to document in invertebrates that social circumstances influence the length of the male organ. The investigators who carried out this study conclude that ducks are essentially engineering their own phallus in response to environmental social challenges. Fortunately, or not, humans compete in other ways.

J. A. Stockman III, MD

Reference

1. Milius S. Natural male enhancement: ducks' penises grow longer with increased competition. *Science News*. August 28, 2010:11.

Growth and Development of Male External Genitalia: A Cross-Sectional Study of 6200 Males Aged 0 to 19 Years
Tomova A, Deepinder F, Robeva R, et al (Med Univ, Sofia, Bulgaria; Cedars Sinai Med Ctr, Los Angeles, CA; et al)
Arch Pediatr Adolesc Med 164:1152-1157, 2010

Objective.—To provide estimates of normal variations in penile measurements and testicular volumes, and to establish reference ranges for clinical use.

Design.—Cross-sectional, population-based study.

Setting.—Schools, kindergartens, and child care centers in different parts of Bulgaria.

Participants.—A population of 6200 clinically healthy white males aged 0 to 19 years.

Interventions.—The study physician chose schools, kindergartens, and child care centers randomly and examined children at random until he reached the required number. Each of the 20 age groups (age range, 0-19 years) had an equal number of males (ie, 310).

Main Outcome Measures.—The mean (SD) values and fifth, 50th, and 95th percentiles of height (Siber Hegner anthropometer), weight (beam balance), testicular volume (Prader orchidometer), penile length (rigid tape), and penile circumference (measuring tape) from birth to 19 years of age.

Results.—Testes did not show any increase in size until the onset of puberty at age 11 years, whereas penile growth was gradual after birth. However, both penile and testicular development demonstrated peak growth from 12 to 16 years of age, which coincided with the maximal male pubertal growth spurt. Data indicate an earlier pubertal development for this study population than that for a similar population several decades ago. Significant differences between urban and rural populations regarding penile length were also noticed.

Conclusions.—Our study provides the contemporary reference range values for height, weight, testicular volume, and penile length and circumference of males aged 0 to 19 years. Our data show that, even by the end of 20th century, there is still some acceleration of male pubertal development. For the first time are reported somatic differences in genitalia within a population between urban and rural representatives.

▶ It seems to be an uncommon human trait to want to size everything up. When it comes to testicular size, one would have thought that we had long ago learned what was within normal boundaries at varying ages. The same is true of the size of the human penis. Indeed, assessment of the growth of the external genitalia is an essential component of the physical examination in children. Aberrant growth of the male external genitalia may be the first sign of an underlying biophysiologic or psychosocial illness. Studies have been conducted here and abroad to determine the interindividual variations in the onset and duration of normal puberty. What Tomova et al have done is to establish reference ranges in quite detail of various anthropometric measurements for the male genitalia based on the largest cross-sectional population-based study on male sexual growth and development ever undertaken.

   Tomova et al have examined 6200 white males aged 0 to 19 years from the capital city of Bulgaria (Sofia) and from 4 other regions of Bulgaria. The towns and villages were chosen at random and represented both urban and rural areas of that country. All 6200 males were clinically examined by a single physician, an endocrinologist. Each child had measurements of height, testicular volume, penile length, and penile circumference. The Prader orchidometer was used to measure the volume of the testes. Data were collected separately for the left and right testicles. Although ultrasonography would be the absolute gold standard for measurement of the volume of a testis, there are good data in the literature to indicate that there is an excellent correlation between ultrasound determinations and the Prader orchidometer when it comes to a precise measurement of testicular volume. Fig 1 in the original article illustrates the growth curves representing various growth parameters of external genitalia in these boys, illustrating the fifth centile, the 50th centile, and the 95th centile. In this study, the beginning of pubertal development was marked by an increase in testicular volume at 11 years. This is consistent with the data of Prader who indicated that an increase in testicular volume greater than 2 mL is considered the first perceptible sign of oncoming puberty. The study from Bulgaria showed that with a testicular volume of 5 mL at age 12 years, the pubic hair was already at Tanner stage 2, showing that growth of the testes tends to start before pubic hair development, which is in agreement with other studies. The boys in this study reached a testicular size of 12 mL on average at 15 years, consistent with data from the literature showing progression to a late stage of pubertal development. After 16 years of age, the difference between various age groups was not significant, indicating that puberty was more or less completed by that time. As one can see, however, in Fig 1 in the original article, there are significant differences between the 5th and 95th centiles illustrating relatively large variations in the timing of puberty, which should always be kept in mind when evaluating growth and development in healthy populations. The data from Bulgaria show that the testes of a 19-year-old man have the volume typical for maturity (on average 16.28 mL). The data also indicate earlier pubertal development compared with the same population several decades ago and that even by the end of the 20th century, there was still some acceleration in male pubertal development. This is in line with studies on girls of comparable ages showing 1-year acceleration in the age of menarche at the end of the last century compared with middle of the last century.

The bottom line is that this report, which in fact does represent the largest population-based study on male growth and sexual development conducted by a single investigator, demonstrates that testicles do not show any increase in size until the onset of puberty, whereas penile growth is gradual from birth. For both the penis and the testes, however, peak growth occurs between the ages of 12 and 16 years, coinciding with the onset of the pubertal growth spurt.

This commentary closes with the notation that Dr James Mourilyan Tanner passed from this earth in 2010. Dr Tanner was professor of Growth and Development at Great Ormond Street Hospital in London. Dr Tanner invented the eponymous scale that measures sexual growth and development in childhood and adolescence. Before Tanner, child growth charts were "one size fits all" in nature. The Tanner Growth Curves took into account variations in a child's speed of growth allowing pediatricians to chart a child's growth in relation to the average and see how growth lags and spurts. On the more personal side, Dr Tanner was a runner and in fact was the fastest British runner in the 110-meter hurdles in 1939 and was expected to shine for Great Britain in the 1940 Olympic Games, which were canceled because of the war. In 1940, he won a Rockefeller Foundation scholarship to the University of Pennsylvania in a scheme to help 30 UK medical students finish their studies away from the stresses of war. It was in Philadelphia that he met and married Bernice Alture, a student at Women's Medical College of Philadelphia. He did his internship at Johns Hopkins Hospital and then entered the military shortly before the end of World War II, ultimately settling for a period of time at Oxford University. It was there that he did his first study on child development, charting puberty by measuring genital size and pubic hair quantity from photographs. He was among the very first to use human growth hormone obtained from cadavers. He continued treating children with short stature until it was recognized that human-derived growth hormone was contaminated with prions in 1985. James Tanner died from metastatic prostate cancer and a stroke on August 11, 2010.

J. A. Stockman III, MD

Growth Hormone plus Childhood Low-Dose Estrogen in Turner's Syndrome

Ross JL, Quigley CA, Cao D, et al (Thomas Jefferson Univ, Philadelphia, PA; Lilly Res Laboratories, Indianapolis, IN; et al)
N Engl J Med 364:1230-1242, 2011

Background.—Short stature and ovarian failure are characteristic features of Turner's syndrome. Although recombinant human growth hormone is commonly used to treat the short stature associated with this syndrome, a randomized, placebo-controlled trial is needed to document whether such treatment increases adult height. Furthermore, it is not known whether childhood estrogen replacement combined with growth hormone therapy provides additional benefit. We examined the independent and combined effects of growth hormone and early, ultra-low-dose estrogen on adult height in girls with Turner's syndrome.

Methods.—In this double-blind, placebo-controlled trial, we randomly assigned 149 girls, 5.0 to 12.5 years of age, to four groups: double placebo (placebo injection plus childhood oral placebo, 39 patients), estrogen alone (placebo injection plus childhood oral lowdose estrogen, 40), growth hormone alone (growth hormone injection plus childhood oral placebo, 35), and growth hormone—estrogen (growth hormone injection plus childhood oral low-dose estrogen, 35). The dose of growth hormone was 0.1 mg per kilogram of body weight three times per week. The doses of ethinyl estradiol (or placebo) were adjusted for chronologic age and pubertal status. At the first visit after the age of 12.0 years, patients in all treatment groups received escalating doses of ethinyl estradiol. Growth hormone injections were terminated when adult height was reached.

Results.—The mean standard-deviation scores for adult height, attained at an average age of 17.0 ± 1.0 years, after an average study period of 7.2 ± 2.5 years were -2.81 ± 0.85, -3.39 ± 0.74, -2.29 ± 1.10, and -2.10 ± 1.02 for the double-placebo, estrogen-alone, growth hormone—alone, and growth hormone—estrogen groups, respectively (P<0.001). The overall effect of growth hormone treatment (vs. placebo) on adult height was a 0.78 ± 0.13 increase in the height standard-deviation score (5.0 cm) (P<0.001); adult height was greater in the growth hormone—estrogen group than in the growth hormone—alone group, by 0.32 ± 0.17 standard-deviation score (2.1 cm) (P=0.059), suggesting a modest synergy between childhood low-dose ethinyl estradiol and growth hormone.

Conclusions.—Our study shows that growth hormone treatment increases adult height in patients with Turner's syndrome. In addition, the data suggest that combining childhood ultra-low-dose estrogen with growth hormone may improve growth and provide other potential benefits associated with early initiation of estrogen replacement. (Funded by the National Institute of Child Health and Human Development and Eli Lilly; ClinicalTrials.gov number, NCT00001221.)

▶ This report tells us about the results of a unique placebo-controlled trial of growth hormone treatment (with or without early low-dose ethinyl estradiol) on adult height in Turner syndrome. Turner syndrome, of course, is character-ized by short stature and hypogonadism. The data provided by Ross et al come from a randomized trial that began approximately 25 years ago. There are not many investigators who are so dogged in their pursuit of answers to important questions as this set of authors. The results reported confirm those of previous less rigorous studies showing that treatment with growth hormone significantly increases adult height in patients with Turner syndrome. Interest-ingly, the results also suggest a modest and curious synergism between growth hormone and low-dose estrogen in promoting growth.

Estrogen has been the ultimate growth-suppressive hormone—high-dose estrogen has been used to stifle growth in tall girls—and is necessary and suffi-cient to bring about epiphyseal closure. It should be recognized, however, that the effect of estrogen is 2-fold. Low doses actually can increase height philos-ophy. Estradiol accounts for the normal female growth spurt seen during puberty if given at the right physiologic dose, and at the appropriate age, estra-diol can stimulate pubertal growth in teens with hypogonadism without compromising their height potential. Despite this, it has been common practice in the management of Turner syndrome to delay estrogen replacement therapy until the midteens because of the perceived possibility of interfering with growth. This is despite the potential negative implications of such a delay with respect to bone mineral accrual and age-appropriate psychosocial development.

If one reads the report of Ross et al in detail, one can see that the overall effect of growth hormone treatment is a gain of 0.78 points in the adult height on the standard deviation score, as compared with placebo. This represents a significant gain of about 5.0 cm. The main adult height, even with growth hormone treatment, does remain below the normal range, and not every treated youngster achieves the same results.

In an editorial that accompanied this report, Cuttler and Rosenfield note that the ability to increase height should not be the sole yardstick for assessing benefit in girls with Turner syndrome. For disorders in which final height would be clearly disabling, a gain of 5 to 7.5 cm may prove a practical benefit.[1] It is noted, however, that height did not influence quality of life, social adjust-ment, or self-esteem among patients with Turner syndrome who were treated with growth hormone. Needless to say, such additional growth also comes at significant cost. Calculated in terms of dollars and cents, each centimeter of height gained has an expense of approximately $35 000.

Virtually all girls with Turner syndrome are now treated with growth hormone. This report tells us that such therapy can be assisted by the administration of low-dose estrogen. Cuttler and Rosenfield remind us that when deciding whether to recommend growth-promoting therapy, physicians will take into account subjective factors such as perceptions, beliefs, and attitude as well as physiological data and scientific evidence. We do need to learn more about the functional benefit of a couple of extra inches in final height in those with Turner syndrome.

This commentary closes with an unrelated, but interesting observation having to do with hormones. If you have a new baby and are feeling like you are waist deep in dirty diapers, you might want to forget about diaper collection services and just volunteer your infant for a poop study. Researchers will take your dirty diapers off your hands for free. Dirty diapers, it seems, hold the key for measuring infant hormones.[2] It appears that a baby's stool can be used to assay for biological influences on hormone secretion. Endocrinologists are very interested in the effects of estrogen and estrogen-like substances, for example, in soy formula, plant fertilizer, and even plastics. Few babies will tolerate frequent finger or heel pricks, so little is known about various hormone levels in infants. Diapers can be collected frequently and over a long period of time, perfect for a longitudinal study. A technique has now been developed for extracting hormone levels from baby poop that allows longitudinal studies of various hormones, including estrogen and estrogen-like hormones. The collection technique is simple with respect to its ingredients: a dirty diaper, preferably cotton, a Ziploc bag, and an icepack.

J. A. Stockman III, MD

References

1. Cuttler L, Rosenfield RL. Assessing the value of treatments to increase height. *N Engl J Med.* 2011;364:1274-1276.
2. Editorial comment. Poop scoop. *Science.* 2010;330:1297.

The Effects of Growth Hormone on Body Composition and Physical Performance in Recreational Athletes: A Randomized Trial

Meinhardt U, Nelson AE, Hansen JL, et al (Centre for Pediatric Endocrinology, Zurich, Switzerland; Garvan Inst of Med Res, Sydney, Australia; et al)
Ann Intern Med 152:568-577, 2010

Background.—Growth hormone is widely abused by athletes, frequently with androgenic steroids. Its effects on performance are unclear.

Objective.—To determine the effect of growth hormone alone or with testosterone on body composition and measures of performance.

Design.—Randomized, placebo-controlled, blinded study of 8 weeks of treatment followed by a 6-week washout period. Randomization was computer-generated with concealed allocation. (Australian–New Zealand Clinical Trials Registry registration number: ACTRN012605000508673).

Setting.—Clinical research facility in Sydney, Australia.

Participants.—96 recreationally trained athletes (63 men and 33 women) with a mean age of 27.9 years (SD, 5.7).

Intervention.—Men were randomly assigned to receive placebo, growth hormone (2 mg/d subcutaneously), testosterone (250 mg/wk intramuscularly), or combined treatments. Women were randomly assigned to receive either placebo or growth hormone (2 mg/d).

Measurements.—Body composition variables (fat mass, lean body mass, extracellular water mass, and body cell mass) and physical performance variables (endurance [maximum oxygen consumption], strength [dead lift], power [jump height], and sprint capacity [Wingate value]).

Results.—Body cell mass was correlated with all measures of performance at baseline. Growth hormone significantly reduced fat mass, increased lean body mass through an increase in extracellular water, and increased body cell mass in men when coadministered with testosterone. Growth hormone significantly increased sprint capacity, by 0.71 kJ (95% CI, 0.1 to 1.3 J; relative increase, 3.9% [CI, 0.0% to 7.7%]) in men and women combined and by 1.7 kJ (CI, 0.5 to 3.0 kJ; relative increase, 8.3% [CI, 3.0% to 13.6%]) when coadministered with testosterone to men; other performance measures did not significantly change. The increase in sprint capacity was not maintained 6 weeks after discontinuation of the drug.

Limitations.—Growth hormone dosage may have been lower than that used covertly by competitive athletes. The athletic significance of the observed improvements in sprint capacity is unclear, and the study was too small to draw conclusions about safety.

Conclusion.—Growth hormone supplementation influenced body composition and increased sprint capacity when administered alone and in combination with testosterone.

▶ Despite the fact that the World Anti-Doping Agency prohibits the use of growth hormone by competitive athletes, its illegal use remains widespread. Unfortunately, some athletes believe that growth hormone will enhance performance simply because it increases lean body mass, even in extremely fit individuals, while reducing body fat as well. Athletes frequently use growth hormone along with androgenic-anabolic steroids on the basis of belief from studies of elderly men and men with hypopituitarism that testosterone enhances the effects of growth hormone on body composition. It is fair to say, however, that there are little data to support any pharmacologic improvement in translating body composition changes into improvements in physical performance or whether anabolic steroids actually enhance the effect of growth hormone. For these reasons, Meinhardt et al performed a randomized, placebo-controlled, blinded study of 8 weeks of treatment followed by a 6-week washout period to determine the effect of growth hormone and/or testosterone versus placebo in fit noncompetitive athletes. For obvious reasons, such a study could not be undertaken in currently competitive athletes.

The trial of growth hormone with and without testosterone in athletes had 4 major findings. First, body cell mass at baseline was correlated with all measures of physical performance. Second, growth hormone significantly reduced fat mass, increased lean body mass through an increase in extracellular water, and increased body cell mass when given with testosterone. Third, growth hormone led to statistically significant improvements in sprint capacity that were not maintained after a 6-week washout period in a group of men and women. The improvements were greater when growth hormone was coadministered with testosterone to men. Finally, changes in lean body mass did not correlate with improvement in sprint capacity, except when growth hormone was coadministered with testosterone. These findings are consistent with previous observations that long-term growth hormone treatment in children with the Präder-Willi syndrome increased sprint capacity. Sprint capacity is a measure of power and anaerobic performance, which suggests that growth hormone may have affected muscle power, energy supply, or both. Anabolic effects (power) are unlikely because the improvement in sprint capacity that was observed was not accompanied by a statistically significant increase in lean body mass, the changes in these parameters did not correlate, and the drug had no clear effect on jump height or dynamometry. It should be noted that previous studies have demonstrated no effect of growth hormone on strength or power in athletes or on muscle protein synthesis in weight lifters.

The improvement in sprint capacity with growth hormone administration may alternatively be explained by effects on muscle energy supply. Growth hormone will enhance the use of glucose over fatty acids and will suppress oxidative mitochondrial energy production, suggesting regulation through anaerobic metabolism, enhancing anaerobic performance. The important message here is that the athletic significance of this improvement in sprint capacity is uncertain. If one runs the math, one can speculate that the approximate 4% increase in sprint capacity observed would translate to an improvement of about 0.4 seconds in a 10-second sprint over 100 meters or 1.2 seconds in a 30-second swim over 50 meters. You would have to be the judge of how important these timing differences may be in real life. In any event, 8 weeks of growth hormone treatment does not significantly improve strength, power, or endurance, but it will increase to some small amount sprint capacity, an effect that is greater when coadministered with testosterone. This improvement in sprint capacity is of unclear significance when it comes to illicit growth hormone use, which may be associated with much higher drug dosing.

J. A. Stockman III, MD

Newborn Screening Results in Children with Central Hypothyroidism

Nebesio TD, McKenna MP, Nabhan ZM, et al (Indiana Univ School of Medicine, Indianapolis)
J Pediatr 156:990-993, 2010

Objective.—To investigate newborn screening results in children with congenital hypopituitarism, including central hypothyroidism, and to determine whether there were differences between children who had abnormal results and children with normal newborn screening results.

Study Design.—Medical records of children with central hypothyroidism observed in our pediatric endocrinology clinics from 1990 to 2006 were reviewed.

Results.—Forty-two subjects (22 boys) were identified. Eight children (19%) had a low total thyroxine level (<5.0 mcg/dL) on the newborn screening test. The average total thyroxine level in the remaining 34 subjects was 9.8 ± 3.4 mcg/dL. Thyrotropin levels were within the reference range in all children. No differences were found in the 2 groups for birth history, jaundice (53% overall), hypoglycemia (36% overall), or micropenis (43% of boys). Fifty-seven percent of children had septo-optic dysplasia, and 98% had multiple pituitary hormone deficiencies. Children with an abnormal newborn screening results were initially examined by a pediatric endocrinologist at an average age of 4.6 ± 5.0 months, and children with normal newborn screening results were initially examined at an average age of 16.9 ± 26.7 months ($P = .037$).

Conclusions.—Most children with congenital central hypothyroidism have normal thyroid function at birth. Normal newborn screening results can be falsely reassuring and may contribute to a delay in diagnosis of hypopituitarism despite classic clinical features.

▶ The data from this report are most disturbing in that they suggest that most children with the central forms of congenital hypothyroidism show normal thyroid function at birth and therefore may be missed with standard newborn screening programs. Newborn screening programs in the United States use either primary thyrotropin (TSH) screen with thyroxine (T4) backup, a primary T4 screen with TSH backup, or a combined TSH plus T4 approach. The simultaneous measurement of T4 and TSH is considered to be the ideal screening method because this combination strategy is useful in detecting the causes of central hypothyroidism. As of 2010, 8 states here in the United States were using the combined screening method.

Nebesio et al sought to systematically investigate newborn screening results in children with congenital hypothyroidism, including central hypothyroidism, using data from a 17-year period when combination screening was used. The data from this report are consistent with earlier studies suggesting that congenital central hypothyroidism may not be diagnosed at birth but only detected later after signs and symptoms of pituitary hormone deficiency have occurred. In this report, only 8 of 40 children with central hypothyroidism were detected with the newborn screening. Eighty-one percent of cases had normal results with the combination screening method. This is much higher than has been suggested previously, but the study of Nebesio et al represents the largest cohort of patients with congenital central hypothyroidism. The presence of multiple pituitary hormone deficiencies in this patient population with congenital central hypothyroidism was nearly universal (98%).

A very significant finding from this study was that youngsters with central hypothyroidism who had normal newborn screening results had significantly delayed evaluations by pediatric endocrinologists. This delay occurred despite no differences existing in the prevalence of classic signs and symptoms of hypopituitarism in children with abnormal versus normal newborn screening results, suggesting that normal results on the newborn screening resulted in a false sense of security about pituitary function in these patients. Due in part to the findings from this study, the state of Indiana stopped using combination screening method in September 2007 and now uses TSH as the primary screening test. Long-term studies, as the authors point out, will be needed to determine whether there is an increase in the number of missed cases or delay in diagnosis of central hypothyroidism in upcoming years in Indiana as TSH screening alone is used. An alternative screening method used in Europe includes a 3-tier assessment of T4, TSH, and thyroid-binding globulin. Studies from the Netherlands have found a 3-fold increase in the detection rate of congenital central hypothyroidism with this approach.[1] Some screening programs routinely do a second screen at 2 weeks of life, which could be an alternative as well. The validity of the latter is unproven but would address a theoretical significant maternal contribution of T4 to neonatal thyroxin levels that could result in infants with central hypothyroidism being missed on the initial newborn screening. Needless to say, no one has found the silver bullet to solve the problem of picking up all children with congenital hypothyroidism using newborn screening.

As an aside, in recent years, patients receiving thyroid hormone have been told by pharmacists that the medications should be given on an empty stomach. A recent review of the relationship between food and thyroid hormone administration in infants and children suggests that it is difficult to track down the source of these recommendations.[2] The American Thyroid Association, in their consensus guidelines for the treatment of hypothyroidism, does not recommend that levothyroxine be given on an empty stomach. Rather, the guidelines indicate that absorption of levothyroxine may be influenced by the presence of food and recommend that levothyroxine be taken consistently in both time of day in the presence or absence of food. Dosage then can be adjusted on the basis of routine measurement of TSH to determine the appropriate dosing in this setting. Avoidance of soy and calcium is also recommended. Similarly, the American Academy of Pediatrics and the American Thyroid Association joint statement on the management of congenital hypothyroidism states only that concomitant ingestion of soy, calcium, and iron should be avoided.

One final comment having to do with the relationship between delayed diagnosis and the availability of pediatric endocrinologists when it comes to the treatment of congenital hypothyroidism—a report from Japan clearly documents that a shortage of endocrinologists may be 1 reason for the upward trend in the prevalence of treated patients with congenital hypothyroidism. Although neonatal screening for congenital hypothyroidism in Japan has been performed for over 3 decades and is well supported by medical aid systems, there are some serious pediatric medical problems in Japan, including a shortage of specialists in endocrinology. The shortage and overworking of pediatricians in Japan are reaching critical levels. The pediatrician-to-patient ratio in Japan is about half that of the United States. It is suspected that the increasing prevalence of congenital hypothyroidism may actually represent misdiagnosis/overdiagnosis of congenital hypothyroidism based on the poor availability of endocrinologists to confirm a definitive diagnosis. Some of the nonspecialists making the diagnosis may have, for example, accepted the positive screening test in the newborn period as definitive evidence of congenital hypothyroidism instead of viewing the screening result as an indication for repeat assessment and more detailed evaluation.[3]

J. A. Stockman III, MD

References

1. Lanting CI, van Tijn DA, Loeber JG, Vulsma T, de Vijlder JJ, Verkerk PH. Clinical effectiveness and cost effectiveness of the use of thyroxine/thyroxin-binding globulin ratio to detect congenital hypothyroidism of thyroidal and central origin in neonatal screening program. *Pediatrics.* 2005;116:168-173.
2. Zeitler P, Solberg P. Food and levothyroxine administration in infants and children. *J Pediatr.* 2010;157:13-14.
3. Gu Y-H, Kato T, Harada S, Inomata H, Aoki K. Time, trend and geographic distribution of treated patients with congenital hypothyroidism relative to the number of available endocrinologists in Japan. *J Pediatr.* 2010;157:153-157.

Celiac Disease in Children, Adolescents, and Young Adults with Autoimmune Thyroid Disease

Sattar N, Lazare F, Kacer M, et al (Univ Hosp at Stony Brook, NY)
J Pediatr 158:272-275, 2011

Objective.—To determine the prevalence of antibodies associated with celiac disease and biopsy-proven celiac disease in children with autoimmune thyroid disease.

Study Design.—A total of 302 patients with positive anti-thyroid antibodies were prospectively studied. Total immunoglobulin A (IgA) and tissue transglutaminase-IgA (tTG-IgA) levels were obtained. Those with a positive tTG-IgA titer were offered biopsy for definitive diagnosis of celiac disease.

Results.—A total of 4.6% of subjects with autoimmune thyroid disease had positive tTG-IgA titers. The prevalence of biopsy-confirmed celiac disease was 2.3%. Our population was enriched with patients with type 1 diabetes mellitus (4.3%) and Down syndrome (3.4%). Excluding individuals with these co-morbidities, the prevalence of celiac disease in autoimmune thyroid disease is 1.3%, similar to that of the general population.

The positive predictive value of biopsy-proven celiac disease in patients with autoimmune thyroid disease and positive tTG-IgA titer was 54%.

Conclusion.—The increase in prevalence of celiac disease in auto-immune thyroid disease in our study was largely caused by enrichment with co-morbidities. Without comorbidities or symptoms, screening for celiac disease may not be justified in this population. The specificity of tTG-IgA titer for the diagnosis of celiac disease was decreased in patients with autoimmune thyroid disease compared with the general population.

▶ Everyone knows that celiac disease is a common problem in the United States and in many other places around the globe. It is an immune-mediated enteropathy that develops in genetically susceptible individuals in response to the ingestion of wheat gluten and related proteins found in barley and rye. Importantly, celiac disease is known to occur with a higher prevalence in individuals with certain syndromes and autoimmune disorders. For example, there is an increased prevalence of celiac disease in individuals with Down syndrome and Turner syndrome. Similarly, patients with type 1 diabetes mellitus, also an immune-mediated disorder, have a higher prevalence of celiac disease. The report of Sattar et al tells us a fair amount about a potential association between celiac disease and autoimmune thyroid disease. A study undertaken in Italian children and adolescents known to have autoimmune thyroid disease showed biopsy results positive for celiac disease in 7.7% of affected children, well above the background prevalence of celiac disease of about 1%.[1] Another study conducted in Italy found 10.5% of 324 children with celiac disease had clear-cut evidence of autoimmune thyroid disease.[2]

The purpose of the study of Sattar et al was to determine both the prevalence of antibodies associated with celiac disease and a biopsy-proven celiac disease in children with autoimmune thyroid disease in the United States. Just under 5% of subjects with autoimmune thyroid disease had evidence of positive tissue transglutaminase-IgA (tTG-IgA) levels. The prevalence of biopsy-confirmed celiac disease was 2.3%. It should be noted that the population of patients studied with autoimmune thyroid disease included individuals also with type 1 diabetes mellitus and Down syndrome. With the exclusion of individuals with the latter 2 conditions, the prevalence of celiac disease and autoimmune thyroid disease was just 1.3%, similar to that of the general population. It should also be noted that this study showed that a patient with a positive tTG-IgA titer had a 54% probability of having biopsy-proven celiac disease if they had evidence of autoimmune thyroid disease.

These results show a prevalence of positive tTG-IgA titers in patients with autoimmune thyroid disease that is higher than that seen in the healthy US population. The report also showed an increased prevalence (2.3%) of biopsy-confirmed celiac disease in the patients studied with autoimmune thyroid disease. This is higher than the 0.3% to 1.25% prevalence of celiac disease in the general US pediatric population but not as high as reported in children with autoimmune thyroid disease in Europe. However, most of the increased prevalence was the result of a mixture of patients who had comorbid diseases such as Down syndrome and type 1 diabetes mellitus. In the absence of these comorbidities or gastrointestinal symptoms, the prevalence of celiac disease in autoimmune thyroid disease does not seem to be high enough to justify aggressive screening for celiac disease.

In closing, we reflect on an endocrine-related issue: hermaphrodism and the origin of the word "hermaphrodite." Hermaphroditus in Greek mythology was the son of Hermes and Aphrodite. The water-nymph Salmacis, seeing him in a pool, fell in love with him and prayed that they might never be separated. The gods interpreted her request literally and joined the pair into one body. In both his name and being, therefore, Hermaphroditus combines male and female. The word "hermaphrodite" seems to have entered the late middle English, via Latin from the Greek, in John Trevis's 1398 translation of Bartholomaeus Anglicus' *De proprietatius rerum* (On the Property of Things). Here it described an animal comprising both sexes, male and female. The term subsequently referred to those species of plants or animals in which the coexistence of male and female organs was not an aberration, but a natural state, for example, in flowering plants and some varieties of molluscs and worms. When applied to animals, however, and especially human beings, the word implied "monstrous malformation."

Times have obviously changed in terms of the thinking about medical disorders that can cause hermaphrodism. To read more about this, see the commentary by Seymour.[3]

J. A. Stockman III, MD

References

1. Larizza D, Calcaterra V, De Giacomo C, et al. Celiac disease in children with autoimmune thyroid disease. *J Pediatr.* 2001;139:738-740.
2. Meloni A, Mandas C, Jores RD, Congia M. Prevalence of autoimmune thyroiditis in children with celiac disease and effect gluten withdrawal. *J Pediatr.* 2009;155: 51-55.
3. Seymour J. Hermaphrodite. *Lancet.* 2011;377:547.

7 Gastroenterology

Exposure to *Helicobacter pylori*–positive Siblings and Persistence of *Helicobacter pylori* Infection in Early Childhood

Cervantes DT, Fischbach LA, Goodman KJ, et al (Univ of North Texas Health Science Ctr at Fort Worth; Univ of Alberta, Edmonton, Canada; et al)
J Pediatr Gastroenterol Nutr 50:481-485, 2010

Objectives.—Cross-sectional studies suggest that *Helicobacter pylori* may be transmitted between siblings. The present study aimed to estimate the effect of an *H pylori*–infected sibling on the establishment of a persistent *H pylori* infection.

Materials and Methods.—The authors used data collected from a Texas–Mexico border population from 1998 to 2005 (the "Pasitos Cohort Study"). Starting at age 6 months, *H pylori* and factors thought to be associated with *H pylori* were ascertained every 6 months for participants and their younger siblings. Hazard ratios were estimated from proportional hazards regression models with household-dependent modeling.

Results.—Persistent *H pylori* infection in older siblings always preceded persistent infection in younger siblings. After controlling for mother's *H pylori* status, breast-feeding, antibiotic use, and socioeconomic factors, a strong effect was estimated for persistent *H pylori* infection in an older sibling on persistent infection in a younger sibling (hazard ratio 7.6, 95% confidence interval 1.6–37], especially when the difference in the age of the siblings was less than or equal to 3 years (hazard ratio 16, 95% confidence interval 2.5–112).

Conclusions.—These results suggest that when siblings are close in age, the older sibling may be an important source of *H pylori* transmission for younger siblings.

▶ The mode of transmission for *Helicobacter pylori* is not well understood. Person-to-person transmission is the most likely mode of transfer, and evidence exists that oral-oral, fecal-oral, and gastric-oral may be significant modes of transmission. *H pylori* is one of the most common chronic bacterial infections worldwide, and it is estimated that more than half of the world's population is currently infected with *H pylori*. Such infection can lead to serious disease outcomes such as gastric cancer, peptic ulcer, and other gastrointestinal diseases. In those who become infected, long-term colonization of the stomach generally occurs often for up to decades if not a lifetime, assuming that antibiotic therapy is not given.

The report of Cervantes et al examines to what extent an *H pylori*-infected sibling causes transmission of *H pylori* to be established in a brother or a sister. The findings are consistent with person-to-person transmission occurring from older to younger siblings living in the same household. If an older sibling has *H pylori*, the likelihood of a younger sibling having it is almost 8-fold greater because of transmission from the older child. This is particularly true when the siblings are close in age. The data from this report appear to be accurate. If so, the only way to prevent such transmission is to be an only child.

While on the topic of things that cause dyspepsia, Guariso et al[1] examined the appropriateness of upper gastrointestinal endoscopy in children presenting with dyspeptic symptoms. The term dyspepsia has yet to be given a standard definition, although it is commonly used by clinicians to mean symptoms including epigastric pain, epigastric fullness and regurgitation, upper abdominal discomfort, early satiety, bloating, nausea, and vomiting. The investigation undertaken found that upper gastrointestinal endoscopy was appropriate but not for all children with dyspeptic symptoms. Indications for the procedure included selected features such as family history of peptic ulcer and/or *H pylori* infection, age older than 10 years, symptoms lasting more than 6 months, and symptoms severe enough to affect activities of daily living. Although upper endoscopy is relatively straightforward in this day and age, it still demands particular skill, especially in pediatric patients, and it is not totally without risk.

We close with a historical observation having to do with the gastrointestinal problems that apparently Charles Darwin suffered from. Two hundred years after the birth of Darwin, scientists are putting modern medicine to the test to unravel the mystery of the painful illness that plagued him for much of his life. Darwin was the subject of the 2011 Annual Historical Clinicopathological Conference (CPC) sponsored by the University of Maryland School of Medicine and the Veteran's Hospital (VA Maryland Healthcare System).[2] The conference is devoted to the modern medical diagnosis of disorders that have affected prominent historical figures. Born in 1809, Darwin suffered from chronic vomiting, abdominal pain, and gastrointestinal distress. It did not stop him, however, from fathering 10 children. He did live to be 73 years old, dying of heart failure. Darwin led a relatively healthy life until his late 20s. Around that time, after returning from a trip to South America, the Pacific, the Far East, and Africa, his symptoms began. These included attacks of abdominal pain, nausea, vomiting, and retching. When his symptoms were at their worst, he vomited after nearly every meal. At the CPC, it was concluded that these particular symptoms match very closely the description of an entity we now call cyclic vomiting syndrome. A gastroenterologist attending the CPC also believed that Darwin suffered from Chagas disease, most likely contracted during his five years traveling the globe on the HMS Beagle. Chagas disease can eventually cause heart failure, a disorder that he suffered from later in life and speculated to have eventually caused his death. Some also believe that part of the explanation for his abdominal pain and gastrointestinal distress was infection from *Helicobacter pylori*, the subject of the reports abstracted. To learn more about the historical medical conference at the University of Maryland, see the Web site listed in the references.[2]

J. A. Stockman III, MD

References

1. Guariso G, Meneghel A, Dalla Pozza LV, et al. Indications for upper gastrointestinal endoscopy in children with dyspepsia. *J Pediatr Gastroenterol Nutr.* 2010; 50:493-499.
2. Historical medical conference finds Darwin suffered from various gastrointestinal illnesses. University of Maryland School of Medicine: News and Events. http://somvweb.som.umaryland.edu/absolutenm/templates/?a=1527&z=41. Published May 6, 2011. Accessed August 12, 2011.

Exchange Transfusion as a Possible Therapy for Neonatal Hemochromatosis
Escolano-Margarit MV, Miras-Baldó MJ, Parrilla-Roure M, et al (San Cecilio Hosp, Granada, Spain)
J Pediatr Gastroenterol Nutr 50:566-568, 2010

Neonatal hemochromatosis (NH) is a rare congenital disorder that affects the fetus in late gestation, and it is clinically defined as severe neonatal liver disease associated with both hepatic and extrahepatic iron deposition in a distribution similar to that seen in hereditary hemochromatosis.

Prognosis of the disease is variable; a few cases are reported to have had spontaneous remission, but affected infants rarely survive without treatment, which often includes liver transplantation. Pathogenesis remains unknown; 1 interesting theory is the alloimmune etiology of the disease.

We report a case of confirmed NH that underwent exchange transfusion at an early stage of the disease and subsequently presented a complete cure. ET has never been evaluated as a specific treatment for NH. If the alloimmune etiology of the disease is accepted, then ET may have lessened the severity of liver injury in the case reported here, thus improving the outcome.

▶ All of us learned a bit about hemochromatosis in medical school. Chances are that we have not seen it much in pediatric practice. Neonatal hemochromatosis is an entirely different entity than that seen in older children and adults. It is a rare medical condition presenting as severe liver disease in the newborn period. It should be thought of anytime a newborn develops evidence of severe hepatic inflammation or if there is evidence of unexplained hyperbilirubinemia. The main feature of this syndrome, that is, hepatitic and extrahepatic iron accumulation, is probably the result of a hepatic inflammatory process of incompletely understood etiology. Its severity is variable, ranging from fulminant liver failure to cases with spontaneous recovery. The prognosis of the condition is generally quite poor. Neonatal hemochromatosis is a frequent indication for liver transplantation in the newborn period. A positive family history, high serum ferritin levels, and siderosis demonstrated by histologic examination or magnetic resonance imaging are the clinical criteria usually considered in making a diagnosis of neonatal hemochromatosis. The current medical treatment for the disorder is based on the use of antioxidants and iron chelation, but both of these are largely ineffective and may be associated with significant adverse effects. The use of antioxidants is based on the theory that iron overload-related oxidant burden plays a significant role in determining the liver impairment. However, recent data suggest that the iron overload is really only an epiphenomenon of the liver disease itself. In fact, mounting evidence indicates that some cases have an alloimmune origin. Neonatal hemochromatosis could be caused by the transplacental passage of antifetal liver antigen immunoglobulin G to the fetus from neonatal hemochromatosis-sensitized mothers, leading to fetal liver damage and iron mishandling.

Obviously, this form of hemochromatosis based on a theory akin to Rh sensitization is very different from the type of hemochromatosis seen in older children and adults in which the iron overload is actually the cause of liver damage. The immunologic theory would also explain the 80% of recurrence in subsequent pregnancies after an index case has been described. The prevention trial by Whitington and Hibbard[1] with high-dose immunoglobulin during gestation, based on the alloimmune model, was a breakthrough because it reduced the severity of the disease in affected newborns dramatically. In a recent report, 52 of 55 newborns born to treated pregnancies survived with medical treatment. The 3 failures were from causes other than neonatal hemochromatosis. Ninety-two percent of untreated pregnancies resulted in intrauterine fetal demise, neonatal death, or liver failure requiring transplantation. The rub, of course, is affected first pregnancies where there is no clue that a mother has been or is being sensitized by neonatal hepatic antigens against which she produces antibodies.

The report by Escolano-Margarit et al represents one of the first experiences on the successful use of exchange transfusion in the newborn period for management of neonatal hemochromatosis. This procedure, associated or not with immunoglobulin administration, appears to be a promising approach to the rare and scarcely understood condition. Given the concerns related to liver transplantation in the neonatal period and the lack of both efficacy and safety of previously accepted treatments including iron chelators and antioxidants, a convincing and codified medical treatment would represent a turning point in the management of this serious problem of the newborn. Stay tuned for further studies confirming this emerging and encouraging approach to management.

This commentary closes with an observation on a report from a team of scientists from Massachusetts General Hospital that has developed a cell-free matrix that can be used to grow liver grafts that may be useful for transplantation.[2] The technique involves flushing liver cells out of a liver's natural matrix of connective tissue and blood vessels. After the cells are removed, the lobular structure of the liver and its extracellular matrix remain, containing biochemical signals that direct newly introduced liver cells to migrate and resume function. Engineered liver grafts created in this way support liver-specific functions including albumin secretion, urea synthesis, and other functions. These grafts, when transplanted into rats, have supported liver cell function and do so with minimal damage. This study provides a proof of principle for the generation of a transplantable liver graft as a potential treatment for liver disease. Science is amazing!

J. A. Stockman III, MD

References

1. Whitington PF, Hibbard JU. High-dose immunoglobulin during pregnancy for recurrent neonatal hemachromatosis. *Lancet.* 2004;364:1690-1698.
2. Uygun BE, Soto-Gutierrez A, Yaji H, et al. Organ reengineering through development of a transplantable recellularized liver graft using decellularized liver matrix. *Nat Med.* 2010;16:814-820.

Evidence for a Novel Blood RNA Diagnostic for Pediatric Appendicitis: The Riboleukogram

Muenzer JT, Jaffe DM, Schwulst SJ, et al (Washington Univ School of Medicine, St Louis, MO)
Pediatr Emerg Care 26:333-338, 2010

Objective.—To test the hypothesis that gene expression analysis of circulating white blood cells and/or plasma cytokines could be used to improve diagnostic accuracy in children being evaluated for appendicitis.

Methods.—We recruited 28 children being evaluated for abdominal pain from a tertiary pediatric emergency department. Twenty patients were used as a training cohort and 8 patients as a validation cohort. After consent was obtained, blood was processed for plasma cytokine analysis and RNA gene expression. Alvarado and pediatric appendicitis scores were obtained. Principal components analysis was used to explore global differences in gene expression. The random forest method was used to classify patients into those with and without appendicitis in the prospective cohort. Comparisons were made evaluating clinical scoring systems, cytokine analysis, and gene expression analysis to accurately predict appendicitis.

Results.—The random forest method accurately predicted appendicitis in 4 of 5 patients in the prospective cohort. Cytokine analysis was not as accurate as gene expression analysis; however, it did accurately rule out all 3 patients in the prospective cohort. Pediatric appendicitis scores and Alvarado scores were not useful for predicting appendicitis.

Conclusions.—Our findings provide proof of technical feasibility and support the diagnostic potential of plasma cytokines to rule out and riboleukograms to rule in the diagnosis of appendicitis.

▶ Before reading this interesting report out of St Louis, I was not aware of the term *riboleukogram*. The background of this report is fairly straightforward. The differential diagnosis of abdominal pain in children, specifically as it relates to the potential diagnosis of appendicitis, can be complex. Various systems have been developed to help create a greater sensitivity and specificity in the diagnosis of appendicitis using score-based recommendations for further diagnostic testing such as CT scanning or ultrasound, but independent validation of these scoring systems suggests a predictive accuracy as low as 42%. Recently, high-throughput multiplexed RNA assays have provided evidence for additional blood diagnostic modalities for a variety of acute infectious diseases. For example, micro-assay gene expression analysis has helped in the differentiation of sepsis in animal models of various forms of infection. The authors of this report have used circulating leukocyte gene expression profiles in the diagnosis of sepsis in the creation of what are known as riboleukograms. Many feel that this form of blood testing, which measures inflammatory responses at the cytokine level, may hold significant promise in the field of advanced clinical diagnostics for inflammatory and infectious diseases.

What Muenzer et al have done is to examine 28 children being evaluated for abdominal pain and have added to the clinical assessment of these patients plasma cytokine analysis and gene expression analysis (blood tests) to diagnose pediatric appendicitis in the emergency department. The aggregate data constitute a riboleukogram when added to information gathered from analysis of plasma cytokine levels. Although the number of patients looked at was quite small, in 5 patients who were ultimately diagnosed with appendicitis, 4 were correctly assigned this diagnosis preoperatively.

The concept of using a riboleukogram as an aid in the diagnosis of infectious and other inflammatory states is moving along quite quickly. It also shows some promise in other areas such as monitoring the host response to infection in the critically ill. The findings from this report provide what is known as a proof of principle, motivating more definitive prospective studies that will need to include larger sample sizes and more detailed comparisons with existing clinical classification systems. The proof of principle, however, shows that it is technically feasible in real time to create a riboleukogram as a potential tool for diagnosis of conditions such as acute appendicitis.

While on the topic of appendicitis, if you look at Wikipedia, you will find 9 signs that can be used to assist in the diagnosis of this gastrointestinal problem.[1] These include:

- Psoas sign: right lower quadrant pain that is produced or worsens with passive extension of the patient's right hip.
- Obturator sign: if an inflamed appendix is in contact with the obturator internus muscle, spasm of the muscle can be demonstrated by flexing and internal rotation of the hip. This maneuver will cause pain in the vagina as well.
- Dunphy's sign: increased pain in the right testicle when coughing.
- Kocher's sign: the appearance of pain in the epigastric region or about the stomach at the beginning of the disease with a subsequent shift to the right iliac region.
- Sitkovskiy's sign: increased pain in the right iliac region as a patient lies on his/her left side.
- Bartomier-Michelson's sign: increased pain on palpation at the right iliac region as the patient lays on his/her left side compared to when the patient is in the supine position.

- Aure-Rozanova's: increased pain on palpation with finger in right petit triangle (typical in retrocecal position of the appendix).
- Blumberg sign: also referred to as rebound tenderness. Deep palpation of the viscera over the suspected inflamed appendix followed by sudden release of the pressure causes severe pain on the site, indicating a positive Blumberg sign and peritonitis.

The above is probably more than you ever wanted to know about the signs and symptoms of appendicitis. It is what the public now knows as the result of Wikipedia. Do not exhibit ignorance if you get a call from a parent of a child with abdominal pain when the parent complains of their youngster having a positive Blumberg sign. The stockmarket is not tanking.

J. A. Stockman III, MD

Reference

1. Wikipedia. Appendicitis. http://en.wikipedia.org/wiki/Appendicitis. Accessed August 12, 2011.

Predictive indicators for bowel injury in pediatric patients who present with a positive seat belt sign after motor vehicle collision
Paris C, Brindamour M, Ouimet A, et al (Centre Hospitalier Universitaire Sainte-Justine, Montréal, Quebec, Canada)
J Pediatr Surg 45:921-924, 2010

Purpose.—Abdominal wall bruising (AWB) is a frequent finding in children wearing seat belts involved in motor vehicle collision (MVC) and is highly suspicious but not indicative of intestinal injury. The aim of this study was to find objective clinical and radiologic predictors for the need of an abdominal exploration in these children.

Materials and Methods.—A retrospective chart review of children admitted from 1998 and 2008 with AWB after MVC was conducted. Demographics, vital signs, physical examinations, radiologic investigations, associated injuries, management, and outcome were extracted. Univariate and multivariate statistical analyses were done.

Results.—Fifty-three children with a median age of 9 years (range, 3-16 years) were included. Forty-four patients (83%) had abdominal pain on arrival, and 25 (47%) had free intraabdominal fluid on ultrasound/scan. Intraabdominal injuries were noted in 29 patients (55%), and the most common were mesenteric or bowel injuries (25%), splenic injuries (13%), and hepatic injuries (8%). Ten patients (19%) needed therapeutic laparotomy, and all were victims from collision involving 2 moving vehicles, had abdominal pain, free intraabdominal fluid, and tachycardia. Five patients (50%) operated on had lumbar fracture compared to only 4 patients (9%) in the nonoperative group. Pulse rate higher than 120 ($P = .048$), lumbar fracture ($P = .008$), and free intraabdominal fluid

$(P \leq .001)$ were significant predictors for intestinal perforation. Overall survival was 98% with 1 death because of head trauma.

Conclusion.—Intraabdominal injuries in children with AWB after MVC are frequent. Associated lumbar fracture, the presence of free intraabdominal fluid, and pulse rate higher than 120 are significant predictors of intestinal injuries. An abdominal exploration should be considered in these patients.

▶ With the introduction of lap-type seat belts into automobiles in the United States in the 1960s, we saw a dramatic decrease in the incidence of deaths related to motor vehicle accidents. Also, there were changes in mortality causes in such accidents with a decreasing number of severe head traumas as a cause of death shifting to other causes including the seat belt syndrome, the latter consisting of lumbar spine fractures and abdominal wall/intra-abdominal injuries.

The report abstracted from Canada reminds us how difficult it is to make an early diagnosis of intra-abdominal injury to the mesentery, spleen, or bowel and what to look for as a tip-off to such problems. The investigators in Montreal examined the charts of all patients with abdominal wall bruising following auto accidents between the period June 1998 and October 2008. Some 53 children were admitted during this study period with abdominal wall bruising secondary to a motor vehicle accident. Approximately half of these children were boys and half were girls. The significant majority were rear seat passengers. Forty percent of the patients had used 2-point (abdominal) seat belts with the remainder using 3-point belts. Intra-abdominal injuries were seen in 55% of the patients with abdominal wall bruising. Intra-abdominal organs most frequently injured were the mesentery or bowel in 25%, the spleen in 13%, and the liver in 8%. Associated other injuries included musculoskeletal injuries (60%), of which lumbar spine fractures were fairly prominent (17%). Thirty percent of the patients also had head trauma. One in 5 patients developed a hollow viscus perforation requiring therapeutic laparotomy with bowel resection and primary anastomosis. Statistical analysis showed that a pulse rate higher than 120 per minute, the presence of free intra-abdominal fluid, and an associated lumbar fracture were significant predictors for intestinal perforation.

Seat belts were never specifically designed for children. Lap belts tend not to be apposed correctly on children, leading to a tendency to migrate from the immature iliac crest toward the abdomen. Injuries reported as being part of the seat belt syndrome are abdominal wall contusions, intra-abdominal injuries to both solid and hollow organs, and fractures, particularly of the lumbar spine most often from L2 to L4. The mechanism of this constellation of findings is rapid deceleration resulting in compression of the lower abdomen and sudden hyperflexion of the upper torso around the seat belt, leading to crushing of the abdominal contents against the spine. It is estimated that the incidence of seat belt syndrome is roughly 1 per 1000 children injured in a motor vehicle collision. Hollow viscus injuries in the setting of blunt trauma are among the most difficult types of injuries to identify because of the limits of radiologic testing. All caring for a child with a potential intra-abdominal injury should have a high degree of suspicion about this being on the differential diagnosis.

The authors of this report strongly suggest, based on the information they have gathered, that intra-abdominal injuries be suspected in the presence of any abdominal wall bruising following a motor vehicle accident. Moreover, the presence of associated lumbar spine fracture, a pulse rate greater than 120 per minute, and intra-abdominal free fluid on ultrasound or CT scan should raise the suspicion to an even higher degree. These findings are highly predictive of intestinal injuries in children with abdominal wall bruising. Abdominal exploration should be considered in these patients.

J. A. Stockman III, MD

Rifaximin Therapy for Patients with Irritable Bowel Syndrome without Constipation

Pimentel M, for the TARGET Study Group (Cedars—Sinai Med Ctr, Los Angeles, CA; et al)
N Engl J Med 364:22-32, 2011

Background.—Evidence suggests that gut flora may play an important role in the pathophysiology of the irritable bowel syndrome (IBS). We evaluated rifaximin, a minimally absorbed antibiotic, as treatment for IBS.

Methods.—In two identically designed, phase 3, double-blind, placebo-controlled trials (TARGET 1 and TARGET 2), patients who had IBS without constipation were randomly assigned to either rifaximin at a dose of 550 mg or placebo, three times daily for 2 weeks, and were followed for an additional 10 weeks. The primary end point, the proportion of patients who had adequate relief of global IBS symptoms, and the key secondary end point, the proportion of patients who had adequate relief of IBS-related bloating, were assessed weekly. Adequate relief was defined as self-reported relief of symptoms for at least 2 of the first 4 weeks after treatment. Other secondary end points included the percentage of patients who had a response to treatment as assessed by daily self-ratings of global IBS symptoms and individual symptoms of bloating, abdominal pain, and stool consistency during the 4 weeks after treatment and during the entire 3 months of the study.

Results.—Significantly more patients in the rifaximin group than in the placebo group had adequate relief of global IBS symptoms during the first 4 weeks after treatment (40.8% vs. 31.2%, P=0.01, in TARGET 1; 40.6% vs. 32.2%, P=0.03, in TARGET 2; 40.7% vs. 31.7%, P<0.001, in the two studies combined). Similarly, more patients in the rifaximin group than in the placebo group had adequate relief of bloating (39.5% vs. 28.7%, P=0.005, in TARGET 1; 41.0% vs. 31.9%, P=0.02, in TARGET 2; 40.2% vs. 30.3%, P<0.001, in the two studies combined). In addition, significantly more patients in the rifaximin group had a response to treatment as assessed by daily ratings of IBS symptoms, bloating, abdominal pain, and stool consistency. The incidence of adverse events was similar in the two groups.

Conclusions.—Among patients who had IBS without constipation, treatment with rifaximin for 2 weeks provided significant relief of IBS symptoms, bloating, abdominal pain, and loose or watery stools. (Funded by Salix Pharmaceuticals; ClinicalTrials.gov numbers, NCT00731679 and NCT00724126.)

▶ There is a lot written these days about purported techniques/therapies to treat irritable bowel syndrome (IBS). This disorder affects both adults and children and represents a functional gastrointestinal problem associated with recurring abdominal pain, bloating, and altered bowel function, all in the absence of structural, inflammatory, or biochemical abnormalities. Treatment for IBS historically has been a failure. Treatments have included dietary and lifestyle modifications, fiber supplementation, psychological therapy, and various pharmacologic therapies. Unfortunately, because no reliable biologic or structural markers have been identified, the effects of such therapies are typically assessed by asking a patient whether they are better or worse off as a result of the therapy. A simple yes or no response is generally all you get.

Recently, however, much attention has been paid to the antibiotic management of IBS. Many patients with IBS have alterations in their intestinal flora. Some have wondered whether targeting intestinal microbiota for the treatment of this condition might be helpful. In the report abstracted, the antibiotic rifaximin was used to determine its benefits in subjects with IBS. Rifaximin is a poorly absorbed antibiotic that targets a wide range of gut flora. All participants received 3 pills per day for 2 weeks without knowing whether they were getting the active drug. Over the next 4 weeks, 41% of those getting rifaximin had clear improvement in their symptoms in at least 2 of those 4 weeks, compared with 32% of those getting a placebo, a statistically significant difference. Although the benefits did not extend to all patients, or even a majority, the report does appear to be good news for people with IBS. The benefits of rifaximin lingered for about 10 weeks after the 2-week treatment. Although the percentage of people reporting improved IBS symptoms dropped off gradually, the average scores of people taking the drug remained better than those who were given placebo.

Rifaximin is poorly absorbed through the intestines, a drawback for the treatment of systemic diseases, but perhaps it's a blessing for the management of bowel specific problems. It has been suggested that rifaximin may be valuable for the management of traveler's diarrhea.

As of this writing, the US Food and Drug Administration is considering licensing rifaximin for the treatment of IBS. The drug is sold as Xifaxan by its manufacturer, Salix Pharmaceuticals, which funded the research appearing in *The New England Journal of Medicine.*

J. A. Stockman III, MD

VSL#3 Improves Symptoms in Children With Irritable Bowel Syndrome: A Multicenter, Randomized, Placebo-Controlled, Double-Blind, Crossover Study

Guandalini S, Magazzù G, Chiaro A, et al (Univ of Chicago Section of Pediatric Gastroenterology, IL; Univ of Messina, Italy; et al)
J Pediatr Gastroenterol Nutr 51:24-30, 2010

Background and Objectives.—Irritable bowel syndrome (IBS) is a common problem in pediatrics, for which no safe and effective treatment is available. Probiotics have shown some promising results in adult studies, but no positive study has been published on pediatric age. We aimed at investigating the efficacy of VSL#3 in a population of children and teenagers affected by IBS, in a randomized, double-blind, placebo-controlled, crossover study conducted in 7 pediatric gastroenterology divisions.

Patients and Methods.—Children 4 to 18 years of age, meeting eligibility criteria, were enrolled. The patients were assessed by a questionnaire for a 2-week baseline period. They were then randomized to receive either VSL#3 or a placebo for 6 weeks, with controls every 2 weeks. At the end, after a "wash-out" period of 2 weeks, each patient was switched to the other group and followed for a further 6 weeks.

Results.—A total of 59 children completed the study. Although placebo was effective in some of the parameters and in as many as half of the patients, VSL#3 was significantly superior to it ($P < 0.05$) in the primary endpoint, the subjective assessment of relief of symptoms; as well as in 3 of 4 secondary endpoints: abdominal pain/discomfort ($P < 0.05$), abdominal bloating/gassiness ($P < 0.05$), and family assessment of life disruption ($P < 0.01$). No significant difference was found ($P = 0.06$) in the stool pattern. No untoward adverse effect was recorded in any of the patients.

Conclusions.—VSL#3 is safe and more effective than placebo in ameliorating symptoms and improving the quality of life in children affected by IBS.

▶ All too many children (and a fair number of adults) suffer from the irritable bowel syndrome (IBS). In recent years, the definition of IBS has become much sharper with most pediatric gastroenterologists diagnosing it according to the Rome II criteria.[1] The predominant symptomatologies in patients with IBS include abdominal pain, abdominal bloating/gassiness, and stool changes (either constipation or diarrhea). In general, most feel that there is no safe and effective pharmacological or dietetic treatment available to manage IBS. However, one of the most promising developments in our understanding of IBS, and thus of its possible treatment, is the recognition that many episodes of IBS can be traced back to intestinal infections and that disturbances of intestinal microbiota resulting in low numbers of lactobacilli and bifidobacteria can be detected in a substantial percentage of patients with IBS.

Based on the suspicion that alterations in intestinal flora may underlie some cases of IBS, Guandalini et al studied the effects of a mixture of probiotics known as VSL#3. VSL#3 is produced by VSL Pharmaceuticals, Inc (Gaithersburg,

MD). Patients receiving VSL#3 had it administered in a sachet once a day for children 4 to 11 years of age and twice a day for those 12 to 18 years of age or older. A placebo that was identical in look and taste was given to a control group of children. A global assessment of relief was obtained based on the patient's symptomatology. While not a cure-all, VSL#3 statistically had definitive benefits in comparison to placebo in this patient population.

Unfortunately, the mechanisms underlying the possible beneficial effects of probiotic use in children with IBS are not known. Given the fact that probiotic treatments are largely benign and the fact that this report documents a statistically significant effectivity in improving the overall perception of symptoms related to the severity and frequency of abdominal pain, abdominal bloating, and caregivers assessment of overall well being, it seems reasonable to at least consider a trial of probiotics in those with IBS. The authors of this report conclude that probiotics are a welcomed addition to the remarkably poor armamentarium of therapeutic strategies available for children and teens with IBS. We look forward to further studies using this interesting approach.

J. A. Stockman III, MD

Reference

1. Rasquine-Weber A, Hyman P, Cucchiara S, et al. Childhood functional gastrointestinal disorders. *Gut.* 1999;45:II60-II68.

Celiac Disease without Villous Atrophy in Children: A Prospective Study

Kurppa K, Ashorn M, Iltanen S, et al (Univ of Tampere and Tampere Univ Hosp, Finland; et al)

J Pediatr 157:373-380, 2010

Objective.—To establish whether children who are endomysial antibody (EmA) positive and have normal small-bowel mucosal villous morphology are truly gluten-sensitive and may benefit from early treatment with a gluten-free diet.

Study Design.—Children who were EmA positive with normal small-bowel mucosal villi were compared with children who were seropositive with villous atrophy by using several markers of untreated celiac disease. Thereafter, children with normal villous structure either continued on a normal diet or were placed on a gluten-free diet and re-investigated after 1 year. Seventeen children who were seronegative served as control subjects for baseline investigations.

Results.—Normal villous morphology was noted in 17 children who were EmA positive, and villous atrophy was noted in 42 children who were EmA positive. These children were comparable in all measured variables regardless of the degree of enteropathy, but differed significantly from the seronegative control subjects. During the dietary intervention, in children who were EmA positive with normal villi, the disease was exacerbated in children who continued gluten consumption, whereas in all children who started the gluten-free diet, both the gastrointestinal symptoms and abnormal antibodies disappeared.

Conclusions.—The study provided evidence that children who are EmA positive have a celiac-type disorder and benefit from early treatment despite normal mucosal structure, indicating that the diagnostic criteria for celiac disease should be re-evaluated.

▶ More and more is being written about celiac disease, a fairly common disorder with an estimated prevalence of about 1% in our population. The hallmark of the disease has been villous atrophy as determined by small bowel biopsy. With few exceptions, individuals with celiac disease produce antibodies to tissue transglutaminase (TG2) and/or endomysium (EMA). Once diagnosed, it is recommended that affected individuals be on a lifelong strict gluten-free diet. Needless to say, an accurate diagnosis at the start of all this is critical. Currently, the guidelines for diagnosis recommend an intestinal biopsy. The presence of villus blunting is strong evidence of the condition, and the diagnosis is confirmed if complete symptom resolution occurs after the implementation of a gluten-free diet.

In recent years, the question has arisen whether a villous biopsy needs to be performed given the advent of serologic tests, which has expanded our understanding of the protean manifestations of the disease. The report of Kurppa et al describes a group of symptomatic EMA-positive children with either completely normal small bowel histology or very minimally abnormal bowel histology. These children were compared with a symptomatic EMA-positive group diagnosed with celiac disease on the basis of histologic abnormalities as well as with a control group who had symptoms but were EMA negative and had normal intestinal histology (nonceliac controls). This celiac group was started on a gluten-free diet and followed up with repeat celiac serology testing after a year. The gluten-free diet option was also offered to those in the study group. Of the children in the study group who were available for long-term follow-up, the majority chose to remain on a regular diet and the remainder chose a gluten-free diet. All children in this group were followed up with annual repeat celiac serology. Intestinal biopsy analyses were repeated in those who chose to stay on a regular diet. Children in the nonceliac control group were followed up with repeated celiac serologic testing after 1 year. At presentation, there were no differences among the groups in terms of mean age, sex, symptoms, and family history of celiac disease. Most of the children in the celiac group demonstrated improved symptoms and all had decreased or normalized EMA and TG2 titers. The 5 children in the study group who chose the gluten-free diet demonstrated resolution of clinical symptoms and normalization of EMA and TG2 values. All 8 children in the study group who remained on a regular diet had persistent symptoms with positive serologic tests. Seven developed small bowel mucosal atrophy within 1 to 2 years on repeat biopsy. Initiation of a gluten-free diet in these cases resulted in subsequent symptom alleviation and normalization of serologic tests confirming the diagnosis of celiac disease. None of the nonceliac controls had a positive serologic test on repeated testing.

The conclusions of the Kurppa et al report are that the criteria for histologic diagnosis of celiac disease seem to be inadequate. This raises the question of whether biopsy still has a major role in the diagnostic process. On the other hand, some have said that a biopsy is even more important in the circumstances of patients who have gluten sensitivity symptoms relieved by removing gluten from the diet, a phenomenon known as gluten sensitivity. A new concept is arising around this phenomenon of gluten sensitivity not caused by celiac disease. It is considered in individuals with typical symptoms who have positive serologic tests for celiac disease and normal intestinal histology but with symptom improvement after initiation of a gluten-free diet. Some patients with gluten sensitivity are in an early stage of celiac disease and eventually will develop the typical intestinal findings if they continue on a gluten-containing diet. Still, there may be a subset of patients, many with neurologic symptoms including ataxia who do not have classic celiac disease but are responsive to a gluten-free diet.

In an editorial that accompanied the report of Kurppa et al, Hill suggests that distinguishing between celiac disease and other gluten-sensitive conditions that may not be related to celiac disease is important to our understanding of these conditions.[1] If all this seems confusing to you, join the crowd. All that appears to be classic celiac disease may not be, even though the symptoms are relieved with a gluten-free diet.

J. A. Stockman III, MD

Reference

1. Hill ID. Diagnosing celiac disease: how important is the biopsy? *J Pediatr.* 2010; 157:353-354.

Inflammatory Bowel Disease Developing in Paediatric and Adult Age
Guariso G, Gasparetto M, Visonà Dalla Pozza L, et al (Univ of Padua, Italy)
J Pediatr Gastroenterol Nutr 51:698-707, 2010

Background and Objective.—In recent decades, there has been a significant increase in the incidence of inflammatory bowel disease (IBD). It has yet to be established whether the manifestations of IBD are similar in paediatric and adult ages. The objective of this study was to compare the phenotypic expression of the disease between patients with childhood-onset IBD and adulthood-onset cases, all afferent to the same clinical centre.

Patients and Methods.—Descriptive and multivariate analyses were completed on retrospective and prospective data of paediatric-onset and adult-onset consecutive cases who were diagnosed and followed at the same tertiary referral hospital of the University of Padua, Italy, during a period of 14 years (1994–2008). Paediatric-onset patients were further divided into age brackets (0–5, 6–12, and 13–17 year-olds). Analyses were conducted using the SAS package, version 9.1 (SAS Institute Inc, Cary, NC).

Results.—Three hundred twelve patients were analysed. At disease onset, the manifestations which were more frequent among the 133 paediatric patients (50.4% with diagnosis of Crohn disease [CD], 43.6% with ulcerative colitis, and 6% with unclassified IBD) with respect to the adult-onset patients were perianal disease (12.8%) ($P < 0.0001$) and extraintestinal manifestations (14.3%) ($P = 0.043$). Among the 179 adult patients (55.3% with diagnosis of ulcerative colitis, 36.3% with CD, and 8.3% with unclassified IBD) instead, severe abdominal pain ($P = 0.008$), diarrhoea ($P = 0.005$), and anorexia ($P < 0.0001$) were more frequently observed. During the follow-up, the presence of extraintestinal manifestations (50.4%) ($P = 0.005$) and perianal disease (44.8% of the patients with childhood-onset CD) ($P = 0.006$) was observed more often in the paediatric-onset group.

Conclusions.—In our cases, the phenotypic expression of IBD developing in paediatric age differs from that seen in adults.

▶ Most of us recognize, based on personal experience, that there has been a significant increase in the incidence of inflammatory bowel disease (IBD). This experience is somewhat different than our colleagues in internal medicine have observed where there has been a leveling off in the incidence/prevalence of this class of disorders in recent years. It has been somewhat difficult to compare children with adults since most reports come from discrete childhood or adult centers—thus the importance of the information provided by Guariso et al. These investigators pooled information from a single institution: a tertiary referral hospital of the University of Padua, Italy. Fourteen years worth of accumulative data from this pediatric and adult center were reviewed in this report.

What we learn from this Italian study is that IBD can and does develop at any age with about 20% of the population studied in this institution having disease occurring in infancy or childhood. There was an increase in all forms of IBD in young people over the past 20 years. Crohn disease is significantly more prevalent than ulcerative colitis. Significant differences were observed between children and adults in terms of signs, symptoms, and complications. At disease onset, the classical symptoms of IBD (ie, severe abdominal pain, diarrhea) were observed more frequently in adult-onset patients than in pediatric-onset cases and more adult-onset patients needed surgery at disease presentation. Perianal disease, extraintestinal manifestations, and associated diseases were more frequent at the onset of IBD among pediatric age patients. Atypical presentations were also much more common in childhood, making IBD less likely to be suspected at presentation of symptoms. One example of this is that 40% of pediatric age—onset patients have growth deficiency as one of the initial manifestations. Needless to say, those kids presenting in their midteens tended to more closely resemble the situation seen in adult-onset patients (with severe abdominal pain and a greater likelihood of needing surgery at presentation). Children at any age were much more likely to have inflammation above the terminal ileum.

These data from Italy are very similar to information being learned about here in the United States. Abramson et al, for example, have shown that over a recent

11-year period, the annual incidence per 100 000 children increased from 2.2 to 4.3 for Crohn disease and from 1.8 to 4.9 for ulcerative colitis.[1] Curiously, Hispanic and Asian children were more likely to develop ulcerative colitis than Crohn disease by a significant margin.

J. A. Stockman III, MD

Reference

1. Abramson O, Durant M, Mow W, et al. Incidence, prevalence and time trends of inflammatory bowel disease in northern California, 1996–2006. *J Pediatr.* 2010; 157:233-239.

Extraintestinal Manifestations of Pediatric Inflammatory Bowel Disease and Their Relation to Disease Type and Severity

Dotson JL, Hyams JS, Markowitz J, et al (Nationwide Children's Hosp, Columbus, OH; Connecticut Children's Med Ctr, Hartford; North Shore Long Island Jewish Health System, New Hyde Park, NY; et al)
J Pediatr Gastroenterol Nutr 51:140-145, 2010

Objectives.—Although it is known that extraintestinal manifestations (EIMs) commonly occur in pediatric inflammatory bowel disease (IBD), little research has examined rates of EIMs and their relation to other disease-related factors in this population. The purpose of this study was to determine the rates of EIMs in pediatric IBD and examine correlations with age, sex, diagnosis, disease severity, and distribution.

Patients and Methods.—Data were prospectively collected as part of the Pediatric IBD Collaborative Research Group Registry, an observational database enrolling newly diagnosed IBD patients <16 years old since 2002. Rates of EIM (occurring anytime during the period of enrollment) and the aforementioned variables (at baseline) were examined. Patients with indeterminate colitis were excluded from the analysis given the relatively small number of patients.

Results.—One thousand nine patients were enrolled (mean age 11.6 ± 3.1 years, 57.5% boys, mean follow-up 26.2 ± 18.2 months). Two hundred eighty-five (28.2%) patients experienced 1 or more EIMs. Eighty-seven percent of EIM occurred within the first year. Increased disease severity at baseline (mild vs moderate/severe) was associated with the occurrence of any EIM ($P < 0.001$), arthralgia ($P = 0.024$), aphthous stomatitis ($P = 0.001$), and erythema nodosum ($P = 0.009$) for both Crohn disease (CD) and ulcerative colitis (UC) during the period of follow-up. Statistically significant differences in the rates of EIMs between CD and UC were seen for aphthous stomatitis, erythema nodosum, and sclerosing cholangitis.

Conclusions.—EIMs as defined in this study occur in approximately one quarter of pediatric patients with IBD. Disease type and disease severity were commonly associated with the occurrence of EIMs.

▶ Limited data in the pediatric literature suggest that somewhere between a quarter to almost half of pediatric patients with inflammatory bowel disease (IBD) experience at least 1 extraintestinal manifestation of IBD at the time of diagnosis. Such manifestations include arthritis, aphthous stomatitis, primary sclerosing colitis, growth failure, anemia, pyoderma gangrenosum, and arthralgias. We see in this report of Dotson et al just how common such extraintestinal manifestations are.

Using strict definitions, extraintestinal manifestations of IBD were noted in a quarter of pediatric-onset patients with IBD. If these manifestations were more broadly defined to include other systemic effects such as growth delay, nutritional deficiency, anemia, decreased bone mineral density, and fatigue, the actual rate of extraintestinal manifestations would in fact approach 100%. For these reasons, it is perhaps more appropriate to actually catalog the individual rates of extraintestinal manifestations to make some sense of the literature.

If the data by Dotson et al are broken down, we see that arthralgias are present in 17% of patients with IBD. True arthritis is seen in 4%. Aphthous stomatitis was noted in 8% of cases. The latter was much more common in Crohn disease than ulcerative colitis. Table 2 illustrates the specific prevalence of the various extraintestinal manifestations reported in this series of patients. The data represent extraintestinal manifestations that are observed within 2.5 years from the time of diagnosis, not necessarily those signs/symptoms present at the original diagnosis. You will note that differences do exist in the prevalences of the extraintestinal manifestations between Crohn disease and

TABLE 2.—Extraintestinal Manifestations Reported in Pediatric Patients with Inflammatory Bowel Disease and Statistically Significant Differences Among Disease Type (N = 1009)

	Total	CD	UC
Total	1009	728	281
Any EIM[a]	285 (28.2%)	218 (29.9%)	67 (23.8%)
Arthralgia	166 (16.5%)	124 (17%)	42 (14.9%)
AS	81 (8%)	72 (9.9%)*	9 (3.2%)*
Arthritis	37 (3.7%)	32 (4.4%)	5 (1.8%)
EN	28 (2.8%)	26 (3.6%)[#]	2 (0.71%)[#]
PSC	15 (1.5%)	7 (1%)[^]	8 (2.8%)[^]
Pancreatitis	9 (0.9%)	5 (0.7%)	4 (1.4%)
Chronic active hepatitis	6 (0.6%)	2 (0.3%)	4 (1.4%)
I/U	7 (0.7%)	6 (0.8%)	1 (0.4%)
Ankylosing spondylitis	4 (0.4%)	4 (0.5%)	0
PG	3 (0.3%)	3 (0.4%)	0

[a]=individual subjects ≥1 EIM. AS = aphthous stomatitis; CD = Crohn disease; EN = erythema nodosum; I/U = iritis/uveitis; PG = pyoderma gangrenosum; PSC = primary sclerosing cholangitis; UC = ulcerative colitis.
*$P < 0.001$.
[#]$P = 0.010$.
[^]$P = 0.039$.

ulcerative colitis when looking at 3 specific problems: aphthous stomatitis, primary sclerosing colitis, and erythema nodosum.

J. A. Stockman III, MD

Pediatric Inflammatory Bowel Disease and Imaging-related Radiation: Are We Increasing the Likelihood of Malignancy?
Fuchs Y, Markowitz J, Weinstein T, et al (North Shore-Long Island Jewish Health System, NY)
J Pediatr Gastroenterol Nutr 52:280-285, 2011

Background and Aims.—Increasing use of diagnostic radiography has led to concern about the malignant potential of ionizing radiation. We aimed to quantify the cumulative effective dose (CED) from diagnostic medical imaging in children with inflammatory bowel disease (IBD) and to identify which children are at greatest risk for high amounts of image-related radiation exposure.

Patients and Methods.—A retrospective chart review of pediatric IBD patients seen between January 1 and May 30, 2008 was conducted. The effective dose of radiation received from all of the radiology tests performed during the course of each patient's treatment was estimated using typical effective doses and our institution's computed tomography dose index. A CED ≥50 mSv was considered high.

Results.—Complete records were available for 257 of 372 screened subjects. One hundred seventy-one had Crohn disease (CD) and 86 had ulcerative colitis (UC). The mean CED was 17.56 ± 15.91 mSv and was greater for children with CD than for those with UC (20.5 ± 17.5 vs 11.7 ± 9.9 mSv, $P < 0.0001$). Fifteen children (5.8%) had a CED ≥50 mSv, including 14 of 171 (8.2%) with CD and 1 of 86 (1.2%) with UC ($P = 0.02$). In children with CD, factors associated with high CED per multivariate analysis were any IBD-related surgery (odds ratio 42, 95% confidence interval 8–223, $P < 0.0001$) and platelet count (odds ratio 16, 95% confidence interval 1.5–175, $P = 0.02$).

Conclusions.—Although all doses of ionizing radiation have some malignancy-inducing potential, a small but important percentage of children with IBD are exposed to particularly high doses of ionizing radiation from diagnostic tests and procedures. Physicians caring for such patients must seek to limit radiation exposure whenever possible to lessen the lifetime risk of malignancy.

▶ The initial evaluation as well as the management of complications related to inflammatory bowel disease (IBD) often involve imaging studies, particularly abdominal CT and radiographic small bowel series. These studies involve an appreciable amount of radiation. In recent years, there has been a marked increase in concern about the long-term oncologic effects of such studies. Data suggest that the relative risk of malignancy persists throughout one's life, is greater in girls than in boys, and is highest for those exposed during childhood. Radiation in an amount as low as 50 mSv from imaging-related exposure has been implicated in the development of certain solid tumors, particularly of the large bowel and bladder. It has been estimated that as much as 2% of all malignancies that are seen these days are the result of diagnostic medical radiation.[1]

One should be concerned about an increased risk of malignancy related to imaging-associated radiation in those with IBD. IBD itself is considered a risk factor for certain cancers including colorectal carcinoma. Also, common medications used to treat IBD, immunosuppressives in particular, are associated with a risk of lymphoma. There is also an increasing use these days of CT enteroclysis in those with IBD. This is a new technique that combines CT with fluoroscopy-guided infusion of contrast into the small bowel. This technique has been heralded as a preferred method of depicting mucosal abnormalities, bowel thickening, fistulae, and extraintestinal manifestations of Crohn disease. This technique, however, comes at the cost of increased radiation exposure.[2]

Fuchs et al undertook a study to quantify the cumulative doses of radiation from diagnostic medical procedures in children with IBD. Very few other reports have attempted to do such quantification in this patient population. The authors reviewed the charts of youngsters with IBD who were seen between January 1 and May 30, 2008. A small but significant proportion of these children were exposed to radiation in excess of 50 mSv during that short time interval. Such radiation dosing is considered potentially malignancy inducing. The authors strongly suggest that it is important for physicians caring for children with IBD to consider comparable tests with little or no radiation exposure whenever possible. Fortunately, a number of imaging modalities such as MRI, ultrasound, and capsule endoscopy are becoming viable options in many centers. Magnetic resonance enterography is particularly useful in providing information regarding disease activity and can aid in distinguishing inflammation from fibrosis in areas of bowel wall thickening. Unfortunately, most children younger than 7 years require general anesthesia for prolonged and multiple sequences, thus limiting the use of this technique. On the other hand, in the hands of an experienced radiologist, ultrasound can be highly accurate for the detection of IBD and can identify disease complications such as small bowel obstruction and abscess formation. Capsule endoscopy has the benefit of providing direct images of small bowel mucosa, and the recent development of the patency capsule has lessened concerns about capsule retention in a strictured segment.

The bottom line here is that children are not little adults and are at much greater risk of the development of long-term complications, malignancy in particular, related to diagnostic imaging radiation. It has been proposed that anyone undergoing diagnostic imaging that carries a radiation risk should have cumulative dosing records kept of their procedures. This seems like a wise recommendation, particularly for children who are possibly going to have a lifelong disease requiring repeated studies.

J. A. Stockman III, MD

References

1. Berrington de González A, Darby S. Risk of cancer from diagnostic x-rays: estimates for the United Kingdom and 14 other countries. *Lancet.* 2004;363:345-351.
2. Sailer J, Peloschek P, Schober E, et al. Diagnostic value of CT enteroclysis compared with conventional enteroclysis in patients with Crohn's disease. *AJR Am J Roentgenol.* 2005;185:1575-1581.

Familial Adenomatous Polyposis in Children and Adolescents
Alkhouri N, Franciosi JP, Mamula P (Cleveland Clinic, OH; Cincinnati Children's Hosp Med Ctr, OH; The Children's Hosp of Philadelphia)
J Pediatr Gastroenterol Nutr 51:727-732, 2010

Background.—Familial adenomatous polyposis (FAP) is the most common inherited polyposis syndrome characterized by the development of hundreds of colorectal adenomatous polyps. The aim of this study was to review cases of FAP diagnosed at The Children Hospital of Philadelphia in a 16-year period.

Methods.—Medical records of patients diagnosed as having FAP between 1990 and 2005 were reviewed. The collected data included disease presentation, genetic profile, extraintestinal manifestations, surveillance, and treatment.

Results.—We identified 12 patients with FAP. The age range at presentation was 7 to 18 years. Seven (68%) patients presented due to symptoms, the most common of which was rectal bleeding (6 patients, 86%). The youngest age at which polyps were detected was 7 years. Eight patients (67%) had positive family history. Three patients had Gardner syndrome and 1 presented in infancy with hepatoblastoma. Four patients had adenomatous polyposis coli gene mutation identified. One patient was diagnosed as having rectal carcinoma in situ. Six patients (50%) had gastric fundic gland polyposis and 6 had duodenal adenomatous changes. Capsule endoscopy was performed in 3 patients; 1 had multiple polyps in the duodenum and the jejunum. Seven patients (58%) underwent total colectomy with no serious complications.

Conclusions.—FAP is a rare condition but with significant risk of cancer and comorbidity. In this series, patients commonly presented to medical attention due to their symptoms. The youngest patient with polyps detected was 7 years old. We identified 1 patient with rectal cancer in situ and high proportion of patients with duodenal adenomatous lesions. Majority of patients underwent early colectomy.

▶ All pediatricians should be familiar with the familial adenomatous polyposis (FAP) syndrome, an autosomal dominant condition that is characterized by the development of large numbers of colorectal adenomatous polyps that inevitably lead to the development of colorectal cancer. FAP is caused by an inactivating germline mutation in the adenomatous polyposis coli tumor suppressor gene located at chromosome 5q21. It is estimated that between 1:5000 and

1:17 000 newborns are born into the world with this mutation, which represents the most common inherited polyposis syndrome in man. Unless a careful family history is taken, most youngsters with FAP are not diagnosed because they are largely symptomatic in childhood. Although the average age of colorectal cancer diagnosis in patients with FAP is 42 years, colonic polyps begin to appear at an average age of 16 years. There are case reports, however, of adenomatous polyps and cancer developing in the first decade of life. Current recommendations suggest initiation of colonic screening with a flexible sigmoidoscopy or colonoscopy at 12 years of age. Ultimately, colectomy is the recommended preventative treatment to decrease the risk of colorectal cancer in patients with FAP. The age at which colectomy should be undertaken is controversial and largely based on disease burden and psychosocial factors.

Even with prophylactic colectomy, there is a risk of the occurrence of duodenal adenomas. FAP covers an increased risk of 3% to 4% of progression of the duodenal adenomas to duodenal and periampullary carcinoma. Most gastroenterologists recommend upper endoscopic surveillance of the stomach, duodenum, and periampullary region during the third decade of life, although the start of age of surveillance is also controversial. In addition to intestinal polyps and associated problems, there are numerous extraintestinal manifestations of FAP. These include an increased risk of brain, thyroid, hepatic, and pancreatic malignancies. The risk of hepatoblastoma is 850 times greater in patients with FAP than in the general population. Nonmalignant associations include desmoid tumors, epidermoid cysts, osteomas, congenital hypertrophy of the retinal pigment epithelium, fibromas, and lipomas. The combination of FAP with colonic polyps and extraintestinal tumors is known as Gardner syndrome.

The report of Alkhouri et al represents an analysis identifying pediatric patients diagnosed with FAP over a 16-year period with special attention paid to disease presentation, genetic profile, extraintestinal manifestations, treatment, and long-term surveillance. The study is a review of cases of FAP diagnosed at the Children's Hospital of Philadelphia. In this Philadelphia series, unfortunately, more than half of patients presented with symptoms requiring medical attention rather than a diagnosis based on a positive family history. One of the patients, who was 18 years old, initially presented having a rectal carcinoma in situ. For patients with a strong family history, the diagnosis can be excluded with genetic testing. This study also showed that among family members with FAP, the finding of retinal involvement establishes a diagnosis of FAP 100% of the time. Data from this study have suggested that annual colonoscopy should be performed beginning at 10 years of age. In the Philadelphia series, half of patients who underwent upper gastrointestinal (GI) endoscopy had evidence of stomach polyps and fundic gland polyposis, and two-thirds had evidence of duodenal adenomatous changes. No high-grade dysplasia or cancer was identified in the upper GI tract. Interestingly, one patient who had hepatoblastoma diagnosed in infancy was found to have a diagnosis of FAP 18 years later. In families with FAP, some recommend yearly screening with α-fetoprotein levels and hepatic ultrasounds from birth through 5 years of age.

The authors of this report do recognize that the only treatment for reducing a colorectal cancer risk in a patient with FAP is colectomy. The timing of surgery the authors indicate is best decided on a patient-by-patient basis. One approach is to delay colectomy until after adolescence when patients can more actively participate in the decision-making process. In Philadelphia, the approach is to offer early surgical intervention to minimize the risk of cancer. Once colectomy is performed, however, patients continue to be at risk of developing adenomas and cancer in the small bowel pouch. Some have suggested the risk of this problem runs as high as 23% 5 years after a colectomy. It is recommended that endoscopic surveillance of a colectomy pouch be undertaken yearly. There are drugs (sulindac and celecoxib) that will reduce the numbers of adenomatous polyps, but drug therapy is no substitute for definitive surgical intervention.

Although FAP is not a common disorder, it is one that the average pediatrician will run across sometime during his or her lifetime of practice. We should all be generally familiar with the entity, its diagnosis, and potential treatments.

J. A. Stockman III, MD

Direct Medical Costs of Constipation From Childhood to Early Adulthood: A Population-based Birth Cohort Study
Choung RS, Shah ND, Chitkara D, et al (Mayo Clinic, Rochester, MN; UNC Ctr for Functional GI and Motility Disorders, Chapel Hill, NC)
J Pediatr Gastroenterol Nutr 52:47-54, 2011

Background.—Although direct medical costs for constipation-related medical visits are thought to be high, to date there have been no studies examining whether longitudinal resource use is persistently elevated in children with constipation. Our aim was to estimate the incremental direct medical costs and types of health care use associated with constipation from childhood to early adulthood.

Methods.—A nested case-control study was conducted to evaluate the incremental costs associated with constipation. The original sample consisted of 5718 children in a population-based birth cohort who were born during 1976 to 1982 in Rochester, MN. The cases included individuals who presented to medical facilities with constipation. The controls were matched and randomly selected among all noncases in the sample. Direct medical costs for cases and controls were collected from the time subjects were between 5 and 18 years of age or until the subject emigrated from the community.

Results.—We identified 250 cases with a diagnosis of constipation in the birth cohort. Although the mean inpatient costs for cases were $9994 (95% Confidence interval [CI] 2538−37,201) compared with $2391 (95% CI 923−7452) for controls ($P = 0.22$) during the time period, the mean outpatient costs for cases were $13,927 (95% CI 11,325−16,525) compared with $3448 (95% CI 3771−4621) for controls ($P < 0.001$) during the same time period. The mean annual number of emergency department visits for cases was 0.66 (95% CI 0.62−0.70) compared with 0.34 (95% CI 0.32−0.35) for controls ($P < 0.0001$).

Conclusions.—Individuals with constipation have higher medical care use. Outpatient costs and emergency department use were significantly greater for individuals with constipation from childhood to early adulthood.

▶ The report by Maffai and Vicentini told us about how one can use wheat bran to manage constipation in children.[1] Now we see what the actual costs are of having a child who is constipated. Choung et al undertook a study to evaluate the incremental cost associated with constipation in childhood. Chronic constipation is certainly one of the most common reasons for ambulatory visits by children. Of the 3 most common gastrointestinal complaints seen by primary care pediatricians (constipation, gastroesophageal reflux disease, and abdominal pain of unknown origin), chronic constipation is the most prevalent. It is 7 times more prevalent than asthma in children and 3 times more prevalent than migraine headaches.

Choung et al studied children born in Olmstead County, Minnesota, a rural area some 90 miles southeast of Minneapolis. This county keeps very accurate census data, and a number of studies have been undertaken of children born in that county. In this study, the overall incidence of constipation in children aged between 5 and 21 years was estimated to be 45 per 1000 person-years. Those with a diagnosis of constipation had consistently higher health care costs from childhood into early adulthood. The annual medical cost for care of these children was approximately twice that of their peers without constipation. Youngsters with a diagnosis of constipation younger than 5 years have about a 2 to 5 times higher incidence of subsequent medical visits for constipation compared with the incidence rate among children without an early medical presentation.

This is not the first report to look at the cost of childhood constipation in the United States. Liem et al have studied the health care use and the cost effect of constipation showing that children with constipation use more health care services than children without constipation. This results in significantly higher costs: $3430 per year versus $1099 per year.[2] If one runs the math, this amounts to an additional cost of $3.9 billion per year for children with constipation. In the report of Choung et al, total incremental cost per year for subjects with constipation was $630. By comparison, asthmatic children generate annual charges of $1004.

Thus, we need to get moving in getting bowel movements going. A few billion dollars here, a few billion dollars there saved could help the economy quite a bit.

J. A. Stockman III, MD

References

1. Maffei HV, Vicentini AP. Prospective evaluation of dietary treatment in childhood constipation: high dietary fiber and wheat bran intake are associated with constipation amelioration. *J Pediatr Gastroenterol Nutr.* 2011;52:55-59.
2. Liem O, Harman J, Benninga M, Kelleher K, Mousa H, Di Lorenzo C. Health utilization and cost impact of childhood constipation in the United States. *J Pediatr.* 2009;154:258-262.

Prospective Evaluation of Dietary Treatment in Childhood Constipation: High Dietary Fiber and Wheat Bran Intake Are Associated With Constipation Amelioration

Maffei HVL, Vicentini AP (UNESP-São Paulo State Univ, Botucatu, SP—Brazil)
J Pediatr Gastroenterol Nutr 52:55-59, 2011

Objectives.—The aim of the study was to evaluate, over 24 months, the intake of dietary fiber (DF) and the bowel habit (BH) of constipated children advised a DF-rich diet containing wheat bran.

Patients and Methods.—BH and dietary data of 28 children with functional constipation defined by the "Boston criteria" were obtained at visit 1 (V1, n = 28) and at 4 follow-up visits (V2—V5, n = 80). At each visit the BH was rated BAD (worse/unaltered; improved but still complications) or RECOVERY (REC) (improved, no complications; asymptomatic), and a food intake questionnaire was applied. DF intake was calculated according to age (year)+5 to 10 g/day and bran intake according to international tables. Nonparametric statistics were used.

Results.—Median age (range) was 7.25 years (0.25—15.6 years); 21 children underwent bowel washout (most before V1/V2), and 14 had the last visit at V3/V4. DF intake, bran intake, and the BH rate significantly increased at V2 and remained higher than at V1 through V2 to V5. At V1, median DF intake was 29.9% below the minimum recommended and at the last visit 49.9% above it. Twenty-four children accepted bran at 60 visits, at which median bran intake was 20 g/day and median proportion of DF due to bran 26.9%. Children had significantly higher DF and higher bran intake at V2 to V5 at which they had REC than at those at which they presented BAD BH. DF intake >age+ 10 g/day was associated with bran acceptance and REC. At the last visit 21 children presented REC (75%); 20 of them were asymptomatic and 18 were off washout/laxatives.

Conclusions.—High DF and bran intake are feasible in constipated children and contribute to amelioration of constipation.

▶ Just about everybody knows that dietary fiber can be used to help manage constipation in children. Wheat bran and cocoa husk are the most commonly available insoluble fibers. In theory, insoluble fiber is better for treatment of constipation than soluble fiber. Wheat bran, with high pentose content, seems to work better than cocoa husk whose main component is cellulose. Rarely, however, have diets that included wheat bran been advocated for children. The report abstracted is from Brazil where wheat bran is cheap, can be mixed up into usual foods, and is generally considered to be a safe product. On the other hand, processed whole-grain foods containing wheat are relatively expensive by comparison. The investigators from Brazil undertook a prospective evaluation of dietary fiber/wheat bran acceptance and its effects on the bowel habits of children with functional constipation. Children were given a bran intake of approximately 20 g/day with a median proportion of dietary bran fiber of 26.9%.

Approximately three-fourths of children treated with the high-fiber diet described had resolution of their constipation. The authors concluded that a diet rich in wheat bran is both feasible and cheap for treating constipated children in everyday clinical settings. Bran acceptance seemed to be quite good, and the administration was certainly easy. It should be noted that the protocol used did start with a brief bowel wash out involving disimpaction enemas followed by laxatives.

J. A. Stockman III, MD

Cow's-Milk–free Diet as a Therapeutic Option in Childhood Chronic Constipation

Irastorza I, Ibañez B, Delgado-Sanzonetti L, et al (Hosp de Cruces, Bilbao, Spain; Basque ndation for Health Innovation and Res, Bilbao, Spain; et al)
J Pediatr Gastroenterol Nutr 51:171-176, 2010

Objectives.—It has been reported that a number of children with constipation respond to a diet free of cow's-milk (CM) proteins, although evidence is lacking to support an immunoglobulin E—mediated mechanism.

Patients and Methods.—We performed an open-label crossover study comparing CM and rice milk in 69 children who fulfilled Rome III criteria for chronic constipation. Clinical, physical, and immunologic parameters of patients who responded (R) and who did not respond (NR) to a CM-free diet were compared.

Results.—Thirty-five of the 69 children (51%) improved during the first CM-free diet phase, 8 of these did not develop constipation when CM was reintroduced, and 27 children (39%) developed constipation during the CM challenge and improved during the second CM-free diet phase (R group). Thirty-four children (49%) did not improve during the first CM-free diet phase (NR group). Bowel movements per week among R children significantly increased compared with NR children (R: 2.8–7.7 vs NR: 2.6–2.7) ($P < 0.001$). Seventy-eight percent of the children with developmental delay responded to the CM-free diet ($P = 0.007$). No significant statistical difference was found between the R and NR children in terms of fiber and milk consumption; atopic or allergic history; full-blood eosinophil count and percentage, and lymphocyte populations; immunoglobulins, immunoglobulin (Ig)G subclasses, total IgE; and serum-specific immunoglobulin E for CM proteins.

Conclusions.—A clear association between CM consumption and constipation has been found in more than one third of children. However, analytical parameters do not demonstrate an immunoglobulin E-mediated immunologic mechanism.

▶ The poor cow is being blamed for so many things these days. Now we see more evidence that perhaps the milk of a cow is one of the major contributory factors to constipation in children. In fact, the link between cow milk congestion and constipation is hardly a new concept for many of us. Carraccio et al in 2006 suggested an intriguing relationship between constipation and food hypersensitivity that included the possibility of a linkage of the sluggish bowel to cow milk ingestion.[1] More recently, it has been suggested that cow's milk proteins could play a direct role in the genesis of constipation through an immune-mediated mechanism.[2] Resolution of histologic and manometric abnormalities when put on a cow's milk—free diet underscores the possible link between cow's milk and constipation in some children.

What Irastorza et al have done is to describe historical relationships in children with chronic constipation and then to evaluate the usefulness of a cow's milk—free diet as a treatment. Just over half of the children with chronic constipation when put on a cow's milk—free diet showed significant improvement in constipation-related symptoms. Most of these children redeveloped worsening constipation when put back on cow's milk. The data seem to support the hypothesis that cow's milk plays a significant role in many children with constipation. The authors also observed another interesting finding. Many children with developmental delay experience long-term problems with constipation. These investigators, however, show that 98% of children with developmental delay who have constipation respond to a cow's milk—free diet.

So if there is a link between a cow's milk congestion and constipation, what is the mechanism? It has been suggested that children who drink significant amounts of cow's milk are not receiving diets with sufficient bulk residue, a reason for the constipation. In the report, however, from Spain, dairy and fiber consumption was similar in children who improved and in those who did not respond after a cow's milk—free diet, suggesting that dairy products and fiber intake are not predictors in and of themselves to a cow's milk—free diet. Also, these investigators did not find a recognizable pattern of immune deviation in children with cow's milk—sensitive constipation when various immune mediators were looked at in detail.

Needless to say, a trial of dairy products seems to make sense for children who have constipation significant enough to warrant management. However, it would be nice to see further studies of this type, perhaps in larger numbers of children to verify the findings.

This commentary started with the observations that cows are being blamed for everything these days. The summer of 2010 was an exceptionally hot one across the United States. One can be sure that this was likely due to global warming, secondary to the methane that cows produce, wearing out our ozone layer. If only that methane could be recycled for more useful purposes.

J. A. Stockman III, MD

References

1. Carraccio A, Iacono G. Review article: Chronic constipation and food hypersensitivity—an intriguing relationship. *Aliment Pharmacol Ther.* 2006;24: 1295-1304.
2. Iacono G, Cavataio F, Montalto G, et al. Intolerance of cow's milk and chronic constipation in children. *N Engl J Med.* 1998;339:1100-1104.

Creation and Initial Evaluation of a Stool Form Scale for Children

Chumpitazi BP, Lane MM, Czyzewski DI, et al (Baylor College of Medicine, Houston, TX; et al)
J Pediatr 157:594-597, 2010

Objective.—To develop a pediatric stool form rating scale and determine its interrater reliability, intrarater reliability, and agreement among pediatric gastroenterologists.

Study Design.—An ordinal stool scale with 5 categorical stool form types was created on the basis of the Bristol Stool Form Scale, and 32 color 2-dimensional stool photographs were shown to 14 pediatric gastroenterologists. Each gastroenterologist rated the stool form depicted in each photograph with the modified stool scale. Ten gastroenterologists agreed to rerate the stool form depicted in each photograph a minimum of 6 months after the first rating.

Results.—A total of 448 ratings were completed; 430 (94%) of all ratings were within at least 1 category type of the most common (modal) rating for each photograph. Eight (25%) stool photographs had complete agreement among all raters. Interrater and intrarater reliability was high with a single measure intraclass correlation of 0.85 (95% confidence interval: 0.78-0.91; $P < .001$) and 0.87 (95% confidence interval: 0.81-0.92; $P < .001$), respectively.

Conclusion.—A modified pediatric Bristol Stool Form Scale provided a high degree of interrater reliability, intrarater reliability, and agreement among pediatric gastroenterologists (Fig).

▶ This is not the first report that attempts to establish a rating system for the way children form stools. An often used measure of stool form is the Bristol Stool Form Scale (BSFS). BSFS classifies stool form into 7 different types ranging from separate hard lumps like nuts (type 1) to watery, no solid pieces, entirely liquid (type 7), with everything in between. BSFS, it should be noted, has been validated in adults as a measure of stool transit rather than a means of identifying stool form, but it has been used in a number of clinical studies of adults with diarrhea related to human immunodeficiency virus infection and functional bowel disorders. Other rating systems have been proposed, but none of these have been validated either. What Chumpitazi et al have done is to develop a scale for stool form use in both adults and children and have assessed its interrater reliability, intrarater reliability, and agreement when used by expert stool examiners (whatever the latter is). The study was performed largely at the Baylor College of Medicine, Texas Children's Hospital. Because there already are dibs on "BSFS" and the Chumpitazi report has no nomenclature with it, we will call it the Texas Stool Form Scale (TSFS). For ease of poop identification, the investigators decided on 5 variations of stools to be assessed (Fig). Using the images in the Fig for comparative purposes, a panel of stool experts was individually shown 32 color, 2-dimensional photographs of stools ranging from liquid to formed to hard pellets, all obtained from public domains on the Internet. One wonders if the study would have been

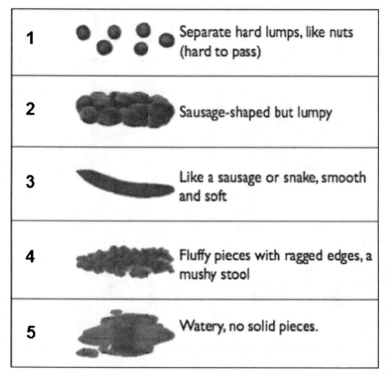

1		Separate hard lumps, like nuts (hard to pass)
2		Sausage-shaped but lumpy
3		Like a sausage or snake, smooth and soft
4		Fluffy pieces with ragged edges, a mushy stool
5		Watery, no solid pieces.

FIGURE.—Modified stool form scale that was used during the study. There are 5 ordinal categories. (Reprinted from Journal of Pediatrics, Chumpitazi BP, Lane MM, Czyzewski DI, et al. Creation and initial evaluation of a stool form scale for children. *J Pediatr.* 2010;157:594-597. Copyright 2010 with permission from Elsevier.)

enhanced with 3D images. The review included 14 pediatric gastroenterologists who had a median of 17.5 years of clinical experience at looking at poop. The bottom line is that the modified pediatric BSFS, which we are calling the TSFS, has a high degree of overall interrater reliability, intrarater reliability, and agreement.

The TSFS, having only 5 variations, should be easier to use than the BSFS with its 7 variations. Needless to say, those who actually are taking care of patients most likely will have other sensory input, including smell, in addition to visual cues as to what a stool is all about. No one has developed a stool scale involving senses such as smell, touch, or taste (thank goodness). Thank goodness no one has developed a scale that involves listening to a stool as it is being passed.

In closing, here is a question to test your knowledge of the gastrointestinal literature. The question is: describe the Rapunzel syndrome. The answer is that the Rapunzel syndrome describes a condition in which swallowed hair forms a trichobezoar in the stomach that has a "tail" extending into the small bowel that may lead to partial or complete intestinal obstruction. The typical presentations of Rapunzel syndrome are abdominal pain and nausea/vomiting.

Less common presentations may include weight loss and/or intussusception. Halitosis may result from bacterial overgrowth within the bezoar. Rapion (*Campanula rapunculus*) is a plant that is characterized by its long stems of stiff white "hairs." It inspired the name for the heroine of the German fairytale "Rapunzel," written by the Grimm brothers in the early 1800s. Rapunzel was imprisoned by a witch in a tall tower for many years. She was only able to meet her prince after she lowered her long locks of hair from her window, allowing him to climb to her aid. As an aside, the term bezoar comes from the Arabic term *bāzahr*, meaning "counter poison." Bezoars can be composed of a variety of substances and are found in the gastrointestinal tract of both humans and animals. They were once thought of as containing antidotes to certain poisons and also to having magical properties. These beliefs are still held by some eastern cultures today.[1] This is more than you ever wanted to know about Rapunzel syndrome and bezoars.

J. A. Stockman III, MD

Reference

1. Williams RS. The fascinating history of bezoars. *Med J Aust.* 1986;145:613-614.

8 Genitourinary Tract

Risk of Nephropathy After Consumption of Nonionic Contrast Media by Children Undergoing Cardiac Angiography: A Prospective Study
Ajami G, Derakhshan A, Amoozgar H, et al (Shiraz Univ of Med Sciences, Iran)
Pediatr Cardiol 31:668-673, 2010

Despite increasing reports on nonionic contrast media-induced nephropathy (CIN) in hospitalized adult patients during cardiac procedures, the studies in pediatrics are limited, with even less focus on possible predisposing factors and preventive measures for patients undergoing cardiac angiography. This prospective study determined the incidence of CIN for two nonionic contrast media (CM), iopromide and iohexol, among 80 patients younger than 18 years and compared the rates for this complication in relation to the type and dosage of CM and the presence of cyanosis. The 80 patients in the study consecutively received either iopromide (group A, $n = 40$) or iohexol (group B, $n = 40$). Serum sodium (Na), potassium (K), and creatinine (Cr) were measured 24 h before angiography as baseline values, then measured again at 12-, 24-, and 48-h intervals after CM use. Urine samples for Na and Cr also were checked at the same intervals. Risk of renal failure, Injury to the kidney, Failure of kidney function, Loss of kidney function, and End-stage renal damage (RIFLE criteria) were used to define CIN and its incidence in the study population. Accordingly, among the 15 CIN patients (18.75%), 7.5% of the patients in group A had increased risk and 3.75% had renal injury, whereas 5% of group B had increased risk and 2.5% had renal injury. Whereas 33.3% of the patients with CIN were among those who received the proper dosage of CM, the percentage increased to 66.6% among those who received larger doses, with a significant difference in the incidence of CIN related to the different dosages of CM ($p = 0.014$). Among the 15 patients with CIN, 6 had cyanotic congenital heart diseases, but the incidence did not differ significantly from that for the noncyanotic patients ($p = 0.243$). Although clinically silent, CIN is not rare in pediatrics. The incidence depends on dosage but not on the type of consumed nonionic CM, nor on the presence of cyanosis, and although CIN usually is reversible, more concern is needed for the prevention of such a complication in children.

▶ This report reminds us that even straightforward diagnostic studies can have serious complications. Iodinated contrast media have been used for years as diagnostic tools in the performance of certain X-ray procedures. Over the last half century, we have recognized the potential of such media to cause kidney damage. This risk diminished with the development of nonionic contrast media, which have lower osmolality and tonicity. These are now iso-osmolar to plasma. This report from Iran tells about the incidence of contrast media—induced nephropathy in children undergoing cardiac catheterization procedures.

The findings from this report show that almost 20% of children undergoing cardiac angiography will show some evidence of contrast media—induced nephropathy as defined by changes in serum creatinine level or glomerular filtration rate. Fortunately, these laboratory findings were associated with clinically silent presentations, and the laboratory findings were transient. The data in children are virtually identical to data that have been derived from adult studies.

The likelihood of developing nephropathy from the use of contrast media is directly related to the amount of contrast media used. Also, patients with any degree of dehydration and those who already have renal dysfunction are at greater risk for the development of nephropathy. More often than one would like, the volume of contrast media administered during the angiographic procedures described was not being carefully monitored. Dosing should not exceed the dosage recommended by the manufacturer at any time. One way to minimize the risk of nephropathy is to ensure adequate hydration with intravenous fluid administration. The authors of this report also suggest that in some instances the administration of acetazolamide or N-acetylcysteine should be considered.

While on the topic of side effects of commonly used radiographic procedures, it is recognized that the average dose of radiation to which persons in the United States are exposed has doubled over the past 30 years.[1] Although the average dose from natural background sources has not changed, the average radiation dose from medical imaging has increased more than 6-fold. Medical imaging now contributes to about 50% of the overall radiation dose to the US population, compared with about 15% in 1980. The largest contributor to this dramatic increase in population radiation exposure is the CT scan. In 1980, fewer than 3 million CT scans were performed, but the annual number now approaches 80 million and is increasing by approximately 10% per year. Because CT scanning involves acquiring multiple images, CT scans result in a far larger radiation dose to the patient than most other common radiographic procedures such as chest X-rays or mammograms. Other radiation sources from testing are also increasing (nuclear medicine procedures, positron emission tomography-CT, etc).

Several studies suggest that 20% to 40% of CT scans could be avoided if clinical decision guidelines were followed more carefully.[2] To read more about radiation exposure from medical imaging, see the excellent commentary on this topic by Brenner and Hricak.[3]

J. A. Stockman III, MD

References

1. Brenner DJ, Hall EJ. Computed tomography–an increasing source of radiation exposure. *N Engl J Med.* 2007;357:2277-2284.

2. Lehnert PE, Bree RL. Analysis of appropriateness of outpatient CT and MRI referred from primary care clinics at an academic medical center: how critical is the need for improved decision support? *J Am Coll Radiol.* 2010;7:192-197.
3. Brenner DJ, Hricak H. Radiation exposure from medical imaging: time to regulate? *JAMA.* 2010;304:208-209.

Glomerular filtration rate, proteinuria, and the incidence and consequences of acute kidney injury: a cohort study

James MT, Hemmelgarn BR, Wiebe N, et al (Univ of Calgary, Alberta, Canada; Univ of Alberta, Edmonton, Canada)

Lancet 376:2096-2103, 2010

Background.—Low values of estimated glomerular filtration rate (eGFR) predispose to acute kidney injury, and proteinuria is a marker of kidney disease. We aimed to investigate how eGFR and proteinuria jointly modified the risks of acute kidney injury and subsequent adverse clinical outcomes.

Methods.—We did a cohort study of 920 985 adults residing in Alberta, Canada, between 2002 and 2007. Participants not needing chronic dialysis at baseline and with at least one outpatient measurement of both serum creatinine concentration and proteinuria (urine dipstick or albumin-creatinine ratio) were included. We assessed hospital admission with acute kidney injury with validated administrative codes; other outcomes were all-cause mortality and a composite renal outcome of end-stage renal disease or doubling of serum creatinine concentration.

Findings.—During median follow-up of 35 months (range 0—59 months), 6520 (0·7%) participants were admitted with acute kidney injury. In those with eGFR 60 mL/min per 1·73 m^2 or greater, the adjusted risk of admission with this disorder was about 4 times higher in those with heavy proteinuria measured by dipstick (rate ratio 4·4 vs no proteinuria, 95% CI 3·7—5·2). The adjusted rates of admission with acute kidney injury and kidney injury needing dialysis remained high in participants with heavy dipstick proteinuria for all values of eGFR. The adjusted rates of death and the composite renal outcome were also high in participants admitted with acute kidney injury, although the rise associated with this injury was attenuated in those with low baseline eGFR and heavy proteinuria.

Interpretation.—These findings suggest that information on proteinuria and eGFR should be used together when identifying people at risk of acute kidney injury, and that an episode of acute kidney injury provides further long-term prognostic information in addition to eGFR and proteinuria.

▶ The report by Ajami et al tells us about the role of assessing albumin in the urine of patients with chronic renal disease.[1] The report of James et al tells us how we can use the assessment of proteinuria, when added to glomerular filtration rate determination, to identify those at greatest risk who have sustained acute renal injury.

James et al have used a province-wide sample of nearly 1 million adult Canadians to show the independent association between estimated glomerular filtration rate (eGFR), proteinuria, and the incidence of acute kidney injury. Moreover, they provide evidence to show that the risks of death and progression to end-stage renal disease that are associated with acute kidney injury vary with levels of eGFR and proteinuria. These investigators found that patients with normal eGFR values ($\geq$60 mL/min/1.73 m^2) and mild proteinuria (urine dipstick trace to 1+) have 2.5 times the risk of hospital admission with acute kidney injury than do patients with no urinary protein; this risk was increased by 4.4-fold in patients with heavy proteinuria (urine dipstick $\geq$2+). These findings confirm and expand on reports suggesting that both eGFR and albuminuria are potent risk factors for subsequent acute kidney injury.

We are seeing more and more cases these days of acute renal injury in both adults and children. Many of these cases are iatrogenic and preventable. Drug-induced nephrotoxicity accounts for a good proportion of acute kidney injury in both adults and children. Contrast-induced nephropathy is another well-described and potentially avoidable cause. The use of intravenous contrast has increased substantially in the last decade or two. Many procedures that involve contrast administration are elective. More accurate identification of high-risk patients might allow timely implementation of preventive measures when undertaking such studies. Although a serum creatinine is commonly checked before a contrast is administered, a few think to check a urine dipstick. Perhaps we should be doing this routinely.

To read more about proteinuria and the risk of acute kidney injury, see the excellent commentary by Grams and Coresh.[2]

J. A. Stockman III, MD

References

1. Ajami G, Derakhshan A, Amoozgar H, et al. Risk of nephropathy after consumption of nonionic contrast media by children undergoing cardiac angiograph: A prospective study. *Pediatr Cardiol.* 2010;31:668-673.
2. Grams M, Coresh J. Proteinuria and risk of acute kidney injury. *Lancet.* 2010;376:2046-2048.

Using Proteinuria and Estimated Glomerular Filtration Rate to Classify Risk in Patients With Chronic Kidney Disease: A Cohort Study
Tonelli M, for the Alberta Kidney Disease Network (Univ of Alberta, Edmonton, Canada; et al)
Ann Intern Med 154:12-21, 2011

Background.—The staging system for chronic kidney disease relies almost exclusively on estimated glomerular filtration rate (eGFR), although proteinuria is also associated with adverse outcomes.

Objective.—To validate a 5-category system for risk stratification based on the combination of eGFR and proteinuria.

Design.—Retrospective cohort study.

Setting.—A provincial laboratory registry in Alberta, Canada, and a representative sample of noninstitutionalized U.S. adults.

Patients.—A derivation data set of 474 521 adult outpatients, 2 independent internal validation cohorts with 51 356 and 460 623 patients, and an external validation cohort of 14 358 patients.

Measurements.—Glomerular filtration rate, estimated by using the Modification of Diet in Renal Disease Study equation, and proteinuria, measured by using urine albumin-to-creatinine ratio or dipstick urinalysis. Outcomes included all-cause mortality and a composite renal outcome of kidney failure or doubling of serum creatinine level.

Results.—Over a median follow-up of 38 months in the internal validation cohorts, higher risk categories (indicating lower eGFR or more proteinuria) were associated with a graded increase in the risk for the composite renal outcome. The projected number of U.S. adults assigned to risk categories 3 and 4 in the alternate system was 3.9 million, compared with 16.3 million assigned to stage 3 and 4 in the current staging system. The alternate system was more likely to correctly reclassify persons who did not develop the renal outcome than those who did, although some persons developed the renal outcome despite reclassification to a lower category. However, all analyses of patients reclassified to a lower category showed that substantially fewer such patients developed the renal outcome than did not. Correct reclassification by the alternate system was more likely when proteinuria was measured by using albumin-to-creatinine ratio than with dipstick testing, and also more likely for the composite renal outcome than for mortality.

Limitation.—The study had a short follow-up time.

Conclusion.—Using proteinuria in combination with eGFR may reduce unnecessary referrals for care at the cost of not referring or delaying referral for some patients who go on to develop kidney failure.

▶ This report was undertaken in adults, but you can bet that the information provided by this report will creep down into the care of children with renal disease fairly quickly. If one looks at the overall population of the United States, approximately 23 million adults have chronic kidney disease (CKD), for a prevalence of 11.5%. Obviously this prevalence is much less in children, but we use the same criteria laboratory-wise to define degrees of renal failure. CKD is a term that is quite heterogeneous for various disorders of kidney structure and function. The severity of CKD is traditionally classified according to glomerular filtration rates, but a number of studies have shown that a higher level of proteinuria (as ascertained by an albumin-creatinine ratio or dipstick protein testing) is a risk factor for CKD progression and mortality independent of estimated glomerular filtration rate (GFR).

Tonelli et al undertook a study in Edmonton, Alberta, Canada, to see if adding information about proteinuria to estimated GFR would help to better classify patients with CKD. These investigators showed that using proteinuria in combination with estimated GFR does reduce unnecessary referrals for care, at least in adults.

The ultimate goal of a classification system for CKD should be to facilitate clinical decisions that improve patient outcomes. Correct diagnosis, concurrent complications, and prognosis are key factors in clinical decision making. Important adverse outcomes include not only CKD progression and mortality but also infections, impairment of cognitive and physical function, and medical errors. Tonelli et al have provided a rigorous evaluation of incorporating more detailed information on proteinuria for prognosis and for guiding referral. While the data referred to mostly adults with chronic renal disease, we learn a lot about how to better estimate prognosis in children. Adding albuminuria to estimated GFR enables a better description of CKD for both prognosis and management. Fig 1 in the original article shows the current National Kidney Foundation's guidelines for determining the stages of CKD based on glomerular filtration rate alone. This is the staging system as it exists now in the United States.

J. A. Stockman III, MD

Time for Initial Response to Steroids Is a Major Prognostic Factor in Idiopathic Nephrotic Syndrome

Vivarelli M, Moscaritolo E, Tsalkidis A, et al (Bambino Gesù Children's Hosp and Res Inst, Rome, Italy; Univ Hosp of Alexandroupolis, Greece)
J Pediatr 156:965-971, 2010

Objective.—To identify early prognostic factors for idiopathic nephrotic syndrome (INS) in childhood.

Study Design.—A retrospective analysis of 103 patients with INS at onset, all treated in a single center with the same induction protocol, was conducted. Minimum length of follow-up was 2 years; median length of follow-up was 43 months. Survival data were assessed with Cox-Mantel analysis. Predictive values were estimated with receiver operating characteristic curves.

Results.—The median time of response to steroid therapy was 7 days. A significant association was found between the interval from onset of steroid therapy to remission and the risk of relapsing within 3 months after steroid therapy discontinuation ($P < .0001$). A similar association was found between the time to achieve remission and the risk of developing frequent relapsing or steroid-dependent nephrotic syndrome ($P < .0001$), the prescription of maintenance steroid therapy ($P < .003$), and the prescription of all other non-steroid drugs ($P < .0001$) during follow-up. Patients with non-relapsing and infrequent relapsing nephrotic syndrome had a median time to achieve remission <7 days; in patients with frequent relapsing and steroid-dependent nephrotic syndrome, this median was >7 days.

Conclusion.—The interval from onset of steroid therapy to remission is an accurate early prognostic factor in INS.

▶ Virtually every child with idiopathic nephrotic syndrome (INS) will be treated with steroids. Obviously, those youngsters who fail to respond to treatment have a much poorer prognosis. What has not been looked at before, however, is whether the time to remission on steroids is a solid prognostic factor. As we see from this report of Vivarelli et al, it is an important predictive variable. In this report, just over 100 patients presenting with INS were treated with standard doses of steroids and were followed up for their clinical outcome. The data from the report defined 3 separate groups of patients on the basis of initial response to steroids: response within the first week, the second week, or after more than 2 weeks of treatment. Patients who are fast responders (within 7 days) have a significantly higher chance of remaining in remission after steroid discontinuation and a lower chance of requiring additional medication with time, suggesting that they may be treated with a relatively short interval of steroids. However, patients who respond later would probably benefit from a prolonged initial course of steroids with gradual tapering extending as long as 4 to 6 months. Whether this approach should be applied in clinical practice was not studied in this report and is something that should be followed up with more extensive investigation.

It also seems clear from this report that late responders who require more than 2 weeks of treatment to achieve initial remission do represent a difficult prognostic category. Not only do these patients relapse rapidly but they require early addition of a second drug. They also tend to relapse during the induction period. The authors of this report suggest that lengthening the initial steroid course would be unlikely to achieve a prolonged remission in such patients and that treatment should probably be intensified during the first weeks after diagnosis. Whether this would include a high-dose steroid given parenterally or the addition of a second drug has not been studied extensively.

All those caring for children with INS should be aware of the importance of assessing time to initial remission and its relationship to prognosis. Failure to go into a prompt remission within 7 days is definitely not a good sign.

J. A. Stockman III, MD

Everolimus in Patients with Autosomal Dominant Polycystic Kidney Disease

Walz G, Budde K, Mannaa M, et al (Univ Hosp, Freiburg, Germany; Charité Universitätsmedizin Berlin Campus Mitte; Charité Universitätsmedizin Berlin, Campus Virchow; et al)
N Engl J Med 363:830-840, 2010

Background.—Autosomal dominant polycystic kidney disease (ADPKD) is a slowly progressive hereditary disorder that usually leads to end-stage renal disease. Although the underlying gene mutations were identified several years ago, efficacious therapy to curtail cyst growth and prevent renal failure is not available. Experimental and observational studies suggest that the mammalian target of rapamycin (mTOR) pathway plays a critical role in cyst growth.

Methods.—In this 2-year, double-blind trial, we randomly assigned 433 patients with ADPKD to receive either placebo or the mTOR inhibitor everolimus. The primary outcome was the change in total kidney volume, as measured on magnetic resonance imaging, at 12 and 24 months.

Results.—Total kidney volume increased between baseline and 1 year by 102 ml in the everolimus group, versus 157 ml in the placebo group (P = 0.02) and between baseline and 2 years by 230 ml and 301 ml, respectively (P = 0.06). Cyst volume increased by 76 ml in the everolimus group and 98 ml in the placebo group after 1 year (P = 0.27) and by 181 ml and 215 ml, respectively, after 2 years (P = 0.28). Parenchymal volume increased by 26 ml in the everolimus group and 62 ml in the placebo group after 1 year (P = 0.003) and by 56 ml and 93 ml, respectively, after 2 years (P = 0.11). The mean decrement in the estimated glomerular filtration rate after 24 months was 8.9 ml per minute per 1.73 m^2 of body-surface area in the everolimus group versus 7.7 ml per minute in the placebo group (P = 0.15). Drug-specific adverse events were more common in the everolimus group; the rate of infection was similar in the two groups.

Conclusions.—Within the 2-year study period, as compared with placebo, everolimus slowed the increase in total kidney volume of patients with ADPKD but did not slow the progression of renal impairment. (Funded by Novartis; EudraCT number, 2006-001485-16;ClinicalTrials. gov number, NCT00414440.).

▶ Autosomal dominant polycystic kidney disease (ADPKD) is a common enough inherited cause of renal failure that all of us should be familiar with. It affects approximately 1 in 1000 persons and is characterized by the progressive formation of renal cysts that leads to end-stage renal disease in middle adulthood in at least 50% of affected patients. It also results in a number of other complications, including massive renal enlargement, chronic pain, and hypertension. Some will have recurrent urinary tract infection and renal stones. The significant majority of patients with ADPKD will have mutations in the *PKD1* gene. The remainder of cases (about 15%) have the *PKD2* gene mutations and generally milder manifestations. The products of these genes make up what is known as the polycystin protein complex. These complexes are located in the primary nonmotile cilium, a microtubular organelle present on most cells of the body. This protein complex translates mechanochemosensory signals. It is thought that dysregulation of the mammalian target of rapamycin (mTOR) kinase promotes cyst formation and disease progression. This kinase enzyme coordinates cell growth and proliferation, processes that are dysregulated in patients with PKD. It has been shown in mice that the mTOR inhibitor sirolimus is effective in ameliorating cyst growth and preserving renal function in mice with the mouse model of PKD. Clinical trials with this enzyme inhibitor are obviously hampered by the long natural history of ADPKD with gradual cyst growth over decades, coupled with a gradual decline in renal function. Thus, clinical trials relying on traditional end points such as serum creatinine levels are impractical because years of follow-up would be required to detect any benefit. This is where the Consortium for Radiologic Imaging Studies of Polycystic Kidney Disease (CRISP) comes into play. CRISP has studied any degree of renal enlargement as a surrogate for early kidney disease. CRISP studies have shown that total kidney and cyst volumes increase exponentially (approximately 5% annually) and that MRI studies can reproducibly detect such changes.[1]

Recognizing that it was possible to use MRI findings as a surrogate for progression of end-stage renal disease in patients with ADPKD, Walz et al have described the results of a 2-year placebo-controlled trial of another mTOR inhibitor, everolimus. This study involved 433 patients with ADPKD with stage II or stage III chronic kidney disease and an average baseline renal volume of greater than 1500 mL. Most interestingly, although everolimus appeared to slow the increase in total kidney volume, this change did not correlate with improvement in the estimated glomerular filtration rate. In fact, after transient improvement, the estimated glomerular filtration rate declined more rapidly in the everolimus group than in the placebo group, leading the authors to conclude that smaller may not necessarily be better when it comes to the management of ADPKD.

The same issue in *The New England Journal of Medicine* reported a study by Serra et al[2] on this topic. In the latter study, sirolimus itself was compared with placebo in 100 patients between the ages of 18 and 40 years who had early stage ADPKD. In contrast to the study of Walz et al, Serra et al found that treatment with sirolimus for 18 months did not slow kidney disease as measured by MRI. Because the study was conducted in patients with early stage disease, there was no difference in glomerular filtration rates between the 2 groups. The bottom line in these 2 studies together tell us that mTOR inhibitors are not the magic bullet for the management of ADPKD, at least at this point. Unanswered is the question of whether the patients in the Walz study were too far along to show improvement in renal function or to slow a decline in renal function and whether the patients in the Serra et al study may have received insufficient amounts of sirolimus. The challenge of achieving adequate mTOR suppression without dose-limiting toxic effects remains to be investigated. As many as one-third of patients in the study of Walz et al were unable to complete the study protocol because of drug-related adverse events. Some of the adverse effects, if allowed to continue, would be very problematic since they included chronic proteinuria and hyperlipidemia. Why some patients have a significant reduction in progression of cyst formation yet no improvement in renal function is also a mystery.

Those interested in the topic of PKD may wish to read the excellent editorial on this topic by Watnick and Germino.[3] It is quite clear that we need better tools for assessing the effects of therapeutic interventions on renal function in humans. This is a problem for the study of almost every form of chronic renal disease and as noted in the editorial, one that urgently needs a solution.

J. A. Stockman III, MD

References

1. Grantham JJ, Torres VE, Chapman AB, et al. Volume progression in polycystic kidney disease. *N Engl J Med.* 2006;354:2122-2130.
2. Serra AL, Poster D, Kistler AD, et al. Sirolimus and kidney growth in autosomal dominant polycystic kidney disease. *N Engl J Med.* 2010;363:820-829.
3. Watnick T, Germino GG. mTOR inhibitors in polycystic kidney disease. *N Engl J Med.* 2010;363:879-881.

The Association Between Age and Nephrosclerosis on Renal Biopsy Among Healthy Adults

Rule AD, Amer H, Cornell LD, et al (Mayo Clinic, Rochester, MN)
Ann Intern Med 152:561-567, 2010

Background.—Chronic kidney disease is common with older age and is characterized on renal biopsy by global glomerulosclerosis, tubular atrophy, interstitial fibrosis, and arteriosclerosis.

Objective.—To see whether the prevalence of these histologic abnormalities in the kidney increases with age in healthy adults and whether histologic findings are explained by age-related differences in kidney function or chronic kidney disease risk factors.

Design.—Cross-sectional study.

Setting.—Mayo Clinic, Rochester, Minnesota, from 1999 to 2009.

Patients.—1203 adult living kidney donors.

Measurements.—Core-needle biopsy of the renal cortex obtained during surgical implantation of the kidney, and medical record data of kidney function and risk factors obtained before donation.

Results.—The prevalence of nephrosclerosis (≥ 2 chronic histologic abnormalities) was 2.7% (95% CI, 1.1% to 6.7%) for patients aged 18 to 29 years, 16% (CI, 12% to 20%) for patients aged 30 to 39 years, 28% (CI, 24% to 32%) for patients aged 40 to 49 years, 44% (CI, 38% to 50%) for patients aged 50 to 59 years, 58% (CI, 47% to 67%) for patients aged 60 to 69 years, and 73% (CI, 43% to 90%) for patients aged 70 to 77 years. Adjustment for kidney function and risk factor covariates did not explain the age-related increase in the prevalence of nephrosclerosis.

Limitation.—Kidney donors are selected for health and lack the spectrum or severity of renal pathologic findings in the general population.

Conclusion.—Kidney function and chronic kidney disease risk factors do not explain the strong association between age and nephrosclerosis in healthy adults.

► It may seem a bit strange including an article about the association between age and nephrosclerosis found on renal biopsy among healthy adults in this series. This report, however, is important to our understanding of renal transplantation in children because a healthy adult is frequently a kidney donor source for youngsters. These adults are usually selected as volunteer donors on the basis of having had normal kidney function. Age is the strongest predictor of chronic kidney disease as assessed by the presence of nephrosclerosis on renal biopsy and/or decreased glomerular filtration rate (GFR). Chronic kidney disease is reported to be present among 47% of adults who are 70 years or older, compared with 4% of adults who are 20 to 39 years of age.[1] The underlying cause of chronic kidney disease is often unclear. The cost, discomfort, illness, and lack of perceived benefit restrict the use of renal biopsy to determine the cause of chronic renal disease in the average adult. The reduction in GFR is suspected to be age related and may reflect chronic histologic abnormalities on renal biopsy, changes that might include global glomerulosclerosis, tubular atrophy, interstitial fibrosis, and arteriosclerosis, which together are frequently described as nephrosclerosis. These histologic abnormalities are clearly associated with reduced GFR and risk for kidney failure among patients with clinically diagnosed chronic renal disease and transplant recipients. Mild nephrosclerosis is also known to occur with aging in autopsy series, but whether nephrosclerosis occurs in older adults with normal kidney function and without chronic renal disease risk factors is unknown. The important aspect of this is that it would be good to know whether a kidney that is being transplanted from an adult into another adult or a child from a donor who presumably has normal kidney function, in fact, might or might not already have evidence of nephrosclerosis.

This report from the Mayo Clinic provides significant insights into this issue. Living kidney donors provide the unique opportunity to relate clinical changes in kidney function to renal histologic findings. Since kidney donors are selected on the basis of good health, the spectrum and severity of renal pathologic findings has been limited. What the investigators from the Mayo Clinic have done is to determine whether the prevalence of histologic abnormalities in the kidney increases with age in otherwise healthy adult kidney donors and whether these findings are explained by age-related differences in kidney function or chronic kidney risk factors. Core-needle biopsies of a donor kidney were undertaken at the time of transplant. These donors all had GFRs that were greater than the lower limit of normal (5th percentile) and had no evidence of microalbinuria. Excluded were potential donors with diabetes mellitus or those with glucose intolerance. Among these otherwise healthy adult donors, the prevalence of nephrosclerosis increased linearly from 2.7% for those 18 to 29 years of age to 73% for those aged 70 to 77 years. These findings reveal a subclinical age-related nephropathy that is not detected by existing clinical tests other than renal biopsy.

So what is the bottom line here? The bottom line has importance for both the donor and the recipient of a kidney transplant. Without doubt, there is an association between age and nephrosclerosis in otherwise healthy adults with normal GFRs who are donating kidneys. This phenomenon is not explained by differences in chronic renal disease risk factors, urinary albumin excretion, or GFR itself. While it is probably not reasonable to biopsy in vivo an otherwise normal adult kidney donor prior to removal of the kidney for transplant purposes, the data from this report do raise some interesting questions. What happens to an adult who has a kidney removed who already has evidence of nephrosclerosis? Will this donor over time develop chronic renal disease in a more accelerated manner than the person who has 2 kidneys? What happens to a kidney recipient who receives a less than perfect kidney from an adult with normal renal function if that kidney already manifests evidence of nephrosclerosis? There are no answers to these questions at this time, but thanks to the work of the folks at Mayo Clinic, we now have a heads up on what to look for in both the donor and the recipient.

J. A. Stockman III, MD

Reference

1. Coresh J, Selvin E, Stevens LA, et al. Prevalence of chronic kidney disease in the United States. *JAMA*. 2007;298:2038-2047.

Meta-analysis: Erythropoiesis-Stimulating Agents in Patients With Chronic Kidney Disease

Palmer SC, Navaneethan SD, Craig JC, et al (Univ of Otago, Christchurch, New Zealand; Cleveland Clinic, OH; Univ of Sydney and George Inst for International Health, Sydney, Australia; et al)
Ann Intern Med 153:23-33, 2010

Background.—Previous meta-analyses suggest that treatment with erythropoiesis-stimulating agents (ESAs) in chronic kidney disease (CKD) increases the risk for death. Additional randomized trials have been recently completed.

Purpose.—To summarize the effects of ESA treatment on clinical outcomes in patients with anemia and CKD.

Data Sources.—MEDLINE (January 1966 to November 2009), EMBASE (January 1980 to November 2009), and the Cochrane database (to March 2010) were searched without language restriction.

Study Selection.—Two authors independently screened reports to identify randomized trials evaluating ESA treatment in people with CKD. Hemoglobin target trials or trials of ESA versus no treatment or placebo were included.

Data Extraction.—Two authors independently extracted data on patient characteristics, study risks for bias, and the effects of ESA therapy.

Data Synthesis.—27 trials (10 452 patients) were identified. A higher hemoglobin target was associated with increased risks for stroke (relative risk [RR], 1.51 [95% CI, 1.03 to 2.21]), hypertension (RR, 1.67 [CI, 1.31 to 2.12]), and vascular access thrombosis (RR, 1.33 [CI, 1.16 to 1.53]) compared with a lower hemoglobin target. No statistically significant differences in the risks for mortality (RR, 1.09 [CI, 0.99 to 1.20]), serious cardiovascular events (RR, 1.15 [CI, 0.98 to 1.33]), or end-stage kidney disease (RR, 1.08 [CI, 0.97 to 1.20]) were observed, although point estimates favored a lower hemoglobin target. Treatment effects were consistent across subgroups, including all stages of CKD.

Limitations.—The evidence for effects on quality of life was limited by selective reporting. Trials also reported insufficient information to allow analysis of the independent effects of ESA dose on clinical outcomes.

Conclusion.—Targeting higher hemoglobin levels in CKD increases risks for stroke, hypertension, and vascular access thrombosis and probably increases risks for death, serious cardiovascular events, and end-stage renal disease. The mechanisms for harm remain unclear, and meta-analysis of individual-patient data and trials on fixed ESA doses are recommended to elucidate these mechanisms.

▶ This is another report emanating from adult studies that could have an influence on the care of children with chronic renal disease. Almost 20 years ago we began to see early clinical trials first evaluating the use of recombinant human erythropoietin replacement therapy in patients with chronic renal disease. These early trials did demonstrate dose-dependent increases in hemoglobin levels and the avoidance of red blood cell transfusions, but they also began to report an increased incidence of hypertension and vascular thrombosis. Subsequent studies over the years have concluded that erythropoietin treatment is associated with some improvement in quality of life but at the expense of an increased risk of hypertension and vascular thrombosis. The review of Palmer et al summarizes the benefits and harms of treating uremia with an erythropoietin-stimulating agent using cumulative data in the form of a meta-analysis. The results are quite compelling.

Palmer et al identify 27 randomized clinical trials of patients with chronic kidney disease who were being treated with erythropoiesis-stimulating agents to achieve certain levels of hemoglobin. The authors found that treatment with either erythropoietin or darbepoetin to higher target hemoglobin levels in patients with chronic kidney disease at any stage increases the risk for stroke, worsens hypertension, and carries a greater risk of vascular access thrombosis, compared with treatment to lower hemoglobin targets. The authors found no statistically significant differences between higher and lower hemoglobin targets for the risk of all-cause mortality, serious cardiovascular complications, or end-stage kidney disease but estimates for all outcomes favored a lower hemoglobin target and effectively excluded the likelihood of any clinically relevant benefit for a higher hemoglobin target. Targeting a higher hemoglobin level was linked to a reduction in need for blood transfusions but a greater demand for intravenous iron therapy. Most importantly, there were no clinically important effects of erythropoiesis-stimulating agents on quality of life.

Thus it is, when it comes to adults, evidence for harm when targeting higher hemoglobin values in chronic kidney disease patients has now been available for more than 2 decades, and this evidence is being incorporated into adult care guidelines and clinical practice. Children are much less likely to die of complications such as hypertension causing stroke in comparison with adults, but they certainly can develop vascular access problems related to thrombosis of catheters. We should pay careful attention to these adult studies to see what is important to the care of children.

J. A. Stockman III, MD

A Randomized, Controlled Trial of Early versus Late Initiation of Dialysis

Cooper BA, for the IDEAL Study (Univ of Sydney, NSW, Australia; et al)
N Engl J Med 363:609-619, 2010

Background.—In clinical practice, there is considerable variation in the timing of the initiation of maintenance dialysis for patients with stage V chronic kidney disease, with a worldwide trend toward early initiation. In this study, conducted at 32 centers in Australia and New Zealand, we examined whether the timing of the initiation of maintenance dialysis influenced survival among patients with chronic kidney disease.

Methods.—We randomly assigned patients 18 years of age or older with progressive chronic kidney disease and an estimated glomerular filtration rate (GFR) between 10.0 and 15.0 ml per minute per 1.73 m² of body-surface area (calculated with the use of the Cockcroft–Gault equation) to planned initiation of dialysis when the estimated GFR was 10.0 to 14.0 ml per minute (early start) or when the estimated GFR was 5.0 to 7.0 ml per minute (late start). The primary outcome was death from any cause.

Results.—Between July 2000 and November 2008, a total of 828 adults (mean age, 60.4 years; 542 men and 286 women; 355 with diabetes) underwent randomization, with a median time to the initiation of dialysis of 1.80 months (95% confidence interval [CI], 1.60 to 2.23) in the early-start group and 7.40 months (95% CI, 6.23 to 8.27) in the late-start group. A total of 75.9% of the patients in the late-start group initiated dialysis when the estimated GFR was above the target of 7.0 ml per minute, owing to the development of symptoms. During a median follow-up period of 3.59 years, 152 of 404 patients in the early-start group (37.6%) and 155 of 424 in the late-start group (36.6%) died (hazard ratio with early initiation, 1.04; 95% CI, 0.83 to 1.30; P = 0.75). There was no significant difference between the groups in the frequency of adverse events (cardiovascular events, infections, or complications of dialysis).

Conclusions.—In this study, planned early initiation of dialysis in patients with stage V chronic kidney disease was not associated with an improvement in survival or clinical outcomes. (Funded by the National Health and Medical Research Council of Australia and others; Australian New Zealand Clinical Trials Registry number, 12609000266268.)

▶ This report obviously emanates from a study of adults with renal failure. Although the data referred to patients aged 18 years or older with progressive chronic renal disease, there is a lot to be learned that perhaps can be applied to children as well.

It has been more than half a century since renal replacement therapy for end-stage renal disease has been a matter of routine. Still, the optimal timing for the initiation of dialysis remains highly debated. In recent times, there has been a trend toward initiating dialysis at a relatively high estimated glomerular filtration rate (GFR), based on the assumption that starting dialysis early may avert the many medical and social problems associated with advanced uremia. The decision when to initiate dialysis is even more nebulous in children because some of the manifestations of uremia in childhood are not seen in adults, such as growth retardation. Fifteen years ago, in the adult population, only 1 in 5 patients would begin renal dialysis if the GFR was higher than 10 ml per minute per 1.73 m² of body surface area, but within 10 years, a good half of adults with renal failure would have dialysis initiated at this level. Given the fact that care for patients with end-stage renal disease requires a massive economic commitment of human resources for dialysis purposes, premature initiation of renal replacement therapy has a major impact on societal costs and on the daily life of a patient, given the personal burden of dialysis. Thus the defining of the optimal timing for initiation of dialysis is extremely important.

Cooper et al report results from the Initiating Dialysis Early And Late (IDEAL) study, a multicenter, randomized, and controlled trial in which those aged 18 years and older who had progressive end-stage renal disease and were already receiving care in nephrology units were assigned to planned initiation of hemodialysis or peritoneal dialysis when the estimated GFR was either 10 mL to 14 mL per minute per 1.73 m^2 (early start) or 5 mL to 7 mL per minute per 1.73 m^2 (late start). The patients in these 2 study groups were well matched with respect to baseline characteristics, including other diseases or complications of renal failure. After a period of about 3.5 years follow-up, patient survival and the frequency of adverse events were not significantly different between the 2 groups; however, there was a 6-month separation between the groups in the start of dialysis. The important conclusion of the study was that waiting to initiate dialysis until signs of uremia appear does not jeopardize the patient and that starting renal-replacement therapy on the basis of a predefined estimated GFR value does not necessarily improve outcome. Because the IDEAL study considered both estimated GFR and symptoms, the results of the study are difficult to compare with those of previous registry studies in which the decision to start dialysis early or late was based on estimated GFR alone, not on the presence of symptoms of uremia.

The main conclusion of this important study—that asymptomatic patients with renal replacement therapy can be delayed by an average of 6 months—should be placed in perspective. This is commented upon in an editorial by Lameire and van Biesen.[1] An important prerequisite for a wait-and-see policy is careful clinical follow-up of each patient to avoid some of the life-threatening complications of uremia that may necessitate immediate renal replacement therapy. The study protocol explicitly advocated that the method of dialysis be selected ahead of time and a functioning peritoneal or vascular access be prepared in advance, a policy that permits the immediate initiation of dialysis if the patient becomes symptomatic. Temporary and urgently placed dialysis catheters have a much higher risk of infection and stenosis.

The IDEAL trial supports the practice of many adult nephrologists who start patients on renal replacement therapy on the basis of clinical factors rather than solely on numerical criteria such as an estimated GFR alone. While these data are difficult to apply to children, one wonders if a similar philosophy applies and whether a clinical study, if one is possible, of the same sort in children should be undertaken.

We close this commentary related to endstage renal disease with an observation reported in 2011 in the *British Medical Journal* related to comments made by the United Kingdom's Chief Rabbi, Jonathan Sacks. Rabbi Sacks issued an edict that carrying donor cards is unacceptable and that the current organ donor system is incompatible with Jewish law. The ruling comes after years of debate among rabbinical authorities over the definition of death and when an organ may be removed for transplant purposes. The statement says that organs may be removed for transplantation only at the point of cardiorespiratory failure, rather than at brain stem death. In Great Britain, recent data show that 66% of donations came from donors after brain death and 34% from donors after cardiovascular death. Rabbi Sacks' statement did indicate that a living person may donate an organ, such as a kidney, to save someone else's life, providing that the donor does not put his or her own life at major risk. Jewish law also permits donation after death as long as the organ is needed for immediate transplantation. To read more about this topic, including that the numbers of patients in Israel who die while waiting for a transplant has risen at a time when the number of transplantations fell by 20%, see the discussion of these topics that appeared this past year in the *British Medical Journal.*[2,3]

J. A. Stockman III, MD

References

1. Lameire N, Van Biesen W. The initiation of renal-replacement therapy—just-in-time delivery. *N Engl J Med.* 2010;363:678-680.
2. Wise J. Rabbi says brain stem death is not enough for organ donation. *BMJ.* 2011; 342:d275.
3. Traubmann T. Transplantations fall in Israel as new law complicates procedures. *BMJ.* 2011;342:d332.

Regulated Payments for Living Kidney Donation: An Empirical Assessment of the Ethical Concerns
Halpern SD, Raz A, Kohn R, et al (Univ of Pennsylvania School of Medicine and Philadelphia Veterans Affairs Med Ctr)
Ann Intern Med 152:358-365, 2010

Background.—Although regulated payments to encourage living kidney donation could reduce morbidity and mortality among patients waiting for a kidney transplant, doing so raises several ethical concerns.

Objective.—To determine the extent to which the 3 main concerns with paying kidney donors might manifest if a regulated market were created.

Design.—Cross-sectional study of participants' willingness to donate a kidney in 12 scenarios.

Setting.—Regional rail and urban trolley lines in Philadelphia County, Philadelphia, Pennsylvania.

Participants.—Of 550 potential participants, 409 completed the questionnaire (response rate, 74.4%); 342 of these participants were medically eligible to donate.

Intervention.—Across scenarios, researchers experimentally manipulated the amount of money that participants would receive, the participants' risk for subsequently developing kidney failure themselves, and who would receive the donated kidney.

Measurements.—The researchers determined whether payment represents an undue inducement by evaluating participants' sensitivity to risk in relation to the payment offered or an unjust inducement by evaluating participants' sensitivity to payment as a function of their annual income. The researchers also evaluated whether introducing payment would hinder altruistic donations by comparing participants' willingness to donate altruistically before versus after the introduction of payments.

Results.—Generalized estimating equation models revealed that participants' willingness to donate increased significantly as their risk for kidney failure decreased, as the payment offered increased, and when the kidney recipient was a family member rather than a patient on a public waiting list ($P < 0.001$ for each). No statistical interactions were identified between payment and risk (odds ratio, 1.00 [95% CI, 0.96 to 1.03]) or between payment and income (odds ratio, 1.01 [CI, 0.99 to 1.03]). The proximity of these estimates to 1.0 and narrowness of the CIs suggest that payment is neither an undue nor an unjust inducement, respectively. Alerting participants to the possibility of payment did not alter their willingness to donate for altruistic reasons ($P = 0.40$).

Limitation.—Choices revealed in hypothetical scenarios may not reflect real-world behaviors.

Conclusion.—Theoretical concerns about paying persons for living kidney donation are not corroborated by empirical evidence. A real-world test of regulated payments for kidney donation is needed to definitively show whether payment provides a viable and ethical method to increase the supply of kidneys available for transplantation.

▶ The ethical issues surrounding whether we should or should not be paying living kidney donors for their kidney donation have been around for some time. Given the fact that there is an insufficient supply of transplantable kidneys from traditional donors after neurologic determination of death, other donor sources have been sought. Such donors have included donors after circulatory determination of death, donors with risk factors for harboring transmittable infections, expanded-criteria donors (that is, those with risk factors such as older age or hypertension), and living donors related or unrelated to the recipient. Despite these efforts to increase the pool of kidneys, the median time to transplantation, number of patients on the waiting list, and number of patients who die while waiting for an organ continue to increase. For these reasons, ethicists and members of the transplant community have debated paying healthy persons to become living donors. International black markets in organs are almost universally condemned because safeguards to protect donors are largely absent, brokers rather than donors may commandeer most of the payments, and such systems almost invariably entail wealthy travelers purchasing organs from poor natives.

So should there be a regulated national market for kidneys in which donors receive payments according to a fixed and transparent schedule where organs are allocated according to standard criteria, and standards are set and monitored to ensure appropriate longitudinal care for donors? In a purely monetary sense, paying a donor to obtain a kidney makes sense because the payment cost is far offset by decreased medical expenses on the part of the recipient who has to be maintained on dialysis for a longer period of time. Even payments as high as $100 000 are estimated to be cost effective.

What is the rub with paying a potential kidney donor for his/her kidney? At least 3 concerns have been raised by ethicists. The first is that payments may represent undue inducements; payments might alter a person's perception of the risks associated with donation thereby preventing a fully informed decision to sell a kidney. Second, payments may represent unjust inducements; payments might preferentially induce lower income people, thereby creating a market in which organs are acquired from poor people and provided to those with sufficient financial and social resources to be listed for transplantation. Third, payments may dissuade altruistic donation or cause potential altruistic donors to request payment. Halpern et al used empirical methods to determine the extent to which these concerns might manifest if a regulated market for kidneys was established in the United States. The researchers surveyed people using Philadelphia-area public transportation about whether they would donate a kidney under a range of scenarios that did and did not include various payments. Responses suggested that payment would not create undue or unjust incentives for donation or alter a person's willingness to donate or to help another person without payment. Some 550 passengers on the rail system in and around Philadelphia were asked to participate in this survey. Specifically, the investigators found that providing payments did not dull a person's sensitivity to the risk associated with donor nephrectomy, suggesting that payment does not represent an undue inducement—one that would make rational choice difficult. It also appeared that providing a payment would not preferentially motivate a poor person to sell a kidney. Interestingly, it was noted that poor persons were more willing to donate a kidney independent of payment. Also, there was no evidence found that introducing monetary incentives would crowd out a person's altruistic incentives to donate.

The authors of this report caution that the participants' responses to hypothetical offers may not reflect the decisions they would make if they were actually offered payment for kidney. Nonetheless, the study adds evidence to what has been largely a theoretical debate about the propriety of paying people to become kidney donors. The results both corroborate predictions that payments could effectively increase the supply of transplantable kidneys and cast doubts on intuitions that payments would be undue or unjust or would undermine a person's otherwise altruistic behaviors.

Interestingly, Israel is taking a somewhat different approach to increasing the donor pool of kidneys. Israel's parliament passed a law that became effective in January 2010 that granted donor-card holders priority in organ allocation, with the aim of increasing the number of organ donations and reducing the length of the transplantation waiting list. Anyone willing to sign a donor card, should that person ultimately need an organ themselves later in life, would receive some preferential treatment. Not only does the person with the donor card receive such treatment, but also first-degree relatives would get priority in organ allocation.[1]

One final comment about organ donation, this regarding new rules in Great Britain. Until recently, it has not been possible in England for a donor to specifically name someone who wants to receive their organs. This was based on the fundamental principle of the United Kingdom donation program, which is that organs are given freely, voluntarily, and unconditionally. The belief has been that donation must not depend on whether the donors are wanting their organs to go to a specific relative or friend; instead organs had to be donated on the understanding that they would go to whoever was most in need—even though a complete stranger might be the recipient, rather than a family member who was in need. With the new regulations, a targeted donation can be made. The change in the rules follows a case in 2008 when a mother, who needed a kidney replacement after developing complications from diabetes, could not use the organs from her daughter who had died during an asthma attack. The daughter had indicated that should anything happen to her she wished her kidneys to be given to her mother. Instead, when the 21-year-old passed away, her kidneys went to others on the transplant list deemed to have more urgent need. According to the current law, an individual with a super urgent heart or liver transplant need who would not live past 72 hours would still get priority over any request to donate an organ to family or close friends.[2]

This commentary closes with an observation about a subject raised earlier in this chapter: medical donations of body parts. The great recession has changed the way many people live, and the repercussions appear to be altering how some people have chosen to die. At least 2 prominent tissue banks have seen an increase in the number of individuals who are interested in donating their bodies to research in exchange for a break in funeral cost. The Banner Sun Health Research Institute near Phoenix typically receives some 1000 inquiries every year about making donations. That number has increased by 15% since the beginning of the 2008 recession and a list of donors has lengthened. It appears that with devaluation of retirement funds, home values, etc, some are looking at alternative ways of financing their funeral arrangements. Savings from forgoing even a cremation can range from $1000 to $1500. The Anatomy Gifts Registration, a nonprofit in Glen Burnie, Maryland, that supplies tissue for medical research has seen donor calls increase from 150 per month to as many as 400, largely related to people trying to offset high funeral costs. To read more about this trend, see the editorial by Stix.[3]

J. A. Stockman III, MD

References

1. Lavee J, Ashkenazi T, German G, Steinberg D. A new law for allocation of donor organs in Israel. *Lancet.* 2010;375:1131-1133.
2. Eaton L. New guidance allows donors to name who receives their organs when they die. *BMJ.* 2010;340:778.
3. Stix G. Donate your brain, save a buck: Hard times are making tissue donation more appealing. *Scientific American.* January 4, 2011:29.

Dextranomer/Hyaluronic Acid for Pediatric Vesicoureteral Reflux: Systematic Review

Routh JC, Inman BA, Reinberg Y (Children's Hosp Boston, MA; Duke Univ Med Ctr, Durham, NC; Children's Hosps and Clinics of Minnesota, Minneapolis)
Pediatrics 125:1010-1019, 2010

Objective.—Published success rates of dextranomer/hyaluronic acid (Dx/HA) injection for pediatric vesicoureteral reflux (VUR) vary widely.

Our objective of this study was to assess whether underlying patient or study factors could explain the heterogeneity in reported Dx/HA success rates.

Methods.—We searched the Cochrane Controlled Trials Register and Medline, Embase, and Scopus databases from 1990 to 2008 for reports in any language, along with a hand search of included study bibliographies. Articles were assessed and data abstracted in duplicate, and differences were resolved by consensus. Conflict of interest (COI) was determined by published disclosure. Meta-regression was performed to adjust for patient as well as study-level factors.

Results.—We identified 1157 reports, 89 of which were reviewed in full with 47 included in the pooled analysis. Of 7303 ureters that were injected with Dx/HA, 5633 (77%) were successfully treated according to the authors' definition. Injection success seemed to vary primarily on the basis of the preoperative reflux grade. After adjustment for VUR grade, other factors, such as the presence or absence of COI disclosure, were not significant. Studies were markedly heterogeneous overall.

Conclusions.—The overall per-ureter Dx/HA success rate was 77% after 3 months, although success rates varied widely among studies. Increased VUR grade negatively affected success rates, whereas COI, patient age, and injected Dx/HA volume were not significantly associated with treatment outcome after adjustment for VUR grade. There is a significant need for improved reporting of VUR treatments, including comparative studies of Dx/HA and other VUR treatments.

▶ This is not the first report to tell us about dextranomer/hyaluronic acid (Dx/HA) copolymer use for endoscopic injection in children with grade 2 to 4 vesicoureteral reflux (VUR). Dx/HA has been around since 2001, when the Food and Drug Administration approved its use for VUR. When injected into the right place in a ureter, this synthetic product is capable of diminishing the degree of reflux that a patient may have. As a result of the minimally invasive nature of Dx/HA treatment, its use has rapidly increased. Indeed, the reported low morbidity of Dx/HA injection has prompted some investigators to recommend it as a first-line alternative to traditional therapeutic standards of antibiotic prophylaxis or ureteroneocystostomy in spite of the lack of good data to support its use.

Routh et al have undertaken a systematic review to evaluate the accumulated literature on the surgical treatment of pediatric VUR by using Dx/HA. As part of this review they also attempted to determine the extent to which reported success rates were influenced by VUR grade, other underlying patient- or study-level factors, and any stated conflicts of interests of the urologists reporting results. The importance of conflicts of interest has not been addressed to any degree in the setting of pediatric urologic research. A number of authors of studies using Dx/HA stated openly and transparently potential conflicts of interests when reporting their data. More than 1100 reports were reviewed as part of the systematic review, and of 7303 ureters that were injected with Dx/HA, 77% were stated to have been successfully managed. The only variable that influenced success rates was the degree of VUR. Other factors, such as the stated presence of conflicts of interest, did not influence the success rate in these reports.

It does appear that when used sensibly and in seasoned hands, Dx/HA endoscopic injection may be the safe way to go to manage the average patient with VUR, assuming guidelines are met for the grade of VUR treated.

J. A. Stockman III, MD

Risk of Renal Scarring in Children With a First Urinary Tract Infection: A Systematic Review
Shaikh N, Ewing AL, Bhatnagar S, et al (Univ of Pittsburgh School of Medicine, PA)
Pediatrics 126:1084-1091, 2010

Background.—To our knowledge, the risk of renal scarring in children with a urinary tract infection (UTI) has not been systematically studied.

Objective.—To review the prevalence of acute and chronic renal imaging abnormalities in children after an initial UTI.

Methods.—We searched Medline and Embase for English-, French-, and Spanish-language articles using the following terms: "Technetium ^{99m}Tc dimercaptosuccinic acid (DMSA)," "DMSA," "dimercaptosuccinic," "scintigra*," "pyelonephritis," and "urinary tract infection." We included articles if they reported data on the prevalence of abnormalities on acute-phase (≤15 days) or follow-up (>5 months) DMSA renal scans in children aged 0 to 18 years after an initial UTI. Two evaluators independently reviewed data from each article.

Results.—Of 1533 articles found by the search strategy, 325 full-text articles were reviewed; 33 studies met all inclusion criteria. Among children with an initial episode of UTI, 57% (95% confidence interval [CI]: 50—64) had changes consistent with acute pyelonephritis on the acute-phase DMSA renal scan and 15% (95% CI: 11—18) had evidence of renal scarring on the follow-up DMSA scan. Children with vesicoureteral reflux (VUR) were significantly more likely to develop pyelonephritis (relative risk [RR]: 1.5 [95% CI: 1.1—1.9]) and renal scarring (RR: 2.6 [95% CI: 1.7—3.9]) compared with children with no VUR. Children with VUR grades III or higher were more likely to develop scarring than children with lower grades of VUR (RR: 2.1 [95% CI: 1.4—3.2]).

Conclusions.—The pooled prevalence values provided from this study provide a basis for an evidence-based approach to the management of children with this frequently occurring condition.

► This report represents a systematic review of the literature that examines the prognosis of children with urinary tract infections (UTIs), providing guidelines to allow for evidence-based decisions when caring for children with UTI. One of the most frequently asked questions with a youngster's first UTI is whether that youngster is likely to have any long-term consequences, specifically renal scarring.

One of the areas reviewed in this report was the prevalence of acute-phase dimercaptosuccinic acid (DMSA) scan abnormalities occurring with a first UTI. Overall, 57% of children with an initial episode of UTI had evidence of DMSA scan abnormalities consistent with pyelonephritis. Children with vesicourethral reflux (VUR) were 1.5 times more likely than children with no VUR to exhibit findings consistent with acute pyelonephritis. We also learn from this report that the overall incidence of UTI recurrence per year runs 8% and that the overall prevalence of renal scarring 5 to 24 months after an initial episode of UTI is 18%. Long-term renal scarring was 2.1 times more likely in children with grades III to V VUR than among children with grades I and II VUR (53% vs 25%). Approximately 25% of children with a first UTI had VUR, 2.5% had high grade (IV or V) VUR, and less than 1% had preexisting renal scarring and/or dysplasia. Approximately 15% of children overall with a first UTI showed evidence of renal scarring 5 to 24 months later.

The authors of this report remind us that although they found that the identification of VUR is important, VUR is neither necessary nor sufficient for the development of renal scarring. In fact, their analysis clearly shows that most acute pyelonephritis and renal scarring occur in children with no VUR. The authors strongly remind us that because VUR is not the only risk factor for renal scarring, a sole focus on VUR, as has been the dominant strategy for decades, is unlikely to result in large reductions in rates of renal scarring. We can also see from this report that the low rate of preexisting abnormalities suggests that the yield of routine ultrasonography in children who present with an initial UTI and who have no known genitourinary abnormalities on prenatal ultrasonography is likely to be low, which is in agreement with a great deal of recent literature, indicating that ultrasonography modifies management in less than 1% of cases. Although routine voiding cystourethrograms are quite accurate in identifying children with VUR, they are both expensive and invasive and will miss a significant proportion of children who are at risk for renal scarring. DMSA scans are expensive and invasive and expose children to radiation and therefore should be used quite wisely. Furthermore, although 57% of all children with UTIs in this series had positive DMSA scan results, indicating the presence of acute pyelonephritis, most of these children (85%) will not scar, thus diminishing any predictive value of the DMSA scan.

Although this report does not provide us with any clear pathway to firmly manage children with initial UTI, the report is loaded with important new information. Fortunately, the prevalence of long-term renal scarring appears to be diminishing over time, which is most likely the result of the early detection of certain renal abnormalities on prenatal ultrasound. This still leaves us with the problem of children who have no known anatomical disease who will go on to develop both UTIs and renal scarring.

This commentary closes with the interesting observation that scientists have now engineered autologous urethras for patients in need of reconstructive surgery. Complex urethral problems can occur as a result of injury, disease, or congenital defects and treatment options are often limited. Urethras, similar to other long tubularized tissues, can stricture after reconstruction. Investigators from North Carolina and Mexico City have assessed the effectiveness of tissue-engineered urethras using patient's own cells in individuals who need urethral reconstruction. Five boys who had urethral defects were included in the study. A tissue biopsy was taken from each patient, and the muscle and epithelial cells were expanded and seeded onto tissue engineered tubularized scaffolds. Patients then underwent urethral reconstruction with the tubularized urethras. Urethral biopsies taken long after the surgery showed that the engineered grafts had developed a normal-appearing architecture essentially 3 months after implantation and functioned well for up to 6 years of follow-up.[1]

J. A. Stockman III, MD

Reference

1. Raya-Rivera A, Esquiliano DR, Yoo JJ, Lopez-Bayghen E, Soker S, Atala A. Tissue-engineered autologous urethras for patients who need reconstruction: an observational study. *Lancet.* 2011;377:1175-1182.

Laparoscopic inguinal hernia repair in the pediatric age group—experience with 437 children

Parelkar SV, Oak S, Gupta R, et al (King Edward Memorial Hosp, Parel, Mumbai, India)
J Pediatr Surg 45:789-792, 2010

Background/Purpose.—A retrospective analysis of prospectively collected data of pediatric patients that underwent laparoscopic inguinal hernia repair.

Material and Methods.—A retrospective review was performed of the prospectively collected data of 576 laparoscopic internal ring closures in 437 children (age, 30 days-11 years; median, 1.9 years) from June 1999 to February 2009. The internal ring was closed with a 3-0 nonabsorbable suture. Both extracorporeal and intracorporeal methods of knotting were used. All patients were asked to return at 1 week and 6 weeks postoperatively for routine follow-up.

Results.—A contralateral patent processus vaginalis was present in 13% (45/352) of boys and 15% (12/83) of girls on the right side, and 7% (25/352) of boys and 6% (5/83) of girls on the left side. Follow-up range was from 1 week postoperatively to 108 months. There were 14 recurrences (2.4 % [14/576], 11 in boys and on the right side and 3 in girls) and 2 hydroceles 0.35% (2/576). Mean operating time was 23 minutes for unilateral and 29 minutes for bilateral inguinal hernia. There was neither metachronus hernia nor testicular atrophy observed during follow-up.

Conclusion.—Laparoscopic inguinal hernia repair is technically easier, as there is no need to dissect the vas deferens and vessels. The risk of metachronous hernia is reduced, and we believe the cosmetic result is better. Although recurrences were more common early in the series, currently they are much less frequent. Laparoscopic inguinal hernia repair appears to have less morbidity than open herniotomy and can be used as routine procedure in the pediatric age group.

▶ Increasingly, we are reading reports about the use of laparoscopic techniques being widely used in a variety of various common pediatric surgical conditions. Questions have been raised about the pros and cons of laparoscopy versus open surgical techniques. Concerns have centered on whether the laparoscopic procedure is more time consuming. Does it pose a risk to the patient since, in certain procedures such as hernia repair, it violates the peritoneal cavity, and does it result in a higher recurrence rate? This report from India helps address some of these issues, looking at more than 500 inguinal hernia repairs performed laparoscopically over a 10-year period. The recurrence rate with this technique was found to be just 2.4% in boys and much less in girls. A very small percentage (0.35%) resulted in hydrocele formation. The mean operating time was just 23 minutes for unilateral and 29 minutes for bilateral inguinal hernia.

In a related article, Lee et al[1] examined the cost effectiveness of doing a laparoscopic examination of the opposite groin when performing a hernia repair. The answer was yes. It appears that transinguinal laparoscopy at the time of unilateral inguinal hernia repair is both safe and effective as a method of exploring the contralateral groin. This method is superior to open contralateral inguinal exploration, as it minimizes the risk of damaging the spermatic cord and obviously eliminates the need for a second operation to repair a contralateral inguinal hernia. The authors of the report offer this to the parents of all patients undergoing laparoscopic inguinal hernia repair. It adds only a few minutes to the operating time.

In conclusion, we highlight recent recommendations that have emanated from the US Preventive Services Task Force related to screening for testicular cancer. The Task Force makes recommendations about preventative care services. It bases its recommendations on systematic reviews of evidence of the benefits and harms and an assessment of the net benefit of the service. In its most recent recommendations on screening for testicular cancer, as reported in 2011, the Task Force recommended against screening for testicular cancer in adolescent or adult males. The recommendation recognizes that there is inadequate evidence that screening asymptomatic patients by means of self-examination or clinician examination has greater yield or accuracy for detecting testicular cancer at more curable stages. Currently, regardless of disease stage, more than 90% of all newly diagnosed cases of testicular cancer will be cured. Screening by self-examination or clinician examination is unlikely to offer meaningful health benefits, given the very low incidence and high cure rate of even advanced testicular cancer. Potential harms include false-positive results, anxiety, and harm from diagnostic tests or procedures. Even before this report appeared, the American Academy of Family Physicians recommended against routine screening for testicular cancer in asymptomatic adolescent and adult males. The American Academy of Pediatrics does not include screening for testicular cancer in its recommendations for preventive care. Finally, the American Cancer Society does not recommend testicular self-examination. To read more about screening for testicular cancer, see the US Preventive Task Force Report.[2]

J. A. Stockman III, MD

References

1. Lee SL, Sydorak RM, Lau ST. Laparoscopic contralateral groin exploration: is it cost effective? *J Pediatr Surg.* 2010;45:793-795.
2. U.S. Preventive Services Task Force. Screening for testicular cancer: U.S. Preventive Services Task Force reaffirmation recommendation statement. *Ann Intern Med.* 2011;154:483-486.

9 Heart and Blood Vessels

HDL cholesterol and residual risk of first cardiovascular events after treatment with potent statin therapy: an analysis from the JUPITER trial
Ridker PM, for the JUPITER Trial Study Group (Brigham and Women's Hosp, Boston, MA; et al)
Lancet 376:333-339, 2010

Background.—HDL-cholesterol concentrations are inversely associated with occurrence of cardiovascular events. We addressed, using the JUPITER trial cohort, whether this association remains when LDL-cholesterol concentrations are reduced to the very low ranges with high-dose statin treatment.

Methods.—Participants in the randomised placebo-controlled JUPITER trial were adults without diabetes or previous cardiovascular disease, and had baseline concentrations of LDL cholesterol of less than 3·37 mmol/L and high-sensitivity C-reactive protein of 2 mg/L or more. Participants were randomly allocated by a computer-generated sequence to receive rosuvastatin 20 mg per day or placebo, with participants and adjudicators masked to treatment assignment. In the present analysis, we divided the participants into quartiles of HDL-cholesterol or apolipoprotein A1 and sought evidence of association between these quartiles and the JUPITER primary endpoint of first non-fatal myocardial infarction or stroke, hospitalisation for unstable angina, arterial revascularisation, or cardiovascular death. This trial is registered with ClinicalTrials.gov, number NCT00239681.

Findings.—For 17 802 patients in the JUPITER trial, rosuvastatin 20 mg per day reduced the incidence of the primary endpoint by 44% (p<0·0001). In 8901 (50) patients given placebo (who had a median on-treatment LDL-cholesterol concentration of 2·80 mmol/L [IQR 2·43–3·24]), HDL-cholesterol concentrations were inversely related to vascular risk both at baseline (top quartile *vs* bottom quartile hazard ratio [HR] 0·54, 95% CI 0·35–0·83, p=0·0039) and on-treatment (0·55, 0·35–0·87, p=0·0047). By contrast, among the 8900 (50%) patients given rosuvastatin 20 mg (who had a median on-treatment LDL-cholesterol concentration of 1·42 mmol/L [IQR 1·14–1·86]), no significant relationships were noted between quartiles of HDL-cholesterol concentration and vascular risk either at baseline (1·12, 0·62–2·03, p=0·82) or on-treatment (1·03, 0·57–1·87, p=0·97). Our analyses for apolipoprotein A1 showed an equivalent strong relation to frequency of primary outcomes in the placebo group but little association in the rosuvastatin group.

Interpretation.—Although measurement of HDL-cholesterol concentration is useful as part of initial cardiovascular risk assessment, HDL-cholesterol concentrations are not predictive of residual vascular risk among patients treated with potent statin therapy who attain very low concentrations of LDL cholesterol.

▶ This report emanating from the Justification for the Use of Statins in Primary Prevention: An Intervention Trial Evaluating Rosuvastatin (JUPITER) Trial Study Group represents a study done in adults, but such studies have important implications for children in terms of our better understanding of what the long-term outcomes are for those managed with statin therapy. JUPITER represents a randomized, double-blind, placebo-controlled trial to investigate whether a statin (rosuvastatin, 20 mg/d) would decrease the rate of first-ever cardiovascular events compared with placebo in over 17 000 apparently healthy men and women. The study challenges whether high-density lipoprotein (HDL) cholesterol concentrations in fact are predictive of cardiovascular risk when a patient has low concentrations of HDL cholesterol.

Of 17 802 patients in the JUPITER clinical trial who had increased C-reactive protein, but who did not have cardiovascular disease or diabetes, treatment with a statin reduced major adverse cardiovascular events by 44% at 2 years. There was no increased risk of cardiovascular events in those in whom HDL cholesterols were very low (1.4 mmol/L). This suggests that in this group of patients, HDL cholesterol concentrations are not major determinants of residual cardiovascular risk.

If one extrapolates the data from this study to any age group, the implications are straightforward. As of now, there are no good ways to pharmacologically increase HDL levels in those who have low HDL concentrations, a known cardiovascular risk factor. It would appear, however, that in such patients, if you can really drive down the low-density lipoprotein (LDL) cholesterol concentrations, patients will be protected. Whether increasing HDL cholesterol in patients with very low LDL cholesterol has any beneficial effects at all on cardiovascular risk remains to be seen in future large randomized trials.

The bottom line here is that for those adequately managed with statins who have low HDL levels, we might be able to breathe a little easier. This does not mean that lifestyle changes, including more aerobic exercise, weight loss, etc, should not be undertaken to increase HDL cholesterol. Teens should be carefully warned against smoking as well. New drugs are currently being evaluated to raise HDL levels. The most promising are inhibitors of cholesterylester-transfer protein. The most widely studied agent to date, torcetrapib, has had a number of problems associated with its use when used in adults and therefore is not recommended as of this writing.

This commentary concludes with Part I of *Name that Murmur—Eponyms for the Astute Auscultician.* After the introduction of the stethoscope by René Laennec in 1819, the art of auscultation gained popularity as a group of early adopters described the heart murmurs they were able now to hear. A robust crop of eponyms was born for use by future generations of physicians and medical trainees. This chapter will have sprinkled within it eponyms for the astute auscultician. To read more about the murmurs described, see the occasional notes by Ma and Tierney.[1]

Eponyms for the *Astute Auscultician,* Part I: Austin Flint Murmur: Austin Flint was an American physician practicing in the early mid-19th century and a true pioneer in medical education. He cofounded 2 medical schools: Buffalo Medical College (now State University of New York at Buffalo) and Bellview Medical College (which later joined the New York University College of Medicine). He published more than 200 articles in his professional career. The Austin Flint murmur is a mid-diastolic rumbling sound present in selected cases of nonrheumatic aortic regurgitation. The sound is indistinguishable from mitral stenosis.[2]

J. A. Stockman III, MD

References

1. Ma I, Tierney LM. Name that murmur—eponyms for the astute auscultician. *N Engl J Med.* 2010;363:2164-2168.
2. Flint A. On cardiac murmur. *Am J Med Sci.* 1862;44:29-54.

Safety and efficacy of long-term statin treatment for cardiovascular events in patients with coronary heart disease and abnormal liver tests in the Greek Atorvastatin and Coronary Heart Disease Evaluation (GREACE) Study: a post-hoc analysis

Athyros VG, for the GREACE Study Collaborative Group (Aristotle Univ of Thessaloniki, Greece; et al)
Lancet 376:1916-1922, 2010

Background.—Long-term statin treatment reduces the frequency of cardiovascular events, but safety and efficacy in patients with abnormal liver tests is unclear. We assessed whether statin therapy is safe and effective for these patients through post-hoc analysis of the Greek Atorvastatin and Coronary Heart Disease Evaluation (GREACE) study population.

Methods.—GREACE was a prospective, intention-to-treat study that randomly assigned by a computer-generated randomisation list 1600 patients with coronary heart disease (aged <75 years, with serum concentrations of LDL cholesterol >2·6 mmol/L and triglycerides <4·5 mmol/L) at the Hippokration University Hospital, Thessaloniki, Greece to receive statin or usual care, which could include statins. The primary outcome of our post-hoc analysis was risk reduction for first recurrent cardiovascular event in patients treated with a statin who had moderately abnormal liver tests (defined as serum alanine aminotransferase or aspartate aminotransferase concentrations of less than three times the upper limit of normal) compared with patients with abnormal liver tests who did not receive a statin. This risk reduction was compared with that for patients treated (or not) with statin and normal liver tests.

Findings.—Of 437 patients with moderately abnormal liver tests at baseline, which were possibly associated with nonalcoholic fatty liver disease, 227 who were treated with a statin (mainly atorvastatin 24 mg per day) had substantial improvement in liver tests (p<0·0001) whereas 210 not treated with a statin had further increases of liver enzyme concentrations. Cardiovascular events occurred in 22 (10%) of 227 patients with abnormal liver tests who received statin (3·2 events per 100 patient-years) and 63 (30%) of 210 patients with abnormal liver tests who did not receive statin (10·0 events per 100 patient-years; 68% relative risk reduction, p<0·0001). This cardiovascular disease benefit was greater (p=0·0074) than it was in patients with normal liver tests (90 [14%] events in 653 patients receiving a statin [4·6 per 100 patient-years] *vs* 117 [23%] in 510 patients not receiving a statin [7·6 per 100 patient-years]; 39% relative risk reduction, p<0·0001). Seven (<1%) of 880 participants who received a statin discontinued statin treatment because of liver-related adverse effects (transaminase concentrations more than three-times the upper limit of normal).

Interpretation.—Statin treatment is safe and can improve liver tests and reduce cardiovascular morbidity in patients with mild-to-moderately abnormal liver tests that are potentially attributable to non-alcoholic fatty liver disease.

▶ This study describing abnormal liver function studies in patients receiving statins was performed in adults. A pediatric study comparable to this is crying out to be done. One of the concerns any medical care provider has when starting statins is the effect of such drugs on liver function tests. If liver function tests are already elevated when one is thinking about starting statins, red flags go up. What Athyros et al have done is to perform an analysis from a randomized trial of the efficacy and safety of a statin in patients with baseline increases in alanine aminotransferase (ALT) concentrations that were elevated by less than 3 times the upper limit of normal. Needless to say, these patients were thought to have fatty liver or nonalcoholic steatohepatitis (NASH). It was found that in those patients who had fatty liver or NASH, serious increases in ALT in those given statins occurred no more often than in a similar group who were not given statins. Moreover, with time, ALT improved or normalized in patients who were given statins, whereas in the group not given statins, liver tests continued to worsen. Most importantly, patients who started the trial with elevated liver function tests derived the greatest cardiovascular benefit of any group.

Interestingly, the findings of this report, showing uniformed improvement of liver function tests for patients who started with abnormal liver functions who were then treated with statins, are consistent with findings in subjects with hepatitis C who were given statins who also showed improvement in liver function tests.

There are no studies to document how many individuals at any age are denied statins because they have preexisting changes in liver function tests or how many patients have statins discontinued when ALT increases. The data from this report from the United Kingdom call into question the need for monitoring liver function studies in those taking statins. In the United States, the price tag of such monitoring runs about $10 billion per year.

So is statin-induced hepatotoxicity a myth? The authors of this report definitely say yes as does the author of a commentary that accompanied this report.[1] Indeed, large trials of statins have showed no difference in the frequency or degree of ALT increases between treatment and placebo groups, but these studies have uniformly been carried out in an older population. Again, a study of a similar nature begs to be done in children. It may very well be that those with elevated ALTs are in fact those who are most in need of statin therapy. Despite the lack of definitive literature in this regard, a recent survey in the United States showed that 50% of academic physicians would be reluctant to give a statin to a patient who presents with an ALT of more than 1.5 times the upper limit of normal. More than 40% say they would deny a statin to patients with chronic hepatitis C (2% of the general population here in this country).[2] It has been suggested that drug companies delete the serious warnings on their package inserts about the relationship between statins and liver damage.[1]

Please note that coronary artery—related heart disease is not a new phenomenon. While Ancient Egyptian tomb paintings of the Nile Valley suggest that occupants were lithe, beautiful, and healthy, new research suggests otherwise. Cardiologists from Cairo have performed detailed cardiac CT scans on a number of mummies. Of 44 that still possess cardiovascular tissue, 45% had definite or probable atherosclerosis of their coronary arteries. Their average age was just 40 years. Although Ancient Egyptians did not smoke, they did enjoy relatively high calorie—rich fare such as cakes sweetened with honey and were exposed to a number of chronic infections resulting in inflammation that could increase their risk of hardening of the arteries. To read more about this, see the references.[3] Clearly the more things change the more they stay the same.

J. A. Stockman III, MD

References

1. Bader T. Liver tests are irrelevant when prescribing statins. *Lancet.* 2010;376: 1882-1883.
2. Rzouq FS, Volk ML, Hatoum HH, Talluri SK, Mummadi RR, Sood GK. Hepatotoxicity fears contribute to underutilization of statin medications by primary care physicians. *Am J Med Sci.* 2010;340:89-93.
3. Pringle H. The curse of the mummies' arteries. *Science.* http://news.sciencemag. org/sciencenow/2011/04/the-curse-of-the-mummies-arteries.html?ref=hp. Published April 3, 2011. Accessed August 17, 2011.

Cholesterol Efflux Capacity, High-Density Lipoprotein Function, and Atherosclerosis

Khera AV, Cuchel M, de la Llera-Moya M, et al (Univ of Pennsylvania, Philadelphia, PA; Children's Hosp of Philadelphia, PA; et al)

N Engl J Med 364:127-135, 2011

Background.—High-density lipoprotein (HDL) may provide cardiovascular protection by promoting reverse cholesterol transport from macrophages. We hypothesized that the capacity of HDL to accept cholesterol from macrophages would serve as a predictor of atherosclerotic burden.

Methods.—We measured cholesterol efflux capacity in 203 healthy volunteers who underwent assessment of carotid artery intima–media thickness, 442 patients with angiographically confirmed coronary artery disease, and 351 patients without such angiographically confirmed disease. We quantified efflux capacity by using a validated ex vivo system that involved incubation of macrophages with apolipoprotein B–depleted serum from the study participants.

Results.—The levels of HDL cholesterol and apolipoprotein A-I were significant determinants of cholesterol efflux capacity but accounted for less than 40% of the observed variation. An inverse relationship was noted between efflux capacity and carotid intima–media thickness both before and after adjustment for the HDL cholesterol level. Furthermore, efflux capacity was a strong inverse predictor of coronary disease status (adjusted odds ratio for coronary disease per 1-SD increase in efflux capacity, 0.70; 95% confidence interval [CI], 0.59 to 0.83; P<0.001). This relationship was attenuated, but remained significant, after additional adjustment for the HDL cholesterol level (odds ratio per 1-SD increase, 0.75; 95% CI, 0.63 to 0.90; P = 0.002) or apolipoprotein A-I level (odds ratio per 1-SD increase, 0.74; 95% CI, 0.61 to 0.89; P = 0.002). Additional studies showed enhanced efflux capacity in patients with the metabolic syndrome and low HDL cholesterol levels who were treated with pioglitazone, but not in patients with hypercholesterolemia who were treated with statins.

Conclusions.—Cholesterol efflux capacity from macrophages, a metric of HDL function, has a strong inverse association with both carotid intima-media thickness and the likelihood of angiographic coronary artery disease, independently of the HDL cholesterol level. (Funded by the National Heart, Lung, and Blood Institute and others.)

▶ There are abundant data, both clinical and epidemiologic, that have consistently shown that low levels of high-density lipoprotein (HDL) cholesterol are strongly associated with an increased risk of coronary artery disease. Moreover, hypercholesterolemic mice with genetic defects in HDL metabolism are markedly atherosclerotic, providing compelling evidence that HDL is a key modulator of the disease in animal models. These observations, put together with the large residual disease risk among patients with coronary artery disease who are treated with statins, have triggered intense interest in therapies to raise HDL cholesterol. Unfortunately, certain drugs, such as fibric acid derivatives and nicotinic acid, that elevate HDL cholesterol levels have shown inconsistent clinical benefit. Moreover, it is unclear how HDL in humans interacts with the artery wall to influence the progression or regression of atherosclerosis. A central theory is that HDL promotes cholesterol efflux from macrophage foam cells in atheromatous vessels, decreasing the cholesterol burden and macrophage-driven inflammation. This is where the report of Khera et al comes in.

Khera et al have measured the ability of human serum HDL to promote cholesterol efflux from cultured macrophage foam cells. The association was found to be inverse, consistent with studies in animals that show that HDL is atheroprotective because it promotes cholesterol efflux from macrophages. These data provide important evidence that the ability of HDL to promote cholesterol efflux from macrophage foam cells is a key property that explains in part the inverse relationship between HDL and the risk of atherosclerotic coronary artery disease in humans. Khera et al found that the ability of serum HDL to promote cholesterol efflux from macrophages was not determined simply by measuring HDL cholesterol levels and that the association between efflux capacity and the risk of coronary disease remains significant after adjustment for levels of HDL cholesterol and apolipoprotein A-I, the major protein component of HDL. These observations suggest that HDL efflux capacity is a measure of HDL function not just amount. The observations also support the proposal that this functional HDL contributes to the risk of coronary artery disease. It has been suggested that inflammation and other disorders that increase the risk of coronary artery disease involve the conversion of HDL to a dysfunctional form that is no longer cardioprotective.

An understanding of the deleterious effects of dysfunctional HDL may lead to new diagnostic and therapeutic approaches to the prevention and treatment of atherosclerosis, understandings that may trickle down to the care of youngsters in the pediatric population. The ability to measure the efflux capacity of HDL as shown by Khera et al may thus be a useful tool in the further investigation of HDL function.

To read more about this interesting topic relating HDL and cardiovascular disease risk, including new ways of thinking about all this, see the excellent commentary by Heinecke.[1]

Name that Murmur—Eponyms for the Astute Auscultician, Part 2: Barlow's murmur[2]: South African physician John Barlow was the first to describe mitral-valve prolapse. After considerable debate, the manuscript representing this disorder was published in 1968 and as of this past year, Barlow's work is the 13th most cited research paper in the cardiology literature. In his paper, Barlow described the features of mitral valve prolapse in 90 patients with non-ejection clicks, late systolic murmurs, or a combination of the 2.[3]

J. A. Stockman III, MD

References

1. Heinecke J. HDL and cardiovascular-disease risk—time for a new approach? *N Engl J Med.* 2011;364:170-171.

2. Ma I, Tierney LM. Name that murmur—eponyms for the astute auscultician. *N Engl J Med.* 2010;363:2164-2168.
3. Chen TO, John B. Barlow: Master clinician and compleat cardiologist. *Clin Cardiol.* 2000;23:66-67.

Endothelial Abnormalities in Adolescents with Type 1 Diabetes: A Biomarker for Vascular Sequelae?

DiMeglio LA, Tosh A, Saha C, et al (Indiana Univ School of Medicine, Indianapolis; Univ of Missouri School of Medicine, Columbia)

J Pediatr 157:540-546, 2010

Objective.—To evaluate whether counts of circulating colony forming unit-endothelial cells (CFU-ECs), cells co-expressing CD34, CD133, and CD31 (CD34+CD133+CD31+), and CD34+CD45- cells are altered in adolescents with type 1 diabetes and if the changes in counts correlate with endothelial dysfunction.

Study Design.—Adolescents with diabetes (ages 18 to 22 years) and race- and sex-matched control subjects were studied. We assessed circulating CFU-ECs, using colony assays, and CD34+CD133+CD31+ and CD34+ CD45- cells, using poly-chromatic flow cytometry. CFU-ECs and CD34+ CD133+CD31+ are hematopoietic-derived progenitors that inversely correlate with cardiovascular risk in adults. CD34+CD45- cells are enriched for endothelial cells with robust vasculogenic potential. Vascular reactivity was tested by laser Doppler iontophoresis.

Results.—Subjects with diabetes had lower CD34+CD133+CD31+ cells, a trend toward reduced CFU-ECs, and increased CD34+CD45- cells compared with control subjects. Endothelium-dependent vasodilation was impaired in subjects with diabetes, which correlated with reductions in circulating CD34+CD133+CD31+ cells.

Conclusions.—Long-term sequelae of type 1 diabetes include vasculopathies. Endothelial progenitor cells promote vascular health by facilitating endothelial integrity and function. Lower CD34+CD133+CD31+ cells may be a harbinger of future macrovascular disease risk. Higher circulating CD34+CD45- cells may reflect ongoing endothelial damage. These cells are potential biomarkers to guide therapeutic interventions to enhance endothelial function and to prevent progression to overt vascular disease.

▶ There is much being written these days about markers of early cardiovascular disease, markers that hopefully can predict long-term outcomes in patients who have certain risk factors, such as diabetes mellitus or obesity. All of us know that atherosclerosis begins in childhood. In fact, autopsy studies performed in children who die of unrelated causes show early vascular fibrous plaques in children as young as 8 years of age.[1] In the pediatric population, we have to look for surrogate markers for later onset of cardiovascular disease since children rarely show absolute risk factors for detectable cardiovascular events such as heart attack or stroke during childhood. Thus we look to measures of vascular function and arterial atherosclerotic load such as brachial reactivity, augmentation index, and carotid intima media thickness in children. Although not without problems, such surrogates seem to remain the best available methods for assessing vascular function and atherosclerosis development.

Di Meglio et al have used polychromatic flow cytometry to measure circulating endothelial cells in young individuals with type 1 diabetes mellitus and have compared their findings with values seen in healthy control subjects. It turns out that adolescents with type 1 diabetes mellitus have increased levels of circulating endothelial progenitor cells (CD34$^+$CD133$^+$CD31$^+$). Such cells promote endothelial integrity and may be important in vascular repair. In adults, such endothelial progenitors are inversely related to cardiovascular risk. Conversely, circulating angiogenic macrophages (CD34$^+$CD45$^-$) correlate with the presence of coronary artery disease and have been observed in higher numbers in adolescents with type 1 diabetes mellitus. Such macrophages promote new blood vessel growth and may indicate ongoing vascular injury.

The study of Di Meglio et al provides insight into a new way to evaluate the biology of vascular injury in at-risk youth. The association between circulating endothelial cells with multiple cardiovascular risk factors and the finding that a number of endothelial cells predict cardiovascular events, regardless of lipid levels and blood pressure, make such studies an attractive means of assessing cardiovascular risk in children. Similar findings were seen in a report of Kelly et al showing that vascular endothelium is in fact activated in relation to excess adiposity, particularly in severely obese children.[2]

Name that Murmur—Eponyms for the Astute Ausculician, Part 3: Cabot-Locke murmur[3]: Richard Cabot was an American physician and a trailblazing educator. He introduced case analysis at Harvard medical School and founded Case Histories of the Massachusetts General Hospital, the case series that continues to be published regularly in the *New England Journal of Medicine*. Cabot, collaborating with his colleague Frank Locke, published a series describing 3 cases of severe anemia with diastolic murmur in patients who had been given a diagnosis of valvular heart disease but found to have normal heart valves on autopsy. The Cabot-Locke murmur is a diastolic murmur that sounds similar to aortic insufficiency, but does not have a decrescendo; it is heard best at the left sternal border and resolves completely with treatment of anemia.[4]

J. A. Stockman III, MD

References

1. Berenson GS, Sathanur R, Bao W, Newman WP 3rd, Tracy RE, Wattigney WA. Association between multiple cardiovascular risk factors and atherosclerosis in children and young adults. The Bogalusa heart study. *N Engl J Med.* 2003;338:1650-1656.
2. Kelly AS, Hebbel RP, Solovey AN, et al. Circulating activated endothelial cells in pediatric obesity. *J Pediatr.* 2010;157:547-551.
3. Ma I, Tierney LM. Name that murmur-eponyms for the astute ausculician. *N Engl J Med.* 2010;363:2164-2168.
4. Cabot RC, Locke EA. On the occurrence of diastolic murmurs without lesions of the aortic or pulmonary valves. *Bull Johns Hopkins Hospital.* 1903;14:115-120.

Preclinical Noninvasive Markers of Atherosclerosis in Children and Adolescents with Type 1 Diabetes Are Influenced by Physical Activity

Trigona B, Aggoun Y, Maggio A, et al (Univ Hosps of Geneva and Univ of Geneva, Switzerland)
J Pediatr 157:533-539, 2010

Objectives.—To measure preclinical noninvasive markers of atherosclerosis in youth with type 1 diabetes (T1DM), and to determine their associations between physical activity level and cardiorespiratory fitness (maximal oxygen consumption [Vo_2max]).

Study Design.—This was a cross-sectional study including 32 patients with T1DM and 42 healthy subjects aged 6 to 17 years. Main outcome measures included arterial flow-mediated dilation (FMD) and intima-media thickness with high-resolution ultrasonography; physical activity by accelerometer (valid 26 patients with T1DM, 35 healthy subjects) and Vo_2max.

Results.—Compared with healthy control subjects, patients with T1DM had higher intima-media thickness (mean 0.50 mm [0.48-0.52, 95% CI] vs 0.48 [0.47-0.49], $P = .02$) and reduced FMD (4.9% [4.1%-5.7%] vs 7.3 [6.4-8.1], $P = .001$), Vo_2max (45.5 mL/kg/min [43.0-48.0] vs 48.7 [46.7-50.6], $P \leq .001$), total (567.1 [458.6-675.6] vs 694.9 [606.6-883.2] counts per minute, $P = .001$) and moderate-to-vigorous physical activity. Patients with T1DM who did more than 60 min/day^{-1} of moderate-to-vigorous physical activity had similar FMD compared with relatively inactive healthy subjects, but not as high as active control subjects.

Conclusion.—Youth with T1DM present early signs of atherosclerosis, as well as low physical activity level and cardiorespiratory fitness. Endothelial function is enhanced in patients who practice more than 60 min/day^{-1} of moderate-to-vigorous physical activity.

▶ The commentary on the article by DiMeglio et al provides information about noninvasive markers of atherosclerosis in children and adolescents, particularly those with type 1 diabetes.[1] Such assessments of risk are fairly meaningless unless there are ways to deal with the vascular abnormality uncovered by such assessments. The report by Trigona et al evaluates children with type 1 diabetes mellitus and compares the data with those of control subjects who are otherwise normal in order to determine the effects of varying degrees of exercise on endothelial function by measuring brachial artery reactivity and arterial response to nitroglycerine. The authors also measured carotid intima media thickness (CIMT) with ultrasound. It was not surprising that youngsters with diabetes mellitus at baseline showed lower vascular reactivity, higher blood pressure, and greater CIMT in control subjects. When the data were broken down, however, those youngsters with diabetes mellitus who had participated in 60 minutes or more of moderate to vigorous exercise daily had better vascular reactivity than children who were sedentary. The children studied were aged between 6 and 17 years and abnormalities were present even in the prepubertal children and before the onset of clinically evident cardiovascular risk factors such as elevated blood lipid levels.

The bottom line from the report of Trigona et al is that diabetes mellitus can wreak havoc even on a young person's cardiovascular system, and the data show that there are beneficial effects of exercise in either retaining or in improving vascular function. The benefits of exercise on vascular distensibility make daily moderate to vigorous activity an important component of diabetes care. This translates into a prescription for at least 60 minutes of exercise per day as part of educating these youngsters and their families on diabetes management. To read more about coronary artery disease in youngsters with diabetes mellitus, see the excellent editorial by Silverstein and Haller.[2]

Name that Murmur—Eponyms for the Astute Auscultician, Part 4: Carey Coombs Murmur[3]: The Englishman Carey Coombs was a rheumatic fever specialist. In 1924 he published a book on rheumatic heart disease. The Carey Coombs murmur is a short mid-diastolic murmur caused by active rheumatic carditis with mitral-valve inflammation. The murmur is soft and low pitched, best heard at the apex. The murmur is frequently transient with onset during acute rheumatic mitral valvulitis and improves or resolves with recovery of the acute illness.[4]

J. A. Stockman III, MD

References

1. DiMeglio LA, Tosh A, Saha C, et al. Endothelial abnormalities in adolescents with type 1 diabetes: a biomarker for vascular sequelae? *J Pediatr.* 2010;157:540-546.
2. Silverstein J, Haller M. Coronary artery disease in youth: present markers, future hope? *J Pediatr.* 2010;157:523-524.
3. Ma I, Tierney LM. Name that murmur—eponyms for the astute auscultician. *N Engl J Med.* 2010;363:2164-2168.
4. Coombs CF. *Rheumatic heart disease.* New York: William Wood; 1924.

Ventricular Tachyarrhythmias after Cardiac Arrest in Public versus at Home

Weisfeldt ML, for the Resuscitation Outcomes Consortium (ROC) Investigators (Johns Hopkins Univ, Baltimore, MD; et al)
N Engl J Med 364:313-321, 2011

Background.—The incidence of ventricular fibrillation or pulseless ventricular tachycardia as the first recorded rhythm after out-of-hospital cardiac arrest has unexpectedly declined. The success of bystander-deployed automated external defibrillators (AEDs) in public settings suggests that this may be the more common initial rhythm when out-of-hospital cardiac arrest occurs in public. We conducted a study to determine whether the location of the arrest, the type of arrhythmia, and the probability of survival are associated.

Methods.—Between 2005 and 2007, we conducted a prospective cohort study of out-of-hospital cardiac arrest in adults in 10 North American communities. We assessed the frequencies of ventricular fibrillation or pulseless ventricular tachycardia and of survival to hospital discharge for arrests at home as compared with arrests in public.

Results.—Of 12,930 evaluated out-of-hospital cardiac arrests, 2042 occurred in public and 9564 at home. For cardiac arrests at home, the incidence of ventricular fibrillation or pulseless ventricular tachycardia was 25% when the arrest was witnessed by emergency-medical-services (EMS) personnel, 35% when it was witnessed by a bystander, and 36% when a bystander applied an AED. For cardiac arrests in public, the corresponding rates were 38%, 60%, and 79%. The adjusted odds ratio for initial ventricular fibrillation or pulseless ventricular tachycardia in public versus at home was 2.28 (95% confidence interval [CI], 1.96 to 2.66; P<0.001) for bystander-witnessed arrests and 4.48 (95% CI, 2.23 to 8.97; P<0.001) for arrests in which bystanders applied AEDs. The rate of survival to hospital discharge was 34% for arrests in public settings with AEDs applied by bystanders versus 12% for arrests at home (adjusted odds ratio, 2.49; 95% CI, 1.03 to 5.99; P=0.04).

Conclusions.—Regardless of whether out-of-hospital cardiac arrests are witnessed by EMS personnel or bystanders and whether AEDs are applied by bystanders, the proportion of arrests with initial ventricular fibrillation or pulseless ventricular tachycardia is much greater in public settings than at home. The incremental value of resuscitation strategies, such as the ready availability of an AED, may be related to the place where the arrest occurs. (Funded by the National Heart, Lung, and Blood Institute and others.)

▶ Weisfeldt et al report that ventricular fibrillation is identified less frequently during sudden cardiac arrest when the latter occurs at home than in public places, even when the arrest is witnessed. The authors summarize that age and coexisting illnesses are responsible and that the location of sudden cardiac arrest may be a surrogate for underlying disease severity. In addition, poorer outcomes were observed with the use of automated external defibrillator (AED) at home, as compared with public AED use. The authors conclude that perhaps AEDs should be reserved for public locations and cardiopulmonary resuscitation (CPR) should be taught more broadly as the better path to improving survival from sudden cardiac arrest. Needless to say, this research is controversial in a number of ways.

So what are the problems with the findings of this report? One can legitimately ask the question, does this study really show that ventricular fibrillation in sudden cardiac arrest occurs less often at home than in public? Without electrocardiographic data regarding the onset of the event, we really cannot know for certain. What we do know is that untreated ventricular fibrillation will deteriorate to asystole over a period of minutes and probably more rapidly in patients with more advanced cardiac disease. After 25 minutes, nearly all patients are in asystole. Although primary bradyarrhythmias as the cause of sudden cardiac arrest are becoming more common, most instances of bradyarrhythmia, specifically asystole, follow ventricular fibrillation. These considerations would alter the interpretation of the findings that Weisfeldt et al report. If the home rescuer takes just 60 seconds longer to call 911 as compared with the public witness, then the findings could be explained simply as a matter of response speed. The home use of AEDs for sudden cardiac arrest trial showed that spouses confronted with the sudden collapse of a loved one commonly exhibit emotional distress and confusion, thus delaying the effective response.

So the next question is how much time actually elapses between witnessing and assessing the sudden cardiac arrest and dialing 911? Does the interval differ between the home and the public setting? Does it differ between those who have CPR training and those who do not? Knowing the answers to these questions has broad implications. The greater number of bystanders who witness sudden cardiac arrest in public makes calling 911 more likely to occur closer to the time of the collapse. Moreover, those who have completed CPR courses know that they should call 911 promptly. Because seconds matter, even a modest delay in the 911 call could lead to differences in outcome. Consequently, the lone rescuer at home, who is probably less aware of the critical importance of speed, would lose the race to a public bystander.

What about AED use in the home? Certainly at present, no grounds exist to broadly promote publicly financed home AEDs. However, this policy assessment should not dissuade persons from purchasing their own AEDs. The dismissal of home AEDs is premature, and other than the personal expense, there is no known downside to such a purchase. Moreover, many home rescuers do indeed act quickly and can save a life. Perhaps the presence of AEDs at home would prompt a more rapid response and shave off valuable seconds to minutes improving outcomes of arrests at home.

In an interesting editorial that accompanied the report of Weisfeldt, Bardy makes a heretical postulate and that is that perhaps in this modern age, no CPR is as good as CPR if there is ready and rapid access to an AED.[1] First, he notes that improvement in resuscitation (eg, at airports and in casinos) has been driven by the prompt availability of AEDs, not CPR. Second, the broad national outcomes after sudden cardiac arrest have remained essentially unchanged for the past 40 years. Despite a national awareness and acceptance of CPR, we still have 300 000 deaths a year with a dismal overall survival rate to hospital discharge running about 8%, even with emergency-medical-services assessment. Third, it could be that the perceived benefit of CPR represents merely a more prompt 911 call made by a bystander with CPR training, resulting in the greater likelihood that the patient has a shockable rhythm. Fourth, Bardy notes that we should not ignore the financial incentives in maintaining the proposition that CPR is useful. The lion's share of the budget of many nonprofit organizations, including the American Heart Association, comes from teaching and licensing CPR courses. Several corporations exist solely because of CPR. Bardy also notes that CPR is not harmless. Coronary arteries can be crushed, livers lacerated, and esophagi ruptured. Aspiration is nearly a universal occurrence with mouth-to-mouth ventilation. Mediastinal hemorrhage is common. As many as 3% of patients have abdominal and visceral or esophageal ruptures. Almost 10% have pericardial bleeding, coronary air emboli, or laceration of the great vessels and myocardia. Last, it is noted, but not proven, that the CPR performed during organized rhythms after a shock has been administered will actually reinduce ventricular fibrillation in about one-fourth of patients with sudden cardiac arrest.

Maybe it is time to reassess the overall value of CPR in the age of AEDs. Such an evaluation would require an extraordinary amount of thoughtfulness in terms of study design given the entrenched way in which we think about resuscitation. Is it time for many more of us to buy AEDs and keep them in our cars or home? Talk about profits for private companies!

Name that Murmur—Eponyms for the Astute Auscultician, Part 5: Dock's Murmur[2]: In his New York Times obituary, the American physician William Dock was remembered as a devoted career academic and visionary. Many of his thinkings bumped convention, including the questioning of the value of prolonged rest in hospitalized patients in the 1930s and a decade later, cautioning that high-fat diets could lead to clogged arteries. Dock described the murmur that bears his name in 1967 in a case report of a patient with heart failure resulting from hypertension. The patient had no apparent valvular disease, but did have a continuous diastolic murmur with early and late accentuation in a sharply demarcated highly localized area, 4 cm left of the sternum in the third intercostal space, detectable only when the patient was sitting upright. The patient's autopsy revealed that the descending branch of the left coronary artery was markedly stenosed whereas the heart valves, great vessels, and other coronary arteries were normal. The murmur represents a flow murmur across a stenosis of the left anterior descending artery and is almost diagnostic of the latter's condition—a real pearl for internists on rounds.[3]

J. A. Stockman III, MD

References

1. Bardy GH. A critic's assessment of our approach to cardiac arrest. *N Engl J Med.* 2011;364:374-375.
2. Ma I, Tierney LM. Name that murmur-eponyms for the astute auscultician. *N Engl J Med.* 2010;363:2164-2168.
3. Dock W, Zoneraich S. A diastolic murmur arising in a stenosed coronary artery. *Am J Med.* 1967;42;617-619.

Compression-Only CPR or Standard CPR in Out-of-Hospital Cardiac Arrest
Svensson L, Bohm K, Castrèn M, et al (Karolinska Institutet at Södersjukhuset, Stockholm, Sweden; et al)
N Engl J Med 363:434-442, 2010

Background.—Emergency medical dispatchers give instructions on how to perform cardiopulmonary resuscitation (CPR) over the telephone to callers requesting help for a patient with suspected cardiac arrest, before the arrival of emergency medical services (EMS) personnel. A previous study indicated that instructions to perform CPR consisting of only chest compression result in a treatment efficacy that is similar or even superior to that associated with instructions given to perform standard CPR, which consists of both compression and ventilation. That study, however, was not powered to assess a possible difference in survival. The aim of this prospective, randomized study was to evaluate the possible superiority of compression-only CPR over standard CPR with respect to survival.

Methods.—Patients with suspected, witnessed, out-of-hospital cardiac arrest were randomly assigned to undergo either compression-only CPR or standard CPR. The primary end point was 30-day survival.

Results.—Data for the primary analysis were collected from February 2005 through January 2009 for a total of 1276 patients. Of these, 620 patients had been assigned to receive compression-only CPR and 656 patients had been assigned to receive standard CPR. The rate of 30-day survival was similar in the two groups: 8.7% (54 of 620 patients) in the group receiving compression-only CPR and 7.0% (46 of 656 patients) in the group receiving standard CPR (absolute difference for compression-only vs. standard CPR, 1.7 percentage points; 95% confidence interval, −1.2 to 4.6; $P = 0.29$).

Conclusions.—This prospective, randomized study showed no significant difference with respect to survival at 30 days between instructions given by an emergency medical dispatcher, before the arrival of EMS personnel, for compression-only CPR and instructions for standard CPR in patients with suspected, witnessed, out-of-hospital cardiac arrest. (Funded by the Swedish Heart—Lung Foundation and others; Karolinska Clinical Trial Registration number, CT20080012.)

▶ This report from Sweden complements the report of Rea et al from the United States.[1] It is nice to see 2 large studies independently performed across the pond that show the same findings. The report from Sweden, a nationwide randomized study of witnessed out-of-hospital cardiac arrest, demonstrates that giving instructions for compression-only cardiopulmonary resuscitation (CPR) before the arrival of emergency medical services (EMS) personnel produces similar outcomes when compared with standard CPR with mouth-to-mouth rescue breathing. For all the reasons mentioned in the commentary on Weisfeldt et al,[2] compression-only CPR results in more compressions per minute than standard CPR and can be started more rapidly. It is also far simpler to perform. The bottom line is that this study and the one from the United States provide further support to the hypothesis that compression-only CPR, which is easier to learn and perform, should be considered the preferred method for CPR performed by bystanders in patients with sudden cardiac arrest.

In addition to the information we are learning now about compression-only CPR, we are seeing reports about the value, or lack of value, of the use of drugs as part of resuscitation protocols in the field. For decades we have relied on trained professionals to administer drugs during sudden cardiac arrest, yet this approach has never been critically evaluated in a randomized controlled trial. Recently, a group of investigators from Oslo, Norway, performed such a trial.[3] The trial randomized more than 900 patients with out-of-hospital sudden cardiac arrest to EMS care that involved the standard advanced cardiac life support protocol (including intubation, defibrillation, and intravenous drugs) or a protocol that omitted the use of such drugs. The trial found no significant difference in survival to hospital discharge between the 2 groups (10.5% in the standard care group vs 9.2% in the no-drugs group). Importantly, the investigators found no significant difference in the quality of CPR during resuscitation care between the 2 groups. The results rightly call into question the value of drugs in sudden cardiac arrest.

It is clear from the report from Norway that whether drugs truly improve the outcome of sudden cardiac arrest or not, their effect on survival is modest at best. Conversely, a growing body of work suggests that the consistent provision of high-quality CPR may have a much larger effect on outcomes. A recent out-of-hospital retrospective study in Arizona has documented that by delaying intubation and focusing on early continuous chest compressions and defibrillation, survival to discharge after sudden cardiac arrest actually triples.[4] This finding has been replicated in other EMS settings.

The bottom line, at least for adults, is less is more when it comes to drugs for resuscitation after cardiac arrest in the nonhospital setting. Again, caution should be applied to translating this information to the care of infants, children, and adolescents who suffer cardiac arrest in the nonhospital setting, but we already know from experience that compression alone, without drugs, seems to be the way to go.

This commentary closes with the observation that a single vodka binge can induce myocardial injury. Two researchers from Germany persuaded 23 healthy young adults to simulate a vodka binge so they could assess the potential damage that might be done to the myocardium by excessive alcohol consumption. The volunteers drank enough vodka over a few hours to generate quite a high alcohol level. One day later, they underwent cardiac magnetic resonance (MR) imaging (all had a hangover that day). Compared with baseline scans, the new scan showed measurable myocardial edema (T2 signal intensity) and hyperemia (global relative enhancement). The vodka had no discernable effect on left ventricular function although 3 of the volunteers did develop small pericardial effusions. Fifty percent of the volunteers had raised serum concentrations of cardiac troponin I, suggesting subtle cardiac injury. All changes on MR resolved 1 week later. These findings suggest that binge drinking can induce reversible changes in the myocardium. The researchers also indicate that there is no evidence that a single episode of binge drinking would trigger an acute cardiac event, at least in a healthy volunteer. The story may be different if the binge drinking continues.[5] Many alcoholics die of a broken heart. Now we know why!

J. A. Stockman III, MD

References

1. Rea TD, Fahrenbruch C, Culley L, et al. CPR with chest compression alone or with rescue breathing. *N Engl J Med.* 2010;363:423-433.
2. Weisfeldt ML, Everson-Stewart S, Sitlani C, et al. Ventricular tachyarrhythmias after cardiac arrest in public versus at home. *N Engl J Med.* 2011;364:313-321.
3. Olasveengen TM, Sunde K, Brunborg C, Thowsen J, Steen PA, Wik L. Intravenous drug administration during out-of-hospital cardiac arrest: a randomized trial. *JAMA.* 2009;302:2222-2229.

4. Bobrow BJ, Clark LL, Ewy GA, et al. Minimally interrupted cardiac resuscitation by emergency medical services for out-of-hospital cardiac arrest. *JAMA*. 2008; 299:1158-1165.

5. One vodka binge induces subtle myocardial injury. *BMJ*. 2010;341:696.

Chest Compression—Only CPR by Lay Rescuers and Survival From Out-of-Hospital Cardiac Arrest

Bobrow BJ, Spaite DW, Berg RA, et al (Arizona Dept of Health Services, Phoenix; Univ of Arizona, Tucson; Children's Hosp of Philadelphia, PA; et al)
JAMA 304:1447-1454, 2010

Context.—Chest compression-only bystander cardiopulmonary resuscitation (CPR) may be as effective as conventional CPR with rescue breathing for out-of-hospital cardiac arrest.

Objective.—To investigate the survival of patients with out-of-hospital cardiac arrest using compression-only CPR (COCPR) compared with conventional CPR.

Design, Setting, and Patients.—A 5-year prospective observational cohort study of survival in patients at least 18 years old with out-of-hospital cardiac arrest between January 1, 2005, and December 31, 2009, in Arizona. The relationship between layperson bystander CPR and survival to hospital discharge was evaluated using multivariable logistic regression.

Main Outcome Measure.—Survival to hospital discharge.

Results.—Among 5272 adults with out-of-hospital cardiac arrest of cardiac etiology not observed by responding emergency medical personnel, 779 were excluded because bystander CPR was provided by a health care professional or the arrest occurred in a medical facility. A total of 4415 met all inclusion criteria for analysis, including 2900 who received no bystander CPR, 666 who received conventional CPR, and 849 who received COCPR. Rates of survival to hospital discharge were 5.2% (95% confidence interval [CI], 4.4%-6.0%) for the no bystander CPR group, 7.8% (95% CI, 5.8%-9.8%) for conventional CPR, and 13.3% (95% CI, 11.0%-15.6%) for COCPR. The adjusted odds ratio (AOR) for survival for conventional CPR vs no CPR was 0.99 (95% CI, 0.69-1.43), for COCPR vs no CPR, 1.59 (95% CI, 1.18-2.13), and for COCPR vs conventional CPR, 1.60 (95% CI, 1.08-2.35). From 2005 to 2009, lay rescuer CPR increased from 28.2% (95% CI, 24.6%-31.8%) to 39.9% (95% CI, 36.8%-42.9%; $P < .001$); the proportion of CPR that was COCPR increased from 19.6% (95% CI, 13.6%-25.7%) to 75.9% (95% CI, 71.7%-80.1%; $P < .001$). Overall survival increased from 3.7% (95% CI, 2.2%-5.2%) to 9.8% (95% CI, 8.0%-11.6%; $P < .001$).

Conclusion.—Among patients with out-of-hospital cardiac arrest, layperson compression-only CPR was associated with increased survival compared with conventional CPR and no bystander CPR in this setting with public endorsement of chest compression-only CPR.

▶ The report by Aufderheide et al[1] tells us about a new technique for cardiopulmonary resuscitation (CPR), whereby once medical personnel arrive, devices are used to compress and decompress the chest wall during resuscitation in such a way as to create a larger negative intrathoracic pressure during the decompression phase of the resuscitation. The nice part about the data from this report is that it increases survival (end point of out-of-hospital survival) by some 50% (6% for controls vs 9% for the compression-decompression technique).[1] The report of Bobrow et al tells us what can be done before proper medical assistance arrives when one has a sudden cardiac arrest out-of-hospital. This, of course, involves what bystanders initiate first.

For more than a decade, CPR using only chest compressions, forgoing ventilations by rescued breathing, has been described as an operation in the out-of-hospital management of sudden cardiac arrest when bystanders are unwilling or unable to provide standard CPR that combines chest compressions with rescued breathing. The American Heart Association has promulgated CPR techniques that do involve chest compressions coordinated with ventilation by mouth. These guidelines note that laymen who are unable or unwilling to provide rescue breaths should be encouraged to provide compression-only CPR to individuals experiencing out-of-hospital cardiac arrest. These recommendations followed a 1997 American Heart Association's signed statement that was the first document to propose compression-only CPR as a reasonable alternative to standard CPR by bystanders. There is a good rationale for this latter suggestion for alternative CPR. It is clearly easier to teach and remember than standard CPR, particularly for those who do not work in health care professions. It also removes the hesitancy many have or will have of putting their mouth to the face of a stranger. Also, and perhaps most compellingly, an increasing body of evidence suggests that interruptions in chest compression, even for such seemingly important interventions as providing artificial ventilation, are detrimental. Forward flow of blood ceases very soon after chest compressions are halted, and several compressions are needed to reestablish profusion when compressions are resumed. The "push hard, push fast, don't stop" mantra of current CPR teaching is designed to reinforce the need for minimal interruptions in chest compressions to maintain some degree of perfusion until more definitive therapy (such as defibrillation) can be delivered.

Bobrow et al report the results of an important observational study of compression-only CPR, the first to show a survival benefit associated with this technique. The authors describe a multifaceted statewide effort in Arizona to teach, encourage, and endorse compression-only CPR as the standard intervention for bystanders to use and as the resulting natural experiment among 4415 adults who sustained out-of-hospital cardiac arrest comparing those who received no bystander CPR, those who received standard CPR, and those who received compression-only CPR. The overall likelihood of survival to hospital discharge was higher among those receiving compression-only CPR than those receiving standard CPR (13.3% vs 7.8%, respectively; odds ratio of 1.60). However, there was no difference between the standard CPR group and the compression-only CPR group in the proportion of survivors with good neurologic status at the time of discharge from hospital. These data can be interpreted in a positive way, however, to say that it is reassuring that compression-only CPR intervention is not associated with an increased incidence of neurologic impairment with survival.

At the time the Bobrow report was published, the American Heart Association considered standard CPR and compression-only CPR to be equivalent. Readers should check to see what these latest recommendations are at present. They should also check to see if there has been any change at all in the recommendations regarding the bystander resuscitation of infants, toddlers, children, and adolescents.

Add another risk to the list of things that can damage your coronary arteries: working long hours. Kivimaki et al undertook a study of working hours and the relationship to risk of coronary heart disease and death.[2] Participants in this study included 7095 adults aged 39 to 62 years who were working full time and who had no evidence of heart disease at baseline. During an observation period (over 12 years), 192 participants had a coronary event. After adjustment for other factors, participants working 11 hours or more per day had a 1.7-fold increased risk for coronary heart disease compared with participants working just 7 to 8 hours a day. After reading this, I decided to take a nap.

J. A. Stockman III, MD

References

1. Aufderheide TP, Frascone RJ, Wayne MA, et al. Standard cardiopulmonary resuscitation versus active compression-decompression cardiopulmonary resuscitation with augmentation of negative intrathoracic pressure for out-of-hospital cardiac arrest: a randomised trial. *Lancet.* 2011;377:301-311.
2. Kivimaki M, Batty GD, Hamer M, et al. Using additional information on working hours to predict coronary heart disease: a cohort study. *Ann Intern Med.* 2011; 154:457-463.

CPR with Chest Compression Alone or with Rescue Breathing

Rea TD, Fahrenbruch C, Culley L, et al (Emergency Med Services Division of Public Health for Seattle and King County, WA; et al)
N Engl J Med 363:423-433, 2010

Background.—The role of rescue breathing in cardiopulmonary resuscitation (CPR) performed by a layperson is uncertain. We hypothesized that the dispatcher instructions to bystanders to provide chest compression alone would result in improved survival as compared with instructions to provide chest compression plus rescue breathing.

Methods.—We conducted a multicenter, randomized trial of dispatcher instructions to bystanders for performing CPR. The patients were persons 18 years of age or older with out-of-hospital cardiac arrest for whom dispatchers initiated CPR instruction to bystanders. Patients were randomly assigned to receive chest compression alone or chest compression plus rescue breathing. The primary outcome was survival to hospital discharge. Secondary outcomes included a favorable neurologic outcome at discharge.

Results.—Of the 1941 patients who met the inclusion criteria, 981 were randomly assigned to receive chest compression alone and 960 to receive chest compression plus rescue breathing. We observed no significant difference between the two groups in the proportion of patients who survived to hospital discharge (12.5% with chest compression alone and 11.0% with chest compression plus rescue breathing, P = 0.31) or in the proportion who survived with a favorable neurologic outcome in the two sites that assessed this secondary outcome (14.4% and 11.5%, respectively; P = 0.13). Prespecified subgroup analyses showed a trend toward a higher proportion of patients surviving to hospital discharge with chest compression alone as compared with chest compression plus rescue breathing for patients with a cardiac cause of arrest (15.5% vs. 12.3%, P = 0.09) and for those with shockable rhythms (31.9% vs. 25.7%, P = 0.09).

Conclusions.—Dispatcher instruction consisting of chest compression alone did not increase the survival rate overall, although there was a trend toward better outcomes in key clinical subgroups. The results support a strategy for CPR performed by laypersons that emphasizes chest compression and minimizes the role of rescue breathing. (Funded in part by the Laerdal Foundation for Acute Medicine and the Medic One Foundation; ClinicalTrials.gov number, NCT00219687.)

▶ This report came as a shot across the bow of traditional cardiopulmonary resuscitation (CPR) approaches for those who have sudden cardiac arrest since the data so clearly seem to minimize the value of rescue breathing as opposed to chest compression alone. The conclusions obviously refer to information garnered in adults, but the information would logically seem to apply to the resuscitation of infants, children, and adolescents.

By way of background, 2010 saw the 50th anniversary of modern CPR. When first described, Kouwenhoven et al proposed external chest compression to provide circulation of blood to the brain and heart after cardiac arrest.[1] What has evolved since then is known as the chain of survival paradigm, a stepwise set of actions that includes prompt recognition of arrest and notification of emergency medical system personnel, immediate delivery of CPR, electrical defibrillation if appropriate, and rapid delivery of the patient to health care professionals who can administer advance cardiac life support. The latter involves the use of airway management, ventilation and supplemental oxygen, and the administration of drugs such as adrenaline, atropine, or amiodarone. Shortly after the first descriptions of CPR, mouth-to-mouth rescue breathing was adopted as an essential addition to this lifesaving procedure, and since that time, there has been very little fundamental change in the method or manner of CPR. We do know after 50 years of experience that survival is improved if CPR is administered by bystanders rather than being provided only by emergency medical services (EMS) because it takes time for the latter staff to arrive. Furthermore, the use of automated external defibrillators by bystanders also has been documented to improve outcomes in patients with cardiac arrest. It has taken 50 years, however, to examine the individual components of the initial resuscitation process to determine their real value, thus the importance of the report of Rea et al. Animal studies have shown that interruption of chest compression to provide ventilation actually results in lower coronary perfusion pressure and presumably less myocardial blood flow during CPR. Also, an increased frequency of positive pressure ventilation additionally reduces survival rates in animal models. The latter most likely results from both the interruption of compression and the obstruction of venous return to the central circulation because of high intrathoracic pressure during ventilation. Based on these findings, the American Heart Association began to advocate hands-only CPR for bystanders not trained or competent in full CPR with rescue breathing.

In the report of Rea et al, we see a study that took advantage of EMS dispatchers' instruction to bystanders to administer CPR. In this study, patients with out-of-hospital cardiac arrest were randomly assigned to undergo 1 of 2 types of CPR performed by a bystander: either continuous chest compression without any attempts at ventilation or chest compression with interruptions for rescue breathing by bystanders (the current standard recommended approach). The data from the report are perfectly clear. Continuous chest compression without active ventilation results in a survival rate similar to that with chest compression with rescued breathing. Since the technique is much more simple to perform, one can expect a greater likelihood of a bystander effectively performing this CPR and increasing the chances of survival after cardiac arrest. Most bystanders find mouth-to-mouth rescue breathing far more difficult than proper chest compression, even leaving aside the potential for mouth-to-mouth to be distasteful to some bystanders who may have concern about transmission of disease by this technique. In many instances, mouth-to-mouth ventilation is performed so poorly by a bystander that the interruption of chest compressions for this form of ventilation is a waste of precious time in allowing maximal blood flow to the heart and to the brain.

The obvious concern of not performing mouth-to-mouth resuscitation is that one is perfusing less well-oxygenated blood. In fact, there are some studies to suggest that well-oxygenated blood during recovery from cardiac arrest is actually detrimental. Studies of isolated cardiac tissue specimens have raised the possibility that initial reperfusion with hypoxemic blood may in fact result in fewer injurious oxygen-free radicals and less reperfusion injury.[2]

Again, it is not entirely possible to translate the information from this report to the care of infants, children, and adolescents. Sudden cardiac arrest in an uncontrolled environment is relatively infrequent in most circumstances associated with cardiac arrest in this age group. If, however, a 9-year-old little leaguer suddenly collapses after a baseball hits his/her chest, it is likely that the information provided from this report of Rea et al would apply.

This commentary closes with a query: Do you know what made cardiologist Frank Pantridge famous? The answer is that he invented the cardiac defibrillator. The first prototype for a defibrillator weighed 70 kg and in fact gained a fair amount of credibility and support in the United States when it was used to treat a collapsed former President Lyndon B. Johnson in his daughter's home in 1972. Unfortunately, it took a number of years for the US Food and Drug Administration to agree that low voltage shocks could save lives and finally approved Dr. Pantridge's invention.[3]

J. A. Stockman III, MD

References

1. Kouwenhoven WB, Jude JR, Knickerbocker GG. Closed-chest cardiac massage. *JAMA*. 1960;173:1064-1067.
2. Kilgannon JH, Jones AE, Shapiro NI, et al. Association between arterial hyperoxia following resuscitation from cardiac arrest and in-hospital mortality. *JAMA*. 2010; 303:2165-2171.
3. Editorial comment. The cardiac defibrillator. *BMJ*. 2009;339:1092.

Standard cardiopulmonary resuscitation versus active compression-decompression cardiopulmonary resuscitation with augmentation of negative intrathoracic pressure for out-of-hospital cardiac arrest: a randomised trial

Aufderheide TP, Frascone RJ, Wayne MA, et al (Med College of Wisconsin, Milwaukee; Regions Hosp, St Paul, MN; St Joseph Med Ctr, Bellingham, WA; et al)
Lancet 377:301-311, 2011

Background.—Active compression-decompression cardiopulmonary resuscitation (CPR) with decreased intrathoracic pressure in the decompression phase can lead to improved haemodynamics compared with standard CPR. We aimed to assess effectiveness and safety of this intervention on survival with favourable neurological function after out-of-hospital cardiac arrest.

Methods.—In our randomised trial of 46 emergency medical service agencies (serving 2·3 million people) in urban, suburban, and rural areas of the USA, we assessed outcomes for patients with out-of-hospital cardiac arrest according to Utstein guidelines. We provisionally enrolled patients to receive standard CPR or active compression-decompression CPR with augmented negative intrathoracic pressure (via an impedance-threshold device) with a computer-generated block randomisation weekly schedule in a one-to-one ratio. Adults (presumed age or age ≥18 years) who had a nontraumatic arrest of presumed cardiac cause and met initial and final selection criteria received designated CPR and were included in the final analyses. The primary endpoint was survival to hospital discharge with favourable neurological function (modified Rankin scale score of ≤3). All investigators apart from initial rescuers were masked to treatment group assignment. This trial is registered with ClinicalTrials.gov, number NCT00189423.

Findings.—2470 provisionally enrolled patients were randomly allocated to treatment groups. 813 (68%) of 1201 patients assigned to the standard CPR group (controls) and 840 (66%) of 1269 assigned to intervention CPR received designated CPR and were included in the final analyses. 47 (6%) of 813 controls survived to hospital discharge with favourable neurological function compared with 75 (9%) of 840 patients in the intervention group (odds ratio 1·58, 95% CI 1·07–2·36; p=0·019]. 74 (9%) of 840 patients survived to 1 year in the intervention group compared with 48 (6%) of 813 controls (p=0·03), with equivalent cognitive skills, disability ratings, and emotional-psychological statuses in both groups. The overall major adverse event rate did not differ between groups, but more patients had pulmonary oedema in the intervention group (94 [11%] of 840) than did controls (62 [7%] of 813; p=0·015).

Interpretation.—On the basis of our findings showing increased effectiveness and generalisability of the study intervention, active compression-decompression CPR with augmentation of negative intrathoracic pressure should be considered as an alternative to standard CPR to increase long-term survival after cardiac arrest.

▶ This is another report appearing in the recent literature telling us that there are alternatives to standard cardiopulmonary resuscitation (CPR) techniques including active compression-decompression CPR with decreased thoracic pressure in the decompression phase. It is the latter technique that is reported by Aufderheide et al.

In this report, a randomized multicenter trial in 7 geographic regions was undertaken in the United States. Adults aged 18 years and older with out-of-hospital cardiac arrest were eligible for the study. The study itself was approved by the US Food and Drug Administration using standard research protocol guidelines. Patients received either standard CPR or compression-decompression CPR. The latter involved the use of a handheld device consisting of a suction cup that was attached to the chest with a handle and an audible metronome set to 80 beats per minute and a force gauge to guide the compression depth and chest wall recoil. This CPR technique requires the operator to compress to the same depth as standard CPR and then to lift upward to fully decompress the chest. An impedance-threshold device, with an inspiratory resistance of 16 cm H_2O and less than 5 cm H_2O expiratory impedance, was connected to a face mask or advanced airway. The impedance threshold device lowered intrathoracic pressure during the decompression phase by impeding passive inspiratory gas exchange during the chest recoil phase, yet allowing periodic positive pressure ventilation. The CPR device (ResQPump, also called CardioPump) and impedance-threshold device (ResQPOD) were manufactured by Advanced Circulatory Systems (Roseville, MN).

The first basic or advanced life support emergency medical service provider to arrive started chest compressions as soon as possible for both study groups. Standard CPR, defibrillation, and advanced life support treatment were done in accordance with local policy and the American Heart Association guidelines. The compression to ventilation ratio was 30 to 2 during basic life support for both CPR techniques. For the intervention protocol, rescuers provided CPR at 80 compressions per minute as soon as possible, with the active compression-decompression CPR device force gauge used to help achieve the recommended compression depth and complete chest recoil. For this group, rescuers initially attached the impedance-threshold device between the ventilation bag and face mask, and the device was subsequently relocated to the advanced airway. The impedance-threshold device was removed if the patient had return of spontaneous circulation and reapplied if rearrest occurred. The device included a face mask for the study intervention group (or face mask alone for the standard CPR group). CPR efforts in both groups were encouraged for at least 30 minutes on scene before resuscitation attempts were stopped. The study intervention, if in progress, was stopped on arrival to hospital and replaced with traditional CPR, if warranted. The prespecified primary study end point was survival to hospital discharge with favorable neurologic function.

The results of this study show that treatment with active compression-decompression CPR with enhancement of negative intrathoracic pressure during the decompression phase significantly increased survival to hospital discharge with favorable neurologic outcome compared with standard CPR after out-of-hospital cardiac arrest of presumed cardiac cause. The investigators have shown that the physiological changes underlying the synergistic effects of combination of acute compression-decompression CPR with an impedance-threshold device do add benefit. Active compression-decompression CPR by itself transforms the human chest into an active bellows; ventilation was increased to 13.5 L per minute (standard deviation [SD], 5.5) compared with 7.8 L per minute (SD, 5.3) for standard CPR. Interestingly, intrathoracic pressures remain much the same with standard CPR and active compression-decompression CPR unless the endotracheal tube was blocked with the impedance device, thereby preventing respiratory gas from entering the lungs during the decompression phase. The mechanical and physiological advantages associated with a lowering of the intrathoracic pressure by impedance of inspiration (apart from when active pressure ventilation was provided) had been confirmed in various studies of animals and people. Impedance of inspiration lowers intrathoracic pressure and results in increased cardiac output, vital organ blood flow, and survival in animals and in human beings.

These authors have shown for the first time a new technique in CPR and have documented that the technique does increase satisfactory outcomes when looked at the time of hospital discharge. These outcomes are increased by almost 50%. It should be noted what the raw data show, however. The raw data show that with standard CPR, only 6% of patients who experience out-of-hospital cardiac arrest will leave the hospital with good neurologic outcomes. This percentage increases to 9% with the techniques described. Not bad, but not perfect.

Please note that children were not included in this study. The physiology related to cardiac arrest in children may very well be quite different, but you can be sure as shooting that there will be investigations of this type done in children. Such investigations are extremely difficult to undertake with the end point being valid conclusions because of the infrequency of the problem in children. Perhaps we will have to rely on what we learn from adults and call it quits with that. The article by Wang et al tells about compression-only CPR by lay rescuers and ultimate survival from out-of-hospital cardiac arrest.[1]

On an unrelated cardiology topic, there may be a new test available soon that helps clinicians know whether a heart that has been transplanted is being rejected. About 4000 people worldwide get a new heart each year and at least 40% to 50% of them experience 1 episode of acute organ rejection, most often within a year of the transplant. Usually patients must undergo regular biopsies of their new organs to monitor its health. The procedure is both painful and expensive, but a new test now may obviate the need for such invasive procedures. Investigators at Stanford University have developed a test that monitors fragments of DNA that are released into the bloodstream when cells from the transplanted tissue are broken down. When a transplant goes well, organ owner—DNA typically makes up just about 1% of free-DNA in a recipient's blood. During a rejection event, that fraction increases to an average of 3%. Researchers hope that this test can eliminate the need for regular biopsies as a means of rejection monitoring. The new test is likely to be available in the not-too-distant future.[2]

J. A. Stockman III, MD

References

1. Wang YC, Cheung AM, Bibbins-Domingo K, et al. Effectiveness and cost-effectiveness of blood pressure screening in adolescents in the United States. *J Pediatr.* 2011; 158:257-264.
2. Carpenter J. Sensing organ rejection. Science. http://news.sciencemag.org/sciencenow/2011/03/sensing-organ-rejection.html. Published March 28, 2011. Accessed August 17, 2011.

Effectiveness and Cost-Effectiveness of Blood Pressure Screening in Adolescents in the United States

Wang YC, Cheung AM, Bibbins-Domingo K, et al (Columbia Univ Med Ctr, NY; the Univ Health Network, Toronto, Ontario, Canada; Univ of California, San Francisco; et al)
J Pediatr 158:257-264, 2011

Objective.—To compare the long-term effectiveness and cost-effectiveness of 3 approaches to managing elevated blood pressure (BP) in adolescents in the United States: no intervention, "screen-and-treat," and population-wide strategies to lower the entire BP distribution.

Study Design.—We used a simulation model to combine several data sources to project the lifetime costs and cardiovascular outcomes for a cohort of 15-year-old U.S. adolescents under different BP approaches and conducted cost-effectiveness analysis. We obtained BP distributions from the National Health and Nutrition Examination Survey 1999—2004 and used childhood-to-adult longitudinal correlation analyses to simulate the tracking of BP. We then used the coronary heart disease policy model to estimate lifetime coronary heart disease events, costs, and quality-adjusted life years (QALY).

Results.—Among screen-and-treat strategies, finding and treating the adolescents at highest risk (eg, left ventricular hypertrophy) was most cost-effective ($18 000/QALY [boys] and $47 000/QALY [girls]). However, all screen-and-treat strategies were dominated by population-wide strategies such as salt reduction (cost-saving [boys] and $650/QALY [girls]) and increasing physical education ($11 000/QALY [boys] and $35 000/QALY [girls]).

Conclusions.—Routine adolescents BP screening is moderately effective, but population-based BP interventions with broader reach could potentially be less costly and more effective for early cardiovascular disease prevention and should be implemented in parallel.

▶ No one can argue with the fact that pediatric hypertension is associated with short- and long-term problems, including premature atherosclerosis and vascular changes. Current recommendations for hypertension management in children and adolescents include universal and screen and treat approaches. These recommendations pursue a more sweeping societal change to diagnose and prevent the long-term complications of hypertension. Unfortunately, the relative cost-effectiveness of such a strategy has not been established, thus the value of the report of Wang et al, who used a simulation model to determine the population benefit and cost-effectiveness of 3 strategies to address adolescent hypertension in a theoretical cohort of 15-year-old subjects. These strategies included (1) traditional screen and treat strategies based within primary care practices; (2) population-based approaches including widespread education, including universal physical education in schools; and (3) no screening or treatment.

The authors used estimates from longitudinal pediatric cohorts to determine the impact of each intervention on blood pressure at the age of 35 years. As would be expected, the average change in quality-adjusted life-years (QALYs) per individual person was negligible but very large when summed across the population as a whole. Overall, average cost-effectiveness ratios for universal screening options compared with no treatment were higher than traditional thresholds (range, $60 000-$66 000/QALY for boys and $116 000-$135 000/QALY for girls), with the exception of pharmacologic therapy for patients with secondary hypertension or left ventricular hypertrophy: $18 000/QALY for boys and $47 000/QALY for girls. Population-based interventions including individual exercise programs and salt reduction programs for all adolescents resulted in the greatest benefit of life-years but at significant cost. On the other hand, increasing physical education classes for all adolescents also increased life-years dramatically and was cost effective compared with no screening or treatment ($8000/QALY for boys and $29 000/QALY for girls). A salt reduction campaign was also extremely cost saving in and of itself for both boys and girls (< $1000/QALY).

Modeling studies have well-recognized limitations. The correct models need to be selected. The strategies selected must account for the universe of truly realistic options available to address the issue. Despite these limitations, the information provided by Wang et al does give us strong empirical evidence that population-based interventions including salt reduction and increased physical education are cost-effective means to reduce the burden of cardiovascular disease related to hypertension in teens. Small changes in modifiable risk factors across large populations can indeed lead to significant improvements in the population burden of disease.

A device for measuring blood pressure has been field tested for use in low resource settings. The device is manufactured according to World Health Organization criteria and is an inexpensive, semi-automated, solar-powered instrument. It was successfully validated against a European protocol and later tested in Uganda and Zambia, where it was found to be valid for systolic blood pressure. Agreement between the solar-powered device and a sphygmomanometer for systolic blood pressure was 93.7%. Patients actually preferred the new device, which requires no batteries.[1]

J. A. Stockman III, MD

Reference

1. Parati G, Kilama MO, Faini A, et al. A new solar-powered blood pressure measuring device for low-resource settings. *Hypertension*. 2010;56:1047-1053.

Comparison of Shunt Types in the Norwood Procedure for Single-Ventricle Lesions
Ohye RG, for the Pediatric Heart Network Investigators (Univ of Michigan Med School, Ann Arbor; et al)
N Engl J Med 362:1980-1992, 2010

Background.—The Norwood procedure with a modified Blalock–Taussig (MBT) shunt, the first palliative stage for single-ventricle lesions with systemic outflow obstruction, is associated with high mortality. The right ventricle–pulmonary artery (RVPA) shunt may improve coronary flow but requires a ventriculotomy. We compared the two shunts in infants with hypoplastic heart syndrome or related anomalies.

Methods.—Infants undergoing the Norwood procedure were randomly assigned to the MBT shunt (275 infants) or the RVPA shunt (274 infants) at 15 North American centers. The primary outcome was death or cardiac transplantation 12 months after randomization. Secondary outcomes included unintended cardiovascular interventions and right ventricular size and function at 14 months and transplantation-free survival until the last subject reached 14 months of age.

Results.—Transplantation-free survival 12 months after randomization was higher with the RVPA shunt than with the MBT shunt (74% vs. 64%, P = 0.01). However, the RVPA shunt group had more unintended interventions (P = 0.003) and complications (P = 0.002). Right ventricular size and function at the age of 14 months and the rate of nonfatal serious adverse events at the age of 12 months were similar in the two groups. Data collected over a mean (±SD) follow-up period of 32 ± 11 months showed a nonsignificant difference in transplantation-free survival between the two groups (P = 0.06). On nonproportional-hazards analysis, the size of the treatment effect differed before and after 12 months (P = 0.02).

Conclusions.—In children undergoing the Norwood procedure, transplantation-free survival at 12 months was better with the RVPA shunt than with the MBT shunt. After 12 months, available data showed no significant difference in transplantation-free survival between the two groups. (ClinicalTrials.gov number, NCT00115934.) (Figs 1 and 2).

▶ When I was a resident in training in the early 1970s, if a diagnosis of hypoplastic left heart syndrome was made, it was only a matter of time before a newborn with that complex form of congenital heart disease would die. However, in the early 1980s, Norwood and colleagues at the Children's Hospital of Philadelphia pioneered a 3-stage surgical intervention for hypoplastic left heart syndrome that led to survival rates exceeding 60%. The goal of that surgical team was to establish a right-heart-based systemic circulation, using the Fontan procedure to create a separate pulmonary circulation, in which venous blood returns passively to the lungs. The first-stage procedure, known as the Norwood procedure, is the most difficult to perform and is associated with a high risk of death; it must be undertaken soon after birth to save the infant's life and prevent damage to the right side of the heart and the pulmonary vasculature. The procedure involves excising the atrial septum, so that oxygenated blood entering the left atrium crosses to the right heart; remodeling the ascending aorta, which is then patched into the proximal pulmonary artery, allowing the right ventricle to drive the systemic circulation; and establishing a separate conduit to deliver blood from the right ventricle to the pulmonary circulation. In the original Norwood procedure (stage I), a systemic-pulmonary shunt (the modified Blalock-Taussig shunt) connects the brachiocephalic artery to the pulmonary artery. The stage II procedure (performed when the infant is 4 months to 6 months old) and stage III procedure (at 2 to 4 years of age) complete the separation of the pulmonary circulation from the systemic circulation by switching the connections of the superior and inferior vena cava from the right heart to the pulmonary arteries (with the removal of the Norwood shunt). Fortunately, mortality is much lower with the stage II and stage III operations than with the stage I procedure.

While few infants survived the rigors of these surgeries in the early 1980s, by the new millennium, with improvements in surgical techniques and supportive care, survival rates have approached 65% to 75% with the 3-stage procedure at major surgical centers in the United States. These outcomes have not come without cost. Follow-up data on the quality of life of children who have undergone this surgery are limited, but it appears that about three-quarters of school-age survivors have reduced exercise capacity, and 1 in 4 have some degree of cognitive or neurologic impairment. It is hoped that the latter outcomes will show improvement over time with the adoption of regional cerebral profusion techniques during aortic reconstruction. In any event, improvements in survival rates with the 3-stage reconstructive procedures have been so great that neonatal cardiac transplantation—the only alternative approach for children

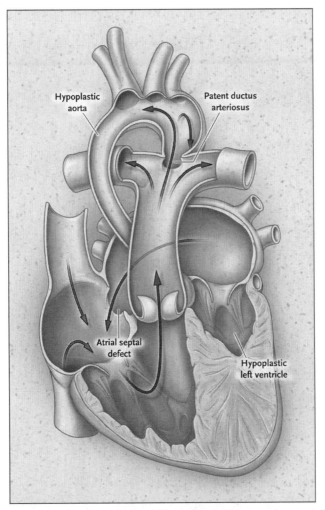

FIGURE 1.—Hypoplastic Left Heart Syndrome. The hypoplastic left heart syndrome and related disorders involving the single right ventricle are characterized by a total admixture lesion. As in the normal heart, deoxygenated blood returns to the right atrium. Oxygenated blood returning from the left atrium crosses an atrial septal defect to join the deoxygenated blood in the right atrium. This mixed blood is then ejected by the right ventricle into the pulmonary artery. A portion of the blood in the pulmonary artery proceeds as normal to the lungs, as well as to the aorta through a patent ductus arteriosus, to supply the systemic circulation. (Reprinted from Ohye RG, for the Pediatric Heart Network Investigators. Comparison of shunt types in the Norwood procedure for single-ventricle lesions. *New Engl J Med.* 2010;362:1980-1992. Copyright 2010 Massachusetts Medical Society. All rights reserved.)

with hypoplastic left heart syndrome—has been largely relegated for those infants in whom surgical reconstruction has not been successful.

We see in this report of Ohye et al further developments in attempts to refine the Norwood procedure. Surgeons have been tinkering with various aspects of the Norwood procedure ever since it was first described, but unfortunately,

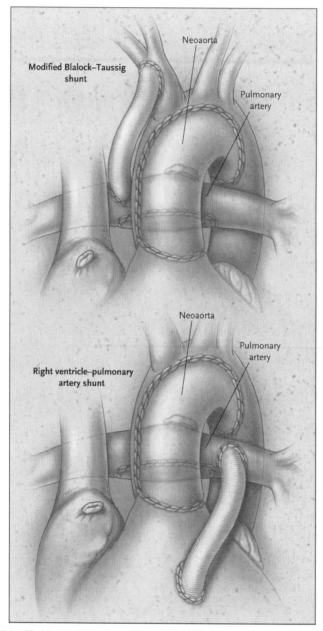

FIGURE 2.—The Norwood Procedure with a Modified Blalock—Taussig Shunt and a Right Ventricle—Pulmonary Artery Shunt. In the completed Norwood procedure, one can see the reconstructed aorta (neoaorta) and the isolated pulmonary artery. Pulmonary blood flow is supplied by either a modified Blalock—Taussig shunt (top) or a right ventricle—pulmonary artery shunt (bottom). (Reprinted from Ohye RG, for the Pediatric Heart Network Investigators. Comparison of shunt types in the Norwood procedure for single-ventricle lesions. *New Engl J Med*. 2010;362:1980-1992. Copyright 2010 Massachusetts Medical Society. All rights reserved.)

there have been no large-scale studies to show what alterations in the procedure might be of benefit to patients. A case in point involves a controversy over the relative benefits of the Blalock-Taussig shunt as used in the original Norwood procedure compared with the recently introduced right ventricle-pulmonary artery (RVPA) shunt, which connects the right ventricle directly to the pulmonary circulation through a right ventriculotomy. The RVPA shunt appears to improve perfusion of the coronary arteries and vital organs, owing to higher diastolic pressures and a better balance of pulmonary and systemic circulation. However, there has been concern that the ventriculotomy might impair myocardial and tricuspid-valve function and increase the risk of ventricular arrhythmias. In a very few small studies involving historical controls, it has been suggested that the RVPA shunt is of greater benefit in comparison to the standard Norwood procedure. To compare these 2 procedures, a randomized controlled trial was designed and implemented by the Pediatric Heart Network with 15 participating centers providing a more than adequate sample of over 500 infants. The results are reported in the article by Ohye et al. The major outcome of the study was transplantation-free survival at 1 year. In this study, there was a significant advantage of the RVPA shunt (transplantation-free survival rate, 74% vs 64%). The potential for harmful effects of the right ventriculotomy proved to be unwarranted, although additional, unplanned interventions were performed in the RVPA shunt group to maintain shunt patency. Long-term follow-up will be needed to assess the benefits beyond this 12-month period that was assessed in the trial.

It is likely that the Pediatric Heart Network will continue to refine and improve the surgical treatment methods that are being used to manage infants with congenital heart disease. The story with the Norwood procedure is not over yet, as already new methods to refine this procedure beyond those described in the Ohye et al report are being undertaken. It will not be long before we see these youngsters grow into adulthood and learn how well their pump is holding up.

To read more about the hypoplastic left heart syndrome, see the superb editorial on this topic by Bondy.[1]

Last, *Name that Murmur—Eponyms for the Astute Auscultician*, Parts 6 and 7: Gibson's Murmur and Graham Steell Murmur[2]: George Gibson was a committed teacher and academic who practiced in London at the turn of the 20th century. It was Gibson who described the persistent murmur of patent ductus arteriosus. The murmur is continuous, beginning after the first heart sound and extending through the second heart sound and is distinctly audible over the unbroken rushing of the murmur. Although the murmur is audible over the entire base of the heart, Gibson noted that it is best heard over the left upper sternal border.[3] Graham Steell was a Scottish cardiologist and an avid horseman and iconoclast, known for his illegible notes, brevity of speech, and excellent bedside teaching. For his healthier patients he recommended horseback riding as the best form of exercise. Although the murmur of pulmonary insufficiency bears Graham Steell's name, it was first described by others, notably George Balfour, for whom Steell worked as a house officer at the Edinburgh Royal Infirmary in 1873. Nonetheless, it was Steell who published numerous articles describing the murmur. The Graham Steell murmur is a soft, blowing, decrescendo diastolic murmur, running off an accentuated second heart sound that mimics the murmur of aortic insufficiency. The murmur is best heard in a localized area at the left upper sternal border.

J. A. Stockman III, MD

References

1. Bondy CA. Hypoplastic left heart syndrome. *N Engl J Med.* 2010;362:2026-2028.
2. Ma I, Tierney LM. Name that murmur—eponyms for the astute auscultician. *N Engl J Med.* 2010;363:2164-2168.
3. Gibson GA. A clinical lecture on persistent ductus arteriosus. *Med Press Circular.* 1906;132:572-574.

Care of the Adult Congenital Heart Disease Patient in the United States: A Summary of the Current System

Patel MS, Kogon BE (Children's Healthcare of Atlanta, GA; Emory Univ School of Medicine, Atlanta, GA)
Pediatr Cardiol 31:511-514, 2010

With improvements in care, there has been exponential growth in the population of adult congenital heart disease (ACHD) patients. We sought to assess the availability of specialized ACHD care in the United States. We analyzed the Adult Congenital Heart Association's ACHD clinic directory for information on patient volume, provider training, and other characteristics. The information is self-reported and unverified. The ACHD directory included 72 programs in the United States. Across programs, the majority of patients (33%) seen were between 21 and 30 years old. Program directors had between 2 and 50 years (median 15) of ACHD experience and had dedicated between 10 and 100% (median 30%) of their clinical time to ACHD. There were 2,800 ACHD operations performed per year, ranging from 0 to 230 (median 28) per program. There were between 0 and 5 cardiac surgeons (median 2) involved per program. Each surgeon averaged 20 ACHD operations per year. The growing ACHD population is a largely underserved group. Few programs in the United States provide specialized care, and this care is variably conducted within pediatric and/or adult facilities. These data should serve as a stimulus to improving accessibility of services for this vulnerable population.

▶ There are now more adults with congenital heart disease (CHD) being cared for in society than there are children. Unfortunately, many of these adults are not receiving optimal care because of our health care system's inability to properly transition care from pediatric providers to adult providers. Based on recommendations from the 32nd Bethesda Conference, adults with moderately severe to greatly complex CHD (including those who have had complex CHD repaired in the past) should be followed up in a regional adult CHD (ACHD) center at least once or twice a year. This does not include the support that should be ongoing by a local cardiologist. This report reminds us that the ACHD population is growing by about 9000 patients a year largely based on the successes achieved by pediatric cardiologists and pediatric cardiovascular surgeons. Current estimates are that there are between 1 million and 1.5 million adult patients with CHD in the United States now. Unfortunately, as this review of Patel et al shows, a large proportion of the ACHD population here in the United States has little or no access to comprehensive care. No one will argue that ACHD patients are better served in adult facilities, including access to adult cardiologists, comfortable with management of adult-onset acquired heart disease and other adult comorbidities, and most importantly, access to adult-oriented primary care. The US health care system, however, falls short in all of these categories. In the best of all worlds, it would be ideal for ACHD clinics to be housed within adult facilities with cooperating engagement by pediatric congenital heart surgeons and pediatric cardiologists. All too often, it is the other way around with the care being stitched together under the umbrella of pediatric services for way too long than is ideal in a patient's life.

One final comment about CHD. The United States is beginning to suffer from a shortage of properly trained congenital heart disease surgeons. Part of the problem lies with the fact that the entry path to the training of congenital heart surgeons is via training in adult thoracic surgery. Training in adult and pediatric cardiac surgery is undergoing major change. In recent years, nearly one-third of the training positions in adult cardiothoracic surgery have gone unfilled. The reasons that are usually cited include a shrinking patient pool (mostly because of percutaneous coronary interventions), the perception of a poorer quality of life for cardiothoracic surgeons (compared with other specialties), declining reimbursements and salaries, long training requirements, a shrinking job market, increased legal challenges, and increased scrutiny by professional societies, payers, and government. While congenital pediatric heart surgery has been somewhat protected from these changes, recruits into these disciplines have traditionally come from the general ranks of cardiothoracic surgery trainees, a diminishing breed. In a recent survey, nearly one-quarter of cardiothoracic surgery training program graduates reported that they would not choose a career in cardiothoracic surgery again, and more than half would not strongly recommend cardiothoracic surgery to potential trainees.[1] Training surgeons to competency in congenital heart surgery is not an easy task. Recognizing that the classic model of 5 years in general surgery, 2 years of cardiothoracic surgery, and 1 year of congenital heart surgery training is outmoded, the American Board of Thoracic Surgery recently revised its required standards for training and has dropped the core requirement for being certified first in general surgery, thus allowing for a more focused and longer training in cardiothoracic surgery at the expense of time spent in general surgery rotations. This move in fact has become quite critical in view of the restricted number of work hours allowed now for training. Focused training on maximizing what time is available therefore is the mantra of residency program directors.

This commentary closes with a historical observation having to do with how ancients viewed the importance of the heart. A review of Ancient Greek philosophical and medical text notes that early primitive societies attributed great significance to the heart. This probably accounted for cannibalistic behaviors in early societies such as possessing and eating the hearts of the defeated enemies. Mental functions such as thinking and feeling at the time were attributed to the heart, rather than the brain. The role of the brain was severely underestimated (and thus sparing the brain from being eaten) probably because it was "silent" compared with the beating heart—even after Galan discovered the course of cranial and spinal nerves.[2]

J. A. Stockman III, MD

References

1. Kogon BE. The training of congenital heart surgeons. *J Thorac Cardiovasc Surg.* 2006;132:1280-1284.
2. Lykouras E, Poulakou-Rebelakou E, Ploumpidis DM. Searching the seat of the soul in Ancient Greek and Byzantine medical literature. *Acta Cardiologica.* 2010;65:619-626.

Intermediate-Term Effects of Transcatheter Secundum Atrial Septal Defect Closure on Cardiac Remodeling in Children and Adults

Kaya MG, Baykan A, Dogan A, et al (Erciyes Univ School of Medicine, Kayseri, Turkey)
Pediatr Cardiol 31:474-482, 2010

The study aimed to investigate the intermediate-term effects of transcatheter atrial septal defect (ASD) closure on cardiac remodeling in children and adult patients. Between December 2003 and February 2009, 117 patients (48 males, 50 adults) underwent transcatheter ASD closure with the Amplatzer septal occluder (ASO). The mean age of the patients was 15 years, and the mean follow-up period was 25.9 ± 12.4 months. New York Heart Association (NYHA) class, electrocardiographic parameters, and transthoracic echocardiographic (TTE) examination were evaluated before the ASD closure, then 1 day, 1 month, 6 months, 12 months, and yearly afterward. Transcatheter ASD closure was successfully performed for 112 (96%) of the 117 patients. The mean ASD diameter measured by transesophageal echocardiography (TEE) was 14.0 ± 4.2 mm, and the mean diameter stretched with a sizing balloon was 16.6 ± 4.8 mm. The mean size of the implanted device was 18.6 ± 4.9 mm. The Qp/Qs ratio was 2.2 ± 0.8. The mean systolic pulmonary artery pressure was 40 ± 10 mmHg. At the end of the mean follow-up period of 2 years, the indexed right ventricular (RV) end-diastolic diameter had decreased from 36 ± 5 to 30 ± 5 mm/m^2 ($p = 0.005$), and the indexed left ventricular (LV) end-diastolic diameter had increased from 33 ± 5 to 37 ± 6 mm/m^2 ($p = 0.001$), resulting in an RV/LV ratio decreased from 1.1 ± 0.2 to 0.8 ± 0.2 ($p = 0.001$). The New York Heart Association (NYHA) functional capacity of the patients was improved significantly 24 months after ASD closure (1.9 ± 0.5 to 1.3 ± 0.5; $p = 0.001$). At the 2-year follow up electrocardiographic examination, the P maximum had decreased from 128 ± 15 to 102 ± 12 ms

$(p = 0.001)$, the P dispersion had decreased from 48 ± 11 to 36 ± 9 ms $(p = 0.001)$, and the QT dispersion had decreased from 66 ± 11 to 54 ± 8 ms $(p = 0.001)$. Five of six patients experienced resolution of their preclosure arrhythmias, whereas the remaining patient continued to have paroxysmal atrial fibrillation. A new arrhythmia (supraventricular tachycardia) developed in one patient and was well controlled medically. Transcatheter ASD closure leads to a significant improvement in clinical status and heart cavity dimensions in adults and children, as shown by intermediate-term follow-up evaluation. Transcatheter ASD closure can reverse electrical and mechanical changes in atrial myocardium, resulting in a subsequent reduction in P maximum and P dispersion times.

▶ Most of us tend to think that atrial septal defect (ASD) as a manifestation of congenital heart disease is a quite benign condition. Indeed it is if handled correctly and diagnosed early on and managed. ASD accounts for as much as 10% of all forms of congenital heart disease and frequently remains asymptomatic until adult age. Early diagnosis is crucial. If the diagnosis is missed for too long, the patient is at added risk for potential complications such as pulmonary hypertension, right-sided heart failure, atrial arrhythmias, and paradoxical embolism.

Although surgical closure of an ASD is frequently stated to be a low-risk procedure, it is associated with certain morbidities including postpericardotomy syndrome, arrhythmia, pericardial-pleural effusion, blood transfusion risk, and scar formation. Transcatheter closure of ASD has become an important alternative to surgical repair in the management of patients with secundum-type ASD. With either approach, when an ASD is corrected, the right side of the heart is protected from volume load, leading to reductions in pulmonary artery pressure. Thus significant symptomatic improvement with a decrease in arrhythmic events is expected. Major problems encountered in patients with ASD are arrhythmias and primarily atrial fibrillation. Data on children have looked at the short-term effects of percutaneous closure of ASD. This report from Turkey looks over a longer period of time to determine the intermediate-term effects of percutaneous ASD closure on cardiac remodeling, electrocardiogram parameters, and exercise capacity in both children and adults. The findings show a significant reduction in right ventricular diameter and significant improvement in the electrocardiograms of these patients. In addition, intermediate-term follow-up shows clinically significant improvement in exercise capacity. Some of these findings are quite interesting since open heart surgery results in 50% to 70% of adults and children having persistent right ventricular enlargement for some time, presumably a consequence of functional abnormalities related to cardiopulmonary bypass and also the direct effect of opening the heart itself.

Thus it is that transcatheter ASD closure is capable of reversing electrical and mechanical changes in the heart, at least when looked at in the short and intermediate term. One can suspect that in those patients eligible for noninvasive management, we will be seeing more and more transcatheter closures.

Name that Murmur—Eponyms for the Astute Auscultician, Parts 8 and 9: Key-Hodgkin Murmur and Roger's Murmur[1]: Charles Aston Key was one of the most prominent surgeons of the early 19th century, working in London. He was a contemporary of Thomas Hodgkin, the physician for whom Hodgkin lymphoma is named. Hodgkin lectured intermittently at Guy's Hospital where Key was a staff surgeon. Key is credited with first drawing Hodgkin's attention to the problem of aortic incompetence. Subsequently, Hodgkin wrote the first case series that both described aortic incompetence and included theories on its cause. Syphilitic aortitis was at the time the leading cause of aortic regurgitation. The Key-Hodgkin murmur is a diastolic murmur of aortic regurgitation having a raspy quality, similar to the sound of a saw cutting through wood. Henri Louis Roger was a pediatrician working in Paris. He recognized that holes in the interventricular wall were associated with murmurs. Roger murmur of the ventricular septal defect is holosystolic and heard best at the left upper sternal border. The murmur is loud and its sound has been compared with that of a rushing waterfall. The smaller the ventricular septal defect, the louder the murmur.[2,3]

J. A. Stockman III, MD

References

1. Ma I, Tierney LM. Name that murmur—eponyms for the astute auscultician. *N Engl J Med.* 2010;363:2164-2168.
2. Hodgkin T. On retroversion of the valves of the aorta. *Lond Med Gaz.* 1828;3:433-443.
3. Henri-Louis. Rogers (1809-1891): Roger's disease. *JAMA.* 1970;213:456-457.

Outcome of Isolated Bicuspid Aortic Valve in Childhood

Mahle WT, Sutherland JL, Frias PA (Sibley Heart Ctr at Children's Healthcare of Atlanta and Dept of Pediatrics of Emory Univ School of Medicine, GA)
J Pediatr 157:445-449, 2010

Objective.—To evaluate the outcomes associated with isolated bicuspid aortic valve (BAV) during childhood and adolescence.

Study Design.—Analysis of a large single institutional cohort of children (n = 981) with isolated BAV was undertaken to determine the prevalence of significant ascending aortic dilation and risk of cardiac events. Subjects with known genetic disorders, critical aortic stenosis (intervention required in infancy), or additional lesions such as coarctation of the aorta were excluded. Aortic dimensions were derived from echocardiography, and values were plotted as Z scores. Clinical outcomes included death, aortic dissection, balloon aortic valvuloplasty, or cardiac surgery.

Results.—The median age of the subjects at diagnosis was 8.3 years. At the time of the last pediatric follow-up, 7% of the subjects had moderate aortic regurgitation or greater, and the median Z score for the ascending aorta was +2.31. There were 9427 patient years of follow-up. Primary cardiac events occurred in 38 subjects, yielding an event rate of 0.004 per patient year. Eleven subjects (1.1%) underwent aortic valve surgery. Thirty subjects (3.0%) underwent balloon dilatation of the aortic valve.

There was a single case of endocarditis. There were no cardiac-related deaths and no cases of aortic dissection.

Conclusions.—The incidence of primary cardiac events in children with BAV is relatively low, approximately 3-fold lower than in young adults, and is generally related to aortic stenosis amenable to balloon dilatation. Although mild ascending aortic dilation is common in children, the clinical course is relatively benign. In this series, aortic dissection did not occur. Whether elective surgery for the dilated aorta has a role in children remains unknown.

▶ While bicuspid aortic valve (BAV) is indeed the most common congenital anomaly in children, most of us do not think too much about it because it rarely causes significant difficulty during childhood. In its severest form, it can be associated with critical aortic stenosis and can require emergent intervention in the neonatal period. BAV is reported to be present in approximately 1% of the population, whereas the birth prevalence of true aortic stenosis is just 3 per 10 000 live births. While the natural history of critical aortic stenosis has been described in great detail, the natural history of BAV in childhood, however, has been much less well cataloged. In the authors' experience, for subjects with isolated BAV in the absence of critical aortic stenosis, the annual incidence rate for any cardiac event/intervention was just 0.004, a rate much lower than the rate reported in young adults.

Adolescents and children with BAV can develop dilatation of the aorta, most markedly of the ascending aorta. It should be noted, however, that the clinical implications of dilated ascending aorta in BAV remain controversial. The presence of BAV is thought to increase the risk of aortic dissection 2- to 5-fold. The mechanism of this increased risk is believed to be related in part to inherent abnormalities in the aortic wall itself, although this remains a subject of some debate. Most do agree that the risk of aortic dissection is related to the degree of aortic dilatation. It seems reasonable to say that children with dilatation of the ascending aorta would be at some increased risk of aortic dissection, although the occurrence of this latter event during childhood is extremely unlikely. There have been cases reported of aortic dissection in adolescents who have BAV, but as the authors of this report note, in all the postmortem series published to date there have been other associated lesions such as repaired coarctations or significant aortic stenosis that would otherwise have met the criteria for surgical or transcatheter intervention.

The authors of this report conclude that BAV is not known to be a risk factor for aortic dissection in and of itself. They do admonish us that further studies are needed to understand what role aortic aneurysm surgery plays in this population and whether some children with BAV should be restricted from sport participation. While this is being sorted out, families should understand that the risks of complications from isolated BAV in childhood are quite small. The same is not true in adults with this congenital anomaly.

This commentary closes with the observation that there is now a new iPhone app that is quite innovative and perhaps useful in the field of cardiology. The iStethoscope application monitors the heartbeat through sensors in the

phone and has been downloaded in droves since a free version was introduced.[1] Try it. You might like it.

J. A. Stockman III, MD

Reference

1. iPhone app to replace the stethoscope. The Telegraph. www.telegraph.co.uk/
technology/apple/7971950/iPhone-app-to-replace-the-stethoscope.html. Published
August 31, 2010. Accessed August 17, 2011.

Percutaneous Repair or Surgery for Mitral Regurgitation

Feldman T, for the EVEREST II Investigators (NorthShore Univ Health System,
Evanston, IL; et al)
N Engl J Med 364:1395-1406, 2011

Background.—Mitral-valve repair can be accomplished with an investigational procedure that involves the percutaneous implantation of a clip
that grasps and approximates the edges of the mitral leaflets at the origin
of the regurgitant jet.

Methods.—We randomly assigned 279 patients with moderately severe
or severe (grade 3+ or 4+) mitral regurgitation in a 2:1 ratio to undergo
either percutaneous repair or conventional surgery for repair or replacement of the mitral valve. The primary composite end point for efficacy
was freedom from death, from surgery for mitral-valve dysfunction, and
from grade 3+ or 4+ mitral regurgitation at 12 months. The primary safety
end point was a composite of major adverse events within 30 days.

Results.—At 12 months, the rates of the primary end point for efficacy
were 55% in the percutaneous-repair group and 73% in the surgery group
(P=0.007). The respective rates of the components of the primary end
point were as follows: death, 6% in each group; surgery for mitral-valve
dysfunction, 20% versus 2%; and grade 3+ or 4+ mitral regurgitation,
21% versus 20%. Major adverse events occurred in 15% of patients in
the percutaneous-repair group and 48% of patients in the surgery group
at 30 days (P<0.001). At 12 months, both groups had improved left
ventricular size, New York Heart Association functional class, and
quality-of-life measures, as compared with baseline.

Conclusions.—Although percutaneous repair was less effective at
reducing mitral regurgitation than conventional surgery, the procedure
was associated with superior safety and similar improvements in clinical
outcomes. (Funded by Abbott Vascular; EVEREST II ClinicalTrials.gov
number, NCT00209274.)

▶ Before this report appeared, I was not familiar with just how common mitral
valve regurgitation was. Eighty percent of us in fact have some normal valve
leakage detectable on echocardiography. Fortunately, for most of us, mitral
regurgitation is well tolerated and rarely leads to overt clinical disease. Both

children and adults, however, can have more significant mitral regurgitation that overloads the left ventricle as blood is pumped both backward across the mitral valve and forward to the systemic circulation. Given enough time, volume overload results in ventricular dilatation and eventual contractile dysfunction. At least in adults, left atrial pressure can lead to atrial fibrillation and pulmonary hypertension. If bad enough, these same problems can occur in children. Left alone, these physiological changes can lead to heart failure symptoms and reduce survival, but prevention is possible with corrective intervention if done early enough.

Currently, the choices for intervention for mitral regurgitation are surgical mitral valve repair or replacement, with repair preferred wherever possible because it has a low postoperative mortality (2%), restores mitral valve function, and provides excellent long-term outcomes. Some causes of mitral regurgitation can be managed medically. For example, in those who have this problem related to dilated cardiomyopathy, regurgitation severity often improves with medical therapy. Similarly, in those who have the problem as the result of coronary artery disease, regurgitation can improve after revascularization.

Feldman et al report the results of a randomized prospective trial of a percutaneously inserted mitral valve clip for the treatment of severe regurgitation. The idea that regurgitation might be treated with a nonsurgical approach is exciting, particularly if the new procedure effectively reduces the severity of regurgitation with a low procedural risk. At 30 days postprocedure, the mitral valve clip was associated with a lower rate of complications, but it is disappointing that 1 year after the procedure, 20% of patients in the percutaneous treatment group required surgery for mitral valve dysfunction compared with just 2% in the surgical group requiring repeat surgery. Of particular concern is the finding that substantial residual regurgitation (grade 2+ or more) was present in 46% of patients in the percutaneous treatment group as compared with 17% in the surgical group at 12 months.

The study of Feldman et al did not include children or adolescents. This age group does have a population of patients with mitral valve regurgitation, some of whom require surgical intervention. It will be interesting to see how the adult story plays out so we know whether noninvasive procedures would be helpful in the management of youngsters with this problem.

Name that Murmur: Eponyms for the Astute Auscultician, Part 10: Still's Murmur. George Frederic Still is considered the father of British Pediatrics and is best known for his eponymous rheumatic disorders: a juvenile febrile arthritis and a more typhoidal illness in adults, both called Still disease. During his long career he published several textbooks and in the twilight of his career he even became physician to Princess Elizabeth (who would become Queen Elizabeth II of the United Kingdom) and her sister, Princess Margaret. He was knighted in 1937. Most often seen in children, Still murmur is a medium to long systolic ejection murmur with a musical quality; it is heard over the left lower sternal border and apex. This murmur is completely benign and is described as "twangy," similar to that of a string being plucked. The murmur increases in intensity with fever, anxiety, or exercise. Its cause is unknown although it has been suggested that the source may be vibration of the cordae tendineae in the left ventricle or the sound of blood gushing into the aorta.[1]

J. A. Stockman III, MD

Reference

1. Hamilton EB. George Frederic Still. *Ann Rheum Dis.* 1986;45:1-5.

Effect of celiprolol on prevention of cardiovascular events in vascular Ehlers-Danlos syndrome: a prospective randomised, open, blinded-endpoints trial

Ong K-T, Perdu J, De Backer J, et al (Hôpital Européen Georges Pompidou, Paris, France; Ghent Univ Hosp, Belgium; et al)

Lancet 376:1476-1484, 2010

Background.—Vascular Ehlers-Danlos syndrome is a rare severe disease that causes arterial dissections and ruptures that can lead to early death. No preventive treatment has yet been validated. Our aim was to assess the ability of celiprolol, a β_1-adrenoceptor antagonist with a β_2-adrenoceptor agonist action, to prevent arterial dissections and ruptures in vascular Ehlers-Danlos syndrome.

Methods.—Our study was a multicentre, randomised, open trial with blinded assessment of clinical events in eight centres in France and one in Belgium. Patients with clinical vascular Ehlers-Danlos syndrome were randomly assigned to 5 years of treatment with celiprolol or to no treatment. Randomisation was done from a centralised, previously established list of sealed envelopes with stratification by patients' age (≤ 32 years or >32 years). 33 patients were positive for mutation of collagen 3A1 (*COL3A1*). Celiprolol was uptitrated every 6 months by steps of 100 mg to a maximum of 400 mg twice daily. The primary endpoints were arterial events (rupture or dissection, fatal or not). This study is registered with ClinicalTrials.gov, number NCT00190411.

Findings.—53 patients were randomly assigned to celiprolol (25 patients) or control groups (28). Mean duration of follow-up was 47 (SD 5) months, with the trial stopped early for treatment benefit. The primary endpoints were reached by five (20%) in the celiprolol group and by 14 (50%) controls (hazard ratio [HR] 0.36; 95% CI $0.15-0.88$; p=0.040). Adverse events were severe fatigue in one patient after starting 100 mg celiprolol and mild fatigue in two patients related to dose uptitration.

Interpretation.—We suggest that celiprolol might be the treatment of choice for physicians aiming to prevent major complications in patients with vascular Ehlers-Danlos syndrome. Whether patients with similar clinical presentations and no mutation are also protected remains to be established.

▶ Clinical manifestations of Ehlers-Danlos syndrome can certainly present in childhood. The syndrome actually represents a group of heterogeneous inherited connective tissue disorders. The most severe form is associated with vascular dissection or rupture of hollow organ (uterus, intestine), both of which are caused by fragility of connective tissue. The median survival is 40 to 50 years, but the first complications of the disorder are usually seen no later than the teenage years. Virtually all patients will have a major event by 40 years of age. The disease results from heterogeneous mutations in the *COL3A1* gene. These mutations cause structural defects in collagen and are characterized by decreased thermal stability, reduced secretion, and abnormal proteolytic processing. The most serious form of Ehlers-Danlos syndrome, the vascular type, is transmitted as an autosomal dominant trait. To date, no treatment has been proven to prevent clinical events.

Ong et al present encouraging results from a multicenter randomized trial in 53 patients with the clinical diagnosis of vascular Ehlers-Danlos syndrome who were randomly assigned to celiprolol, a long-acting β1 antagonist with partial β2 agonist properties used in hypertension versus no treatment. This drug decreased the incidence of arterial rupture or dissection by 3-fold, over a median follow-up period of 47 months (27% in the celiprolol vs 50% in the control group). There were no untoward side effects directly related to the drug treatment.

More research is needed on the mechanism of action of celiprolol in the prevention of cardiovascular events in Ehlers-Danlos syndrome. The report of Ong et al do, however, represent a substantial breakthrough in the evidence-based management of the syndrome. The drug is an inexpensive well-tolerated agent available to treat any patient with the disorder and perhaps with related disorders. To read more about Ehlers-Danlos syndrome and the theories around the action of celiprolol, see the excellent commentary on this topic by Brooke.[1]

J. A. Stockman III, MD

Reference

1. Brooke BS. Celiprolol therapy for vascular Ehlers-Danlos syndrome. *Lancet.* 2010; 376:1443-1444.

Noncanonical TGFβ Signaling Contributes to Aortic Aneurysm Progression in Marfan Syndrome Mice

Holm TM, Habashi JP, Doyle JJ, et al (Johns Hopkins Univ School of Medicine, Baltimore, MD; et al)
Science 332:358-361, 2011

Transforming growth factor—β (TGFβ) signaling drives aneurysm progression in multiple disorders, including Marfan syndrome (MFS), and therapies that inhibit this signaling cascade are in clinical trials. TGFβ can stimulate multiple intracellular signaling pathways, but it is unclear which of these pathways drives aortic disease and, when inhibited, which result in disease amelioration. Here we show that extracellular signal—regulated kinase (ERK) 1 and 2 and Smad2 are activated in a mouse model of MFS, and both are inhibited by therapies directed against TGFβ. Whereas selective inhibition of ERK1/2 activation ameliorated aortic growth, Smad4 deficiency exacerbated aortic disease and caused premature death in MFS mice. Smad4-deficient MFS mice uniquely showed activation of Jun N-terminal kinase−1 (JNK1), and a JNK antagonist ameliorated aortic growth in MFS mice that lacked or retained full Smad4 expression. Thus, noncanonical (Smad-independent) TGFβ signaling is a prominent driver of aortic disease in MFS mice, and inhibition of the ERK1/2 or JNK1 pathways is a potential therapeutic strategy for the disease.

▶ This may seem like a very obtuse, if not obscure, report to include. In fact, it may be but the information provided based on animal model studies has real implications for human disease, specifically Marfan syndrome. It was only about half a dozen years ago that a pediatric cardiologist set in motion a new treatment for Marfan syndrome that upended the field of pediatric and adult cardiology. Prior to that time, most patients with Marfan syndrome were managed with β-blocker drugs to help prevent the development and progression of aneurysms, a major cause of death. β-blockers are an imperfect treatment, with more than half of Marfan patients eventually requiring surgery for this problem. In the middle of this past decade, however, it was found that a blood pressure drug called losartan virtually erased the risk of aneurysms when tested in mice. This then has been translated into clinical trials in humans that, at the time of the report of Holm et al, were still ongoing.

The authors of this report are the group that back in 2006 discovered that losartan would block transforming growth factor β, stopping the enlargement and weakening of the aorta in the mouse model. They now further explore this issue by looking for links between transforming growth factor β and aortic aneurysm at the cellular and tissue level. They have partnered with the US National Institutes of Health Chemical Genomics Center, which screens molecules for potential drug application. They found a protein driven by transforming growth factor β to be activated and have discovered an inhibiting drug that in a mouse model completely eliminates aneurysm development, just like losartan has done. It will be some time before these investigational drugs are studied in humans, and we certainly need to see what effect losartan has in current clinical trials. The largest trial of the latter drug finished enrolling patients in 2010. It has 608 participants, and results are still a few years off. Cardiologists are cautious about betting on losartan's success since the trial has not been halted as yet, suggesting that it might have been if losartan had proven extraordinarily effective. If it turns out that losartan is not the magic bullet for prevention and control of aneurysms in those with Marfan syndrome, other alternatives, such as noted in this report, are certainly welcomed.

This commentary closes with the observation that soon we may be seeing "off-the-shelf blood vessels" being used in humans rather than using a patient's own blood vessels in heart bypass surgery, for dialysis patients, etc. All too frequently, it becomes very difficult to find suitable blood vessels for these purposes. Investigators at Humacyte, a biotechnology company in Morrisville,

North Carolina, have developed a process to seed human smooth muscle cells taken from donated cadavers onto a tubular scaffold made from a biodegradable polymer called polyglycolic acid. As the cells grow to cover the scaffold, they produce collagen and other extracellular matrix proteins that replace the degrading scaffold. Researchers then used detergent to remove the cells, leaving a cell-free blood vessel that can be stored for months, one that does not initiate an immune reaction in the recipient. Such blood vessels have been transplanted into the arms of baboons quite successfully. Perhaps it will not be in the too distant future before we see this application for humans.[1]

J. A. Stockman III, MD

Reference

1. Vogel G. Off-the-Shelf Blood Vessels. Science. http://news.sciencemag.org/science now/2011/02/off-the-shelf-blood-vessels.html?ref=hp. Published February 2, 2011. Accessed August 18, 2011.

10 Infectious Diseases and Immunology

The accuracy of clinical symptoms and signs for the diagnosis of serious bacterial infection in young febrile children: prospective cohort study of 15 781 febrile illnesses

Craig JC, Williams GJ, Jones M, et al (Univ of Sydney, Australia; et al)
BMJ 340:c1594, 2010

Objectives.—To evaluate current processes by which young children presenting with a febrile illness but suspected of having serious bacterial infection are diagnosed and treated, and to develop and test a multivariable model to distinguish serious bacterial infections from self limiting non-bacterial illnesses.

Design.—Two year prospective cohort study.

Setting.—The emergency department of The Children's Hospital at Westmead, Westmead, Australia.

Participants.—Children aged less than 5 years presenting with a febrile illness between 1 July 2004 and 30 June 2006.

Intervention.—A standardised clinical evaluation that included mandatory entry of 40 clinical features into the hospital's electronic record keeping system was performed by physicians. Serious bacterial infections were confirmed or excluded using standard radiological and microbiological tests and follow-up.

Main Outcome Measures.—Diagnosis of one of three key types of serious bacterial infection (urinary tract infection, pneumonia, and bacteraemia), and the accuracy of both our clinical decision making model and clinician judgment in making these diagnoses.

Results.—We had follow-up data for 93% of the 15 781 instances of febrile illnesses recorded during the study period. The combined prevalence of any of the three infections of interest (urinary tract infection, pneumonia, or bacteraemia) was 7.2% (1120/15 781, 95% confidence interval (CI) 6.7% to 7.5%), with urinary tract infection the diagnosis in 543 (3.4%) cases of febrile illness (95% CI 3.2% to 3.7%), pneumonia in 533 (3.4%) cases (95% CI 3.1% to 3.7%), and bacteraemia in 64 (0.4%) cases (95% CI 0.3% to 0.5%). Almost all (>94%) of the children with serious bacterial infections had the appropriate test (urine culture, chest radiograph, or blood culture). Antibiotics were prescribed acutely in 66%(359/543) of children with urinary tract infection, 69%

(366/533) with pneumonia, and 81% (52/64) with bacteraemia. However, 20% (2686/13 557) of children without bacterial infection were also prescribed antibiotics. On the basis of the data from the clinical evaluations and the confirmed diagnosis, a diagnostic model was developed using multinomial logistic regression methods. Physicians' diagnoses of bacterial infection had low sensitivity (10-50%) and high specificity (90-100%), whereas the clinical diagnostic model provided a broad range of values for sensitivity and specificity.

Conclusions.—Emergency department physicians tend to underestimate the likelihood of serious bacterial infection in young children with fever, leading to undertreatment with antibiotics. A clinical diagnostic model could improve decision making by increasing sensitivity for detecting serious bacterial infection, thereby improving early treatment.

▶ In the largest single study to date of clinical predictors of serious infection, Craig et al examined 15 781 febrile illnesses in 12 807 children younger than 5 years presenting to a teaching hospital in Australia. There, emergency department doctors recorded 40 clinical features and followed children for up to 14 days to ascertain clinical outcomes. Most illnesses, as expected, were not due to bacterial infections (86%) and were presumed to be mostly nonspecific viral illnesses. However, 7.2% of youngsters were diagnosed with bacterial infections (eg, abscess, impetigo, mastoiditis, and periorbital cellulitis). Serious bacterial infection occurred in 7.2% (1120) of the cases of febrile illnesses, of which urinary tract infection (543, 3.4%) and pneumonia (533, 3.4%) were the most common, followed by bacteremia (64, 0.4%). Just 12 children had osteomyelitis, and 8 had septic arthritis. Six children had meningitis.

What is unique about the study by Craig et al is that the authors developed a diagnostic model that used 28 variables to discriminate children with serious bacterial infection from those with no bacterial infection or a clinically diagnosed infection. This approach of dichotomizing outcomes (serious vs not serious) is common to many diagnostic studies but overlaps the important group of children that lie somewhere between these 2 extremes, the ones that clinicians have the most difficulty deciding how to manage. That having been said, the diagnostic accuracy of the models derived, expressed as area under the curve, ranges from 0.8 to 0.9 for pneumonia, urinary tract infection, and bacteremia, suggesting a good predictive value. The strongest positive predictors of serious bacterial infection are a generally unwell appearance, high temperature, chronic disease, and prolonged capillary refill time. For children with pneumonia, other predictors include coughing, difficulty breathing, abnormal chest sounds, and to a significantly lesser extent tachypnea, chest crackles, and tachycardia. For urinary tract infection, the presence of urinary symptoms is by far the strongest indicator, whereas for bacteremia, tachycardia and crying are also strong indicators.

Because the findings of Craig et al were analyzed after these youngsters' visits to the emergency room, the opportunity existed to see what physicians did absent the results of this study. It was noted that among the children with serious bacterial infections, just 66% to 81% were given antibiotics during their visit to the emergency department. Thus, somewhere between one-fifth and one-third of the children were missed as having serious bacterial illness.

In a commentary that accompanied the report of Craig et al, we are told what we might do differently now having the information from this study.[1] The suggestion is that this study strongly reinforces the importance of measuring vital signs and assessing a child's overall state of illness. No surprise here. When evaluating children with serious difficulty in breathing, the commentary noted that many of us rely on observing the chest for increased work of breathing, but the findings of Craig et al suggest that auscultation for crackles or altered breath sounds is still valuable. Crucially though, before relying on these signs in clinical practice, more specific definitions of these predictors and evidence of their interrater reliability are needed.

We close this commentary with an observation having to do with the transmission of infectious diseases. A recent review suggests that wearing short or long sleeves makes no difference in the rate of bacterial contamination of a physician's wrist. Specifically, doctors wearing long-sleeved outfits have no greater risk of bacterial contamination around their wrists than those wearing short sleeves, according to a study of doctors in the United States. The findings question guidelines, particularly those in Great Britain, requiring physicians to be "bare below the elbows." The study randomly allocated 50 physicians working at Denver Health—a university hospital in Colorado—to wear freshly laundered, short-sleeved uniforms and another 50 to wear their own long-sleeved white coats, which were infrequently laundered. Cultures were taken from the physicians' wrists, cuffs, and pockets at the end of an 8-hour day after working in internal medicine departments. The results showed no significant difference in overall bacterial or in methicillin resistant *Staphylococcus aureus* (MRSA) contamination between physicians in the short-sleeved uniform and those in the long-sleeved coats.[2] It was in 2007 that the Department of Health in England introduced guidelines banning healthcare workers from wearing white coats or other long-sleeved garments as part of efforts to reduce nosocomial bacterial transmission. It will be interesting to see if the report from the United States in any way diminishes the desire for physicians in Great Britain to be as relatively unclothed as is socially acceptable.

J. A. Stockman III, MD

References

1. Thompson MJ, Van den Bruel A. Diagnosing serious bacterial infection in young febrile children: measuring vital signs and assessing a child's overall state of illness are the priority. *BMJ.* 2010;340:986-987.
2. Burden N, Cervantes L, Weed D, Keniston A, Price CS, Albert RK. Newly claimed physician uniforms and infrequently washed white coats have similar rates of bacterial contamination after an 8-hour workday: a randomized controlled trial. *J Hosp Med.* 2011;6:177-182.

Extreme leucocytosis and the risk of serious bacterial infections in febrile children
Brauner M, Goldman M, Kozer E (Assaf Harofeh Med Ctr, Zerifin, Israel; Tel Aviv Univ, Israel)
Arch Dis Child 95:209-212, 2010

Objective.—To determine the clinical significance of extreme leucocytosis (white blood cell (WBC) count > 25 000/mm^3) as a predictor of serious bacterial infection (SBI) in children.

Patients and Methods.—A retrospective case—control study was conducted in a paediatric emergency department in Israel. The study evaluated children aged 3—36 months admitted to the emergency department with fever (>38°C) who had a complete blood count (CBC). Children with extreme leucocytosis were identified through the laboratory database. Further, for each case patient two consecutive febrile patients with WBC counts of 15 000—24 999/mm^3 (moderate leucocytosis) served as controls (a case—control ratio of 1:2).

Results.—During the study, 146 patients with extreme leucocytosis were identified and compared with 292 patients with moderate leucocytosis. SBI was found in 57 (39%) patients with extreme leucocytosis compared with 45 (15.4%) control patients (p < 0.001). The most commonly found SBI was segmental or lobar pneumonia, which was diagnosed in 41 (28%) patients in the case group compared with 27 (9.2%) patients in the control group (p < 0.001, OR 3.83, 95% CI 2.25 to 6.52). Children with extreme leucocytosis were more often treated with antibiotics (52.7% vs 27.7%, p < 0.001) and admitted to hospital (98.6% vs 50.68%, p < 0.001).

Conclusions.—In febrile children aged 3—36 months, the presence of extreme leucocytosis is associated with a 39% risk of having SBIs. The increased risk for SBI is mainly due to a higher risk for pneumonia.

▶ The authors of this report provide some interesting and useful information that you think would have been covered in the literature many times previously. While there have been a number of reports describing the prevalence of serious bacterial complications in those with elevated white blood cell counts, this study from Israel focuses specifically on those with extreme leukocytosis (white blood cell count > 25000/mm^3). No one will argue with such a white count being extremely elevated. The authors of the report found more than 600 children who had significantly elevated white blood cell counts. Of these, 164 had white blood cell counts more than 25000/mm^3. These children were included in the report and were compared with control children whose white blood cell counts were between 15000 and 25000/mm^3. The investigators were looking for evidence of serious bacterial infections defined as bacteremia, bacterial meningitis, bacterial gastroenteritis/urinary tract infection, or pneumonia. In the study report, it was shown that the rate of serious bacterial infection was found to be higher in patients with extreme leukocytosis (39%) compared with the control group who had only moderate leukocytosis (15000-25000/mm^3). The most common serious bacterial infection found in both groups was segmental or lobar pneumonia. No statistical differences were found in the frequency of other serious bacterial infections when comparing the moderate and severe leukocytosis groups.

The authors of this report do remark that there is no clear definition for serious bacterial infection in the literature, although most practitioners know it when they see it. The bottom line from the study, however, is that one might do a chest X-ray to rule out lobar or segmental pneumonia in anyone with a seriously elevated white blood cell count if no other cause of the leukocytosis is found. As almost 40% of these patients may have a serious bacterial infection, one might also consider empirical antibiotic treatment after a thorough evaluation and collection of appropriate cultures.

On a completely unrelated infectious disease topic, please recognize that cockroach brains can kill bacteria. New research finds that the rudimentary brains of cockroaches team with antimicrobial compounds that can do in bacteria such as *Escherichia coli* and other common organisms. Extracts of ground brain and other nervous tissue from the American cockroach, *Periplaneta americanan*, and the desert locust, *Schistocerca gregaria*, killed more than 90% of a type of *E coli* that causes meningitis and also killed methicillin-resistant staph. Nine molecules appear to be responsible for the antimicrobial activity in cockroach and locust tissue. Needless to say, investigators are still working out the details of how to convert this new knowledge into something useful, but it is unlikely that patients will ever know that they are being treated with cockroach brains if the new antimicrobials hit the market.[1]

J. A. Stockman III, MD

Reference

1. Ehrenberg R. Cockroach brains can kill bacteria: insect extracts active against antibiotic-resistant microbes. *Science News.* October 9, 2010;14.

Fidaxomicin versus Vancomycin for *Clostridium difficile* Infection
Louie TJ, for the OPT-80-003 Clinical Study Group (Univ of Calgary, Alberta, Canada; et al)
N Engl J Med 364:422-431, 2011

Background.—*Clostridium difficile* infection is a serious diarrheal illness associated with substantial morbidity and mortality. Patients generally have a response to oral vancomycin or metronidazole; however, the rate of recurrence is high. This phase 3 clinical trial compared the efficacy and safety of fidaxomicin with those of vancomycin in treating *C. difficile* infection.

Methods.—Adults with acute symptoms of *C. difficile* infection and a positive result on a stool toxin test were eligible for study entry. We randomly assigned patients to receive fidaxomicin (200 mg twice daily) or vancomycin (125 mg four times daily) orally for 10 days. The primary end point was clinical cure (resolution of symptoms and no need for further therapy for *C. difficile* infection as of the second day after the end of the course of therapy). The secondary end points were recurrence of *C. difficile* infection (diarrhea and a positive result on a stool toxin test within 4 weeks after treatment) and global cure (i.e., cure with no recurrence).

Results.—A total of 629 patients were enrolled, of whom 548 (87.1%) could be evaluated for the per-protocol analysis. The rates of clinical cure with fidaxomicin were noninferior to those with vancomycin in both the modified intention-to-treat analysis (88.2% with fidaxomicin and 85.8% with vancomycin) and the per-protocol analysis (92.1% and 89.8%, respectively). Significantly fewer patients in the fidaxomicin group than in the vancomycin group had a recurrence of the infection, in both the modified intention-to-treat analysis (15.4% vs. 25.3%, P=0.005) and the per-protocol analysis (13.3% vs. 24.0%, P=0.004). The lower rate of recurrence was seen in patients with non-North American Pulsed Field type 1 strains. The adverse-event profile was similar for the two therapies.

Conclusions.—The rates of clinical cure after treatment with fidaxomicin were noninferior to those after treatment with vancomycin. Fidaxomicin was associated with a significantly lower rate of recurrence of *C. difficile* infection associated with non–North American Pulsed Field type 1 strains. (Funded by Optimer Pharmaceuticals; ClinicalTrials.gov number, NCT00314951.)

▶ Much has been written about *Clostridium difficile* infection recently. Over the last 15 years, the incidence of *C difficile* infection has more than doubled. It has been roughly estimated that there may be up to 3 million cases of infection with this organism annually. If these statistics are correct, this would make *C difficile* infection the most common bacterial cause of diarrhea in our country. In addition to a rising incidence, we are also seeing a greater mortality associated with the disease. It has been suspected that this is related to the increasing virulence of the *C difficile* and also an increasing host vulnerability to this organism. The latter is partially explained by antibiotic use that disturbs intestinal microbiota and coexisting conditions, including immunosuppressive drugs.

Those who are colonized with *C difficile* can have a variety of clinical presentations: short-term colonization, which usually develops when a patient is in a health care facility; acute diarrhea, ranging from mild to severe; fulminant diarrhea that may be associated with pseudomembranous colitis (which in some cases is severe enough to require colectomy); and recurrent *C difficile* infection that typically occurs within 60 days after initial treatment for infection.

Current treatments for *C difficile* infection have been largely inadequate. Metronidazole is an inexpensive treatment that is considered by most authorities to be the standard therapy for nonsevere cases of *C difficile* infection, despite the fact it is not approved by the Food and Drug Administration for this condition. The rub is that metronidazole has unacceptable pharmacokinetic characteristics. It is almost completely absorbed in the gut resulting in very low drug levels in the colon and a high rate of treatment failure. Severe cases of

C difficile infection are usually treated with oral vancomycin. A lack of response to treatment and recurrence of the disease happen with approximately equal frequency after both metronidazole and oral vancomycin treatment. Recurrent disease is seen in 20% to 30% of cases regardless of which of these 2 treatments is used. Unfortunately, a number of people have multiple recurrences over many months or years and are thus exposed to repeated courses of expensive and potentially toxic antibiotics.

The report of Louie et al tells us about the use of fidaxomicin in the treatment of *C difficile* infection. Fidaxomicin is a new macrocyclic antibiotic that has no cross-resistance with other antibiotics and has in vitro activity against strains of *C difficile*. Louie et al report the results of a phase 3 trial involving 629 patients, in which fidaxomicin was compared with vancomycin for the treatment of *C difficile* infection. The rates of clinical cure in the 2 groups turned out to be similar, but *C difficile* infection recurred significantly less with the use of fidaxomicin than in comparison to vancomycin (15% vs 25%). This reduced rate of recurrence represents an important advance in the treatment of *C difficile* infection. Fidaxomicin has several interesting and positive characteristics including low levels of systemic absorption and the potential for a lesser development of resistance among intestinal and extraintestinal bacteria allowing for high levels of active drug in the colon.

As important as this report is, it leaves a number of questions unanswered. For example, fidaxomicin treatment was given for just 10 days. For a spore-forming pathogen such a *C difficile*, 10 days of treatment may not be sufficient for a cure. The recommended duration of treatment of disease caused by spore-forming *Bacillus anthracis* is 2 months. The question that needs to be asked is whether agents used to treat *C difficile* would be better given for significantly longer periods of time.

Although therapy of *C difficile* infection is fraught with many many challenges, fidaxomicin appears to be an important new advance in the management of this disorder. If further studies confirm a favorable clinical response, fidaxomicin could very well become the recommended therapy for *C difficile* infection.

This commentary closes with 2 observations related to transmission of disease by animals that are often around people: the sheep and the frog. Sheep droppings have been blamed for an outbreak of diarrheal illness in mountain bikers in rural Wales. A cyclist event took place in 2008 at the time of a heavy rain. Participants tended to skid off the road more often than perhaps normally and frequently fell from their bikes. Many appeared to have inadvertently ingested mud that was contaminated with sheep droppings containing *Campylobacter*, accounting for the subsequent development of diarrhea.[1] Also, between April 2009 and March 2010, the Centers for Disease Control in Atlanta traced 113 United States *Salmonella* cases to the aquarium-dwelling frog. Three-quarter of the cases were in children under the age of 10. Symptoms ranged from abdominal cramping to severe and bloody diarrhea; about one-third needed hospitalization, but there were no fatalities.[2] Soon we will have no friendly animals or pets allowed to be around us humans.

J. A. Stockman III, MD

References

1. Editorial comment. Sheep droppings blamed for outbreak of diarrheal illness. *BMJ.* 2010;341:c6458.
2. Seppa N. Pet frogs transmit *Salmonella. Science News.* November 20, 2010;9.

Artesunate versus quinine in the treatment of severe falciparum malaria in African children (AQUAMAT): an open-label, randomised trial
Dondorp AM, for the AQUAMAT group (Mahidol Univ, Bangkok, Thailand; et al)
Lancet 376:1647-1657, 2010

Background.—Severe malaria is a major cause of childhood death and often the main reason for paediatric hospital admission in sub-Saharan Africa. Quinine is still the established treatment of choice, although evidence from Asia suggests that artesunate is associated with a lower mortality. We compared parenteral treatment with either artesunate or quinine in African children with severe malaria.

Methods.—This open-label, randomised trial was undertaken in 11 centres in nine African countries. Children (<15 years) with severe falciparum malaria were randomly assigned to parenteral artesunate or parenteral quinine. Randomisation was in blocks of 20, with study numbers corresponding to treatment allocations kept inside opaque sealed paper envelopes. The trial was open label at each site, and none of the investigators or trialists, apart from for the trial statistician, had access to the summaries of treatment allocations. The primary outcome measure was in-hospital mortality, analysed by intention to treat. This trial is registered, number ISRCTN50258054.

Findings.—5425 children were enrolled; 2712 were assigned to artesunate and 2713 to quinine. All patients were analysed for the primary outcome. 230 (8·5%) patients assigned to artesunate treatment died compared with 297 (10·9%) assigned to quinine treatment (odds ratio [OR] stratified for study site 0·75, 95% CI 0·63—0·90; relative reduction 22·5%, 95% CI 8·1—36·9; p=0·0022). Incidence of neurological sequelae did not differ significantly between groups, but the development of coma (65/1832 [3·5%] with artesunate *vs* 91/1768 [5·1%] with quinine; OR 0·69 95% CI 0·49—0·95; p=0·0231), convulsions (224/2712 [8·3%] *vs* 273/2713 [10·1%]; OR 0·80, 0·66—0·97; p=0·0199), and deterioration of the coma score (166/2712 [6·1%] *vs* 208/2713 [7·7%]; OR 0·78, 0·64—0·97; p=0·0245) were all significantly less frequent in artesunate recipients than in quinine recipients. Post-treatment hypoglycaemia was also less frequent in patients assigned to artesunate than in those assigned to quinine (48/2712 [1·8%] *vs* 75/2713 [2·8%]; OR 0·63, 0·43-0·91; p=0·0134). Artesunate was well tolerated, with no serious drug-related adverse effects.

Interpretation.—Artesunate substantially reduces mortality in African children with severe malaria. These data, together with a meta-analysis of all trials comparing artesunate and quinine, strongly suggest that parenteral artesunate should replace quinine as the treatment of choice for severe falciparum malaria worldwide.

▶ Obviously we do not see much malaria in the United States, but it does occur, and as citizens of the world, we should be aware of the global impact that severe malaria has. Malaria is one of the few infections that can kill within hours. It requires swift and effective therapy, which is best delivered intravenously. This is particularly true of cerebral malaria. Unlike other causes of coma, most survivors of cerebral malaria do not have serious sequelae. Mortality depends largely on how soon a patient is treated, but even in expert centers, 1 in 5 dies. The choice of the best antimalarial drug for severe malaria has been unclear, at least until this report from *The Lancet* appeared. This study documents that artesunate is superior to quinine. The Artesunate Versus Quinine in the Treatment of Severe Falciparum Malaria in African Children study group accepts patients in Sub-Saharan Africa. More than 5000 children older than 5 years have been enrolled. Results indicate that intravenous artesunate is now the standard therapy for severe malaria. Infectious disease experts should now end the 400-year use of quinine for severe malaria.

It should be noted that the first promising malaria vaccine continues to make its way through phase 3 clinical trials in Sub-Saharan Africa. The nonprofit organization Malaria Vaccine Initiative and the vaccine's creator GlaxoSmithKline (GSK) Biologicals partnered in 2001 to develop the vaccine for infants and children in Sub-Saharan Africa. The vaccine is known as RTS, S. The origins of this vaccine date back to 1984 when GSK collaborated on preclinical studies with researchers at the Walter Reed Army Institute of Research in Silver Spring, Maryland. Human trials in adults in the United States and Belgium began in 1992. The first African trials were launched in 1995. Since then, several published studies have shown that the vaccine has a favorable safety and efficacy profile. Preliminary information suggests that the risk of *Plasmodium falciparum* infection is reduced by 65% with vaccine use. Tens of thousands of children are now enrolled in clinical efficacy trials. If the phase 3 trials are successful, GSK will ask the European Medicines Agency to review the vaccine and certify it as safe and effective, which would pave the way for GSK to apply to African regulatory authorities for marketing authorization.

The last couple of years have seen a few new insights into the control of malaria in addition to the potential of a new vaccine. In the war against malaria, researchers may have recruited an unlikely ally, a seaweed found in Fiji. In 2005, investigators discovered that a certain seaweed, a red algae called *Callophycus serratus*, contains unusual ring-shaped compounds called bromophycolides that are particularly effective in killing certain fungi. In 2009, these same investigators found that they also kill the parasite malaria in red blood cells. It appears that malarial parasites infect red blood cells with hemoglobin, but as the parasites break down hemoglobin releasing—heme, the latter is toxic to the malarial organism. To protect themselves, the parasites crystalize heme and store it in a separate chamber. It turns out that bromophycolide prevents this crystallization, causing heme to accumulate and poison the parasite. Further testing is underway to see whether or not this turns into a useful mechanism to help manage malaria.[1] Last, be aware that genetically modified male *Aedes aegypti* mosquitoes have been released into the wild in Malaysia in an effort to control dengue. Larva from mating of these male mosquitoes with the female vector produces a self-destructive toxic enzyme. The mosquitoes have been developed by Malaysia's Institute for Medical Research in the United Kingdom biotechnology company Oxitec.

J. A. Stockman III, MD

Reference

1. Pennisi S. Seaweed a source of potential antimalarial drug. Science. http://news.sciencemag.org/sciencenow/2011/02/seaweed-a-source-of-potential.html?ref=hp. Published February 21, 2011. Accessed August 19, 2011.

Probable Zoonotic Leprosy in the Southern United States
Truman RW, Singh P, Sharma R, et al (Louisiana State Univ, Baton Rouge; Global Health Inst, Lausanne, Switzerland; et al)
N Engl J Med 364:1626-1633, 2011

Background.—In the southern region of the United States, such as in Louisiana and Texas, there are autochthonous cases of leprosy among native-born Americans with no history of foreign exposure. In the same region, as well as in Mexico, wild armadillos are infected with *Mycobacterium leprae*.

Methods.—Whole-genome resequencing of *M. leprae* from one wild armadillo and three U.S. patients with leprosy revealed that the infective strains were essentially identical. Comparative genomic analysis of these strains and *M. leprae* strains from Asia and Brazil identified 51 single-nucleotide polymorphisms and an 11-bp insertion−deletion. We genotyped these polymorphic sites, in combination with 10 variable-number tandem repeats, in *M. leprae* strains obtained from 33 wild armadillos from five southern states, 50 U.S. outpatients seen at a clinic in Louisiana, and 64 Venezuelan patients, as well as in four foreign reference strains.

Results.—The *M. leprae* genotype of patients with foreign exposure generally reflected their country of origin or travel history. However, a unique *M. leprae* genotype (3I-2-v1) was found in 28 of the 33 wild armadillos and 25 of the 39 U.S. patients who resided in areas where exposure to armadillo-borne *M. leprae* was possible. This genotype has not been reported elsewhere in the world.

Conclusions.—Wild armadillos and many patients with leprosy in the southern United States are infected with the same strain of *M. leprae*. Armadillos are a large natural reservoir for *M. leprae*, and leprosy may be a zoonosis in the region. (Funded by the National Institute of Allergy and Infectious Diseases and others.)

▶ Who would have thought that Hansen disease is still with us? This disease, perhaps more commonly known as leprosy, is caused by *Mycobacterium leprae*. This disease is often thought of as a disease of antiquity. It was not present in the New World before Columbus discovered the Americas and appears to have been introduced by Europe and Africa during colonization. Early writings show that the disease was well established in the United States in the vicinity of New Orleans by the 1750s.

Leprosy is obviously rare on the shores of the United States. About 150 cases are reported each year. Most of these are reported in individuals who have lived or worked abroad in leprosy-endemic areas, and the disease most likely was acquired therefore overseas. At the same time, however, about one-third of patients in the United States with leprosy report no foreign residence and appear to have acquired their disease locally. Such cases arise mostly in Texas and Louisiana, but the geographic range of acquisition is widening in recent years.

M leprae is a fascinating organism. It is an obligate intracellular pathogen. It cannot be cultivated on artificial laboratory media. The only animal in which leprosy can be used to document infection is the nine-banded armadillo (*Dasypus novemcinctus*). Demonstration of the latter took place back in the 1970s and ever since the armadillo has been the primary animal model for leprosy. Unfortunately, leprosy infection also occurs naturally among some free-ranging armadillos.

The manuscript of Truman et al tells us about the potential risks of infected armadillos to people. This is an important report since in some parts of the south, the natural reservoir for *M leprae* has a prevalence of 20% in armadillos in some locales. Infected armadillos have been reported in Alabama, Arkansas, Louisiana, Mississippi, Texas, and Mexico. Using whole-genome sequencing, single-nucleotide polymorphism typing, and variable-numbered tandem-repeat analysis to compare *M leprae* obtained from wild armadillos and patients in the United States with leprosy, Truman et al have shown that wild armadillos in many patients with leprosy in the southern United States are infected with the exact same strain of *M leprae*, documenting that armadillos are in fact a huge natural reservoir for human disease.

What this report does not tell us is exactly how armadillos and humans interact in such a way that infection is spread from this critter to us. One thing is for sure, and the authors suggest this, and that is that frequent direct contact with armadillos and cooking and consumption of armadillo meat should be discouraged. Most of us were not aware that anyone ate armadillo meat, but at least now we know not to.

One last comment about leprosy: Britain's earliest hospital in Winchester, Hampshire, is now under excavation by archeologists. Analyses of artifacts have provided a date range of AD 960-1030 and show that the hospital was used to treat leprosy. This site predates the Norman conquest of 1066, thought by most historians and archeologists to have been the beginning of hospitals in

Great Britain. An aerial view shows the walls and trenches of an infirmary and its chapel.[1]

J. A. Stockman III, MD

Reference

1. Winchesterarchaeology. http://winchesterarchaeology.wordpress.com. Accessed August 19, 2011.

Detection of prion infection in variant Creutzfeldt-Jakob disease: a blood-based assay
Edgeworth JA, Farmer M, Sicilia A, et al (UCL Inst of Neurology, UK; et al)
Lancet 377:487-493, 2011

Background.—Variant Creutzfeldt-Jakob disease (vCJD) is a fatal neurodegenerative disorder originating from exposure to bovine-spongiform-encephalopathy-like prions. Prion infections are associated with long and clinically silent incubations. The number of asymptomatic individuals with vCJD prion infection is unknown, posing risk to others via blood transfusion, blood products, organ or tissue grafts, and contaminated medical instruments. We aimed to establish the sensitivity and specificity of a blood-based assay for detection of vCJD prion infection.

Methods.—We developed a solid-state binding matrix to capture and concentrate disease-associated prion proteins and coupled this method to direct immunodetection of surface-bound material. Quantitative assay sensitivity was assessed with a serial dilution series of 10^{-7} to 10^{-10} of vCJD prion-infected brain homogenate into whole human blood, with a baseline control of normal human brain homogenate in whole blood (10^{-6}). To establish the sensitivity and specificity of the assay for detection of endogenous vCJD, we analysed a masked panel of 190 whole blood samples from 21 patients with vCJD, 27 with sporadic CJD, 42 with other neurological diseases, and 100 normal controls. Samples were masked and numbered by individuals independent of the assay and analysis. Each sample was tested twice in independent assay runs; only samples that were reactive in both runs were scored as positive overall.

Findings.—We were able to distinguish a 10^{-10} dilution of exogenous vCJD prion-infected brain from a 10^{-6} dilution of normal brain (mean chemiluminescent signal, $1 \cdot 3 \times 10^5$ [SD $1 \cdot 1 \times 10^4$] for vCJD vs $9 \cdot 9 \times 10^4$ [$4 \cdot 5 \times 10^3$] for normal brain; p<0·0001)—an assay sensitivity that was orders of magnitude higher than any previously reported. 15 samples in the masked panel were scored as positive. All 15 samples were from patients with vCJD, showing an assay sensitivity for vCJD of 71·4% (95% CI 47·8−88·7) and a specificity of 100% (95% CIs between 97·8% and 100%).

Interpretation.—These initial studies provide a prototype blood test for diagnosis of vCJD in symptomatic individuals, which could allow development of large-scale screening tests for asymptomatic vCJD prion infection.

▶ A great deal of attention has been paid to variant Creutzfeldt-Jakob disease (CJD), both in Great Britain where most cases have been described as well as in the United States. There are several types of prion disease. These disorders include CJD, Gerstmann-Sträussler-Scheinker disease, fatal familial insomnia, and kuru in men. Other prion diseases include bovine spongiform encephalopathy (BSE) in cattle, chronic wasting disease of deer and elk, and scrapie in sheep. The emergence of variant CJD (vCJD) and the documentation that it arises from exposure to BSE has created a lot of attention in the literature since BSE can be transmitted to humans via endoscopy, surgery, dentistry, organ transplantation, and blood transfusion. vCJD in fact is a human infection in the family of transmissible spongiform encephalopathies/prion diseases. Most cases of vCJD result from the consumption of food infected with the BSE agent, but infection has also been transmitted by blood transfusion and plasma products.

Although vCJD is very rare with just 220 cases of dietary transmission described worldwide and 5 blood-related cases, all reported in the United Kingdom, its effect on blood transfusion medicine everywhere has been enormous. Edgeworth et al now report a new test to identify vCJD-infected blood. The assay detects abnormal prion protein that is commonly associated with vCJD infection. If confirmed, this study is an important breakthrough that opens up a host of possible new studies that could describe exactly how vCJD is transmitted not only in humans but also in animals. The report is a description of the first assay capable of discriminating vCJD-infected blood from the blood of individuals who at the time of sampling were either healthy or affected by non-vCJD neurodegenerative disorders. Whether this test will become routine in blood bank screening has yet to be determined either in Great Britain or elsewhere. A major issue is assay specificity. Clinical assessment will require testing of a large number of blood donations from healthy individuals to assess true initial and repeat false-positive rates. Communication to the public of uncertainty about a positive test result will be challenging and could result in fewer donors as well as causing unnecessary anxiety to those who wind up being deferred as blood donors because of a positive test result. Nonetheless, it is good to know that somewhere down the line we may very well have a test to screen for a rare but lethal disorder that is transmissible by blood products.

J. A. Stockman III, MD

Inhibitory Effect of Breast Milk on Infectivity of Live Oral Rotavirus Vaccines

Moon S-S, Wang Y, Shane AL, et al (Natl Ctrs for Immunization and Respiratory Disease, Atlanta, GA; Emory Univ, Atlanta, GA; et al)
Pediatr Infect Dis J 29:919-923, 2010

Background.—Live oral rotavirus vaccines have been less immunogenic and efficacious among children in poor developing countries compared with middle income and industrialized countries for reasons that are not yet completely understood. We assessed whether the neutralizing activity of breast milk could lower the titer of vaccine virus and explain this difference in vitro.

Methods.—Breast milk samples were collected from mothers who were breast-feeding infants 4 to 29 weeks of age (ie, vaccine eligible age) in India (N = 40), Vietnam (N = 77), South Korea (N = 34), and the United States (N = 51). We examined breast milk for rotavirus-specific IgA and neutralizing activity against 3 rotavirus vaccine strains—RV1, RV5 G1, and 116E using enzyme immunoassays. The inhibitory effect of breast milk on RV1 was further examined by a plaque reduction assay.

Findings.—Breast milk from Indian women had the highest IgA and neutralizing titers against all 3 vaccine strains, while lower but comparable median IgA and neutralizing titers were detected in breast milk from Korean and Vietnamese women, and the lowest titers were seen in American women. Neutralizing activity was greatest against the 2 vaccine strains of human origin, RV1 and 116E. This neutralizing activity in one half of the breast milk specimens from Indian women could reduce the effective titer of RV1 by ∼2 logs, of 116E by 1.5 logs, and RV5 G1 strain by ∼1 log more than that of breast milk from American women.

Interpretation.—The lower immunogenicity and efficacy of rotavirus vaccines in poor developing countries could be explained, in part, by higher titers of IgA and neutralizing activity in breast milk consumed by their infants at the time of immunization that could effectively reduce the potency of the vaccine. Strategies to overcome this negative effect, such as delaying breast-feeding at the time of immunization, should be evaluated.

▶ Given the pervasive nature of rotavirus around the world and the availability of rotavirus vaccines now, this report from the National Centers for Immunization and Respiratory Disease (NCIRD), Centers for Disease Control and Prevention, provides important information about the effectiveness of the rotavirus vaccines in infants who are being breast fed. Rotavirus is indeed the most common cause of severe infectious diarrhea in children in the preschool age group. Data from this report and elsewhere tell us that rotavirus disease is responsible for over half a million deaths per year worldwide, most of these occurring in low-income countries. For reasons that have been unexplained, both of the currently available vaccines have lower immunogenicity and efficacy in low-income countries of both Africa and Asia. While one can expect positive responses from these vaccines in more than 90% of infants in developed countries, only 40% to 60% effectiveness is seen in South Africa, Malawi, Bangladesh, and India. Even on the other side of the Atlantic/Pacific, there is significantly lower vaccine effectiveness in countries such as Nicaragua (60% effectiveness against severe rotavirus disease, considerably lower than the efficacy of > 90% in the United States).

One possible explanation for the lower efficacy of these vaccines in low-income settings is that mothers more frequently breast-feed their infants in clinic, the very time the vaccine is being orally administered. It is possible that mothers in low-income countries have greater natural exposure to rotavirus and therefore have higher titers of neutralizing antibodies in their breast milk and also higher titers of transplacental IgG in their infants, both of which could decrease the effective amount of vaccine virus reaching and replicating in the small intestine, thus rendering the vaccine less effective. The investigators from the NCIRD investigated the various possibilities causing vaccine ineffectiveness by studying whether the neutralizing activity of breast milk could lower the titer of vaccine virus and explain at least part of the problem. Their findings suggest that the neutralizing activity of breast milk could indeed substantially reduce the potency and effectiveness of live oral virus vaccine among infants in low-resource countries where mothers often breast-feed at the time a vaccine is orally administered. A short delay of breast-feeding at the time of immunization might be the least complicated intervention to improve the efficacy of these vaccines. Needless to day, some of the messages from this report have applicability even to the situation in the United States, although it is unlikely that most mothers will have significantly high rotavirus antibodies in their serum and therefore in their breast milk. Still, the vaccine is not effective in every baby in our country, and perhaps we could get a tick-up in vaccine take by recommending that mothers not breast-feed around the time their infants are receiving the oral vaccine.

While on the topic of rotavirus vaccines, a recent report from the Children's Hospital of Philadelphia does document a sustained decline in the frequency of community-acquired rotavirus gastroenteritis, most likely a result of the new rotavirus vaccines.[1] Most rotavirus gastroenteritis appearing now seem to be of the G9 serotype, a serotype that is not included in either currently available vaccine.

This commentary closes with a completely unrelated topic having to do with bats. We generally think of bats as being bad critters, capable of carrying rabies. In fact, bats are voracious predators of nocturnal insects and for this activity are widely valued as protectors of crops and forest damage. Not good for society is the fact that some species of bats are falling precipitously in their numbers to the point of potential extinction. A major cause of this problem is the wind turbine. Why these species are particularly susceptible to self-destruction in the blades of wind turbines remains a mystery. By 2020 it is estimated that over 100 000 bats will have been killed annually by wind turbines in the mid-Atlantic highlands alone. To read more about the economic importance of bats in agriculture, see the editorial by Boyles et al.[2]

J. A. Stockman III, MD

References

1. Clark HF, Lawley D, Matthijnssens J, DiNubile MJ, Hodinka RL. Sustained decline in cases of rotavirus gastroenteritis presenting to the Children's Hospital of Philadelphia in the new rotavirus vaccine era. *Pediatr Infect Dis J.* 2010;29: 699-702.
2. Boyles JG, Cryan PM, McCracken GF, Kunz TH. Economic importance of bats in agriculture. *Science.* 2011;332:41-42.

Dissolving polymer microneedle patches for influenza vaccination
Sullivan SP, Koutsonanos DG, del Pilar Martin M, et al (Wallace H. Coulter
Dept of Biomedical Engineering at Emory Univ and Georgia Tech, Atlanta;
Emory Univ School of Medicine, Atlanta, GA; et al)
Nat Med 16:915-920, 2010

Influenza prophylaxis would benefit from a vaccination method enabling simplified logistics and improved immunogenicity without the dangers posed by hypodermic needles. Here we introduce dissolving microneedle patches for influenza vaccination using a simple patch-based system that targets delivery to skin's antigen-presenting cells. Microneedles were fabricated using a biocompatible polymer encapsulating inactivated influenza virus vaccine for insertion and dissolution in the skin within minutes. Microneedle vaccination generated robust antibody and cellular immune responses in mice that provided complete protection against lethal challenge. Compared to conventional intramuscular injection, microneedle vaccination resulted in more efficient lung virus clearance and enhanced cellular recall responses after challenge. These results suggest that dissolving microneedle patches can provide a new technology for simpler and safer vaccination with improved immunogenicity that could facilitate increased vaccination coverage.

▶ The traditional method for administering influenza vaccination has been by intramuscular (IM) injection, which of course requires hypodermic needles. This process in many creates a phenomenon called hyperdermophobia. In addition to the problem of hyperdermophobia, the process of administering large numbers of intramuscular injections results in a mountain of biohazardous waste. When you think about it, perhaps the most desirable method of vaccine delivery would be transdermal. The skin is a highly active immune organ containing a large population of resident antigen-presenting cells. The actual vaccine dose required for such immunization would theoretically be much lower than that required for IM injection. Transdermal delivery of other medications is essentially innocuous resulting in enhanced compliance. Transdermal injection is far more likely to be better received than intradermal injection. Intradermal immunization is limited by the need for specifically trained personnel. This problem can be counteracted by the use of transdermal microneedles, which are designed to reliably administer antigen at a specific skin depth that maximizes interaction with dermal reactive cells. Anyone should be capable of administering such a delivery method.

What Sullivan et al have done is to use mouse skin for in vivo vaccination experiments using microneedles. These researchers have invented a new vaccine delivery system that replaces 1 big needle with 100 tiny dissolvable ones imbedded in an adhesive patch. The patch can immunize mice against influenza just as effectively as conventional needle vaccination. In a sense, the patch is very much like a Band-Aid with a bunch of tiny needles on the sticky side. Thinner than a nickel's thickness, the microneedles pierced the mouse's skin and dissolved into the surrounding bodily fluid, releasing the vaccine in the process. The whole process of putting the micropatch on takes nanoseconds (you simply slap it on). The dissolution of the vaccine takes anywhere from 30 seconds to 5 minutes. The patch can be stored at room temperature. Medical training and careful handling are not required.

In mice, and perhaps in pigs, the data do show that microneedle transdermal vaccine delivery is possible. Needless to say, this is a very attractive approach, but obviously, more studies are needed before this method will be adopted in humans. If it is adopted successfully, the new patch will prove to be a powerful public health tool, especially in developing countries where electricity to keep liquid vaccines cold is in short supply and trained personnel are scarce. Studies have not been done yet to determine how durable these patches are at room temperature, but the authors of this report suspect that they should be stable for several months.

To read more about this interesting new vaccine approach, see the editorial comment by Sanders.[1]

J. A. Stockman III, MD

Reference

1. Sanders L. Getting the shot without the jab: vaccine patch could make for an ouchless immunization. *Sci News.* August 14, 2010:9. http://www.sciencenewsdigital.org/sciencenews/20100814?pg=11#pg11. Accessed June 29, 2011.

Burden of Seasonal Influenza Hospitalization in Children, United States, 2003 to 2008

Dawood FS, for the Emerging Infections Program (EIP) Network (Ctrs for Disease Control and Prevention, Atlanta, GA; et al)
J Pediatr 157:808-814, 2010

Objectives.—To estimate the rates of hospitalization with seasonal influenza in children aged <18 years from a large, diverse surveillance area during 2003 to 2008.

Study Design.—Through the Emerging Infections Program Network, population-based surveillance for laboratory-confirmed influenza was conducted in 10 states, including 5.3 million children. Hospitalized children were identified retrospectively; clinicians made influenza testing decisions. Data collected from the hospital record included demographics, medical history, and clinical course. Incidence rates were calculated with census data.

Results.—The highest hospitalization rates occurred in children aged <6 months (seasonal range, 9-30/10 000 children), and the lowest rates occurred in children aged 5 to 17 years (0.3-0.8/10 000). Overall, 4015 children were hospitalized, 58% of whom were identified with rapid diagnostic tests alone. Forty percent of the children who were hospitalized had underlying medical conditions; asthma (18%), prematurity (15% of children aged <2 years), and developmental delay (7%) were the most common.

Severe outcomes included intensive care unit admission (12%), respiratory failure (5%), bacterial coinfection (2%), and death (0.5%).

Conclusions.—Influenza-associated hospitalization rates varied by season and age and likely underestimate true rates because many hospitalized children are not tested for influenza. The proportion of children with severe outcomes was substantial across seasons. Quantifying incidence of influenza hospitalization and severe outcomes is critical to defining disease burden.

▶ Seasonal influenza remains a common reason for hospitalization of youngsters in the United States. Many of these youngsters have underlying medical conditions. The report of Dawood et al tells us about the latter. From 2003 through 2008, almost half of all admissions to pediatric services for influenza were associated with underlying medical conditions, the 3 most prominent being asthma, cardiovascular disease, and chronic lung disease. A variety of other chronic conditions made up the remainder of such admissions for seasonal influenza.

Since the data from the report of Dawood et al pretty much speak for themselves, this commentary will focus on some miscellaneous facts about the interesting influenza virus. It was in 2005 that a team of scientists resurrected the 1918 influenza virus from the lungs of a long-frozen victim from the tundra. At the time, the Jurassic Park—like feat was both widely celebrated and sharply criticized. Opponents of the effort worried about the risk of an accidental (or intentional) release of the revived killer, which claimed somewhere between 50 million and 100 million lives in about 15 months and has been dubbed the worse plague in human history. Proponents insisted that the insight gained from a fully reconstructed virus would be instrumental in fighting the next pandemic. The latter appears to have been the situation. Researchers have closed in on a protein called PB1 from the 1918 influenza virus that enables the virus to copy itself. When the 1981 PB1 protein is inserted into a normal influenza virus, the normal virus becomes a super killer replicating quickly and spreading through infected rodent hosts some 8 times faster than normal seasonal influenza. All 20th century pandemic viruses, among them the 2009 swine influenza, have been shown to have avian influenza PB1 genes. Most seasonal influenza viruses have the human influenza PB1 genes, rather than the avian genes. The virus from the permafrost body has allowed scientists to develop new drugs that are targeting PB1 with small molecules that bind to the protein receptors, which prevent the virus from replicating, and may greatly reduce virulence. When combined with existing antivirals such as Tamiflu, PB1-targeted drugs could drastically reduce the spread of resistance, making the approach of the annual influenza season a little less worrisome for everyone.

While on the topic of influenza virus carried by birds, scientists have recently trained mice to detect the scent of duck and goose droppings that are infected with influenza virus. Mice trained on the scent of poop from infected birds correctly choose infected over noninfected feces 90% of the time. It is not known what precise chemical compounds the mice are detecting, but they are pretty good at what they do.[1] It is suspected that mice are tuning into compounds produced by the duck's immune system in response to influenza infection. It should be noted that the research team undertaking this investigation irradiated the duck droppings to be sure that the influenza virus was not infectious, a precaution that may have affected the smell profile of the duck poop. It should be noted that some duck feces (such as those of mallards) excrete much more virus than other birds making the water birds prime disease spreaders via migratory travels or, more often, when ducks are bought and sold in live poultry markets.

One final comment about swine influenza: the colloquial name for the most recent pandemic strain of H1N1 attracted a minor controversy when in April 2009, Israel's Deputy Minister of Health proposed changing the virus name to remove the porcine reference, which he deemed offensive to Jews and Muslims, who regard pigs as unclean. The proposed name was Mexican influenza, to reflect the first recorded outbreak of the disease that appeared in the southern Mexican state of Vera Cruz. Mexico's ambassador to Israel immediately voiced an official complaint and Israel hastily rushed to emphasize that they were never seriously endorsing the name change.[2]

This commentary closes with a clinical situation and asks a question. You receive an important notice from an airline on which you have recently flown from the United States to Australia. The airline wants to let you know that you were seated within 2 rows of 2 passengers who later identified themselves as having active influenza at the time of your flight. The question is, what is your chance of developing influenza in this situation? The answer to this question comes from a report of Baker et al, which investigated passengers seated in the rear section of a Boeing 747—400 long-haul flight to New Zealand in April 2009 and examined the passengers located near where an individual with active influenza was seated. It turns out that no one caught influenza beyond 2 rows disparate from the passenger who was infected. The probability of developing influenza within the 2-row radius sideways and back and forth turned out to be 3.5%.[3]

J. A. Stockman III, MD

References

1. Ehrenberg R. Tracking bird flu using duck poop. *Science News*. September 25, 2010:8.
2. Palmer R. A disease—or gene—by any other name would cause a stink. *Nat Med*. 2010;16:1059.
3. Baker MG, Thornley CN, Mills C, et al. Transmission of pandemic A/H1N1 2009 influenza on passenger aircraft: retrospective cohort study. *BMJ*. 2010;340:c2424.

Use of Screening Dried Blood Spots for Estimation of Prevalence, Risk Factors, and Birth Outcomes of Congenital Cytomegalovirus Infection

Kharrazi M, Hyde T, Young S, et al (California Dept of Public Health, Richmond; Public Health Inst, Oakland, CA; Natl Ctr for Immunization and Respiratory Diseases, Atlanta, GA)
J Pediatr 157:191-197, 2010

Objectives.—To determine the birth prevalence of cytomegalovirus (CMV) in a population-based sample of newborns by use of dried blood spots compared with previous studies that used established detection methods, and to evaluate risk factors and birth outcomes for congenital CMV infection.

Study Design.—A total of 3972 newborn dried blood spots collected for the California Newborn Screening Program were tested for presence of CMV DNA. Demographic and pregnancy data were obtained from linked newborn screening and live-birth records.

Results.—CMV prevalence among newborns by maternal race and ethnicity was 0.9% for blacks, 0.8% for Hispanics, 0.6% for whites, and 0.6% for Asians. Among Hispanics (n = 2053), infants who were infected had younger mothers (23 vs 26 years, $P = .03$), and prevalence was higher for children with no father information provided (2.6% vs 0.6%, $P = .03$). Overall CMV infection was associated with low birth weight (prevalence ratios [95% CI]: 3.4 [1.4-8.5]) and preterm birth (2.7 [1.4-5.1]). CMV viral loads were inversely related to birth weight and gestational age (both $P = .03$).

Conclusions.—CMV prevalence measured with dried blood spots was similar to reports using standard viral culture methods. Dried blood spots may be suitable for detection of CMV infection in newborns and warrant further evaluation. Congenital CMV infection may contribute to low birth weight and preterm birth.

▶ There are pretty good reasons to want to know whether a newborn infant has been exposed to the cytomegalovirus (CMV) or has already become infected with this virus. Although no states currently screen newborns for CMV, it is estimated that somewhere between 20 000 and 40 000 of all newborns in the United States in fact have congenital CMV infection (per year), and at least 10% of these infants, or perhaps slightly more, will have some neurologic sequelae. In the past, the only way to screen for this virus has been by virologic methodologies. These studies have shown that those infants who have no clinical abnormalities still can develop hearing loss. What has been desirable is the development of a cost-effective, specific, and sensitive means to institute newborn screening to obtain more accurate population-based estimates of the importance of congenital CMV infection as a cause of disability. Hearing loss is a significant problem frequently with delayed onset or progression that can be missed by universal newborn hearing screening. For this reason, it would be desirable to screen for congenital CMV infection followed then by repeat hearing testing in those at risk.

In terms of ways of screening for CMV, relatively expensive tests obviously are not useful for this purpose. Such testing includes viral culture of the urine or adaptation of culture with monoclonal antibody detection of infected tissue culture cells. Although polymerase chain reaction (PCR) eliminates the need for cell culture techniques and is quite sensitive, there remains the problem of collecting urine from newborns. Urine collection is hardly an ideal way to screen large populations of newborns. What Kharrazi et al describe is the use of dried blood spots for detection of CMV DNA. The procedure for collecting and processing such samples has been around for many decades, and PCR technology is highly automated in this day and age. We see in California that the rate of congenital CMV infection using PCR screening on dried blood spots runs just under 1%, a figure that one would expect on the basis of published studies screening infants for CMV using urine cultures. Unfortunately, not every newborn with congenital CMV infection will be viremic even by sensitive PCR methods, so we will need follow-up studies to determine what percentage of infants would be missed by blood spot screening. There is one other interesting finding in this report, a finding that confirms previous studies and that is one cannot adequately screen newborn infants with IgM-CMV antibodies. Only 25% of infants who are documented to be CMV infected will have IgM antibodies against the virus in the immediate newborn period, supporting the view that neonatal IgM is not a reliable marker for congenital CMV infection.

We can conclude from this report that it may be feasible to use dried blood spots for universal CMV screening. As of now, however, there are no validated high-throughput methodologies for this purpose or an agreed upon protocol for monitoring children who would be found to be CMV positive. Add to this the psychological cost placed on parents who learn that their infant has been exposed to this virus knowing that only 1 in 5 babies, or fewer, will have any negative sequelae. The flip side, however, is that the potential benefits could be significant. Two of 3 children who will develop some form of neurologic disability are in fact asymptomatic at birth, and screening would potentially be of benefit for these infants. Exactly how much benefit we do not know until treatment protocols for such infants are in place.

J. A. Stockman III, MD

Cytomegalovirus glycoprotein-B vaccine with MF59 adjuvant in transplant recipients: a phase 2 randomised placebo-controlled trial
Griffiths PD, Stanton A, McCarrell E, et al (UCL Med School, London, UK; et al)
Lancet 377:1256-1263, 2011

Background.—Cytomegalovirus end-organ disease can be prevented by giving ganciclovir when viraemia is detected in allograft recipients. Values of viral load correlate with development of end-organ disease and are moderated by preexisting natural immunity. Our aim was to determine whether vaccine-induced immunity could do likewise.

Methods.—We undertook a phase-2 randomised placebo controlled trial in adults awaiting kidney or liver transplantation at the Royal Free Hospital, London, UK. Exclusion criteria were pregnancy, receipt of blood products (except albumin) in the previous 3 months, and simultaneous multiorgan transplantation. 70 patients seronegative and 70 seropositive for cytomegalovirus were randomly assigned from a scratch-off randomisation code in a 1:1 ratio to receive either cytomegalovirus glycoprotein-B vaccine with MF59 adjuvant or placebo, each given at baseline, 1 month and 6 months later. If a patient was transplanted, no further vaccinations were given and serial blood samples were tested for cytomegalovirus DNA by real-time quantitative PCR (rtqPCR). Any patient with one blood sample containing more than 3000 cytomegalovirus genomes per mL received ganciclovir until two consecutive undetectable cytomegalovirus DNA measurements. Safety and immunogenicity were coprimary endpoints and were assessed by intention to treat in patients who received at least one dose of vaccine or placebo. This trial is registered with ClinicalTrials.gov, NCT00299260.

Findings.—67 patients received vaccine and 73 placebo, all of whom were evaluable. Glycoprotein-B antibody titres were significantly increased in both seronegative (geometric mean titre 12 537 (95% CI 6593−23 840) versus 86 (63−118) in recipients of placebo recipients; p<0·0001) and seropositive (118 395; 64 503−217 272) versus 24 682 (17 909−34 017); p<0·0001) recipients of vaccine. In those who developed viraemia after transplantation, glycoprotein-B antibody titres correlated inversely with duration of viraemia (p=0·0022). In the seronegative patients with seropositive donors, the duration of viraemia (p=0·0480) and number of days of ganciclovir treatment (p=0·0287) were reduced in vaccine recipients.

Interpretation.—Although cytomegalovirus disease occurs in the context of suppressed cell-mediated immunity post-transplantation, humoral immunity has a role in reduction of cytomegalovirus viraemia. Vaccines containing cytomegalovirus glycoprotein B merit further assessment in transplant recipients.

▶ Cytomegalovirus (CMV) infection after transplantation of human tissue might originate from the donor or from reactivation in the recipient. Infection may cause either primary infection in recipients who are initially seronegative for the virus or reinfection with a new strain in a seropositive recipient. The most serious clinical effects result from primary infection, followed by reinfection, with reactivation being the least likely to cause end-organ disease. Thus, most end-organ disease arises from donor-derived virus. This pecking order of risk occurs because natural immunity before transplantation provides substantial protection against virus replication after transplantation, and a high viral load is needed to cause end-organ disease. This would suggest that given that natural immunity before transplantation can modulate the pathogenicity of CMV after transplantation, it would be reasonable to believe that if a vaccine worked, it would induce immunity and would replicate this natural immunity.

The data provided by the report of Griffiths et al represents an exciting step forward in the management of transplantation-related CMV infection. The results show, for the first time, that a CMV vaccine administered before solid-organ transplantation can affect the natural history of CMV infection after transplantation. This double-blinded placebo-controlled study assessed a series of 3 doses of vaccine with a recombinant form of the immunodominant envelope glycoprotein B, given with an adjuvant (MF59). Seventy patients seronegative for CMV and 70 seropositive for the virus who were receiving either liver or kidney transplantation were vaccinated or given placebo. Serial CMV polymerase chain reaction measurements were obtained before and after transplantation in these recipients. The results were striking, particularly for seronegative patients who received organs from seropositive donors. In these patients, both the duration of virus in the blood and the total number of days required for antiviral treatment were significantly reduced. The viral load documented in treated patients was less than one-tenth that of those who received placebo vaccine.

Historically, antiviral drugs and the use of immune anti-CMV globulin have not been magic bullets to manage posttransplantation CMV infection. A vaccine to control CMV disease in transplant recipients is a far better way to go. It will be interesting to see how this vaccine, if documented in other studies to be successful, might be used to assist in the prevention of congenitally infected newborn infants.

To read more about the CMV vaccine, see the well-done commentary on this topic by Mark Schleiss.[1]

J. A. Stockman III, MD

Reference

1. Schleiss MR. A cytomegalovirus vaccine tames the troll of transplantation. *Lancet.* 2011;377:1216-1218.

Effect of circumcision of HIV-negative men on transmission of human papillomavirus to HIV-negative women: a randomised trial in Rakai, Uganda
Wawer MJ, Tobian AAR, Kigozi G, et al (Johns Hopkins Univ, Baltimore, MD; et al)
Lancet 377:209-218, 2011

Background.—Randomised trials show that male circumcision reduces the prevalence and incidence of high-risk human papillomavirus (HPV) infection in men. We assessed the efficacy of male circumcision to reduce prevalence and incidence of high-risk HPV in female partners of circumcised men.

Methods.—In two parallel but independent randomised controlled trials of male circumcision, we enrolled HIV-negative men and their female partners between 2003 and 2006, in Rakai, Uganda. With a computer-generated random number sequence in blocks of 20, men were assigned to undergo circumcision immediately (intervention) or after 24 months (control). HIV-uninfected female partners (648 of men from the intervention group, and 597 of men in the control group) were simultaneously enrolled and provided interview information and self-collected vaginal swabs at baseline, 12 months, and 24 months. Vaginal swabs were tested for high-risk HPV by Roche HPV Linear Array. Female HPV infection was a secondary endpoint of the trials, assessed as the prevalence of high-risk HPV infection 24 months after intervention and the incidence of new infections during the trial. Analysis was by intention-to-treat. An as-treated analysis was also done to account for study-group crossovers. The trials were registered, numbers NCT00425984 and NCT00124878.

Findings.—During the trial, 18 men in the control group underwent circumcision elsewhere, and 31 in the intervention group did not undergo circumcision. At 24-month follow-up, data were available for 544 women in the intervention group and 488 in the control group; 151 (27·8%) women in the intervention group and 189 (38·7%) in the control group had high-risk HPV infection (prevalence risk ratio=0·72, 95% CI 0·60—0·85, p=0·001). During the trial, incidence of high-risk HPV infection in women was lower in the intervention group than in the control group (20·7 infections *vs* 26·9 infections per 100 person-years; incidence rate ratio=0·77, 0·63—0·93, p=0·008).

Interpretation.—Our findings indicate that male circumcision should now be accepted as an efficacious intervention for reducing the prevalence and incidence of HPV infections in female partners. However, protection is only partial; the promotion of safe sex practices is also important.

▶ The role of circumcision in the prevention of disease transmission and the beliefs associated with it go back well over a century. It was in 1901 that Braithwaite commented on the low incidence of cervical cancer in Jewish women who were married to men who were circumcised.[1] With the recognition that human papillomavirus (HPV) is causative in the development of cervical cancer and with advances in methodology for the detection of HPV, further studies have supported these early observations that circumcision somewhat protects against HPV infection and cervical cancer in female partners.

Wawer et al undertook a randomized trial that shows that circumcision reduces both the incidence and prevalence of high-risk HPV in female partners of circumcised men. In more than 1200 heterosexual couples, adult male circumcision significantly reduced the prevalence and incidence of HPV in women. The prevalence of high-risk HPV in women was 27.8% in the intervention group and 38.7% in the control group ($P = .001$). These data, originating from a rigorous study design, support original observations for a preventive role of male circumcision and cervical cancer.

As good as the data are from the report of Wawer et al, they clearly are not good enough to recommend universal circumcision solely for the purpose of the prevention of HPV infection in women. The reduction in high-risk HPV infection in women was 25%, hardly a perfect means of preventing HPV infection. It should be noted that an important clinical end point, such as high-grade cervical dysplasia, was not assessed. Nonetheless, it is reasonable to endorse policies that foster male circumcision. To read more about this topic, see the commentary by Giuliano et al.[2]

In conclusion, we have one final comment having to do with the number of new infections related to HIV. From 1999 to 2009, the number of new infections of HIV fell worldwide by 16%. Greater use of effective antiretrovirals has resulted in fewer age-related deaths as well. The fall in new infections between 2001 and 2009 exceeded 25% in 33 countries, including 22 in Sub-Saharan Africa. However, in 7 countries, 5 in Eastern Europe and Central Asia, the incidence of HIV rose by more than 25% in the same period. It is estimated that worldwide 33.3 million people were living with HIV in 2009, up from 26.2 million in 1999. The number of new infections in 2009 was 2.6 million, down from 3.1 million a decade ago. Approximately 1.8 million people died from AIDS-related causes, down from 2.1 million in 2004. It appears that Sub-Saharan Africa still has the highest burden of HIV infection with 22.5 million people with HIV (some 68% of the world total). In 2010, some 5.2 million people in low- and middle-income families had access to antiretrovirals. This represents only 35% of those eligible under new World Health Organization guidelines issued in 2010. To read more about the statistics, see www.unaids.org.[3]

J. A. Stockman III, MD

References

1. Braithwaite J. Excess of salt in the diet: a probable factor in the causation of cancer. *Lancet.* 1901;ii:1578-1580.
2. Giuliano AR, Nyitray AG, Albero G. Male circumcision and HPV transmission to female partners. *Lancet.* 2011;377:183-184.
3. UNAIDS. www.unaids.org. Accessed August 19, 2011.

Vaccine-Induced HIV Seropositivity/Reactivity in Noninfected HIV Vaccine Recipients
Cooper CJ, for the NIAID HIV Vaccine Trials Network (HVTN) Vaccine-Induced Seropositivity (VISP) Task Force (Fred Hutchinson Cancer Res Ctr, Seattle, WA; et al)
JAMA 304:275-283, 2010

Context.—Induction of protective anti–human immunodeficiency virus (HIV) immune responses is the goal of an HIV vaccine. However, this may cause a reactive result in routine HIV testing in the absence of HIV infection.

Objective.—To evaluate the frequency of vaccine-induced seropositivity/reactivity (VISP) in HIV vaccine trial participants.

Design, Setting, and Participants.—Three common US Food and Drug Administration–approved enzyme immunoassay (EIA) HIV antibody kits were used to determine VISP, and a routine diagnostic HIV algorithm was used to evaluate VISP frequency in healthy, HIV-seronegative adults who completed phase 1 (n=25) and phase 2a (n=2) vaccine trials conducted from 2000-2010 in the United States, South America, Thailand, and Africa.

Main Outcome Measure.—Vaccine-induced seropositivity/reactivity, defined as reactive on 1 or more EIA tests and either Western blot–negative or Western blot–indeterminate/atypical positive (profile consistent with vaccine product) and HIV-1–negative by nucleic acid testing.

Results.—Among 2176 participants free of HIV infection who received a vaccine product, 908 (41.7%; 95% confidence interval [CI], 39.6%-43.8%) had VISP, but the occurrence of VISP varied substantially across different HIV vaccine product types: 399 of 460 (86.7%; 95% CI,

83.3%-89.7%) adenovirus 5 product recipients, 295 of 552 (53.4%; 95% CI, 49.2%-57.7%) recipients of poxvirus alone or as a boost, and 35 of 555 (6.3%; 95% CI, 4.4%-8.7%) of DNA-alone product recipients developed VISP. Overall, the highest proportion of VISP (891/2176 tested [40.9%]) occurred with the HIV 1/2 (rDNA) EIA kit compared with the rLAV EIA (150/700 tested [21.4%]), HIV-1 Plus O Microelisa System (193/1309 tested [14.7%]), and HIV 1/2 Peptide and HIV 1/2 Plus O (189/2150 tested [8.8%]) kits. Only 17 of the 908 participants (1.9%) with VISP tested nonreactive using the HIV 1/2 (rDNA) kit. All recipients of a glycoprotein 140 vaccine (n=70) had VISP, with 94.3% testing reactive with all 3 EIA kits tested. Among 901 participants with VISP and a Western blot result, 92 (10.2%) had a positive Western blot result (displaying an atypical pattern consistent with vaccine product), and 592 (65.7%) had an indeterminate result. Only 8 participants with VISP received a vaccine not containing an envelope insert.

Conclusions.—The induction of VISP in HIV vaccine recipients is common, especially with vaccines containing both the HIV-1 envelope and group-specific core antigen gene proteins. Development and detection of VISP appear to be associated with the immunogenicity of the vaccine and the EIA assay used.

▶ There has been a bevy of reports recently about vaccine-induced human immunodeficiency virus (HIV) seropositivity/reactivity in noninfected HIV vaccine recipients. For more than 2 decades now, potential vaccine candidates have been through clinical trials involving tens of thousands of HIV-negative participants. All varieties of vaccines have been used, including protein-DNA, HIV peptide, and viral-vectored vaccines. Specific targets within the virus have been singled out. Several of these candidate vaccines have advanced to large field trials. Nearly everyone given vaccine makes some antibodies to HIV, but while the HIV antibodies have been detected since the 1990s, none have had the properties to serve as a cornerstone around which to build a reliable and effective vaccine.

Recently, scientists have discovered 3 previously unknown human antibodies that neutralize HIV, including 2 that target a broad range of HIV strains.[1] One antibody in particular called VRC01 displays potency and broad coverage against HIV strains. Such recent findings are said to establish a proof of the principle that it is possible for the body to generate these kinds of antibodies, and the trick will be to design an HIV vaccine that elicits the immune system to produce a combination of antibodies. HIV poses a particular challenge for vaccine design because it mutates frequently and is camouflaged from the immune system by sugar molecules.

This commentary closes with an update on current recommendations of the International AIDS Society-USA Panel with respect to initiation of antiretroviral treatment. The recommendations read that therapy is recommended for asymptomatic patients with a CD4 cell count 500/uL for all symptomatic patients and those with specific conditions and comorbidities.[2]

J. A. Stockman III, MD

References

1. Seppa N. Three antibodies shown to block HIV. *Science News.* July 31, 2010:13.
2. Thompson MA, Aberg JA, Cahn P, et al. Antiretroviral treatment of adult HIV infection: 2010 recommendations of the international AIDS society? USA Panel. *JAMA.* 2010;304:321-333.

Preexposure Chemoprophylaxis for HIV Prevention in Men Who Have Sex with Men

Grant RM, for the iPrEx Study Team (Univ of California, San Francisco; et al)
N Engl J Med 363:2587-2599, 2010

Background.—Antiretroviral chemoprophylaxis before exposure is a promising approach for the prevention of human immunodeficiency virus (HIV) acquisition.

Methods.—We randomly assigned 2499 HIV-seronegative men or transgender women who have sex with men to receive a combination of two oral antiretroviral drugs, emtricitabine and tenofovir disoproxil fumarate (FTC−TDF), or placebo once daily. All subjects received HIV testing, risk-reduction counseling, condoms, and management of sexually transmitted infections.

Results.—The study subjects were followed for 3324 person-years (median, 1.2 years; maximum, 2.8 years). Of these subjects, 10 were found to have been infected with HIV at enrollment, and 100 became infected during follow-up (36 in the FTC−TDF group and 64 in the placebo group), indicating a 44% reduction in the incidence of HIV (95% confidence interval, 15 to 63; P=0.005). In the FTC−TDF group, the study drug was detected in 22 of 43 of seronegative subjects (51%) and in 3 of 34 HIV-infected subjects (9%) (P<0.001). Nausea was reported more frequently during the first 4 weeks in the FTC−TDF group than in the placebo group (P<0.001). The two groups had similar rates of serious adverse events (P=0.57).

Conclusions.—Oral FTC−TDF provided protection against the acquisition of HIV infection among the subjects. Detectable blood levels strongly correlated with the prophylactic effect. (Funded by the National Institutes of Health and the Bill and Melinda Gates Foundation; ClinicalTrials.gov number, NCT00458393.)

▶ By the beginning of the last decade, we seemed to have hit a plateau in methods to prevent human immunodeficiency virus (HIV) infection transmission. By 2005 to 2007, a number of studies transformed our thinking, however. These studies show that adult male circumcision, vaccination, or the use of a vaginal microbicide could reduce to some extent the risk of HIV infection. The latest news is provided by Grant et al, who report evidence that antiretroviral medications, specifically the combination of emtricitabine and tenofovir disoproxil fumarate (FTC-TDF), taken orally on a daily basis by men and transgender women (born male) who have sex with men, can provide partial protection from HIV infection. The trial, called the Preexposure Prophylaxis Initiative Study, was a placebo-controlled, double-blind, randomized trial involving 2499 subjects in the Americas, South Africa, and Thailand. Of observed infections, 64 occurred in the placebo group and 36 in the FTC-TDF group, for an estimated efficacy of 44% (95% confidence interval, 15-63). Thus, exposure to FTC-TDF is associated with a reduction in HIV acquisition, which supports the biologic plausibility of the primary result that one can at least partially protect against HIV infection in those who are at high risk from sexual activity. These data represent a significant advance in HIV prevention research in providing proof of concept that a antiretroviral drug combination in widespread clinical use in the treatment of chronic HIV infection will reduce the risk of HIV acquisition in men who have sex with men.

So what is the rub? There are several observations that should be made that potentially counter the argument for routine male prophylaxis. One is the fact that the antiretroviral drug combination, in some individuals, can cause renal insufficiency, a problem if you are otherwise a healthy male. In addition, it is possible that exposure to drug combinations such as FTC-TDF could result in the acquisition of drug resistance should one later become infected. Also, the overall reduction in HIV incidence in the FTC-TDF group was less than 50%. Added to the possibility of the troubling development of secondary antiretroviral resistance and a low but measurable degree of renal toxicity, adherence to a daily regimen would likely be low, nondurable, and difficult to assess without pharmacologic testing. For these reasons, the potential implementation of preexposure prophylaxis with FTC-TDF will probably be considered only for men who have sex with men and who are at very high risk for HIV infection.

While the data from this report would not seem to apply to the pediatric population, they are important for us. Infants are infected with HIV largely because their mothers have become infected from sources that could be minimized with prophylactic measures.

J. A. Stockman III, MD

Antiretroviral Therapies in Women after Single-Dose Nevirapine Exposure
Lockman S, for the OCTANE A5208 Study Team (Brigham and Women's Hosp, Boston, MA; et al)
N Engl J Med 363:1499-1509, 2010

Background.—Peripartum administration of single-dose nevirapine reduces mother-to-child transmission of human immunodeficiency virus type 1 (HIV-1) but selects for nevirapine-resistant virus.

Methods.—In seven African countries, women infected with HIV-1 whose CD4+ T-cell counts were below 200 per cubic millimeter and who either had or had not taken single-dose nevirapine at least 6 months before enrollment were randomly assigned to receive antiretroviral therapy with tenofovir—emtricitabine plus nevirapine or tenofovir-emtricitabine plus lopinavir boosted by a low dose of ritonavir. The primary end point was the time to confirmed virologic failure or death.

Results.—A total of 241 women who had been exposed to single-dose nevirapine began the study treatments (121 received nevirapine and 120 received ritonavir-boosted lopin avir). Significantly more women in the nevirapine group reached the primary end point than in the ritonavir-boosted lopinavir group (26% vs. 8%) (adjusted P=0.001). Virologic failure occurred in 37 (28 in the nevirapine group and 9 in the ritonavir-boosted lopinavir group), and 5 died without prior virologic failure (4 in the nevirapine group and 1 in the ritonavir-boosted lopinavir group). The group differences appeared to decrease as the interval between single-dose nevirapine exposure and the start of antiretroviral therapy increased. Retrospective bulk sequencing of baseline plasma samples showed nevirapine resistance in 33 of 239 women tested (14%). Among 500 women without prior exposure to single-dose nevirapine, 34 of 249 in the nevirapine group (14%) and 36 of 251 in the ritonavir-boosted lopinavir group (14%) had virologic failure or died.

Conclusions.—In women with prior exposure to peripartum single-dose nevirapine (but not in those without prior exposure), ritonavir-boosted lopinavir plus tenofovir—emtricitabine was superior to nevirapine plus tenofovir—emtricitabine for initial antiretroviral therapy. (Funded by the National Institute of Allergy and Infectious Diseases and the National Research Center; ClinicalTrials.gov number, NCT00089505.)

▶ Lockman et al report the results of the Optimal Combination Therapy After Nevirapine Exposure (OCTANE) A5208 trial, in which 241 human immunodeficiency virus (HIV)-infected mothers who had been exposed to a single-dose nevirapine 6 months or more before randomization were assigned to receive ritonavir-boosted lopinavir-based therapy or nevirapine-based therapy. After 2 years, 8% of the women in the ritonavir-boosted lopinavir group had virologic failure (or died) as compared with 26% in the nevirapine group. In the nevirapine group, the proportion of women with resistance mutations detectable at the time of initiation of treatment was small (13%), but these women had the highest failure rate (73%) as compared with 19% among women in the nevirapine group without resistance mutations. In a companion trial involving women who had not been exposed to single-dose nevirapine, failure rates were 14% in both the ritonavir-boosted lopinavir group and the nevirapine group.

So what does this mean? Almost half of HIV-infected pregnant women now receive antiretroviral medications for prevention of mother-to-child transmission. In most instances, the simplest intervention, single-dose nevirapine, is given to the mother during labor and to the infant after birth. Nevirapine will cut in half the risk of peripartum transmission, but the agent persists at clinically significant levels for days, potentially selecting HIV resistance mutations that may negatively affect the efficacy of nevirapine-based therapies when mothers and infected children subsequently receive treatment for their own health. This poses an important public health challenge because nevirapine-based therapies are the most widely available and affordable treatments in resource-limited countries where more than 95% of infections in infants and children occur. This is in fact what the OCTANE study showed, specifically that 6 months or more after exposure to single-dose nevirapine one may see a diminished response to nevirapine-based therapy. These results support the updated World Health Organization recommendations that a regimen based on ritonavir-boosted lopinavir should be used for women and for children younger than 24 months if they have had previous exposure to single-dose nevirapine.

J. A. Stockman III, MD

Antiretroviral Treatment for Children with Peripartum Nevirapine Exposure
Palumbo P, Lindsey JC, Hughes MD, et al (Dartmouth Med School, Lebanon, NH; Harvard School of Public Health, Boston, MA; et al)
N Engl J Med 363:1510-1520, 2010

Background.—Single-dose nevirapine is the cornerstone of the regimen for prevention of mother-to-child transmission of human immunodeficiency virus (HIV) in resource-limited settings, but nevirapine frequently selects for resistant virus in mothers and children who become infected despite prophylaxis. The optimal antiretroviral treatment strategy for children who have had prior exposure to single-dose nevirapine is unknown.

Methods.—We conducted a randomized trial of initial therapy with zidovudine and lamivudine plus either nevirapine or ritonavir-boosted lopinavir in HIV-infected children 6 to 36 months of age, in six African countries, who qualified for treatment according to World Health Organization (WHO) criteria. Results are reported for the cohort that included children exposed to single-dose nevirapine prophylaxis. The primary end point was virologic failure or discontinuation of treatment by study week 24. Enrollment in this cohort was terminated early on the recommendation of the data and safety monitoring board.

Results.—A total of 164 children were enrolled. The median percentage of CD4+ lymphocytes was 19%; a total of 56% of the children had WHO stage 3 or 4 disease. More children in the nevirapine group than in the ritonavir-boosted lopinavir group reached a primary end point (39.6% vs. 21.7%; weighted difference, 18.6 percentage-points; 95% confidence interval, 3.7 to 33.6; nominal P=0.02). Baseline resistance to nevirapine was detected in 18 of 148 children (12%) and was predictive of treatment failure. No significant between-group differences were seen in the rate of adverse events.

Conclusions.—Among children with prior exposure to single-dose nevirapine for perinatal prevention of HIV transmission, antiretroviral treatment consisting of zidovudine and lamivudine plus ritonavir-boosted lopinavir resulted in better outcomes than did treatment with zidovudine and lamivudine plus nevirapine. Since nevirapine is used for both treatment and perinatal prevention of HIV infection in resource-limited settings, alternative strategies for the prevention of HIV transmission from mother to child, as well as for the treatment of HIV infection, are urgently required.

(Funded by the National Institutes of Health; ClinicalTrials.gov number, NCT00307151.)

▶ This report confirms the information provided by the study of Lockman et al, in that the study shows that human immunodeficiency virus (HIV)—infected pregnant women given single-dose nevirapine at delivery are at significantly higher risk of failure to subsequent treatment with this antiviral agent.[1] The study also confirms that it would be better not to use nevirapine as a single agent because of this drug resistance; rather, ritonavir-boosted lopinavir would be a more ideal antiviral combination. Unfortunately, in resource-limited settings where many women still present late for antenatal care and too few are screened for CD4+ cell count, single-dose nevirapine will most likely remain an important component of the toolkit for the prevention of mother-to-child transmission, especially given the significantly lower cost of this single agent.

To read more about preventing mother-to-child transmission of HIV, see the excellent editorial by Lallemant and Jourdain and also recognize that a recent communication from the Centers for Disease Control and Prevention (CDC) reminds us that even with modern screening of blood component products, it is still capable for such products to transmit the HIV and cause AIDS.[2,3] Specifically, a 40-year-old blood donor in Missouri was found to be the source of HIV infection in a blood component recipient. The blood donor was a repeat donor who reported no HIV risk factors on the routine eligibility screening questionnaire. He was also not compensated for his blood donation. His blood donation was screened at a reference laboratory for HIV by enzyme immunoassay and by nucleic acid amplification testing of minipools of plasma specimens. Both tests were negative. When this fellow came back to donate blood a bit later, these tests had become positive. Recipients of the first blood donation were tracked down. One unit of packed red blood cells from the donor had been transfused into a patient during cardiac surgery. This patient died 2 days later from cardiac disease. The other recipient received a unit of fresh frozen plasma during a surgical kidney transplant. That recipient, when followed up, was HIV positive and placed on antiretroviral therapy. This report describes the first US case of transfusion-transmitted HIV infection reported to the CDC since 2002. Despite initially denying any risk factors for HIV, the blood component donor did confess to having multiple paid female and male sex partners. Presumably, the sequence of events in this case was consistent with transmission by transfusion of HIV-contaminated plasma collected from a donor during the eclipse period of acute infection (ie, the interval between infection and the development of detectable concentrations of HIV RNA in plasma). The risk of such HIV transmission via blood products is estimated as 1 in 1 467 000 based on data from 2007 to 2008, which incorporates the highest increased incidence of HIV among blood donors.

J. A. Stockman III, MD

References

1. Lockman S, Hughes MD, McIntyre J, et al. Antiretroviral therapies in women after single-dose nevirapine exposure. *N Engl J Med*. 2010;363:1499-1509.

2. Lallemant M, Jourdain G. Preventing mother-to-child transmission of HIV—protecting this generation and the next. *N Engl J Med.* 2010;363:1570-1572.
3. Centers for Disease Control and Prevention (CDC). HIV transmission through transfusion—Missouri and Colorado, 2008. *MMWR Morb Mortal Wkly Rep.* 2010;59:1335-1339.

Focal Epithelial Hyperplasia Caused by Human Papillomavirus 13
Saunders NR, Scolnik D, Rebbapragada A, et al (Hosp for Sick Children, Toronto, Canada; The Univ of Toronto, Canada; Ontario Agency for Health Protection and Promotion, Toronto, Canada; et al)
Pediatr Infect Dis J 29:550-552, 2010

Focal epithelial hyperplasia is a benign, papulo-nodular disease of the oral cavity. It is rare, affecting primarily Native American populations during childhood. It is closely associated with human papillomavirus 13 and 32. This report describes the diagnosis of 2 cases of focal epithelial hyperplasia in children from southern Guyana. The diagnosis was made using clinical criteria, polymerase chain reaction, and DNA sequencing.

▶ We tend to think of the consequences of papillomaviruses largely as they affect teens and young adults. Indeed, this grouping of viruses can wreak havoc even in the young, as evidenced by the reports of these 8-year-old and 11-year-old youngsters. There is a disorder known as Heck disease, which is a rare disease of the oral mucosa associated with human papillomavirus (HPV). Heck disease causes a focal epithelial hyperplasia (FEH). FEH is manifested by multiple well-circumscribed papulonodular, soft, painless lesions on the mucosal epithelium of the lips and tongue. These lesions affect mostly children and young adults and are usually chronic. The first cases were described in New Mexico in 1965 by Dr John Heck.[1] Biopsy of the lesions can yield viral DNA, usually related to HPV 13 and HPV 32.

The figure demonstrates what these oral lesions look like. Girls seem to be affected about twice as commonly as boys. The condition is felt to be benign. Clinically, FEH presents as multiple well-circumscribed papulonodular, soft, painless lesions with a generally smooth surface ranging in size from 1 mm to 10 mm in diameter, but they can be larger and often coalesce. The lesions can vary in color from white to pink to red or many appear as a normal mucosal color. They can affect both upper and lower lips, the cheeks, and the tongue.

While Heck disease is probably rare in the United States, it does occur, and we should be aware of it. Also be aware that while HPV is well known to be the etiologic agent of cervical cancer, it has been associated with numerous other cancers, including oropharyngeal squamous cell carcinoma. There are virtually no data on the long-term follow-up of patients with Heck disease to see if these lesions evolve into anything more serious.

J. A. Stockman III, MD

Reference

1. González LV, Gaviria AM, Sanclemente G, et al. Clinical histopathological and virological findings in patients with focal epithelial hyperplasia from Columbia. *Int J Dermatol.* 2005;44:274-279.

Efficacy of Quadrivalent HPV Vaccine against HPV Infection and Disease in Males

Giuliano AR, Palefsky JM, Goldstone S, et al (H. Lee Moffitt Cancer Ctr and Res Inst, Tampa, FL; Univ of California San Francisco; Mount Sinai School of Medicine, NY; et al)
N Engl J Med 364:401-411, 2011

Background.—Infection with human papillomavirus (HPV) and diseases caused by HPV are common in boys and men. We report on the safety of a quadrivalent vaccine (active against HPV types 6, 11, 16, and 18) and on its efficacy in preventing the development of external genital lesions and anogenital HPV infection in boys and men.

Methods.—We enrolled 4065 healthy boys and men 16 to 26 years of age, from 18 countries in a randomized, placebo-controlled, double-blind trial. The primary efficacy objective was to show that the quadrivalent HPV vaccine reduced the incidence of external genital lesions related to HPV-6, 11, 16, or 18. Efficacy analyses were conducted in a per-protocol population, in which subjects received all three vaccinations and were negative for relevant HPV types at enrollment, and in an intention-to-treat population, in which subjects received vaccine or placebo, regardless of baseline HPV status.

Results.—In the intention-to-treat population, 36 external genital lesions were seen in the vaccine group as compared with 89 in the placebo group, for an observed efficacy of 60.2% (95% confidence interval [CI], 40.8 to 73.8); the efficacy was 65.5% (95% CI, 45.8 to 78.6) for lesions related to HPV-6, 11, 16, or 18. In the per-protocol population, efficacy against lesions related to HPV-6, 11, 16, or 18 was 90.4% (95% CI, 69.2 to 98.1). Efficacy with respect to persistent infection with HPV-6, 11, 16, or 18 and detection of related DNA at any time was 47.8% (95% CI, 36.0 to 57.6) and 27.1% (95% CI, 16.6 to 36.3), respectively, in the intention-to-treat population and 85.6% (97.5% CI, 73.4 to 92.9) and 44.7% (95% CI, 31.5 to 55.6) in the per-protocol population. Injection-site pain was significantly more frequent among subjects receiving quadrivalent HPV vaccine than among those receiving placebo (57% vs. 51%, P<0.001).

Conclusions.—Quadrivalent HPV vaccine prevents infection with HPV-6, 11, 16, and 18 and the development of related external genital lesions in males 16 to 26 years of age. (Funded by Merck and others; ClinicalTrials. gov number, NCT00090285.)

▶ This is an important report giving us information about the efficacy of a human papillomavirus (HPV) vaccine against HPV infection and disease in men. The report is important because HPV infections contribute to approximately 20 000 cases of invasive cancer in the United States each year. About half of these cancers are cervical cancers, and the rest involve the vagina, vulva, penis, anus, oral cavity, and oropharynx. Currently, less than 1 in 4 of HPV-related cancers occur in men. Some small subgroups, however, such as men who have sex with men, have markedly higher rates of HPV-related diseases such as anal cancer. Oncogenic types of HPV cause nearly all cases of cervical cancer, 90% of cases of anal cancer, and a smaller proportion of the remaining cancers. The majority of these cancers are attributable to just 2 types, HPV-16 and HPV-18. Nononcogenic types, HPV-6 and HPV-11, cause approximately 34 000 cases of genital warts in the United States each year.

There are 2 highly efficacious prophylactic vaccines that target HPV-16 and HPV-18. One of these is a quadrivalent vaccine that also targets HPV-6 and HPV-11. Most data in the literature relate to the efficacy of these vaccines in girls and women. The data presented by Giuliano et al, however, affirm the potential for HPV vaccines to prevent related disease in boys and men. The investigators report the efficacy of quadrivalent HPV vaccine in preventing infections with the HPV types included in the vaccine, as well as external genital lesions, primarily genital warts, in young men aged 16 to 26 years. These data were available to the Food and Drug Administration (FDA) when the latter approved these vaccines for prevention of genital warts in young men in the United States and the subsequent recommendation from the Advisory Committee on Immunization Practices (ACIP) that advises the Centers for Disease Control and Prevention (CDC) for the permissive use of the vaccine in older teens and young men. The ACIP stopped short of supporting routine HPV vaccination in adolescent boys, even though routine vaccination of girls between the ages of 11 and 12 years (and as early as 9 years) has been recommended since 2007. The committee did recommend financial coverage via the CDC Vaccines for Children Program for eligible boys aged 18 years or younger. These decisions were made before newer data appeared that show that the quadrivalent HPV vaccine is effective in preventing anal intraepithelial neoplasia, a precursor to anal cancer, in men, particularly in men who have sex with men. On the basis of this new evidence, the FDA has approved the expanded use of the quadrivalent vaccine to include the prevention of anal lesions and cancer in people of both sexes, a decision that has reignited the debate over the routine HPV vaccination in young men.

As of this writing, there is no universal recommendation for HPV vaccination of adolescent boys. The ACIP elected not to recommend routine vaccination of adolescent boys on the basis of multiple considerations, one of which was the less attractive cost-effectiveness profile. Several cost-effectiveness analyses have indicated that HPV vaccination of both sexes is not cost effective when compared with the vaccination of girls only.

In an editorial that accompanied this report by Kim, it was noted that to maximize the benefit to the population's health from health services and interventions, we have a responsibility to use resources as efficiently as possible.[1] Equally important, however, is our responsibility to revisit policy decisions as influential new data and new technologies become available as they undoubtedly will in the case of prevention and control of HPV-related diseases. The report of Giuliano et al provides important new information and should reopen the debate about the routine vaccination of adolescent boys and young adult men against HPV infection.

J. A. Stockman III, MD

Reference

1. Kim JJ. Focus on research: weighing the benefits and costs of HPV vaccination of young men. N Engl J Med. 2011;364:393-395.

Incidence and clearance of genital human papillomavirus infection in men (HIM): a cohort study
Giuliano AR, Lee J-H, Fulp W, et al (H Lee Moffitt Cancer Ctr, Tampa, FL; et al)
Lancet 377:932-940, 2011

Background.—Human papillomaviruses (HPVs) cause genital warts and cancers in men. The natural history of HPV infection in men is largely unknown, and that information is needed to inform prevention strategies. The goal in this study was to estimate incidence and clearance of type-specific genital HPV infection in men, and to assess the associated factors.

Methods.—Men (aged 18–70 years), residing in Brazil, Mexico, and the USA, who were HIV negative and reported no history of cancer were recruited from the general population, universities, and organised health-care systems. They were assessed every 6 months for a median follow-up of 27·5 months (18·0–31·2). Specimens from the coronal sulcus, glans penis, shaft, and scrotum were obtained for the assessment of the status of HPV genotypes.

Findings.—In 1159 men, the incidence of a new genital HPV infection was 38·4 per 1000 person months (95% CI 34·3–43·0). Oncogenic HPV infection was significantly associated with having a high number of lifetime female sexual partners (hazard ratio 2·40, 1·38–4·18, for at least 50 partners *vs* not more than one partner), and number of male anal-sexual partners (2·57, 1·46–4·49, for at least three male partners *vs* no recent partners). Median duration of HPV infection was 7·52 months (6·80–8·61) for any HPV and 12·19 months (7·16–18·17) for HPV 16. Clearance of oncogenic HPV infection decreased in men with a high number of lifetime female partners (0·49, 0·31–0·76, for at least 50 female partners *vs* not more than one partner), and in men in Brazil (0·71, 0·56–0·91) and Mexico (0·73, 0·57–0·94) compared with the USA. Clearance of oncogenic HPV was more rapid with increasing age (1·02, 1·01–1·03).

Interpretation.—The data from this study are useful for the development of realistic cost-effectiveness models for male HPV vaccination internationally.

▶ Starting in 2005, a team led by Giuliano et al of the H. Lee Moffitt Cancer and Research Institute in Tampa, Florida, recruited more than 4000 men living in Brazil, Mexico, and Florida for a study of human papillomavirus (HPV). The study reports on the first 1159 of these volunteers. Their average age was 32 years; none had been vaccinated against HPV. Swabs of the penis and genital area of each man revealed that 50% were infected with at least 1 HPV type on enrollment. Over a median of 28 months, the group acquired 1572 new HPV infections.

It appears that the human immune system can clear HPV from the body, and the men studied wiped out most of their new infections in an average of 7.5 months. Clearance times did not vary substantially among countries that were part of the study but did vary between HPV types. Some cases lingered as long as 20 months.

It is clear that male circumcision and the use of condoms show little protection against HPV infection. The results from this study provide much needed data about the incidence and clearance of HPV infection in men. These data are essential for the development of realistic cost-effectiveness models for male HPV vaccination, in the United States and internationally. This study shows that although the risk of HPV decreases with increasing age in women, men seem to have a stable risk for acquiring new HPV infections throughout life. In this study, the incidence of HPV infection was constant in men aged 18 to 70 years residing in Brazil, Mexico, and the United States. It will be interesting to see how well a vaccine works in men. The report of Giuliano et al notes faster clearance of oncogenic HPV infections in men with increasing age. The more rapid clearance noted in older men might be related to a higher prevalence of HPV antibodies in this population.

J. A. Stockman III, MD

Human Papillomavirus Vaccination of Males: Attitudes and Perceptions of Physicians Who Vaccinate Females
Weiss TW, Zimet GD, Rosenthal SL, et al (Global Health Outcomes, West Point, PA; Indiana Univ School of Medicine, Indianapolis; Columbia Univ Med Ctr, NY; et al)
J Adolesc Health 47:3-11, 2010

Purpose.—We assessed U.S. physicians' attitudes and perceptions regarding potential human papillomavirus (HPV) vaccination of males.

Methods.—We surveyed a random sample of 2,714 pediatricians and family practitioners identified in administrative claims of a U.S. health plan as HPV vaccinators of females; 595 pediatricians and 499 family practitioners participated.

Results.—Most physicians would recommend HPV vaccination to males aged 11—12 (63.9%), 13—18 (93.4%), and 19—26 (92.7%) years. Physicians agreed that males should be vaccinated to prevent them from getting genital and anal warts (52.9% strongly and 36.0% somewhat) and to protect females from cervical cancer (75.3% strongly and 20.8% somewhat). Physicians agreed that an HPV vaccine recommendation for males would increase opportunities to discuss sexual health with adolescent male patients (58.7% strongly, 35.3% somewhat). Most did not strongly agree (15.4% strongly, 45.4% somewhat) that parents of adolescent male patients would be interested in HPV vaccination for males, that a gender-neutral HPV vaccine recommendation would increase acceptance by adolescent females and their parents (19.6% strongly, 42.0% somewhat), or that a gender-neutral recommendation would improve current female vaccination rates (10.4% strongly, 26.0% somewhat).

Conclusions.—Physicians who currently vaccinate females against HPV supported the concept of vaccinating males for its benefits for both sexes. They agreed that a gender-neutral HPV vaccination recommendation would be appropriate with regard to public health and believed that it would increase opportunities for sexual health discussions, but were less sure that such a recommendation would change patient or parental attitudes toward HPV vaccination or improve current HPV vaccination efforts.

▶ It was in 2006 that Merck's human papillomavirus (HPV) vaccine, Guardasil, and the recommendation of the Advisory Committee on Immunization Practices that it routinely be given to girls starting at 11 or 12 years of age set off a flurry of state-level policy making. This vaccine protects against 4 strains of HPV, the most common sexually transmitted infection in the country and the major cause of cervical and oropharyngeal cancer in nontobacco smokers. Legislators in most states in the United States proposed measures intended to increase uptake of the vaccine, including educational campaigns, public subsidies, and insurance-coverage requirements. The most contentious proposals were those to make the vaccine mandatory for girls attending school. Such bills were introduced in 24 states, and 1 state imposed a school mandate by executive order. The backlash against these legislative efforts was quite enormous, and by the end of 2008, policy makers turned decisively away from the idea that the vaccine should be required for school attendance. At the beginning of 2010, only Virginia and Washington, DC, had enacted mandates with Virginia's legislation allowing for an opt-out provision so broad that it might be a misnomer to refer to the law as a mandate. There were lots of reasons for the pushback. Many in the community felt that the vaccine was so new that premarket clinical trials may have missed serious long-term adverse consequences of the vaccine administration. Social conservatives objected to a compulsory policy because they believed that protecting teenagers against sexually transmitted disease might undermine prevention messages that emphasize abstinence. A vocal portion of the community indicated that requiring a girl to be vaccinated at age 11 or 12 years would force parents to have discussions about sex before they or their children were ready. These concerns were not limited to organized advocacy groups that identified themselves as conservative. Another negative for getting the vaccine into the requirement for school admission was the fact that HPV is not contagious through casual contact in the classroom setting. This argument against the vaccine administration became a distinct theme because many in the community believe that the purpose of vaccination mandates is to prevent the spread of contagious disease in schools and that school attendance should not be used as a lever to achieve other public health goals. The latter concerns were reportedly a major driver in the decision of the Virginia legislature to include a liberal opt-out provision in the legislation.

Another factor that soured many policy makers on mandates was consternation over the involvement of the vaccine's manufacturer, Merck, in the policy process. Merck had undertaken a multifaceted marketing campaign to promote the passage of mandate legislation. Representatives of the company met with legislators and hired political consultants to promote the vaccine. Merck provided unrestricted funds to Women in Government, a national organization of female legislators, and many of the bills to require HPV vaccination were introduced by Women in Government members. While Merck's lobbying was a key catalyst in the initial push for mandates, the approach clearly backfired. It did not help that the cost of the vaccine for a full course of 3 doses ran to approximately $320. There were concerns that the cost of the vaccine would consume a large portion of Medicaid budgets and that private insurance rates would have to go up. Added to all these negatives was the fact that the vaccine was introduced at a time when there was a fairly significant antigovernment pushback with respect to governmental intrusion on individual or parental autonomy.

So what does all this have to do with the report of Weiss et al? If it took a long time to get policy makers, parents, and providers on board with the routine administration of the HPV vaccine for girls, just imagine the situation with boys who will never get cervical cancer but who are involved in the cycle of distribution of HPV and who can get oropharyngeal squamous cell carcinoma, penile cancers, genital warts, and cancers of the anus. What Weiss et al have done is to sample almost 3000 pediatricians and family physicians to ask them their opinion about vaccinating boys against HPV. The results of the survey show that more than 90% of this group of physicians who vaccinate females would recommend HPV vaccination to males aged 13 to 18 years and 19 to 26 years. This same group was less likely to recommend HPV vaccination either to males or females aged 9 to 10 years and 11 to 12 years.

This survey did generate strong opinions about a gender-neutral vaccine recommendation and how it might affect acceptance of HPV vaccination by males and/or their parents. Previous surveys of pediatricians identified parent beliefs as a primary barrier to recommending HPV vaccination, and parent concerns have also been raised as an issue by family physicians. Concern was expressed about convincing boys and their parents of the importance of vaccination. Physicians' perceptions of this issue are corroborated by studies showing that parents value direct benefits to their sons over indirect benefits to their son's partners.

This survey of pediatricians and family physicians provides fairly strong evidence that should there be a mandate to vaccinate boys against HPV, it would likely be supported by these care providers. The barrier to get over would be patient and parent attitudes toward HPV vaccination of boys.

J. A. Stockman III, MD

Fever with Thrombocytopenia Associated with a Novel Bunyavirus in China

Yu X-J, Liang M-F, Zhang S-Y, et al (Chinese Ctr for Disease Control and Prevention (Chinese CDC), Beijing, China; Natl Inst for Viral Disease Control and Prevention, Beijing, China; Natl Inst for Communicable Disease Control and Prevention, Beijing, China; et al)

N Engl J Med 364:1523-1532, 2011

Background.—Heightened surveillance of acute febrile illness in China since 2009 has led to the identification of a severe fever with thrombocytopenia syndrome (SFTS) with an unknown cause. Infection with *Anaplasma phagocytophilum* has been suggested as a cause, but the pathogen has not been detected in most patients on laboratory testing.

Methods.—We obtained blood samples from patients with the case definition of SFTS in six provinces in China. The blood samples were used to isolate the causal pathogen by inoculation of cell culture and for detection of viral RNA on polymerase-chainreaction assay. The pathogen was characterized on electron microscopy and nucleic acid sequencing. We used enzyme-linked immunosorbent assay, indirect immunofluorescence assay, and neutralization testing to analyze the level of virus-specific antibody in patients' serum samples.

Results.—We isolated a novel virus, designated SFTS bunyavirus, from patients who presented with fever, thrombocytopenia, leukocytopenia, and multiorgan dysfunction. RNA sequence analysis revealed that the virus was a newly identified member of the genus phlebovirus in the Bunyaviridae family. Electron-microscopical examination revealed virions with the morphologic characteristics of a bunyavirus. The presence of the virus was confirmed in 171 patients with SFTS from six provinces by detection of viral RNA, specific antibodies to the virus in blood, or both. Serologic assays showed a virus-specific immune response in all 35 pairs of serum samples collected from patients during the acute and convalescent phases of the illness.

Conclusions.—A novel phlebovirus was identified in patients with a life-threatening illness associated with fever and thrombocytopenia in China. (Funded by the China Mega-Project for Infectious Diseases and others.)

▶ It is not common in the practice of medicine to see completely new diseases being described with any great frequency. New and emerging infectious diseases, in particular, tend to capture our imagination. One such infectious disease is that caused by a novel bunyavirus, specifically *Anaplasma phagocytophilum*. This disease, with an initial case fatality rate of approximately 30%, was first termed the severe fever with thrombocytopenia syndrome (SFTS), characterized by fever, gastrointestinal symptoms, thrombocytopenia, and leu-kocytopenia. Patients with this syndrome have been documented to have a virus isolatable from their blood designated as SFTS bunyavirus (SFTSV). SFTSV is a novel phlebovirus in the Bunyaviridae family, most closely related to the Uukuniemi virus. The virus now has been documented to be found in patients in a number of different provinces in China. To date there has been no human-to-human transmission. The virus is most likely transmitted by rodents and arthropods.

In an editorial that accompanied this report, Feldmann notes that China has the greatest potential for the emergence or reemergence of infectious diseases worldwide.[1] This is because of its extraordinarily large population and close proximity to wild and domestic animals living in close proximity to humans. In particular, Chinese animal markets are considered unique places for transmis-sion of pathogens from animals to humans. SARS and influenza have been prominent examples.

The bottom line here is that we all should be paying great attention, medici-newise, to diseases that are emerging from China.

J. A. Stockman III, MD

Reference

1. Feldmann H. Truly emerging—a new disease caused by a novel virus. *N Engl J Med.* 2011;364:1561-1563.

Stem-Cell Gene Therapy for the Wiskott–Aldrich Syndrome

Boztug K, Schmidt M, Schwarzer A, et al (Hannover Med School, Germany)
N Engl J Med 363:1918-1927, 2010

The Wiskott–Aldrich syndrome (WAS) is an X-linked recessive primary immunodeficiency disorder associated with thrombocytopenia, eczema, and autoimmunity. We treated two patients who had this disorder with a transfusion of autologous, genetically modified hematopoietic stem cells (HSC). We found sustained expression of WAS protein expression in HSC, lymphoid and myeloid cells, and platelets after gene therapy. T and B cells, natural killer (NK) cells, and monocytes were functionally cor-rected. After treatment, the patients' clinical condition markedly improved, with resolution of hemorrhagic diathesis, eczema, autoimmu-nity, and predisposition to severe infection. Comprehensive insertion-site analysis showed vector integration that targeted multiple genes controlling growth and immunologic responses in a persistently polyclonal hemato-poiesis. (Funded by Deutsche Forschungsgemeinschaft and others; German Clinical Trials Register number, DRKS00000330.)

▶ Although most of us do not see many, if any, patients with the Wiskott-Aldrich syndrome (WAS), we are or should be very familiar with it. WAS is a very complex primary immunodeficiency disorder. Children with this condition have recurrent infections, thrombocytopenia, eczema, and autoimmunity. WAS is caused by mutations in the *WAS* gene. The gene product of WAS is the WAS protein (WASP). WASP is a principal regulator of actin polymerization in hematopoietic cells. The complex biological features of WAS result in dysfunction of T and B cells, disturbed formation of natural killer cell immunologic function, and impaired migratory responses of white blood cells. Patients with severe WAS generally experience an early death from infection or bleeding. As of now, the only cure for the disorder has been allogeneic hematopoietic stem cell transplantation. Unfortunately, this is associated with considerable risk of death or major complications.

Wouldn't it be nice if there were some form of hematopoietic stem cell gene therapy for WAS? Given that WASP expression is restricted to cells of the hematopoietic system, one would think that WAS is a promising candidate for gene therapy approaches. Indeed, this is what the authors of this report have attempted to do. This report summarizes the result of hematopoietic stem cell gene therapy in 2 young boys with WAS. After treatment, the clinical conditions of these patients markedly improved, with resolution of their bleeding problem, eczema, autoimmunity, and predilection for severe infection. The study provides evidence that gene transfer can correct thrombocytopenia in humans, a major cause of death and complications in patients with WAS.

The way this gene therapy was carried out was fairly traditional. The investigators collected autologous CD34$^+$ hematopoietic stem cells by leukapheresis. The cells then were transduced with WAS-expressing retroviral vectors that were created with gibbon ape leukemia virus envelope protein. The cells were then reinfused 4 days later. Before reinfusion of the cells, busulfan was administered at a dose of 4 mg/kg of body weight per day on days 3 and 2 before the procedure. Except for some mild transient myelosuppression and alopecia, there were no significant side effects.

Gene therapy is a tricky business with lots of landmines. Obviously 2 successful cases do not make a series, but the data from this report are really good news for management of this very difficult syndrome.

J. A. Stockman III, MD

Neonatal diagnosis of severe combined immunodeficiency leads to significantly improved survival outcome: the case for newborn screening
Brown L, Xu-Bayford J, Allwood Z, et al (Great Ormond Street Hosp Natl Health Service Trust, London, UK; et al)
Blood 117:3243-3246, 2011

Severe combined immunodeficiency (SCID) carries a poor prognosis without definitive treatment by hematopoietic stem cell transplantation. The outcome for transplantation varies and is dependent on donor status and the condition of the child at the time of transplantation. Diagnosis at birth may allow for better protection of SCID babies from infection and improve transplantation outcome. In this comparative study conducted at the 2 designated SCID transplantation centers in the United Kingdom, we show that SCID babies diagnosed at birth because of a positive family history have a significantly improved outcome compared with the first presenting family member. The overall improved survival of more than 90% is related to a reduced rate of infection and significantly improved transplantation outcome irrespective of donor choice, conditioning regimen used, and underlying genetic diagnosis. Neonatal screening for SCID would significantly improve the outcome in this otherwise potentially devastating condition.

▶ There has been a great deal of interest in recent years concerning the ability to screen for severe combined immunodeficiency (SCID) at birth. It is now possible to do so. Detection of recent thymic emigrants by quantitative polymerase chain reaction of DNA extracted from neonatal dried blood spots can detect all SCID forms regardless of genetic diagnosis. The obvious potential advantage of SCID newborn screening would be to protect infants at the time of birth from respiratory pathogens, including *Pneumocystis jiroveci* and respiratory viruses (however, particularly adenovirus and parainfluenzae) as well as to undertake a transplantation at an earlier age. To date, there have been no formal comparative data to show that newborn diagnosis would improve survival in patients regardless of the type of donor or conditioning regimen for transplantation used.

What Brown et al have done is to perform a retrospective study of outcomes in a cohort of SCID patients who have been diagnosed antenatally or at birth secondary to a diagnosis of SCID in a previous sibling or family member, comparing this with the outcome in the first presenting person in the family. Similar studies were undertaken to verify the value of newborn cystic fibrosis screening by other investigators.

The data from this report show that compared with the presenting sibling, SCID babies diagnosed at birth do in fact have a significantly decreased number of infections, are transplanted earlier, and have a dramatically improved survival outcome after transplantation, regardless of the donor match, conditioning regimen, or SCID type. We have clear evidence from this report supporting newborn screening for SCID.

It has been a long time since the medical and lay community heard the story of David Vetter, a boy with severe combined immunodeficiency (SCID) syndrome, who lived in a protective bubble from his birth in 1971 until his death in 1984. Therapies have been developed since then to restore immune function enabling children with SCID to lead relatively normal lives, yet many children with this disorder are not identified quickly enough to receive such life-saving treatment. In May 2010, the Secretary of the Department of Health and Human Services, Kathleen Sebelius, included SCID in a panel of 30 genetic disorders for which the Department of Health and Human Services recommends states screen all infants at birth. Wisconsin was the first state to undertake such screening back in 2008 and by 2010 had already identified a child with SCID and several others with related immune deficiencies. Tests in the newborn period for SCID costs $5 to $6 per infant or about $400 000 a year, for example, in Wisconsin. Based on data collected by the Children's Hospital of Wisconsin

in Milwaukee, the medical cost of care for a child with SCID who is not identified at birth runs about $1 million compared with $250 000 to $300 000 for
a child who is identified early and who undergoes a transplant. Based on
these estimates, Wisconsin recovered its cost in the first year and a half of
implementation of screening for SCID. Hopefully all states will undertake this
screening for SCID, which is estimated to run between 1 in 50 000 births to
1 in 100 000 births. In the United States, somewhere between 50 and 100
new cases are identified in an average year. To read more about screening for
SCID, see the editorial by Kuehn.[1]

J. A. Stockman III, MD

Reference

1. Kuehn BM. State, federal efforts under way to identify children with "bubble boy syndrome". *JAMA*. 2010;304:1771-1773.

11 Miscellaneous

Errors of Diagnosis in Pediatric Practice: A Multisite Survey

Singh H, Thomas EJ, Wilson L, et al (Baylor College of Medicine, Houston, TX; Univ of Texas Med School at Houston; et al)
Pediatrics 126:70-79, 2010

Objective.—We surveyed pediatricians to elicit their perceptions regarding frequency, contributing factors, and potential system- and provider-based solutions to address diagnostic errors.

Methods.—Academic, community, and trainee pediatricians ($N = 1362$) at 3 tertiary care institutions and 109 affiliated clinics were invited to complete the survey anonymously through an Internet survey administration service between November 2008 and May 2009.

Results.—The overall response rate was 53% ($N = 726$). More than one-half (54%) of respondents reported that they made a diagnostic error at least once or twice per month; this frequency was markedly higher (77%) among trainees. Almost one-half (45%) of respondents reported diagnostic errors that harmed patients at least once or twice per year. Failure to gather information through history, physical examination, or chart review was the most-commonly reported process breakdown, whereas inadequate care coordination and teamwork was the most-commonly reported system factor. Viral illnesses being diagnosed as bacterial illnesses was the most-commonly reported diagnostic error, followed by misdiagnosis of medication side effects, psychiatric disorders, and appendicitis. Physicians ranked access to electronic health records and close follow-up of patients as strategies most likely to be effective in preventing diagnostic errors.

Conclusion.—Pediatricians reported making diagnostic errors relatively frequently, and patient harm from these errors was not uncommon (Table 2).

▶ A little honesty truly goes a long way, and that is what this report is all about. The health services team at Baylor College of Medicine and the Cincinnati Children's Hospital Medical Center designed a survey to solicit information from pediatricians about the frequency with which they make diagnostic errors that may or may not cause harm to patients. The survey recipients included those in academic practice, community-based practice, and residents in training. Of the various types of possible medical errors, errors in diagnosis were ranked fourth in frequency and third in potential for harm. More than

289

TABLE 2.—Ranking of Clinical Activities Respondents Considered to Be Associated With Frequency of Error and Potential for Harm

	n (%)	Average Ranking
Frequency of error		
Medication-related activities, such as prescribing, dispensing, or administering medications	617 (85)	2.06
Prevention-related activities, such as hand-washing, injury prevention/nutrition counseling, or vaccination status	398 (55)	1.11
Monitoring-related activities, such as follow-up data on growth charts or close follow-up monitoring of acutely or chronically ill children	419 (58)	1.01
Evaluation- and diagnosis-related activities, such as history and physical and/or diagnostic tests and consultations	401 (55)	0.99
Surgery- and anesthesia-related activities that occur in operating room	150 (21)	0.36
Nonsurgical procedure-related activities, such as lumbar puncture or venipuncture[a]	91 (13)	0.17
Potential to harm		
Medication-related activities, such as prescribing, dispensing, or administering medications	653 (90)	2.01
Surgery- and anesthesia-related activities that occur in operating room	514 (71)	1.82
Evaluation- and diagnosis-related activities, such as history and physical and/or diagnostic tests and consultations	312 (43)	0.72
Prevention-related activities, such as hand-washing, injury prevention/nutrition counseling, or vaccination status	208 (29)	0.43
Monitoring-related activities, such as follow-up data on growth charts or close follow-up monitoring of acutely or chronically ill children	186 (26)	0.36
Nonsurgical procedure-related activities, such as lumbar puncture or venipuncture[a]	194 (27)	0.35

The n values refer to the number of participants who selected the item and assigned a rank of first, second, or third, and proportions refer to the proportions of participants who selected a particular item and ranked the item first, second, or third.
[a]Errors potentially could include any type of error in procedure performance (eg, wrong patient or wrong technique).

half of those surveyed (54%) reported that they made a diagnostic error at least once or twice per month. Unfortunately, diagnostic errors that led to harm also were not infrequent. Some 45% of survey respondents reported that diagnostic errors had harmed patients at least once or twice per year. The most frequent diagnostic error was viral illness being diagnosed as bacterial illness followed by misdiagnosis of medication side effects, psychiatric disorders, and appendicitis. As often as not, failures in data gathering including history, examination, and chart review and care delays by patients or care givers were the most frequent process breakdowns leading to harm.

This is an important study. It represents the first investigation to assess diagnostic errors in any setting through a comprehensive well-constructed survey instrument. The type of errors mentioned by the responding clinicians was interestingly not of the type reported commonly as part of malpractice suits. Most pediatricians thought that misdiagnosis of viral illnesses as bacterial illnesses was the most common diagnostic error followed by misdiagnosis of medication side effects and psychiatric diseases. None of these 3 overlap with the top diagnostic errors found in malpractice claim files. In malpractice suits, diagnoses of meningitis, pneumonia, testicular torsion, and appendicitis seem to be prevalent.

There were a number of suggestions by those responding to this survey regarding why errors occur and what might be the best solutions to prevent such errors. All ranked electronic medical records as the best system-based solution. Other suggestions included diagnostic decisions support tools and techniques to ensure timely follow-up evaluation of certain patients. A good many pediatricians also thought that diagnostic errors were contributed to by failure of patients or caregivers to seek care in a timely manner. Patient education programs possibly could help with the latter.

When I was in high school and thinking about going into medicine, my physician, a family practitioner, encouraged me to become a subspecialist if I was not going to be comfortable with diagnostic ambiguity. He confessed that only about half the time was he reasonably certain of the diagnosis of any particular patient but also noted that most of the time, diagnostic accuracy really was not that important given the nature of most problems he was seeing. One wonders if this situation has changed all that dramatically. While a resident in training, I was also taught by Professor Lewis Barness that it was always best to achieve a rapid diagnosis; otherwise, the patient might not get better without such a diagnosis. That wisdom has also proven true.

While on the topic of systems-based practice and other variables that contribute to quality of care, a recent report from Philadelphia and Kansas City tells us that children's hospitals vary substantially in their use of antibiotics to a degree unexplained by patient- or hospital-level factors typically associated with the need for antibiotic therapy.[1] Data obtained by investigators showed that 60% of children admitted to a children's hospital received at least one antibiotic agent during their hospitalization, including more than 90% of patients who had surgery, had central venous catheter placement, underwent prolonged ventilation, or remained in hospital for more than 14 days. When adjusting for all confounding variables, a variation in antibiotic use ranged from 38% to 72% of children admitted to hospital. The number of days children received antibiotics ranged from 368 to 601 antibiotic-days per 1000 patient-days. This 100% variation in antibiotic use is not explained by any rational process.

Perhaps this commentary got a bit nostalgic pondering over the way things "used to be." It seems that many practitioners these days long for the way medicine used to be practiced. In fact, there is a fair amount written in the medical literature about nostalgia. The origins of the word "nostalgia" go back a long way. Searching in 1688 for the perfect word to express the strange emotional and mental symptoms seen in Swiss mercenaries fighting far from home, medical student Johannes Hofer decided to make up his own term for this psychological phenomenon. Looking back to Ancient Greece, the birth place of western European medicine, Hofer settled on the term nostalgia, a combination of the words *nosos* (return to the native land) and *algos* (suffering or grief). Nostalgia was literally the pain that came from the intense but unfulfilled desire to go home and for the next 200 years it remained a constant category in medical writings. As seen in the occupational disease of sailors and soldiers, nostalgia could lead to various mental and physical complaints. Those suffering from the condition avoided contact with others, preferring solitude and silence.

A variety of medical symptoms and signs developed including heart palpitations, loss of appetite, constipation, and troubled sleep. In England in the 18th century, nostalgia was considered a psychiatric diagnosis. By the end of the 19th century, however, nostalgia had lost credibility as a disease category. In 1899, *The Lancet* published an opinion piece defending the decision by Royal College of Physicians to exclude nostalgia from its "Nomenclature of Diseases," arguing it was a purely selfish disorder unworthy of medical classification. Today, of course, nostalgia has shed its original medical trappings, moving instead into the world of imagination and the arts. That does not mean that physicians still do not have nostalgia about how the practice of medicine was just a few decades ago. That aside, it is still the best profession on earth. To read more about the historical keyword nostalgia see the writings of Sullivan.[2]

J. A. Stockman III, MD

References

1. Gerber JS, Newland JG, Coffin SE, et al. Variability in antibiotic use at children's hospitals. *Pediatrics*. 2010;126:1067-1073.
2. Sullivan E. Nostalgia. *Lancet*. 2010;376:585.

Epidemiology and aetiology of paediatric malpractice claims in France
Najaf-Zadeh A, Dubos F, Pruvost I, et al (UDSL, France; et al)
Arch Dis Child 96:127-130, 2011

Objective.—To examine paediatric malpractice claims and identify common characteristics likely to result in malpractice in children in France.

Design and Materials.—First, the authors did a retrospective and descriptive analysis of all paediatric malpractice claims involving children aged 1 month to 18 years, in which the defendant was coded as paediatrician or general practitioner, reported to the Sou Médical-groupe MASCF insurance company during a 5-year period (2003—2007). Then, a comparison of these results with those from the USA was performed.

Results.—The average annual incidence of malpractice claims was 0.8/100 paediatricians. 228 malpractice claims were studied and were more frequent (41%) with more severe outcomes in children younger than 2 years of age (52% deaths or major injuries). Meningitis (n=14) and dehydration (n=13) were the leading causes of claims, with highest mortalities (93% and 92%, respectively). The most common alleged misadventures were diagnosis-related error (47%), and medication error (13%). Malignancy was the most common medical condition incorrectly diagnosed (14%).

Conclusions.—Paediatric malpractice claims are less frequent in France than in the USA, but they share many similarities with those in the USA. These data would enhance the knowledge of high-risk areas in paediatric care that could be targeted to reduce the risk of medical malpractices and to improve patient safety.

▶ This interesting report emanates from France. The authors undertook a retrospective review of all pediatric malpractice claims in that country involving children aged 1 month to 18 years in which the defendant was identified to be either a pediatrician or a general practitioner. The average annual incidence of malpractice claims against pediatricians was 0.8 per 100 pediatricians. The top 10 diagnoses resulting in claims along with the mortality rates associated with the claims may be seen in (Tables 1, 2) demonstrates the alleged sources of the malpractice claims. As is true in the United States, the most frequent diagnosis was meningitis when one looks beyond the neonatal age group.

The largest of the published US studies reported to date related to malpractice claims and pediatricians emanates from the Physician Insurers Association of America (PIAA) database. Of the 214 226 closed claims between 1985 and 2005, some 2.97% of them involved pediatricians. Diagnostic errors were the largest cause (31.9%). Medication errors represented 13% in the French series but just 4.7% in the US series.[1] In the United States, the 5 most prevalent diagnostic categories in the PIAA database were brain-damaged infants, meningitis, routine infant or child health check, neonatal respiratory problems, and appendicitis. The French data include neonatal problems. The most common diagnoses included meningitis, dehydration, malignancy, pneumonia, and appendicitis.

Accompanying this French report was a commentary prepared by Marcovitch.[2] Marcovitch reports on the British experience with malpractice claims. Marcovitch has reviewed more than 700 malpractice claims in Great Britain and notes that the most common failings include the following potential issues (in no particular order):

- Failing to communicate adequately with clinicians or other professionals
- Failing to test diagnostic hypotheses and revise them when found wanting
- Inadequate training and screening maneuvers

TABLE 1.—Prevalence and Mortality of the Top 10 Diagnoses Involved in 228 Paediatric Malpractice Claims*

	No	%*	Death (%)
Meningitis	14	7.1	93
Dehydration	13	6.6	92
Malignancy	13	6.6	Nd[†]
Pneumonia	10	5.1	50
Appendicitis	10	5.1	40
Testicular torsion	9	4.6	0
Upper limb trauma	7	3.6	0
Asthma	6	3.0	66
Lower limb trauma	6	3.0	0
Otitis	6	3.0	0

*There was no medical condition identified in 31 claims. The percentage was calculated among the cases where a medical condition was identified.
†Nd, not defined.

TABLE 2.—Alleged Misadventures in 228 Paediatric Malpractice Claims

	No	%
Diagnosis-related error	106	47
Medication error	30	13
No medical error	22	10
Failure to examine	20	9
Failure to respond appropriately	16	7
Treatment related error	11	5
Improper performance of procedure	10	4
Failure to admit to hospital	7	3
Failure to inform patient	3	1
Failure to report child maltreatment	3	1

- Lack of guidance and/or knowledge in handling rare conditions
- Misunderstanding fluid balance
- Inadequate assessment of the neurological state of young children
- Uncertainty about the relevance of vital signs

The Marcovitch commentary is well worth reading because it attempts to get at the origin of many malpractice occurrences. Many of the problems relate to systems errors. An interesting pearl is that in 2003, just 21 pediatric malpractice lawsuits were accepted by the Court of Justice in Japan.[3] The editor of the journal publishing these data added a footnote: "There are very few lawyers in Japan compared with the United States." Enough said?

J. A. Stockman III, MD

References

1. Carroll AE, Buddenbaum JL. Malpractice claims involving pediatricians: epidemiology and etiology. *Pediatrics.* 2007;120:10-17.
2. Marcovitch H. When are paediatricians negligent? *Arch Dis Child.* 2011;96: 117-120.
3. Ehara A. Lawsuits associated with medical malpractice in Japan: rate of lawsuits was very low in pediatrics, although many children visit emergency rooms. *Pediatrics.* 2005;115:1792-1793.

Googling children's health: reliability of medical advice on the internet
Scullard P, Peacock C, Davies P (Nottingham Univ Hosps Trust, UK)
Arch Dis Child 95:580-582, 2010

Aim.—To assess the reliability and accuracy of medical advice, over a range of types of websites, found using the Google search engine, thus simulating a patient's experience.

Design.—Advice was sought for five common paediatric questions using the Google search engine. The first 100 results of each question were classified as either being consistent or inconsistent with current recommendations or as 'no answer given'. Record of the type of site and its visibility was noted.

Results.—39% of the 500 sites searched gave correct information; 11% were incorrect and 49% failed to answer the question. Where an answer was available, 78% of sites gave the correct information. The accuracy of information varied depending on the topic and ranged from 51% (mumps, measles and rubella and autism) to 100% (breast feeding with mastitis/the sleeping position of a baby). Governmental sites gave uniformly accurate advice. News sites gave correct advice in 55% of cases. No sponsored sites were encountered that gave the correct advice.

Implications.—The authors have shown that the advice on the internet is very variable. Patients are known to use the internet for their own research and as such the authors encourage healthcare workers to recommend government or NHS websites.

▶ It is hard to imagine a world without Google. It is also hard to remember a time when there was no Google, but in fact, prior to 1998, there was no Google. Google Corporation was founded in 1998 by 2 Stanford graduates, Larry Page and Sergey Brin, who developed algorithms that allowed astonishingly rapid searches of vast areas of information with a business model that made it pay. It has been noted that Google has grown into a "symbol not just of the growing power of the Internet, but of the global economy's rapid transformation."[1] Current dictionaries allow Google to be both a noun and a verb.

Many in medicine now Google for medical decision making. With very little effort, Googling will get us to a defined end point quickly. Hopefully a clinician will reject any sources that appear unreliable. Unfortunately, parents and patients may not always be so well equipped. Some 99% of Google's income comes from advertising, largely by promotion of favored Web sites on its search engine. We should therefore not necessarily expect it to be the best source for concerned parents to get information. Despite the availability of other medical search engines, the ubiquity of Google means that most parents are likely to visit its search engine first.

What we see in the report of Scullard et al is that a distinct minority of searches on Google will give accurate and correct information. Just over 10% of the information provided was correct and almost half actually failed to answer the question being posed. Government sites uniformly provided current and accurate information.

One of the interesting findings of the Scullard et al report was that the country from which a Google search originates makes a significant difference. A searcher may unwittingly stray onto sites from other countries that give advice inappropriate to their own health care setting. An example is the advice given in African countries on human immunodeficiency virus transmission via breast milk, which is the opposite of that given in the West. Google, for example, can be accessed in the United Kingdom either through Google.com or Google.co.uk, and the results may be quite different.

The inaccuracy of information on Google is quite lamentable, especially since many medical care providers in poorly resourced countries have to rely on such references given the fact that some large publishers have cut access to journals in poor countries to a significant degree. At the beginning of 2011, for example, researchers in Bangladesh, one of the world's poorest countries, received a letter announcing that 4 big publishers would no longer be allowing free access to their 2500 journals through the Health InterNetwork for Access to Research Initiative (HINARI) system. It emerged later that other countries were equally affected. HINARI was born in 2001 following discussions between the World Health Organization and major publishers. HINARI was never a complete answer to the problem of access to journals and information. Countries such as India did not have access because they were considered to be too rich as a lower middle-income country, despite enormous disparity in the distribution of wealth. Nonetheless, HINARI brought about a transformation for institutions that did use it. Around 4800 institutions in 105 countries have had access to some 7000 journals, including all the most prestigious publications. To learn more about the access to medical journals in poor countries, see the editorial of Smith.[2]

J. A. Stockman III, MD

References

1. Horner D, Guyer J, Mann C, et al. *The Children's Health Insurance Program Reauthorization act of 2009: Overview and Summary.* Washington, DC: Georgetown University Health Policy Institute Center for Children and Families; 2009. 1–20.
2. Koehlmoos TP, Smith R. Big publishers cut access to journals in poor countries. *Lancet.* 2011;377:273-276.

Underinsurance among Children in the United States

Kogan MD, Newacheck PW, Blumberg SJ, et al (Maternal and Child Health Bureau, Rockville, MD; Univ of California at San Francisco; Natl Ctr for Health Statistics, Hyattsville, MD)
N Engl J Med 363:841-851, 2010

Background.—Recent interest in policy regarding children's health insurance has focused on expanding coverage. Less attention has been devoted to the question of whether insurance sufficiently meets children's needs.

Methods.—We estimated underinsurance among U.S. children on the basis of data from the 2007 National Survey of Children's Health (sample size, 91,642 children) regarding parents' or guardians' judgments of whether their children's insurance covered needed services and providers and reasonably covered costs. Data on adequacy were combined with data on continuity of insurance coverage to classify children as never insured during the past year, sometimes insured during the past year, continuously insured but inadequately covered (i.e., underinsured), and continuously insured and adequately covered. We examined the association between this classification and five overall indicators of health care access and quality: delayed or forgone care, difficulty obtaining needed care from a specialist, no preventive care, no developmental screening at a preventive visit, and care not meeting the criteria of a medical home.

Results.—We estimated that in 2007, 11 million children were without health insurance for all or part of the year, and 22.7% of children with continuous insurance coverage — 14.1 million children — were underinsured. Older children, Hispanic children, children in fair or poor health, and children with special health care needs were more likely to be underinsured. As compared with children who were continuously and adequately insured, uninsured and underinsured children were more likely to have problems with health care access and quality.

Conclusions.—The number of underinsured children exceeded the number of children without insurance for all or part of the year studied. Access to health care and the quality of health care are suboptimal for uninsured and underinsured children. (Funded by the Health Resources and Services Administration.)

▶ The health care debate that culminated in legislation in early 2010 underscored the issue of insurance status of children in the United States. During the debate, much emphasis was placed on the need to reduce the number of uninsured children. Uninsured children are those who lack insurance and include those with intermittent health insurance (ie, periods without insurance throughout the year). It is well known that children in either category have a significantly greater risk for delayed care, unmet health care needs, a much diminished well-child care, and they lack a usual source of care, including immunizations. What has not received as much attention has been the problem of underinsurance. This is insurance that while in place does not sufficiently meet a child's need. The major problems causing underinsurance are cost-sharing requirements that are too high, benefits that are significantly limited, and inadequate coverage of specific needed services.

What Kogan et al have done is conduct a study that incorporates the multiple dimensions of insurance adequacy as defined by the American Academy of Pediatrics: adequate coverage for needed services, an adequate choice of providers, and reasonable coverage of cost. Kogan et al used information from the 2007 National Survey of Children's Health, a nationally representative study of almost 100 000 children in order to address the extent of underinsurance among those who have been continuously insured in the pediatric population. What they found was that approximately 20% of children with continuous insurance coverage are in fact underinsured (at least in 2007), actually exceeding the number of children without any insurance at all in the same year. Data derived from the study illustrated that the most common reason for underinsurance was that costs not covered by insurance were considered by families to be sometimes or always unreasonable. A smaller proportion of children had health insurance benefits that were felt to be sometimes or never adequate to meet a child's need or that limited a child's ability to see a needed provider. Hispanic and black children were significantly more likely to be under-insured than non-Hispanic white children, and children in the Midwest were more likely to be underinsured than children in the Northeast. Children who had ongoing health care needs and those with special health care needs were also more likely to be underinsured. All underinsured children were much more likely to be without a medical home, to have delayed or for gone care, or to have had difficulty in obtaining a needed specialist's care.

In an editorial that accompanied this report, Perrin notes that the study of Kogan et al did not compare the benefits of public insurance with that of private insurance for children.[1] In fact, families with higher incomes that allow public insurance are likely to have private insurance that is more inadequate than public insurance.

The Affordable Care Act of 2010 may indeed improve access to needed health care services for those with chronic health conditions, including children. Key private insurance reforms, including the removal of provisions imposing lifetime limits or unreasonable limits on annual benefit, the removal of discrim-inatory premium rates, guaranteed availability of coverage, and dependent coverage for young people up to the age of 26 years, may go a long way toward improving coverage in general. Gaps will remain, however, in public insurance coverage even after the institution of safeguards affecting private coverage. The basic Medicaid program, unlike Medicare, includes long-term care benefits, such as care at home and specialized therapies, and it serves as a vital source of financing for nursing home care. The assumption that most children are healthy, however, has led policy makers to limit long-term care and coverage of a number of other benefits for chronic conditions in other programs for chil-dren. The State Children's Health Insurance Program (SCHIP), created in 1997, provides a less generous benefit package and excludes coverage of services for many chronic conditions (eg, respiratory therapy, speech and language services, and home-based services) on the belief that the SCHIP population would not need such benefits. Research conducted since the enactment of SCHIP has shown that substantial numbers of enrolled children have chronic conditions and would in fact benefit from such services.

Thus, it is likely that the pediatric underinsured population will continue to be underserved in the United States, despite the Affordable Care Act. Kogan et al

TABLE.—When the Price is Right

	USA	India
Angioplasty	98 618	11 000
Heart bypass	210 842	10 000
Single heart-valve replacement	274 395	9500
Hip replacement	75 399	9000
Knee replacement	69 991	8500
Gastric bypass	82 646	11 000
Spinal fusion	108 127	5500
Mastectomy	40 832	16 833

Costs of procedures (US$) in the USA (retail rather than insurers' cost) and India, 2006. Source: Subimo (US rates), and PlanetHospital (India rates).

document, and do so very convincingly, evidence that underinsured children face major problems in obtaining both access to care and an appropriate quality of care. Only time will tell whether the Affordable Care Act will make a significant dent in this problem of underinsurance.

This commentary closes with a few facts about the US Healthcare system. Data from the Commonwealth Fund indicates that the United States spent more than $7500 per capita in 2008, greater than twice on average what other countries spent that covered everyone. A third of US citizens have gone without recommended care because of costs (2009). Compare that with the Netherlands (6%) and the United Kingdom (5%), who have performed the best on the measure of meeting recommended preventative care.[2] Interestingly, we are also seeing a fair amount of medical tourism on the part of US citizens leaving the country to find cheaper healthcare for elective procedures. The Table comes from an editorial on this topic that recently appeared in *The Lancet*.[3]

J. A. Stockman III, MD

References

1. Perrin JM. Treating underinsurance. *N Engl J Med.* 2010;363:881-883.
2. Roehr D. US healthcare continues to lag behind other countries despite double the cost. *BMJ.* 2010;341:c6628.
3. Shetty P. Medical tourism booms in India, but at what cost? *Lancet.* 2010;376: 671-672.

Pediatric Emergency Department Use by Adults With Chronic Pediatric Disorders

McDonnell WM, Kocolas I, Roosevelt GE, et al (Univ of Utah, Salt Lake City; Univ of Colorado, Denver)
Arch Pediatr Adolesc Med 164:572-576, 2010

Objective.—To describe pediatric emergency department use by adults with chronic pediatric disorders, known as transition patients.

Design.—Retrospective descriptive study.

Setting.—The pediatric emergency department of a tertiary care pediatric hospital during calendar year 2005.

Participants.—All patients presenting to the pediatric emergency department during the study period.

Main Outcome Measures.—Association of presenting complaint with the patient's chronic pediatric disorder, emergency department interventions and dispositions, and duration of inpatient admissions.

Results.—Patient encounters totaled 43 621, with 445 (1%) involving adult patients. Transition patients accounted for 197 (44%) of the adult encounters. Eighty-nine transition patient encounters (45%) were for complaints unrelated to the patients' chronic pediatric disorders. Only 14 (7%) transition patient visits did not involve diagnostic studies or procedures. Transition patients were 2.1 times (95% confidence interval,

1.8-2.5; $P < .001$) more likely to require admission than pediatric patients and were 4.5 times (95% confidence interval, 3.3-6.1; $P < .001$) more likely to require intensive care. Median length of stay for admitted transition patients was 4 days (range, 1-35 days) compared with 2 days (range, 1-80 days) for pediatric patients ($P < .001$).

Conclusions.—A substantial number of adult patients with chronic pediatric disorders use the pediatric emergency department and often present with complaints unrelated to their pediatric conditions. They have high rates of hospital and intensive care unit admissions. Pediatric hospitals should be prepared with adequate resources and training to deal with these complex adult patients.

▶ It is quite amazing how much we are hearing about difficulties with transition of patients from pediatric care providers to adult care providers. McDonnell et al describe the problem adult survivors of serious chronic pediatric disorders have as they continue on throughout their lifespan transitioning to care that should be given by those trained in the care of adults. No one will argue that there are barriers to such transition. These barriers include lack of funding for transition services, poor access to trained adult health care providers, lack of clinical guidelines, and deficiencies in coordination and communication between health care providers and various agencies, particularly for youth with special care needs. Part of the problem is also based on the fact that adult survivors of severe chronic childhood illnesses and disabilities are a relatively new population, and society has not quite figured out what to do with these individuals now living in the community at large. Children can rely on their parents, but parents are not around forever.

Compounding the problem is that few residency training programs in family medicine or internal medicine have curricula focused on this transitional age population. There are very few faculty members in these training programs with experience in this area. There are some comprehensive transition programs in the United States, however, in which pediatric- and adult-oriented clinicians comanage patients as a team, such as the Jacksonville Health and Transition Services Clinic, the Center for Youth and Adults with Conditions of Childhood at Indiana University, and the Gillette Lifetime Specialty Healthcare Clinic, St. Paul, Minnesota. Unfortunately, these comprehensive transition programs are few and far between, and no one has figured out how to replicate them in the average community or even in large communities.

Given the successes that are seen in pediatrics, it is no surprise that given the problems of transition to adult care providers, as many as 4% of emergency room (ER) visits in departments of pediatrics relate to the care of transitional age and young adult patients. Fortunately, pediatric emergency medicine training and certification has evolved such that these patients are receiving care, albeit expensive care, in an adequate although not ideal environment. There have to be better ways to manage the solutions to this problem other than by visits to the ER.

J. A. Stockman III, MD

Clinical assessment incorporating a personal genome

Ashley EA, Butte AJ, Wheeler MT, et al (Stanford Univ School of Medicine, CA; et al)
Lancet 375:1525-1535, 2010

Background.—The cost of genomic information has fallen steeply, but the clinical translation of genetic risk estimates remains unclear. We aimed to undertake an integrated analysis of a complete human genome in a clinical context.

Methods.—We assessed a patient with a family history of vascular disease and early sudden death. Clinical assessment included analysis of this patient's full genome sequence, risk prediction for coronary artery disease, screening for causes of sudden cardiac death, and genetic counselling. Genetic analysis included the development of novel methods for the integration of whole genome and clinical risk. Disease and risk analysis focused on prediction of genetic risk of variants associated with mendelian disease, recognised drug responses, and pathogenicity for novel variants. We queried disease-specific mutation databases and pharmacogenomics databases to identify genes and mutations with known associations with disease and drug response. We estimated post-test probabilities of disease by applying likelihood ratios derived from integration of multiple common variants to age-appropriate and sex-appropriate pre-test probabilities. We also accounted for gene-environment interactions and conditionally dependent risks.

Findings.—Analysis of 2·6 million single nucleotide polymorphisms and 752 copy number variations showed increased genetic risk for myocardial infarction, type 2 diabetes, and some cancers. We discovered rare variants in three genes that are clinically associated with sudden cardiac death— *TMEM43*, *DSP*, and *MYBPC3*. A variant in *LPA* was consistent with a family history of coronary artery disease. The patient had a heterozygous null mutation in *CYP2C19* suggesting probable clopidogrel resistance, several variants associated with a positive response to lipid-lowering therapy, and variants in *CYP4F2* and *VKORC1* that suggest he might have a low initial dosing requirement for warfarin. Many variants of uncertain importance were reported.

Interpretation.—Although challenges remain, our results suggest that whole-genome sequencing can yield useful and clinically relevant information for individual patients.

▶ While this report deals with a 40-year-old man, the findings are equally applicable to any pediatric-age patient. The study documents the power of studying the personal genome of an individual. The specific patient was a 40-year-old man who presented with a family history of coronary artery disease and sudden death. His medical history was not clinically significant, and the patient exercised regularly without symptoms. He was taking no prescribed medications and appeared well. Clinical characteristics were within normal limits. Electrocardiography was completely normal as was an echocardiogram. A 4-generation family pedigree (Fig 2) showed atherosclerotic vascular disease with several manifestations and prominent osteoarthritis. The patient's first cousin once removed died suddenly of an unknown cause. A first cousin had a diagnosis of arrhythmogenic right ventricular dysplasia or cardiomyopathy. Elsewhere, the family history showed a prominent background of vascular disease, including aortic aneurysm and coronary artery disease. As part of this 40-year-old's overall assessment, he was offered genetic counseling during which a discussion was entertained about the possibility that one could include personal genome assessment in addition to a clinical assessment to potentially uncover any significant risks of heart disease, recognizing that for some of these there was no treatment. The patient was also told that information regarding a whole host of noncardiac-related disorders might be uncovered by studying his personal genome. Also discussed was the possibility of discrimination on the basis of the genetic findings. The patient agreed to have his entire genome examined.

So what did this fella's personal genome analysis uncover? According to standard adult treatment clinical guidelines, this patient does not currently have major risk factors for coronary artery disease and would need a low-density lipoprotein concentration higher than 4.9 mmol/L to qualify for lipid-lowering therapy. However, with the genome study, it was found that he was borderline for 3 major risk factors related to the development of coronary artery disease, and it seemed wise to offer him, even at age 40 years, a lipid-lowering drug. The genome study predicted a likelihood of benefit for the use of statins,

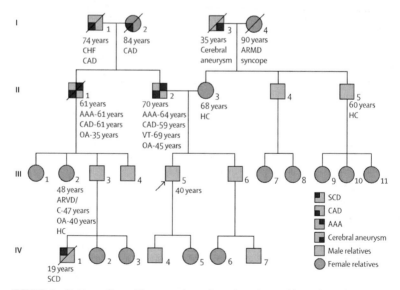

FIGURE 2.—Patient pedigree. The arrow shows the patient. Diagonal lines show relatives who are deceased. Years are age at death or diagnosis. AAA=abdominal aortic aneurysm. ARMD=age-related macular degeneration. ARVD/C=arrhythmogenic rightventricular dysplasia or cardiomyopathy. CAD=coronary artery disease. CHF=congestive heart failure. HC=hypercholesterolaemia. OA=osteoarthritis. SCD=sudden cardiac death (presumed). VT=paroxysmal ventricular tachycardia. (Reprinted from Ashley EA, Butte AJ, Wheeler MT, et al. Clinical assessment incorporating a personal genome. *Lancet.* 2010;375:1525-1535. © 2010, with permission from Elsevier.)

and one aspect of the genome study documented a reduced risk of any adverse effect of statins on skeletal muscle. The genome study also indicated that if future medical therapy was needed with clopidogrel, the drug dosing for this would have to be increased because the gene study showed that this individual would have resistance to this particular drug. At the same time, should this patient ever require warfarin, his genotype suggests that he should take a reduced initial dose of warfarin because he would be very warfarin sensitive. As an aside, the gene study showed that this individual was at risk for having hemachromatosis and that he should be studied for this.

So what is the bottom line here? The bottom line is that this report demonstrates how one can integrate in real time, in a clinical setting, data from analysis of the entire human genome of a specific individual at clinical risk for certain forms of disease. On a June day just over 10 years ago, the leaders of the United States and the United Kingdom, accompanied by the leaders of the public and private teams deciphering the human genome, announced that a draft sequence had been completed. That occasion was rich with promises of new and more powerful ways to understand, diagnose, prevent, and treat disease. There was a cautionary note, suggesting that the full potential of DNA-based transformation of medicine would be realized only over the course of several decades. Indeed, after the first decade only a handful of major changes in patient management have taken place. There have been some gene-specific treatments for a few cancers, some novel therapies for a few Mendelian traits, and some strong genetic markers for assessing drug responsiveness, risk of disease, or risk of disease progression. These findings have entered routine medical practice. As slow as this evolution has been, there is likely to be an acceleration of the incorporation of personal genome knowledge into clinical practice as evidenced by the report of Ashley et al. All of us should learn more about genomic medicine. Readers are referred to the series of articles that relate to this topic in the *New England Journal of Medicine* in 2010.[1] Physicians have practiced personalized medicine since time immemorial, using information about a patient's lifestyle, family history, and environment to inform decisions. Nonetheless, we know that this approach is far from perfect—even for evidence-based medicine, we need to treat many individuals for years to prevent 1 event. Because much of the interindividual variation in disease susceptibility, or therapeutic response, is believed to be genetically determined, only through further application of personalized genomic medicine can we make additional strides. We do know that certain rare mutations in the *BRCA* genes will affect one's breast cancer risk. We do know that one's genes affect the metabolism of a wide variety of medications, including anticoagulants, antiplatelet agents, and lipid-lowering drugs. The first human genome sequence cost approximately $2.7 billion (US). Now with next-generation rapidly sequencing technology, a complete human genome can be sequenced for less than $10 000.00, and in the foreseeable future, this cost is likely to reach as low as $1000.00.[2] The report of Ashley et al stands out as an illustration of the potential that this rapid sequencing technology can have for personalized medicine.

This commentary closes with a quiz question, a clinical curio: What edible has more than twice the number of genes as the human? The next time you crunch down on a crisp apple, consider this: each cell in each bite is packed with 57 000 nuclear genes—more than double the number in humans or a cucumber genome and the highest total gene count to date for any plant. This is because about 40 million years ago, the genome of the apple's ancestor underwent duplication. That is common enough, but more unusually, the apple never lost its extra copies over the years. The genome of the Golden Delicious apple has now been published. Our domesticated apple's closest wild relative is from a species called *Malus sieversii* that was birthed in Central Asia millions of years ago.[3]

J. A. Stockman III, MD

References

1. Feero WG, Guttmacher AE, Collins FS. Genomic medicine—an updated primer. *N Engl J Med.* 2010;362:2001-2011.
2. Waldman M. James Watson's genome sequenced at high speed. *Nature.* 2008;452: 788.
3. Editorial comment. Chock-full of genes. *Science.* September 3, 2010:1131.

Which Pediatricians Are Providing Care to America's Children? An Update on the Trends and Changes During the Past 26 Years

Freed GL, The Research Advisory Committee of the American Board of Pediatrics (Univ of Michigan Health System, Ann Arbor)
J Pediatr 157:148-152, 2010

Objective.—To determine the current proportion of pediatric primary care and specialty visits being conducted by pediatricians versus other providers.

Study Design.—We used data from 1980–2006 National Ambulatory Medical Care Surveys (NAMCS) to examine trends in office visits by patients 0 to 17 years of age. During our years of interest, the total number of visits in NAMCS by children ranged from 2597 to 9220 per year.

Results.—Overall, the percentage of all nonsurgical physician office visits for children 0 to 17 years of age made to general pediatricians increased from 61% in 1996 to 71% in 2006 and those to nonpediatric generalists fell from 28% to 22%. The greatest changes between 2000 and 2006 occurred in the adolescent age group where the proportion of visits to general pediatricians increased from 38% to 53%.

Conclusions.—Pediatricians continue to provide most primary care visits for children in the United States. For the first time, pediatricians now provide most visits for adolescents (Fig 1).

▶ Several years ago, this research group from the Division of General Pediatrics at the University of Michigan Health System reported data on what type of physicians were providing health care to American children.[1] They used information at that time from the National Ambulatory Medical Care Surveys (NAMCS), a survey conducted by the National Center for Health Statistics of the Centers for Disease Control and Prevention. What we see in this report is an update

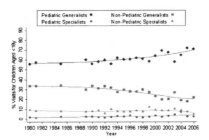

FIGURE 1.—Distribution of visits for children 1 to 17 years of age (all) from 1980–2006, by pediatric generalists, pediatric specialists, nonpediatric generalists, and nonpediatric specialists as published by the National Ambulatory Medical Care Survey. (Reprinted from Journal of Pediatrics, Freed GL, The Research Advisory Committee of the American Board of Pediatrics. Which pediatricians are providing care to America's children? An update on the trends and changes during the past 26 years. *J Pediatr.* 2010;157:148-152. Copyright 2010 with permission from Elsevier.)

showing the trend differences over more than half a decade on who is providing care to American children. NAMCS uses a multistage probability design that includes stratified samples of primary sampling units, physician practices within primary sampling units, and patient visits within practices. Tens of thousands of visits are reported annually as part of NAMCS, allowing profiles of the practices of general and family medicine, osteopathy, internal medicine, pediatrics, general surgery, obstetrics/gynecology, orthopedic surgery, cardiovascular diseases (medical and surgical), dermatology, urology, psychiatry, neurology, ophthalmology, otolaryngology, and a smattering of virtually all other specialty areas.

What we learn from Freed et al is that the trend continues for children (aged 0-17 years) to be seen more and more by pediatricians and less and less by other medical care providers. The percentage of overall visits for children 0 to 17 years provided by general pediatricians rose from 61% in 1996 to 71% in 2006. The percentage of visits to nonpediatric generalists fell from 28% to 22%. If one analyzes the data more closely, one sees some interesting additional trends. While historically most newborn, infant, toddler, and early school age care has been provided by pediatricians, most teens have been seen by family physicians and general medical doctors. The current NAMCS data, however, show that between 2000 and 2006, the provision of care to adolescents by pediatricians increased from 38% to well over 50%.

So what does all this mean? It means that pediatricians are increasingly busy providing care to the full range age spectrum of children, adolescents, and young adults. Importantly, pediatricians and family physicians practice somewhat differently (not meant in a negative way): immunization rates are different; preventive medicine strategies are different; rates of introduction of new therapeutic concepts are different; and referral patterns to pediatric subspecialists and surgical subspecialists are different. In some instances, this does not affect the care of children; in other instances it does.

Some national health care leaders have suggested that the primary care provided by general internal medicine PCPs and pediatricians might better be delivered by family physicians who care for entire families. The data from Freed et al suggest, for whatever reasons, that families are choosing pediatricians for their children's care, even if it means they must have different doctors for different purposes within their family.

Generally speaking, in the United States, we have adequate supplies of primary care pediatricians, albeit with significant discrepancies in rural versus urban distribution. If you think the latter problem is difficult, please see the situation in Canada, where under universal health insurance, access to care by pediatricians in rural areas is truly problematic.[2]

This commentary closes with a query: what is the average monthly income of a general practitioner (GP) in Portugal? The answer is that many Portuguese GPs earn little more than GP trainees. Newly qualified GPs in Portugal earn just 18 Euros more a month than they did during training (€1853/$2580 per month). Only physicians who choose "preferential placements" to areas with shortages of doctors earn an extra "training scholarship" that brings their monthly earnings up a tad.[3]

J. A. Stockman III, MD

References

1. Freed GL, Nahra TA, Wheeler JR. Which physicians are providing healthcare to America's children? Trends and changes during the past 20 years. *Arch Pediatr Adolesc Med.* 2004;158:22-26.
2. Guttmann A, Shipman SA, Lam K, Goodman DC, Stukel TA. Primary care physician supply in children's healthcare use, access and outcomes: findings from Canada. *Pediatrics.* 2010;125:1119-1126.
3. Editorial comment. Many Portuguese GPs earn little more than trainees. *BMJ.* 2010;341:c6334.

Geographic Maldistribution of Primary Care for Children
Shipman SA, Lan J, Chang C-H, et al (Dartmouth Inst for Health Policy and Clinical Practice, Lebanon, NH)
Pediatrics 127:19-27, 2011

Objectives.—This study examines growth in the primary care physician workforce for children and examines the geographic distribution of the workforce.

Methods.—National data were used to calculate the local per-capita supply of clinically active general pediatricians and family physicians, measured at the level of primary care service areas.

Results.—Between 1996 and 2006, the general pediatrician and family physician workforces expanded by 51% and 35%, respectively, whereas the child population increased by only 9%. The 2006 per-capita supply varied by >600% across local primary care markets. Nearly 15 million children (20% of the US child population) lived in local markets with <710 children per child physician (average of 141 child physicians per 100 000 children), whereas another 15 million lived in areas with >4400 children per child physician (average of 22 child physicians per 100 000 children). In addition, almost 1 million children lived in areas with no local child physician. Nearly all 50 states had evidence of similar extremes of physician maldistribution.

Conclusions.—Undirected growth of the aggregate child physician workforce has resulted in profound maldistribution of physician resources. Accountability for public funding of physician training should include efforts to develop, to use, and to evaluate policies aimed at reducing disparities in geographic access to primary care physicians for children.

▶ Whether the United States has an adequate workforce to provide the necessary care for children has been a subject of some significant debate. Shipman et al add useful information to help address this issue. Using data from the National Ambulatory Medical Care Survey and the American Medical Association Physician Masterfile, these investigators were able to map out the distribution of general pediatricians and family physicians by their demographic characteristics. Pediatricians older than 65 years and those with a subspecialty background were excluded. Data from this report show that in 2006 there were 30 981 general pediatricians and 83 081 family physicians in the United States. These values represented a 51% and 35% increase, respectively, in the overall supplies compared with those of 1996. During that same period, the overall child population (younger than 18 years) increased by 9%. With the inclusion of general pediatricians and family physicians (discounting the proportion of their time spent caring for adults), there were 70.4 child physicians per 100 000 children or 1420 children per practicing child physician in the United States in 2006. Of 6542 primary care service areas (PCSAs), 15% had no child physician provider. At the other end of the spectrum, 10% of PCSAs had extraordinarily high supplies of child physician providers, with ≥1 full-time equivalent-adjusted child physician provider for every 661 children. From the standpoint of the overall population, 20% of children living in areas with the highest supplies had an average of 141 child physician providers per 100 000 children (< 710 children per child physician), whereas another 20% lived in areas where there was an average of 22 physician providers per 100 000 children (> 4400 children per child physician). In addition, more than 950 000 children in 47 states lived in regions without any primary care physician provider at all.

Needless to say, the database is used to provide only crude estimates on which to make decisions about workforce supply and demand. Despite this disclaimer, it is fair to say that it is likely that overall the workforce for provision of care to children in the United States is adequate but with the significant problem, a very significant problem, of maldistribution with many undersupplied regions existing, particularly in certain areas such as the deep south, Mississippi being a notable example, ranking number 49 in the country in terms of workforce supply of physician child care providers.

Please note that none of these data apply to the adequacy of the subspecialty workforce in pediatrics. Clearly there have been significant shortages in pediatric subspecialists in a number of disciplines. This is an issue that, hopefully, our free market system will gradually address.

If you think things are bad in the United States with its overall workforce, look to the situation in China. China clearly lacks pediatricians. That country is facing a shortage of 200000 pediatricians after 12 years of insufficient training. Lack of investment and forward planning has led to a major shortfall in children's medical services that hopefully is being addressed in China's next five-year plan.[1]

J. A. Stockman III, MD

Reference

1. Editorial comment. China lacks pediatricians. *Lancet.* 2011;377:322.

Primary Care Pediatricians' Satisfaction with Subspecialty Care, Perceived Supply, and Barriers to Care

Pletcher BA, Rimsza ME, Cull WL, et al (UMDNJ — New Jersey Med School, Newark; Univ of Arizona, Tucson; American Academy of Pediatrics, Elk Grove Village, IL; et al)

J Pediatr 156:1011-1015, 2010

Objectives.—To compare satisfaction with specialty care by primary care pediatricians (PCPs), perceived barriers to care, and adequacy of specialist supply.

Study Design.—A survey of U.S. pediatricians was conducted in 2007. PCPs were asked about satisfaction with specialty care for their patients, as well as supply of specific pediatric subspecialists. Responses of rural and nonrural PCPs were compared regarding 10 potential barriers to care.

Results.—Most PCPs are satisfied with the quality of subspecialty care. However, they were not satisfied with wait times for appointments, and the availability of many pediatric medical subspecialties and several pediatric surgical specialties. Rural PCPs were significantly more likely to report these shortages compared with nonrural pediatricians; these included 9 of the 18 medical and 5 of the 7 surgical specialties. In addition to wait times for appointments, PCPs reported that subspecialists' nonparticipation in health insurance plans and lack of acceptance of uninsured patients were also barriers to obtaining subspecialty care for their patients.

Conclusions.—PCPs provide valuable insight into access to the pediatric subspecialty workforce. This survey of PCPs raises significant concerns about the adequacy of children's access to pediatric subspecialists, especially in rural communities (Tables 2-4).

▶ The American Academy of Pediatrics (AAP) Periodic Survey of Fellows is a powerful tool to provide all in our profession with information across a wide variety of topics. This Periodic Survey is a cross-sectional survey of non-retired US members of the AAP. Periodic Survey 67 from 2007 was used to collect information on the experiences of primary care physicians (PCPs) with subspecialty referrals. Participants in the survey were asked a series of questions regarding satisfaction with subspecialty care provided, availability of subspecialists, and perceived barriers to subspecialty care.

TABLE 2.—Percent of Primary Care Pediatricians Reporting Too Few Medical Subspecialists to Meet the Needs of Patients in Their Practice by Medical Subspecialty Type and Practice Location

Medical Specialty	Total (n = 590)	Non-Rural (n = 514)	Rural (n = 76)
Child/adolescent psychiatry	95.8	95.1	100.0*
Developmental-behavioral pediatrics	86.6	85.9	92.0
Pediatric dermatology	81.6	80.5	89.3
Pediatric rheumatology	68.2	67.3	74.0
Pediatric neurology	66.7	66.1	70.7
Adolescent health	64.2	64.2	64.9
Pediatric endocrinology	58.8	57.2	69.3*
Pediatric gastroenterology	54.5	53.8	59.2
Pediatric emergency medicine	49.2	46.4	68.4*
Pediatric nephrology	48.1	46.2	61.3*
Pediatric genetics	45.1	45.1	44.7
Pediatric pulmonology	41.7	40.2	52.0*
Pediatric infectious disease	36.1	34.4	47.4*
Pediatric allergy and immunology	33.0	31.8	41.3
Pediatric intensive care	23.9	21.7	38.2*
Pediatric hematology and oncology	20.8	19.5	28.9
Pediatric cardiology	17.3	15.9	26.3*
Neonatology	5.5	4.3	13.2*

*Difference between pediatricians from rural and non-rural areas significant at *P* < .05.

TABLE 3.—Percent of Primary Care Pediatricians Reporting Too Few Surgical Subspecialists to Meet the Needs of Patients in Their Practice by Surgical Subspecialty Type and Practice Location

Surgical Specialty	Total (n = 590)	Non-Rural (n = 514)	Rural (n = 76)
Pediatric orthopedics	54.6	52.3	70.7*
Pediatric neurosurgery	49.4	47.9	59.2
Pediatric urology	46.6	44.7	59.2*
Pediatric ophthalmology	42.2	38.5	67.6*
Pediatric otolaryngology	37.9	35.1	55.3*
Pediatric heart surgery	37.2	35.3	50.0*
Pediatric surgery	34.7	33.4	43.4

*Difference between pediatricians from rural and non-rural areas significant at *P* < .05.

The data from the Periodic Survey regarding access to subspecialty care by PCPs were quite interesting. About three-quarters of nonrural PCPs were moderately or completely satisfied with the referral processes for subspecialty care, but just 54% of rural pediatricians rated satisfaction this way. A major concern was waiting times. Sixty-eight percent of rural PCPs and 49% of nonrural PCPs were dissatisfied with waiting times for appointments. More than 65% of rural and only 19% of nonrural PCPs rated the number of subspecialists in their area as poor or fair. It was clear that certain subspecialties appeared to have significant shortages, at least in terms of referral access. A shortage of child/adolescent psychiatrists was reported by 95.8% of all PCPs, and

TABLE 4.—Barriers to Getting Needed Pediatric Subspecialty Care (% Reporting a Moderate or Significant Barrier for Their Patients)

Barrier	Total (n = 586)	Non-Rural (n = 511)	Rural (n = 75)
Long waiting times for appointments	62.4	60.0	79.7*
Subspecialists' nonparticipation in patient's health insurance plan	41.0	39.4	52.1*
Subspecialists not accepting uninsured patients	39.6	38.7	44.0
Length of travel time to subspecialists' office	36.5	29.2	82.7*
Lack of appropriate pediatric subspecialists	33.8	30.6	56.8*
Lack of timely feedback from subspecialists	23.4	22.7	28.0
Inadequate feedback from subspecialists	20.0	19.2	26.7
Subspecialists' lack of adequate resources for effective communication with patients/ parents with limited English proficiency	14.9	13.4	23.0*
Unwillingness of subspecialists to share care	9.0	8.8	9.5
Poor quality of subspecialist's care	3.9	3.3	6.8

*Difference between pediatricians from rural and non-rural areas significant at $P < .05$.

a shortage of neonatologists was reported only by 5.5% of PCPs. Over 80% of PCPs commented on a perceived shortage of developmental-behavioral pediatricians, 81.6% of PCPs indicated pediatric dermatologists were in short supply, 68.2% with respect to pediatric dermatologists, 66.7% with respect to pediatric neurologists, and 64.2% with respect to adolescent health specialists. Table 2 shows the percentage of primary care pediatricians reporting to few medical subspecialists, and Table 3 illustrates the percentage of primary care pediatricians reporting too few surgical subspecialists.

The barriers to getting needed subspecialty care varied significantly by rural and nonrural environments. Clearly the rural PCP experienced longer waiting times for appointments, and significantly fewer numbers of subspecialists were able to participate in their patient's health care plan. Presumably the latter relates to long distances, sometimes out of local geography for patients to be seen by a subspecialist. Table 4 illustrates the barriers to getting needed subspecialty care as perceived by PCPs.

Clearly we need more of certain types of pediatric subspecialists. Fortunately, the number of subspecialty first-year fellows has more than doubled over the last decade, and perhaps we will be seeing more of these individuals leaving the pipeline going into practice soon. Most subspecialists practice within academic environments. This is entirely appropriate, since for most subspecialties, the actual volume of referrals is fairly modest given the rare nature of many subspecialty diseases. This requires subspecialists to aggregate together in academic settings. This is not necessarily true of certain subspecialties such as developmental-behavioral pediatrics and child/adolescent psychiatry where sufficient numbers of patients exist in virtually any moderate-sized community.

The barriers to access cannot be handled with a single brushstroke in terms of solution. Pediatric workforce shortages at the subspecialty level are a complex issue. People, for example, do not go into child/adolescent psychiatry for many reasons, a predominant one being failure of reimbursement in our current payment system.

J. A. Stockman III, MD

Pediatric Nurse Practitioners in the United States: Current Distribution and Recent Trends in Training

Freed GL, for the Research Advisory Committee of the American Board of Pediatrics (Univ of Michigan, Ann Arbor)

J Pediatr 157:589-593, 2010

Objective.—To assess the current distribution and training patterns of pediatric nurse practitioners (PNPs).

Study Design.—Secondary data analysis from the National Association of Pediatric Nurse Practitioners and the 2008 US Census Bureau were used to estimate the distribution of PNPs per 100 000 children. Data on nurse practitioner (NP) graduation and specialty education programs were obtained from the American Association of Colleges of Nursing.

Results.—PNPs have the greatest concentration in the New England and mid-Atlantic regions and a narrow band of Midwestern states. States that allow PNPs to practice or prescribe independently do not consistently have a higher density of PNPs per child population. There has been a slight decrease in the proportion of programs that offer PNP training. In the last decade, the proportion of NP graduates pursuing family nurse practitioner education has increased, and the proportion pursuing PNP education has decreased.

Conclusion.—Workforce planning for the health care of children will require improved methods of assessment of the role of PNPs and the volume of care they provide. Increased use of PNPs in pediatrics will likely require greater effort at recruitment of NPs into the PNP specialty (Figs 1 and 4).

▶ This is an important report providing useful information about recent trends in the United States with respect to the numbers of pediatric nurse practitioners and where such practitioners are located. A report from the American Nurses Credentialing Center (ANCC) that looked at 390 pediatric nurse practitioners currently certified by the ANCC indicated that 76% of such certified pediatric nurse practitioners were employed in areas with more than 50 000 residents, but only 3% were actually practicing in rural areas as defined by less than 2500 residents.[1] The same study showed that 38% of the pediatric nurse practitioners indicated that they were in private practice groups, 26% in outpatient hospital-based practice, 21% in inpatient, 19% in a community/public health agency or rural clinic, and 10% in school/college health. Unfortunately, data from the ANCC are somewhat limited given that most pediatric nurse practitioners are certified by the Pediatric Nursing Certification Board.

One of the most interesting aspects of the report by Freed et al is that the distribution of pediatric nurse practitioners (per 100 000 children) does not

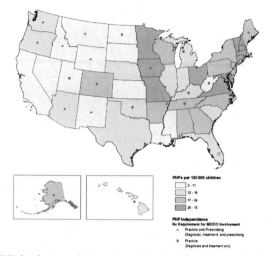

FIGURE 1.—PNP distribution and independence. (Reprinted from Journal of Pediatrics, Freed GL, for the Research Advisory Committee of the American Board of Pediatrics. Pediatric nurse practitioners in the United States: current distribution and recent trends in training. *J Pediatr.* 2010;157:589-593. Copyright 2010 with permission from Elsevier.)

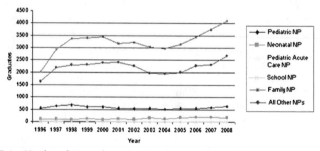

FIGURE 4.—Number of NP graduates by clinical track, 1996 to 2008. (Reprinted from Journal of Pediatrics, Freed GL, for the Research Advisory Committee of the American Board of Pediatrics. Pediatric nurse practitioners in the United States: current distribution and recent trends in training. *J Pediatr.* 2010;157:589-593. Copyright 2010 with permission from Elsevier.)

vary by state on the basis of practice regulation. For example, states that allow more independence in practice for nurse practitioners, reducing prescription and practice barriers, do not necessarily eliminate all impediments for nurse practitioner practice opportunities. States that have populations that could well be served by pediatric nurse practitioners do not seem to have an advantage by having less restrictive regulations in terms of nurse practitioner roles.

In an editorial that accompanied the report of Freed et al, Loman and Clinton comment that medicine and nursing must continue to work together to meet the challenges for optimal health care for children.[2] We need to track in much more detailed data regarding pediatric nurse practitioners and family nurse practitioners, where they practice and how they practice.

J. A. Stockman III, MD

References

1. American Nurses Credentialing Center. *2008 Role Delineation Study: Pediatric Nurse Practitioner—National Results.* Silver Spring, MD: ANCC; 2009.
2. Loman DG, Clinton P. Where are all the PNPs? Pediatric nurse practitioner practice opportunities and challenges. *J Pediatr.* 2010;157:526-527.

The Social Mission of Medical Education: Ranking the Schools
Mullan F, Chen C, Petterson S, et al (George Washington Univ, DC)
Ann Intern Med 152:804-811, 2010

Background.—The basic purpose of medical schools is to educate physicians to care for the national population. Fulfilling this goal requires an adequate number of primary care physicians, adequate distribution of physicians to underserved areas, and a sufficient number of minority physicians in the workforce.

Objective.—To develop a metric called the social mission score to evaluate medical school output in these 3 dimensions.

Design.—Secondary analysis of data from the American Medical Association (AMA) Physician Masterfile and of data on race and ethnicity in medical schools from the Association of American Medical Colleges and the Association of American Colleges of Osteopathic Medicine.

Setting.—U.S. medical schools.

Participants.—60 043 physicians in active practice who graduated from medical school between 1999 and 2001.

Measurements.—The percentage of graduates who practice primary care, work in health professional shortage areas, and are underrepresented minorities, combined into a composite social mission score.

Results.—The contribution of medical schools to the social mission of medical education varied substantially. Three historically black colleges had the highest social mission rankings. Public and community-based medical schools had higher social mission scores than private and non—community-based schools. National Institutes of Health funding was inversely associated with social mission scores. Medical schools in the northeastern United States and in more urban areas were less likely to produce primary care physicians and physicians who practice in underserved areas.

Limitations.—The AMA Physician Masterfile has limitations, including specialty self-designation by physicians, inconsistencies in reporting work addresses, and delays in information updates. The public good provided by medical schools may include contributions not reflected in the social mission score. The study was not designed to evaluate quality of care provided by medical school graduates.

Conclusion.—Medical schools vary substantially in their contribution to the social mission of medical education. School rankings based on the social mission score differ from those that use research funding and subjective assessments of school reputation. These findings suggest that initiatives at

TABLE 1.—Medical School Rankings Based on Social Mission Score*

Rank	School	State	Social Mission Score†	Primary Care Physicians Total, %	Primary Care Physicians Standardized Score‡	Physicians Practicing in HPSAs Total, %	Physicians Practicing in HPSAs Standardized Score‡
Highest 20							
1	Morehouse College	GA	13.98	43.7	1.20	39.1	1.40
2	Meharry Medical College	TN	12.92	49.3	2.00	28.1	0.14
3	Howard University	DC	10.66	36.5	0.19	33.7	0.78
4	Wright State University Boonshoft School of Medicine	OH	5.34	49.2	1.98	28	0.12
5	University of Kansas	KS	4.49	45.2	1.42	43.9	1.96
6	Michigan State University	MI	4.13	43.6	1.20	26.5	-0.05
7	East Carolina University Brody School of Medicine	NC	3.72	51.9	2.36	34.2	0.84
8	University of South Alabama	AL	3.15	42	0.97	52.7	2.97
9	Universidad de Puerto Rico en Ponce	PR	3.02	33	-0.31	43.8	1.94
10	University of Iowa Carver College of Medicine	IA	2.97	37.1	0.28	21	-0.69
11	Oregon Health & Science University	OR	2.93	43.8	1.22	43.8	1.94
12	East Tennessee State University Quillen College of Medicine	TN	2.88	53.5	2.58	32.7	0.67
13	University of Mississippi	MS	2.86	33.5	-0.24	62.5	4.11
14	University of Kentucky	KY	2.61	39.8	0.65	32.5	0.64
15	Southern Illinois University	IL	2.59	45	1.39	46.5	2.26
16	Marshall University Joan C. Edwards University	WV	2.51	46.8	1.64	20.9	-0.70
17	University of Massachusetts Medical School	MA	2.48	45.9	1.52	36.7	1.12
18	University of Illinois	IL	2.27	36.7	0.21	35.7	1.01
19	University of New Mexico	NM	2.25	46.7	1.63	30.7	0.43
20	University of Wisconsin	WI	2.24	35.7	0.07	19.3	-0.87
Lowest 20§							
1	Vanderbilt University	TN	-3.95	21.9	-1.86	20.8	-0.70
2	University of Texas Southwestern Medical Center	TX	-3.64	26.8	-1.18	15.1	-1.36
3	Northwestern University Feinberg School of Medicine	IL	-3.11	24.4	1.51	19.5	-0.86
4	University of California, Irvine	CA	-3.02	32.9	-0.32	14.2	-1.47
5	New York University	NY	-2.65	24.3	-1.53	22.1	-0.55
6	University of Medicine and Dentistry of New Jersey	NJ	-2.46	23.7	-1.61	17.8	-1.05
7	Uniformed Services University of the Health Sciences	MD	-2.36	29.6	-0.78	21.4	-0.64
8	Thomas Jefferson University	PA	-2.34	32.1	-0.42	20.6	-0.72
9	Stony Brook University	NY	-2.21	29.1	-0.85	20.4	-0.76
10	Albert Einstein College of Medicine of Yeshiva University	NY	-2.13	26.1	-1.28	24.8	-0.25

11	Boston University	MA	-2.12	26.7	-1.19	23.3	-0.42
12	Loyola University Chicago Stritch School of Medicine	IL	-2.06	33.7	-0.20	20.7	-0.72
13	University of Pennsylvania	PA	-2.03	19.1	-2.27	20.4	-0.76
14	Medical College of Wisconsin	WI	-2.02	33.5	-0.23	15.9	-1.28
15	University at Albany, State University of New York	NY	-2.00	30.7	-0.63	24.2	-0.32
16	Columbia University	NY	-1.98	20.3	-2.10	31.8	0.57
17	Texas A&M University	TX	-1.95	37	0.26	16.2	-1.24
18	Duke University	NC	-1.91	22.3	-1.82	23.9	-0.34
19	Stanford University	CA	-1.90	27.4	-1.10	16.2	-1.23
20	Johns Hopkins University	MD	-1.90	24.3	-1.53	26.7	-0.02

HPSA = health professional shortage area.

*The ranking of all 141 schools is in the **Appendix**, available at www.annals.org.

†The sum of the primary care, HPSA, and underrepresented minority standardized scores.

‡The standardized value calculated for each measure, with a mean value of 0 (SD, 1).

§Ranked from lowest to highest (i.e., rank 1 is the lowest-performing school).

the medical school level could increase the proportion of physicians who practice primary care, work in underserved areas, and are underrepresented minorities.

▶ Medical schools have a number of missions. They generate new scientific knowledge and are often the home of leading-edge clinical improvement. They also create the teachers of our medical progeny. Medical schools, however, are the only institutions in our society that can produce physicians within our boundaries, yet their performance relative to their mission is rarely calculated in social terms. Routine assessments of medical schools, such as the well known US News & World Report ranking system, often value research funding, school reputation, and student selectivity factors over actual educational output of each school, particularly regarding the number of graduates who enter primary care practice in underserved areas and who are underrepresented minorities. Filling this gap are the data from the report of Mullan et al that rank medical schools based on the percentage of medical school graduates who practice primary care, work in health professional shortage areas (HPSAs), and are underrepresented minorities. Primary care specialty information was obtained from the American Medical Association Physician Masterfile, with primary care being defined as family medicine, general internal medicine, general pediatrics, or internal medicine-pediatrics. HPSAs were based on population-provider ratios, poverty rate, and travel distance or time to the nearest accessible source of care calculated on the percentage of graduates from each medical school with an address in an HPSA. Last, underrepresented minorities were defined as African American, Hispanic, and Native American individuals.

What we learned from this report is encapsulated in the information in Table 1, which shows the 20 schools with the highest and lowest social mission scores and the primary care, HPSA, and underrepresented minority measures on which the schools' composite scores were based. One could go online to find a listing of all 141 schools that were looked at (available at www.annals.org). Compared with allopathic schools, osteopathic schools produce relatively more primary care physicians but fewer trained underrepresented minorities. Public schools scored higher on the composite social mission score and in all 3 component measures, although the differences between public and private schools were not statistically significant for the underserved area and underrepresented minority components. Funding by the National Institutes of Health was inversely associated with social mission score and with a school's output of primary care physicians and physicians practicing in underrepresented areas. The 3 historically black colleges and universities with medical schools (Morehouse College, Meharry Medical College, and Howard University) score at the top of the social mission rankings. These results are not unexpected, as 70% to 85% of each of these schools' graduating classes was underrepresented minorities compared with only 13.5% in all medical schools across the country during the same period. The higher underrepresented minority scores alone significantly increase these schools' social mission scores. However, all these schools also score in the top half of the primary care and underserved output measures.

An important finding from this report is that public schools do seem to be more responsive to the population-based and distributional physician workforce needs. Legislators should pay attention to this since the data suggest that enhanced support for medical education at the state level could address workforce needs more effectively than would investment in private schools. Compared with other US regions, the northeast, with its preponderance of private, traditional, and research-intensive medical schools, had the lowest scores in the primary care and underserved areas components and a distinctly lower social mission score. The size of the metropolitan area in which the schools are located also seems to affect the social mission score. For example, medical schools in less urban areas are more likely to produce primary care physicians and physicians practicing in underserved areas. These findings may be particularly helpful for entities considering building new schools or developing branch campuses of existing schools. One also finds in the data from this report a reinforcement of the known fact that osteopathic schools traditionally focus on primary care and rural practice. At the same time, allopathic schools have recruited more underrepresented minorities than osteopathic schools. Osteopathic medicine has been very creative in establishing new medical schools in nontraditional locations, such as Pikeville, Kentucky, and Harlem, New York, and in developing innovative community programs, such as A. T. Still University in Mesa, Arizona, where all clinical work is based at 10 community health centers. As this commentary is written, a new osteopathic medical school is being considered in the region where this editor lives. That school (Campbell University) would be placed in conjunction with a modest-sized university, which is located halfway between Raleigh and Fayetteville in North Carolina, not a particularly population-dense area of that state.

Obviously there is nothing wrong with a medical school having a research-intensive mission as long as the numbers of such schools are balanced with other schools that are committed to producing highly trained clinicians with diverse racial and ethnic backgrounds who are committed to practicing primary care, hopefully including primary care in underserved areas. It should be noted that no new medical schools were created in the United States during the 1980s and 1990s, primarily because reports issued by federal advisory bodies, the Graduate Medical Education National Advisory Committee in 1980 and the Council on Graduate Medical Education in 1992, projected that the United States would have an excess of physicians by 2000. University governing bodies and state authorities were therefore unwilling to approve the development of new medical schools. How wrong these councils and commissions were! Now we are seeing increasing numbers of medical schools popping up and existing medical schools expanding their class sizes. Before a new medical school can begin to admit students, it must be granted preliminary accreditation by the Liaison Committee on Medical Education (LCME). Between 2006 and 2010, 15 institutions have officially notified the LCME of their intent to start a new medical school. By 2010, 6 of the new schools have already been granted preliminary accreditation; 4 of these (Florida International University College of Medicine, University of Central Florida College of Medicine, Texas Tech University Health Sciences Center Paul L Foster School of Medicine, and Commonwealth Medical College in Pennsylvania) admitted their charter classes in the summer of 2009, one (Virginia Tech Carilion School of Medicine) did so in the summer of 2010, and one (Oakland University William Beaumont School of Medicine, Michigan) did so in the summer of 2011. One additional school (Hofstra University School of Medicine in partnership with North Shore-Long Island Jewish Health System, New York) has submitted the requisite materials for preliminary accreditation and was estimated to be able to admit a charter class in mid-2011. Two other schools (Central Michigan University School of Medicine and Cooper Medical School of Rowan University in New Jersey) have indicated their intent to enroll charter classes in mid-2012. Four institutions (University of South Carolina School of Medicine, Greenville; University of California, Riverside School of Medicine; Western Virginia University; and Palm Beach Medical College) had not by mid-2010 indicated when their charter classes might be enrolled. Two institutions (The Scripps Research Institute and Touro College) had suspended their planning activities in 2010 and at that time seemed unlikely to resume them anytime soon. This process of launching a new medical school is both lengthy and expensive. It takes at least 3 years to get through the accreditation process at a cost of well over 1 million dollars. The planning process typically begins with a feasibility study, which usually requires the availability of discretionary funds within the institution's budget; the cost of the feasibility study depends on whether it is conducted by the institution's staff or outside consultants.

Most of the medical schools that are starting up in the United States are institutions that are likely to have a high social mission. New medical schools are not likely to be research intensive, at least not out of the box. If you wish to read more about new medical schools opening in the United States, see the excellent editorial on this topic by Whitcomb.[1] The newest medical schools in the United States still are not fully up to steam. In the academic year 2009-2010, Florida International University Herbert Wertheim College of Medicine in Miami had just 43 students while the University of Central Florida College of Medicine in Orlando had 41 students enrolled. By comparison, the largest medical school student body resides at the University of Illinois College of Medicine in Chicago with 1303 students enrolled in the academic year 2009-2010. For much in the way of statistics on medical schools in the United States, see the report by Barzansky and Etzel.[2]

J. A. Stockman III, MD

References

1. Whitcomb ME. New medical schools in the United States. *N Engl J Med.* 2010; 362:1255-1258.
2. Barzansky B, Etzel SI. Medical schools in the United States, 2009-2010. *JAMA.* 2010;304:1247-1254.

Online Posting of Unprofessional Content by Medical Students

Chretien KC, Greysen SR, Chretien J-P, et al (George Washington Univ School of Medicine and Health Sciences, DC; Johns Hopkins School of Medicine, Baltimore, MD)
JAMA 302:1309-1315, 2009

Context.—Web 2.0 applications, such as social networking sites, are creating new challenges for medical professionalism. The scope of this problem in undergraduate medical education is not well-defined.

Objective.—To assess the experience of US medical schools with online posting of unprofessional content by students and existing medical school policies to address online posting.

Design, Setting, and Participants.—An anonymous electronic survey was sent to deans of student affairs, their representatives, or counterparts from each institution in the Association of American Medical Colleges. Data were collected in March and April 2009.

Main Outcome Measures.—Percentage of schools reporting incidents of students posting unprofessional content online, type of professionalism infraction, disciplinary actions taken, existence of institution policies, and plans for policy development.

Results.—Sixty percent of US medical schools responded (78/130). Of these schools, 60% (47/78) reported incidents of students posting unprofessional online content. Violations of patient confidentiality were reported by 13% (6/46). Student use of profanity (52%; 22/42), frankly discriminatory language (48%; 19/40), depiction of intoxication (39%; 17/44), and sexually suggestive material (38%; 16/42) were commonly reported. Of 45 schools that reported an incident and responded to the question about disciplinary actions, 30 gave informal warning (67%) and 3 reported student dismissal (7%). Policies that cover student-posted online content were reported by 38% (28/73) of deans. Of schools without such policies, 11% (5/46) were actively developing new policies to cover online content. Deans reporting incidents were significantly more likely to report having such a policy (51% vs 18%; $P = .006$), believing these issues could be effectively addressed (91% vs 63%; $P = .003$), and having higher levels of concern ($P = .02$).

Conclusion.—Many responding schools had incidents of unprofessional student online postings, but they may not have adequate policy in place (Table 2).

▶ This is an interesting and important report that tells us a bit about unprofessional medical student activity in the digital age. It is all too easy to use web 2.0 applications such as Facebook, Twitter, Flickr, YouTube, blogs, wikis, and podcasts, among others, to speak out on what is on one's mind. Words that hit the Internet, however, are like herpes. They are there forever. When a medical student posts something that is unprofessional, words can have real consequences. What Chretien et al have done is to send a survey under the name of the Association of American Medical Colleges Group on Student Affairs to

TABLE 2.—Selected Survey Responses

Survey Questions	No. per Category/Total No. of Respondents (%)	
	Yes	No or Not Sure
Are you aware of any incidents at your school in which medical students have posted unprofessional content online?	47/78 (60)	31/78 (40)
Did any of these incidents in the past year involve violations of patient confidentiality?[a]	6/46 (13)	40/46 (87)
Did any of these incidents in the past year involve conflicts of interest?[a]	2/46 (4)	44/46 (96)
Did any of these incidents involve content that fits into the following categories[a]		
Profanity	22/42 (52)	20/42 (48)
Discriminatory language	19/40 (48)	21/40 (53)
Depicted intoxication	17/42 (40)	25/42 (60)
Sexually suggestive	16/42 (38)	26/42 (62)
Do your school's current professionalism policies cover student-posted online content?	28/73 (38)	45/73 (62)
Does your school's policy specifically address issues of Internet use such as blogs and social networking sites?[b]	5/28 (18)	23/28 (82)
Given your existing policies, do you feel you are able to effectively deal with unprofessional student-posted online content?	58/72 (81)	14/72 (19)
Is there a committee or task force at your school that is responsible for addressing student-posted online content?	14/73 (19)	59/73 (81)
Are you aware of any incidents at other schools in which medical students posted unprofessional content online?	20/75 (27)	55/75 (73)

[a]Answered if the response was yes to "Are you aware of any incidents at your school in which medical students have posted unprofessional content online?".
[b]Answered if the response was yes to "Do your school's current professionalism policies cover student-posted online content?."

designated student affairs deans at each of the 130 US medical schools, asking those deans if they had found instances of student-posted unprofessional online content. The survey asked whether deans were aware of any incidents at their schools in which students posted content including potential violations of patient privacy, use of profanity or frankly discriminatory language, depiction of intoxication or sexual suggestiveness, failure to reveal conflicts of interest (eg, product endorsement without conflict of interest disclosure), and communication about the medical profession or patients in a negative way.

The results of this study show that around 60% of medical school deans responded to the survey, and of those, about 60% reported having incidents involving students posting unprofessional content (Table 2). Student use of profanity, frankly discriminatory language, depiction of intoxication, and sexually suggestive material were more commonly reported. Issues of conflict of interest were rare. Specific examples included 10 open-ended text examples detailing sexually suggestive or explicit content or inappropriate relationships. Examples in this category included sexually provocative photographs of students, requesting inappropriate photographs of students, requesting inappropriate friendships with patients on Facebook, and sexually suggestive comments. Of those deans who reported student dismissal, 1 cited incidents involving patient confidentiality and 1 cited incidents involving conflicts of interest. A third respondent cited multiple incidents involving profanity, frankly discriminatory language, depiction of intoxication, and sexually suggestive material of which 1 infraction resulted in dismissal.

Although some of the incidents identified in the survey appear to be clear cut lapses of professionalism (unintentional violation of patient privacy and photos involving illicit drug use), others fall into more ambiguous categories (using profanity and being sexually suggestive). Certain examples such as negative comments about a student's institution or profession might in fact not be considered unprofessional. The line separating protected first amendment rights and inappropriate postings in fact is unclear. Also, what may be appropriate in one environment may be totally inappropriate in another. For example, medical students frequently write and perform satirical comic strips for student shows, perhaps serving as a coping and stress-release function during difficult training periods. When such shows, however, get posted on YouTube, the boundary may be crossed with respect to professionalism.

What is most surprising about this report is that most of the student dean respondents, while being daily users of the internet for e-mail and similar communications, reported never or rarely using social networking sites, reading blogs, posting on blogs, reading wikis, or writing on wikis, perhaps suggesting a generational divide with the students in the same institutions. Deans of American medical schools should look at an interesting report that appeared in the *British Medical Journal* by Yates and James.[1] The case-controlled study by Yates and James found that male sex, lower estimated social class, and poor early performance at medical school are independent risk factors for subsequent professional misconduct. This is consistent with other evidence that male doctors are overrepresented in cases of professional misconduct, and previous studies in the United States have indicated a link between poor academic record and being disciplined by a medical board.[2] What has not been noted previously is a link between lower social class and future misconduct. This should be looked at very carefully so that the information from the report of Yates and James is not used to discriminate against these students at an undergraduate level. Please be aware that these data were collected overseas and may not have strong relevance to the situation in the United States.

J. A. Stockman III, MD

References

1. Yates J, James D. Risk factors at medical school for subsequent professional misconduct: multicenter retrospective case-controlled study. *BMJ.* 2010;340: c2040.
2. Papadakis MA, Teherani A, Banach MA, et al. Disciplinary action by medical boards and prior behavior in medical school. *N Engl J Med.* 2005;353:2673-2682.

Relationship Between Burnout and Professional Conduct and Attitudes Among US Medical Students

Dyrbye LN, Massie FS Jr, Eacker A, et al (Mayo Clinic College of Medicine, Rochester, MN; Univ of Alabama School of Medicine, Birmingham; Univ of Washington School of Medicine, Seattle; et al)
JAMA 304:1173-1180, 2010

Context.—The relationship between professionalism and distress among medical students is unknown.

Objective.—To determine the relationship between measures of professionalism and burnout among US medical students.

Design, Setting, and Participants.—Cross-sectional survey of all medical students attending 7 US medical schools (overall response rate, 2682/4400 [61%]) in the spring of 2009. The survey included the Maslach Burnout Inventory (MBI), the PRIME–MD depression screening instrument, and the SF-8 quality of life (QOL) assessment tool, as well as items exploring students' personal engagement in unprofessional conduct, understanding of appropriate relationships with industry, and attitudes regarding physicians' responsibility to society.

Main Outcome Measures.—Frequency of self-reported cheating/dishonest behaviors, understanding of appropriate relationships with industry as defined by American Medical Association policy, attitudes about physicians' responsibility to society, and the relationship of these dimensions of professionalism to burnout, symptoms of depression, and QOL.

Results.—Of the students who responded to all the MBI items, 1354 of 2566 (52.8%) had burnout. Cheating/dishonest academic behaviors were rare (endorsed by <10%) in comparison to unprofessional conduct related to patient care (endorsed by up to 43%). Only 14% (362/2531) of students had opinions on relationships with industry consistent with guidelines for 6 scenarios. Students with burnout were more likely to report engaging in 1 or more unprofessional behaviors than those without burnout (35.0% vs 21.9%; odds ratio [OR], 1.89; 95% confidence interval [CI], 1.59-2.24). Students with burnout were also less likely to report holding altruistic views regarding physicians' responsibility to society. For example, students with burnout were less likely to want to provide care for the medically underserved than those without burnout (79.3% vs 85.0%; OR, 0.68; 95% CI, 0.55-0.83). After multivariable analysis adjusting for personal and professional characteristics, burnout was the only aspect of distress independently associated with reporting 1 or more unprofessional behaviors (OR, 1.76; 95% CI, 1.45-2.13) or holding at least 1 less altruistic view regarding physicians' responsibility to society (OR, 1.65; 95% CI, 1.35-2.01).

Conclusion.—Burnout was associated with self-reported unprofessional conduct and less altruistic professional values among medical students at 7 US schools.

▶ In this multi-institutional survey involving 2682 medical students, Dyrbye et al found that just over half of medical students meet the criteria for professional burnout, a measure of emotional exhaustion, depersonalization, and a low sense of personal accomplishment. Interestingly, these investigators hypothesized that medical students undergoing professional distress would be at greater risk for problems with professionalism in general. The authors predicted that professional distress would be more strongly associated with self-reported cheating behaviors, inability to recognize unethical practices in interactions with industry, and less altruistic attitudes related to the care of vulnerable and underserved patients. Indeed, the Dyrbye et al study found that burned-out students did in fact more commonly acknowledge unprofessional behaviors, and, as hypothesized, the investigators did not find as strong an association of personal distress with a lack of professionalism as opposed to professional distress. Because stress is commonly asserted as a principal cause of unprofessional behavior and yet is intuitively associated with depression and mental illness more broadly, the absence of a strong link between personal distress and unprofessionalism represents a valuable understanding. This report is truly worrisome, making one wonder whether such medical students will in fact become poor physicians from the professionalism point of view. The data from this report show that students with burnout are less likely to hold altruistic views regarding physicians' responsibilities to society. Many medical students in this study had opinions about relationships with the pharmaceutical industry inconsistent with well-established policies on conflict of interest.

The bottom line is that the results of this report indicate that medical student burnout is independently associated with self-reporting of unprofessional conduct and less altruistic professional values. What we need now are studies of interventions designed to reduce burnout to see if indeed such interventions can cultivate the type of professional values and behavior we all aspire to as physicians.

J. A. Stockman III, MD

Plagiarism in Residency Application Essays
Segal S, Gelfand BJ, Hurwitz S, et al (Massachusetts General Hosp, Boston)
Ann Intern Med 153:112-120, 2010

Background.—Anecdotal reports suggest that some residency application essays contain plagiarized content.

Objective.—To determine the prevalence of plagiarism in a large cohort of residency application essays.

Design.—Retrospective cohort study.

Setting.—4975 application essays submitted to residency programs at a single large academic medical center between 1 September 2005 and 22 March 2007.

Measurements.—Specialized software was used to compare residency application essays with a database of Internet pages, published works, and previously submitted essays and the percentage of the submission matching another source was calculated. A match of more than 10% to an existing work was defined as evidence of plagiarism.

Results.—Evidence of plagiarism was found in 5.2% (95% CI, 4.6% to 5.9%) of essays. The essays of non—U.S. citizens were more likely to demonstrate evidence of plagiarism. Other characteristics associated with the prevalence of plagiarism included medical school location outside the United States and Canada; previous residency or fellowship; lack of research experience, volunteer experience, or publications; a low United States Medical Licensing Examination Step 1 score; and nonmembership in the Alpha Omega Alpha Honor Medical Society.

Limitations.—The software database is probably incomplete, the 10%-match threshold for defining plagiarism has not been statistically validated, and the study was confined to applicants to 1 institution. Evidence of matching content in an essay cannot be used to infer the applicant's intent and is not sensitive to variations in the cultural context of copying in some societies.

Conclusion.—Evidence of plagiarism in residency application essays is more common in international applicants but was found in those by applicants to all specialty programs, from all medical school types, and even among applicants with significant academic honors (Table 2).

▶ This is a fascinating report giving some insight into the origins of what may turn out to be the first act of unprofessionalism a medical school graduate in the United States might engage in. Virtually every applicant to US residency training programs will complete an original essay known as the personal statement. Some of us are too old to have experienced this rite of passage, but the format of the personal statement is a free-form narrative, the content of which is not specified. Expectations about the statement do vary somewhat by specialty area. Common themes include the motivation for seeking training in a chosen specialty, the factors that affect suitability for a field or program, a critical incident that may have affected the applicant's career choice, and the circumstances that distinguish the applicant from his or her peers. Applicants are warned by the National Resident Matching Program Electronic Residency Application Service (ERAS) that the statements should be only original personal work and that any substantiated findings of plagiarism may result in reporting of such findings to the programs to which an individual may apply now or in the future. The applicant must certify that the work is accurate and original before an ERAS application is complete. What many applicants are not aware of is that there is software that can efficiently and effectively search large databases of previously created content, which can greatly improve the ability to detect plagiarized essays.

What Segal et al have done is to use plagiarism software adapted for application essays analyzing personal statements submitted with residency applications to 5 specialty programs. The design of this investigation was to estimate the prevalence of plagiarism in applicants' personal statements and to determine the association of plagiarism with demographic, educational, and experience-related characteristics of the applicants. The specialized software Turnitin for Admissions (iParadigms, Oakland, California) was used to analyze the essays. This program uses digital fingerprinting to represent groups of characters in

TABLE 2.—Prevalence of Evidence of Plagiarism*

Characteristic[+]	All Applicants, n/N (% [95% CI])	U.S. Citizens, n/N (% [95% CI])	Non–U.S. Citizens, n/N (% [95% CI])
Entire cohort	259/4975 (5.2 [4.5–5.9])	65/3561 (1.8 [1.4–2.3])	194/1414 (13.7 [12.0–15.6])
Specialty			
Anesthesiology	30/675 (4.4 [3.0–6.3])	16/534 (3.0 [1.7–4.8])	14/141 (9.9 [5.5–16.1])
Emergency medicine	10/578 (1.7 [0.8–3.2])	3/519 (0.58 [0.12–1.7])	7/59 (11.9 [4.9–22.9])
Internal medicine	141/2456 (5.7 [4.9–6.7])	23/1652 (1.4 [0.88–2.1])	118/804 (14.7 [12.3–17.3])
Obstetrics and gynecology	44/569 (7.7 [5.7–10.2])	12/398 (3.0 [1.6–5.2])	32/171 (18.7 [13.2–25.4])
General surgery	34/697 (4.9 [3.4–6.8])	11/458 (2.4 [1.2–4.3])	23/239 (9.6 [6.2–14.1])
Citizenship			
U.S. citizen	65/3561 (1.8 [1.4–2.3])	—	—
Permanent resident	48/353 (13.6 [10.0–17.2])	—	—
Foreign national	143/1028 (13.9 [11.9–16.2])	—	—
Other‡	3/33 (9.1 [1.9–24.3])	—	—
Medical school type			
U.S. private	22/1799 (1.2 [0.77–1.9])	21/1712 (1.2 [0.76–1.9])	1/87 (1.1 [0.03–6.2])
U.S. public	15/1443 (1.0 [0.58–1.7])	14/1404 (1.0 [0.55–1.7])	1/39 (2.6 [0.06–13.5])
International	218/1589 (13.7 [12.1–15.5])	26/327 (8.0 [5.3–11.4])	192/1262 (15.2 [13.3–17.3])
Fifth Pathway program and other§	4/144 (2.8 [0.76–7.0])	4/118 (3.4 [0.93–8.5])	0/26 (0 [0–13.2])
Medical school location			
United States or Canada	41/3378 (1.2 [0.87–1.6])	39/3227 (1.2 [0.86–1.6])	2/151 (1.3 [0.16–4.7])
Foreign	218/1597 (13.7 [12.0–15.4])	26/334 (7.8 [5.2–11.2])	192/1263 (15.2 [13.3–17.3])
ECFMG status‖			
Certified	195/1340 (14.6 [12.7–16.6])	17/190 (9.0 [5.3–13.9])	178/1150 (15.5 [13.4–17.7])
Not certified	23/257 (9.0 [5.8–13.1])	9/144 (6.3 [2.9–11.5])	14/113 (12.4 [6.9–19.9])
Sex			
Women	116/2278 (5.1 [4.2–6.1])	39/1737 (2.3 [1.6–3.1])	77/541 (14.2 [11.4–17.5])
Men	142/2693 (5.3 [4.4–6.2])	26/1821 (1.4 [0.93–2.1])	116/872 (13.3 [11.1–15.7])
Mean age at application, y¶			
Plagiarism	259 (29.9 [29.3–30.5])	65 (28.9 [27.6–30.2])	194 (30.2 [29.6–30.9])
No plagiarism	4716 (28.5 [28.3–28.6])	3493 (27.8 [27.7–27.9])	1219 (30.3 [30.1–30.6])
AOA status			
Member	5/526 (0.95 [0.31–2.2])	5/500 (1.0 [0.33–2.3])	0/26 (0 [0–13.2])
Nonmember	254/4449 (5.7 [5.1–6.4])	60/3061 (2.0 [1.5–2.5])	194/1388 (14.0 [12.2–15.9])
Mean USMLE Step 1 score¶			
Plagiarism	94 (216 [213–220])	27 (212 [204–220])	67 (218 [214–222])

(Continued)

TABLE 2. (*continued*)

Characteristic†	All Applicants, n/N (% [95% CI])	U.S. Citizens, n/N (% [95% CI])	Non–U.S. Citizens, n/N (% [95% CI])
No plagiarism	2071 (225 [224–226])	1646 (226 [225–226])	425 (224 [222–226])
Language fluency other than English**			
Yes	232/3451 (6.7 [5.9–7.6])	47/2114 (2.2 [1.6–3.0])	185/1337 (13.8 [12.0–15.8])
No	25/1469 (1.7 [1.1–2.5])	18/1412 (1.3 [0.76–2.0])	7/57 (12.3 [5.1–23.7])
Previous residency or fellowship			
Yes	112/900 (12.4 [10.3–14.6])	12/246 (4.9 [2.6–8.4])	100/654 (15.3 [12.6–18.3])
No	147/4075 (3.6 [3.0–4.2])	53/3315 (1.6 [1.2–2.1])	94/760 (12.4 [10.0–14.7])
Publications			
Yes	142/3122 (4.6 [3.8–5.3])	39/2266 (1.7 [1.2–2.4])	103/856 (12.0 [9.9–14.4])
No	117/1853 (6.3 [5.3–7.5])	26/1295 (2.0 [1.3–2.9])	91/558 (16.3 [13.3–19.6])
Research experience			
Yes	160/3985 (4.0 [3.4–4.7])	50/3076 (1.6 [1.2–2.1])	110/909 (12.1 [10.1–14.4])
No	99/990 (10.0 [8.2–12.0])	15/485 (3.1 [1.7–5.1])	84/505 (16.6 [13.5–20.2])
Volunteer experience			
Yes	181/4290 (4.2 [3.6–4.9])	51/3287 (1.6 [1.2–2.0])	130/1003 (13.0 [10.9–15.2])
No	78/685 (11.4 [9.1–14.0])	14/274 (5.1 [2.8–8.4])	64/411 (15.6 [12.2–19.5])

AOA = Alpha Omega Alpha Honor Medical Society; ECFMG = Educational Commission for Foreign Medical Graduates; IQR = interquartile range; USMLE = United States Medical Licensing Examination.
*Defined as a similarity score ≥10.
†Some applicants applied to more than 1 specialty, and the applicant data were very similar although not identical across the applications from these applicants. For the analyses reported here, each application, rather than the applicant, was treated as the unit of analysis, and the size of a sample (n) given in each analysis refers to the number of applications.
‡Includes conditional permanent residents (n = 24) and refugees, persons seeking asylum, and displaced persons (n = 9).
§Includes students or graduates from Canadian medical schools and U.S. osteopathic medical schools.
‖Non–U.S. medical school applicants.
¶Mean [95% CI] of applicants whose essays had similarity scores ≥10 or <10.
**Includes any language fluency self-reported by candidates.

the source document as numeric sequences, which are sampled in groups of approximately 40 characters. The software then compares the fingerprint of the submitted essay with a database that includes web pages, printed resources, and previously submitted essays. The algorithm in the software efficiently searches for exact or close matches within 40 character strings but rejects very common phrases. The system also ignores material in the submitted essay enclosed in quotation marks. Finally, the software calculates a similarity score between 0 and 100 that represents the percentage of the submitted essay matching a source in the database and then provides a report showing the original source material matching the submitted essay and highlights the matching passages.

Some 5000 applicant files and an almost equal number of essays were analyzed for evidence of plagiarism. Evidence of plagiarism defined as a similarity score of 10 or greater was observed in 5.2% of the applications. Essays from international medical school graduates were more likely to demonstrate evidence of plagiarism. While evidence of plagiarism was seen in just 1.8% of US citizen graduates, foreign graduates had a score suggesting plagiarism in almost 14% of applications. Equal numbers of men and women were represented in the plagiarism category. Student applicants who had achieved Alpha Omega Alpha status represented one-sixth the risk of plagiarism as their nonmember peers. The bottom line, as the authors say, is that "a concerted national effort to detect and deter plagiarism is warranted."

Plagiarism in medicine is no laughing matter. It is truly the cardinal sin of academic life representing both dishonesty and theft. Indeed, plagiarism on a personal statement is a misrepresentation of one's self. It is highly likely that this violation of professionalism is merely the tip of the iceberg of nonprofessionalism both before and after residency application. There is ample evidence that patterns of problematic behavior persist among physicians and that unprofessional behavior during training is a heralding sign of future misbehavior.

Please recognize that a whole industry, not just a cottage industry, has developed to help applicants through the process of getting into the residency they wish to enter. For example, applicants who do not yet have a draft of a personal statement for a medical school application can get help online to begin the writing process (at a cost as much as over $800). Those who already have drafts can hire online consultants and editors for a lesser amount per hour and can receive a complete rushed 10-hour turnaround service for as much as almost $3000. An applicant can hire an online editor to edit a draft of a personal statement on the basis of word count (fee for 251-600 words is $127.95).

The Segal et al study was designed to estimate the prevalence of plagiarism, not to identify predictive variables for it, but the findings tend to unintentionally stigmatize the entire group of non-US citizen applicants, the vast majority of whom do not plagiarize.

One wonders if the personal statement should still be required as part of the medical school application process. Even though we now have techniques to determine frank plagiarism, there is still no way to know whether the statement, even if not plagiarized, was totally written by the applicant or someone else.

Importantly, this component of the application remains despite considerable evidence that the personal statement is not predictive of performance.

I for one would prefer to see the personal statement stay in play as part of residency application. As one who has reviewed many of these, I always find them interesting and at times entertaining. In addition, one can now use software to pick up plagiarism. Thus, even if the personal statement is of no real value to the selection process otherwise, if you do pick up on an incident of plagiarism, at least you have weeded out one bad actor, hopefully permanently, from the profession we all serve.

J. A. Stockman III, MD

12 Musculoskeletal

A Randomized Trial of Tai Chi for Fibromyalgia

Wang C, Schmid CH, Rones R, et al (Tufts Univ School of Medicine, Boston, MA; Mind-Body Therapies, Boston, MA; et al)
N Engl J Med 363:743-754, 2010

Background.—Previous research has suggested that tai chi offers a therapeutic benefit in patients with fibromyalgia.

Methods.—We conducted a single-blind, randomized trial of classic Yang-style tai chi as compared with a control intervention consisting of wellness education and stretching for the treatment of fibromyalgia (defined by American College of Rheumatology 1990 criteria). Sessions lasted 60 minutes each and took place twice a week for 12 weeks for each of the study groups. The primary end point was a change in the Fibromyalgia Impact Questionnaire (FIQ) score (ranging from 0 to 100, with higher scores indicating more severe symptoms) at the end of 12 weeks. Secondary end points included summary scores on the physical and mental components of the Medical Outcomes Study 36-Item Short-Form Health Survey (SF-36). All assessments were repeated at 24 weeks to test the durability of the response.

Results.—Of the 66 randomly assigned patients, the 33 in the tai chi group had clinically important improvements in the FIQ total score and quality of life. Mean ($\pm$SD) baseline and 12-week FIQ scores for the tai chi group were 62.9 ± 15.5 and 35.1 ± 18.8, respectively, versus 68.0 ± 11 and 58.6 ± 17.6, respectively, for the control group (change from baseline in the tai chi group vs. change from baseline in the control group, -18.4 points; P<0.001). The corresponding SF-36 physical-component scores were 28.5 ± 8.4 and 37.0 ± 10.5 for the tai chi group versus 28.0 ± 7.8 and 29.4 ± 7.4 for the control group (between-group difference, 7.1 points; P=0.001), and the mental-component scores were 42.6 ± 12.2 and 50.3 ± 10.2 for the tai chi group versus 37.8 ± 10.5 and 39.4 ± 11.9 for the control group (between-group difference, 6.1 points; P=0.03). Improvements were maintained at 24 weeks (between-group difference in the FIQ score, -18.3 points; P<0.001). No adverse events were observed.

Conclusions.—Tai chi may be a useful treatment for fibromyalgia and merits long-term study in larger study populations. (Funded by the National

Center for Complementary and Alternative Medicine and others; ClinicalTrials.gov number, NCT00515008.)

▶ Fibromyalgia affects not only adults but also children, particularly adolescents. It is a common and poorly understood disorder resulting in pain. Some estimates say that over 200 million or more individuals are affected worldwide.[1] Fibromyalgia is so poorly understood that many believe it doesn't even exist, but just ask any patient with it and you may very well become a believer. Fibromyalgia is a diagnosis of exclusion, with many mimics. Standard treatment regimens have included exercise, sleep, hygiene, and medications. Nonmedication approaches other than exercise include cognitive and behavioral therapies. Pharmacologic agents commonly recommended for fibromyalgia include amitriptyline, cyclobenzaprine, fluoxetine, and several drugs now approved by the Food and Drug Administration, including duloxetine, pregabalin, and milnacipran. Unfortunately, with any or all of these modalities applied to the patient with fibromyalgia, the clinical response is often disappointing. It is not unexpected then that many people with fibromyalgia will seek out less conventional treatments such as tai chi, yoga, massage, and acupuncture.

Wang et al decided to study the efficacy and safety of tai chi as part of the management of fibromyalgia. They report the results of a randomized controlled trial of tai chi as a treatment for the disorder. If you are not familiar with tai chi, it is a gentle meditative exercise that consists of flowing circular movements, balance and weight shifting, breathing techniques, and cognitive tools (eg, imagery and focused internal awareness). Previous investigators have examined the role of tai chi as an intervention for a variety of health issues, including balance impairments and cardiovascular disease. It has been used for the management of rheumatologic conditions such as rheumatoid arthritis and other musculoskeletal conditions such as osteoarthritis and low back pain. Data do suggest that tai chi may be effective for many of these disorders, although rigorous studies with adequate sample sizes have not been performed.

The report of Wang et al attempts to provide more bulletproof data documenting the success or failure of tai chi of 66 randomly assigned patients. Half of the patients in the tai chi group had remarkably clinically important improvements in symptomatology. In an editorial by Yeh et al accompanying the report of the randomized trial of tai chi,[2] it is suggested that with such provocative results being reported with tai chi, the study of Wang et al may have far-reaching implications but that several critical questions remain: how much benefit of tai chi is because of placebo effect and what is the appropriate control for tai chi? The authors dutifully suggest that a true control (sham tai chi intervention) would have been desirable. Ideally, a placebo-control matches all aspects of the therapeutic intervention except for the active element of that intervention, but what is the active element of a complex multicomponent therapy such as tai chi? Is it rhythmic exercise, deliberate and deep breathing, contemplative concentration, group support, relaxing imagery, a charismatic teacher, or some synergistic combination of all these elements? If so, would the matched control include awkward movements, halted breathing, participant isolation, unpleasant imagery, or a tepid teacher? One can see the complexity of trying to control for tai chi.

Despite the potential softness of some of the methodology used in this report, the potential efficacy and lack of adverse effects now make it reasonable for physicians to support patients' interests in exploring tai chi types of exercises, even if it is too early to take out a prescription pad and simply write the words tai chi. One also wonders if other meditative therapies might be effective. How about hypnosis, which has been shown to be possibly effective as part of the management of Tourette syndrome?

The musculoskeletal section often deals with issues related to how to keep our bodies, including our muscles, in shape. We conclude this commentary with an unrelated update on one form of exercise, cycling, and how athletes attempt to beat the odds by doping. A new technique for detecting blood doping in athletes has received a vote of confidence in the sports world. The Court of Arbitration for Sport—considered to be the world's authority on sports disputes—last year upheld the decision by the International Cycling Union (ICU) to bar Italian cyclists Franco Pellizotti and Piatro Caucchioli from competing for 2 years. The 2 cyclists tested positive for doping using ICU's new Athlete Biological Passport (ABP), approved by the World Anti-Doping Agency in 2009. Developed by researchers at the Swiss Laboratories for Doping Analyses in Lausanne, ABP ties an athlete's sex, age, ethnicity, and exposure to altitude to several blood measurements, such as levels of oxygen-binding hemoglobin, which athletes sometimes increase by illegal transfusions or hormone injections. Using previous measurements to establish a personalized baseline, the test flags athletes who have abnormal readings as suspected doping cases. To read more about this new methodology to detect such forms of doping, see the editorial in *Science*.[3]

J. A. Stockman III, MD

References

1. Spaeth M. Epidemiology, cost and the economic burden of fibromyalgia. *Arthritis Res Ther.* 2009;11:117-118.
2. Yeh GY, Kaptchuk TJ, Shmerling RH. Prescribing tai chi for fibromyalgia—are we there yet? *N Engl J Med.* 2010;363:783-784.
3. Editorial comment. New doping test means cyclists can't pull a fast one. *Science.* 2011;331:1373.

Adolescent Chronic Fatigue Syndrome: A Follow-up Study

van Geelen SM, Bakker RJ, Kuis W, et al (Univ Med Ctr Utrecht, the Netherlands)
Arch Pediatr Adolesc Med 164:810-814, 2010

Objective.—To describe the symptomatic and educational long-term outcomes, health care use, and risk factors of nonrecovery in adolescent chronic fatigue syndrome (CFS).

Design.—Follow-up study.

Setting.—Academic pediatric hospital.

Participants.—Sixty adolescents with CFS.

Interventions.—Regular care.

Outcome Measures.—The Checklist Individual Strength, Child Health Questionnaire, and a general questionnaire regarding further symptoms, school attendance, work attendance, and treatment.

Results.—Complete measurements were returned for 54 adolescents (90%). At initial assessment, their mean (SD) age was 16.0 (1.5) years and 20.4% were male. The mean follow-up duration was 2.2 years. At follow-up, the mean (SD) age was 18.2 (1.5) years; 28 adolescents (51.9%) had nearly complete improvement of symptoms but 26 (48.1%) did not experience improvement. Adolescents who attended school (n = 41) had missed an average of 33% of classes during the last month. The rest (n = 13) had worked an average of 38.7% of a full-time job during the last month. A total of 66.7% of subjects were treated by a physiotherapist, 38.9% were clinically treated in rehabilitation, 48.1% had received psychological support, and 53.7% had used alternative treatment.

Conclusions.—About half of the adolescents had recovered from CFS at follow-up. The other half was still severely fatigued and physically impaired. Health care use had been high, and school and work attendance were low. Older age at inclusion was a risk factor, and pain, poor mental health, self-esteem, and general health perception at outcome were associated with an unfavorable outcome. Future research should focus on customizing existing treatment and studying additional treatment options.

▶ For whatever reason, there seems to be an explosion in the literature recently with respect to articles dealing with the chronic fatigue syndrome. This report of van Geelen et al gives us some information about adolescents with this problem. The study describes the long-term outcomes in affected adolescents. We learn that about half of those affected will recover fully but the other half, unfortunately, remain with chronic fatigue, often severe, and are physically impaired.

Included in the recent literature are articles related to a possible viral etiology of the disorder. A recent study linking chronic fatigue syndrome in humans to a family of retroviruses that cause leukemia in mice appears to validate a controversial earlier study.[1,2] Unfortunately, far from settling the debate about the role of viruses in the disease, recent findings simply raise a host of questions about why many scientists, including those in the United States, have failed to find a creditable link between retroviruses and the chronic fatigue syndrome. The cause of chronic fatigue syndrome has long eluded scientists, and it is attractive to think that viruses, such as the xenotropic murine leukemia virus—related virus, found in human prostate cancer cells might be a cause.

It is well established that many cases of chronic fatigue syndrome are preceded by an acute viral infection. There is general consensus that chronic fatigue syndrome is a heterogeneous family of disorders and it seems likely that these disorders arise from a constellation of pathophysiological causes.

With this as a likely given, we are still far from well defining the entity we call chronic fatigue syndrome.

To read more about the biochemical and vascular aspects of pediatric chronic fatigue syndrome, refer to the report of Kennedy et al.[3] This report from the United Kingdom shows, probably for the first time, that oxidative stress and increased white blood cell apoptosis occur in children with the chronic fatigue syndrome. White blood cell apoptosis refers to the early death of neutrophils that has been observed as a marker of an increased cardiovascular risk along with high lipid levels, oxidative stress markers, and inflammatory C-reactive protein. Apoptosis plays a crucial role in developing and maintaining health by eliminating unhealthy cells, old cells, and unnecessary cells. Accelerated apoptosis of neutrophils (which are recruited to the sites of injury within minutes of trauma and are the hallmark of acute inflammation) is observed in patients with infections and other vascular problems. The importance of the report from Great Britain is that it provides somewhat objective documentation of an underlying abnormality in the behavior of immune cells in patients with chronic fatigue syndrome consistent with activated inflammatory processes.

J. A. Stockman III, MD

References

1. Lombardi VC, Ruscetti FW, Das Gupta J, et al. Detection of an infectious retro-virus, XMRV, in blood cells of patients with chronic fatigue syndrome. *Science.* 2009;326:585-589.
2. Kuehn BM. Study reignites debate about viral agents in patients with chronic fatigue syndrome. *JAMA.* 2010;304:1653-1654.
3. Kennedy G, Khan F, Hill A, et al. Biochemical and vascular aspects of pediatric chronic fatigue syndrome. *Arch Pediatr Adolesc Med.* 2010;164:817-823.

Do children who in-toe need to be referred to an orthopaedic clinic?
Blackmur JP, Murray AW (Univ of Edinburgh, UK; Royal Hosp for Sick Children, Edinburgh, UK)
J Pediatr Orthop B 19:415-417, 2010

The objective of this study was to investigate the outcome of in-toeing referrals to a paediatric orthopaedic department. Two hundred and two patients referred to the Royal Hospital for Sick Children, Edinburgh between July 2005 and March 2008 were retrospectively reviewed. Increased femoral anteversion and internal tibial torsion formed the majority of diagnoses. The median age of referral was 4 years. No patient in the audit period required surgery. Eighty-six percent of children were discharged after their first visit. No significant pathology was identified in the 14% reviewed. Management and outcome for these children were not affected by referral to the orthopaedic clinic.

▶ The layperson commonly calls intoeing pigeon feet. While this is a not-so-nice a term, it does adequately describe the nature of the orthopedic issue in affected individuals. Intoeing is a common pediatric problem, and many parents worry about the condition. For whatever reason, they believe that it may lead to long-term musculoskeletal problems or may limit a child's sporting capabilities. From the orthopedic point of view, there are essentially 3 causes of intoeing gait: increased femoral anteversion, internal tibial torsion, and metatarsus adductus. The primary care practitioner should be familiar not only with toeing in but also with each of these 3 causes.

The diagnosis of increased femoral anteversion is specifically made on the basis of increased projection of the femoral neck on the femoral shaft (Fig 2). Specifically, with a child prone and the legs flexed, there will be increased internal rotation, up to 90°, and reduced external rotation. By and large, physical examination is all that is required for this diagnosis of intoeing, and x-rays, ultrasounds, or CT are unnecessary. Please recognize that the condition itself is a developmental norm, with 39° of anteversion at birth, reducing by 1° to 2° every year, up until the adult position of 16° to 24° achieved by skeletal maturity, although only 80% of children reach 10° of the mean angle by 16 years of age. Increased femoral anteversion has never been shown to affect a child's physical ability, and spontaneous correction occurs in more than 80% of cases. If treatment is necessary in someone's mind, nonsurgical techniques (physiotherapy and orthotics) have been shown to be ineffective at either improving outcome or increasing the rate of correction.

With respect to internal tibial torsion (an increased thigh-foot angle), more than 90% of cases resolve spontaneously before skeletal maturity. Again, treatment with wedges, shoes, splints, or orthotics has not been shown to be effective, and the only recommendation for parents is that they avoid their child sleeping in a prone position or from sitting on his/her feet (characteristic positions for children with the condition). While some parents are concerned about the fact that internal tibial torsion may reduce physical ability, it has actually been shown that sprinters tend to have increased internal tibial torsion

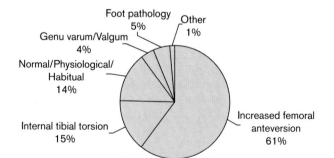

FIGURE 2.—Chart of primary diagnoses for in-toeing. Increased femoral anteversion and internal tibial torsion made up the bulk of the pathology seen. 'Normal/physiological/habitual' in-toeing represents a diagnosis made on the basis of normal walking for the age of that child, or where the child in-toes as a result of habit. The three terms were used interchangeably in the notes. In all these eventualities, there is no pathology to identify. 'Foot pathology' represents pes planus, metatarsus adductus or pronation of the forefoot. 'Other' represents leg length discrepancy, reduced peroneal power or in-toeing after an ankle injury. (Reprinted from Blackmur JP, Murray AW. Do children who in-toe need to be referred to an orthopaedic clinic?. *J Pediatr Orthop B.* 2010;19:415-417.)

compared with control populations. The link between internal tibial torsion and osteoarthritis in the knee is somewhat controversial, but many orthopedic surgeons believe that there is no such link.

True metatarsus adductus is not a particularly common problem, affecting 1 in 1000 live births, with the diagnosis made on the basis of a curved lateral border of the foot. Again, up to 90% of cases resolve before age 1, with only a minority of cases requiring splints or passive stretching. About 5% of affected children will have the condition persisting into adulthood—again, with no increased risk of osteoarthritis or surgical correction.

So why this long background on the report of Blackmur et al? This report summarizes an audit of cases referred by general practitioners of the Royal Hospital for Sick Children in Edinburgh for assessment of toeing in. The average age of a child who was referred was 4 years. In virtually no cases were there any recommendations for different management other than operation. Surgery for femoral anteversion or for internal tibial torsion was considered in a distinct minority of cases and then only rarely when there was severe cosmetic or functional deformity and when there is an anteversion of more than 50° or a thigh-foot angle more than 3 SDs from the mean. The authors of this report say that no surgical treatment should be considered for those younger than 10 years given the risk of surgical complications (such as avascular necrosis).

Thus, we primary care pediatricians need to learn that toeing in is a disorder that, except in very exceptional circumstances, should be managed on our watch and simply with observation. All too often, these kids get to be seen by podiatrists who order orthotics or are seen by physiotherapists who order physical therapy or shoe implants needlessly. The trick here is to figure out how to provide the reassurance families need in order to avoid unnecessary referrals or needless treatments.

This commentary closes with an unrelated brief observation having to do with some very old feet. A tiny 3.2 million-year-old fossil found in East Africa gives Lucy's kind an unprecedented toehold on human-like walking. *Australopithecus afarensis*, an ancient hominid species best known for a partial female skeleton called Lucy, had stiff foot arches like those of people today. A bone from the fourth toe—the first such *A afarensis* fossil on earth—provides crucial evidence that bends in this hominid's feet supported and cushioned a 2-legged stride. The new fossil confirms that members of Lucy's species could have made 3.6 million-year-old footprints previously found in hardened volcanic ash at Laetoli in Tanzania. *A afarensis* lived from about 4 million to 3 million years ago. News of arched feet in these hominids follows a report that a recently discovered *A afarensis* skeleton dubbed Big Man, who, though footless, displays long legs, a relatively narrow chest, and an inwardly curving back—all signs of nearly human-like gait. Thus it is that even as long ago as 4 million years, creatures that may very well have evolved into us stood upright and walked like we do, sort of, and hopefully did so without being pigeon-toed.

J. A. Stockman III, MD

Risk of Injury Associated With Body Checking Among Youth Ice Hockey Players

Emery CA, Kang J, Shrier I, et al (Univ of Calgary, Alberta, Canada; McGill Univ, Montreal, Quebec, Canada; et al)
JAMA 303:2265-2272, 2010

Context.—Ice hockey has one of the highest sport participation and injury rates in youth in Canada. Body checking is the predominant mechanism of injury in leagues in which it is permitted.

Objective.—To determine if risk of injury and concussion differ for Pee Wee (ages 11-12 years) ice hockey players in a league in which body checking is permitted (Alberta, Canada) vs a league in which body checking is not permitted (Quebec, Canada).

Design, Setting, and Participants.—Prospective cohort study conducted in Alberta and Quebec during the 2007-2008 Pee Wee ice hockey season. Participants (N = 2154) were players from teams in the top 60% of divisions of play.

Main Outcome Measures.—Incidence rate ratios adjusted for cluster based on Poisson regression for game- and practice-related injury and concussion.

Results.—Seventy-four Pee Wee teams from Alberta (n = 1108 players) and 76 Pee Wee teams from Quebec (n = 1046 players) completed the study. In total, there were 241 injuries (78 concussions) reported in Alberta (85 077 exposure-hours) and 91 injuries (23 concussions) reported in Quebec (82 099 exposure-hours). For game-related injuries, the Alberta vs Quebec incidence rate ratio was 3.26 (95% confidence interval [CI], 2.31-4.60 [n = 209 and n = 70 for Alberta and Quebec, respectively]) for all injuries, 3.88 (95% CI, 1.91-7.89 [n = 73 and n = 20]) for concussion, 3.30 (95% CI, 1.77-6.17 [n = 51 and n = 16]) for severe injury (time loss, >7 days), and 3.61 (95% CI, 1.16-11.23 [n = 14 and n = 4]) for severe concussion (time loss, >10 days). The estimated absolute risk reduction (injuries per 1000 player-hours) that would be achieved if body checking were not permitted in Alberta was 2.84 (95% CI, 2.18-3.49) for all game-related injuries, 0.72 (95% CI, 0.40-1.04) for severe injuries, 1.08 (95% CI, 0.70-1.46) for concussion, and 0.20 (95% CI, 0.04-0.37) for severe concussion. There was no difference between provinces for practice-related injuries.

Conclusion.—Among 11- to 12-year-old ice hockey players, playing in a league in which body checking is permitted compared with playing in a league in which body checking is not permitted was associated with a 3-fold increased risk of all game-related injuries and the categories of concussion, severe injury, and severe concussion.

▶ Until I read this report, I was not aware of how widespread ice hockey had become as a true phenomenon in North America. More than half a million registered youth are players in Hockey Canada, and almost one-third of a million registered players are in the US Hockey Association as of a couple of years ago. In Canada, hockey injuries account for about 10% of all youth sports injuries. A good many of these injuries are the result of body checking. It is clear from this report and others that children playing ice hockey in leagues that permit body checking have more concussions and other injuries than do youngsters in leagues that prohibit checking.

Checking in hockey is akin to blocking in football. In hockey, it is a defensive hit, in which a player attempts to stop or limit the progress of an offensive player who has the puck. While a check cannot be delivered with the elbows, knees, or a hockey stick, it can still involve a violent collision. Some youth leagues disallow checks altogether among preteens. In Quebec in the late 1980s, the entire province banned checking for all players aged 12 years and younger.

In the report of Emery et al from Canada, we see the frequency of body checking injuries among youth ice hockey players. Participants (aged 11 to 12 years) in Pee Wee leagues were studied. If a youngster played in a league in which body checking was permitted, that youngster had a 3-fold probability of sustaining a game-related injury with concussions being the most common severe injury.

The report of Emery et al is the first prospective cohort study using a validated injury surveillance system to examine the risk of playing in an ice hockey league that permits body checking compared with one that does not. Given all the recent information about the long-term consequences of sustaining concussions, one has to worry about these young kids and how they will function in society 30, 40, or more years later. Coaches in these sports have recently taken a more cautious approach to concussions, keeping players out of subsequent games as a precaution. Also in recent times, the definition of a concussion has changed to include injuries that cause dizziness, brief memory loss, headache, or other symptoms that fall short of a loss of consciousness. Being hit on the head and passing out was once part of playing the game. It is no longer acceptable, particularly in this young age group.

This commentary closes with an observation having to do with another sporting activity: marathon running. A marathoner's worst nightmare—hitting "the wall"—may be completely avoidable if athletes adhere to personalized pace limits. It appears that a 10-second difference in pace per mile could make the difference between success and a dramatic failure. All too often runners push hard early on and then run out of steam in the last few miles of a marathon. To avoid this scenario, a runner has to maintain a pace that conserves carbohydrates, the body's main source of quick-burn energy. Investigators have now calculated the ideal pace from a measure of aerobic fitness using maximum ventilatory capacity and other body measurements in determining how efficiently a body consumes oxygen. Using appropriate calculations, it can be shown that given enough carbs before a race, a man with a VO_2MAX of 60—which after training is attainable only by the top 10% of male runners—can achieve a 3:10 marathon finish time. This time happens to be the cutoff for 18- to 34-year-old men to qualify for the Boston Marathon. VO_2MAX is usually measured with specialized equipment while someone exercises at maximum exertion, but it can be estimated by measuring heart rate at rest or while running at a constant pace. On-the-go snacking helps, but it cannot win races because the body can store only so much fuel, thus the need to be able to predict whether someone can finish a race in a formula-predicted time. To help runners calculate their ideal pace, developers of the predictive model have put a version of their formula online.[1] To read more about all of this, see the editorial by Sanders.[2]

J. A. Stockman III, MD

References

1. Endurance calculator: precision for endurance running. http://endurancecalculator. com/. Accessed August 23, 2011.
2. Sanders L. Making a marathon manageable. *Science News*. November 20, 2010:8.

Escalators, Rubber Clogs, and Severe Foot Injuries in Children

Leong Lim KB, Tey IK, Lokino ES, et al (KK Women's & Children's Hosp, Singapore)
J Pediatr Orthop 30:414-419, 2010

Background.—Reports in the media suggest that escalator-related foot injuries are on the rise. Trendy, bright-colored rubber clogs have been implicated in a significant number of these incidents involving children. We review the children who sustained severe foot injuries on escalators, were wearing rubber clogs at the time of injury, and who were admitted to hospital for emergency surgery.

Methods.—A list of children who sustained foot injuries on escalators was generated from the hospital database and included for study. From clinical chart review, demographic data, footwear type, and injuries sustained were recorded. Inpatient or outpatient treatment rendered was also recorded for each patient.

Results.—Between September 2006 and September 2008, we treated 17 children for escalator-related foot injuries. There were 10 boys and 7 girls who were between 2 and 9 years of age (mean: 5.5). Thirteen children (76.5%) from this group were wearing rubber clogs at the time of injury. Nine of these 13 (69.2%) children sustained severe foot injuries that required admission to hospital for emergency surgery and are the focus of this study. One child had an unsalvageable traumatic amputation of the great toe at the level of the interphalangeal joint. Two children sustained crush injuries to the great toe: 1 with severe degloving and the other with an open fracture of the proximal phalanx. One child had an open fracture-dislocation of the second metatarsophalangeal joint with a comminuted fracture of the second metatarsal. Five children sustained multiple deep lacerations in the foot and 2 of them had associated cut tendons that required repair. In the group not wearing rubber clogs, 3 of 4 children had severe foot injuries. In this series, 4 children with rubber clogs and another child with a different footwear sustained minor injuries; they were treated as outpatients.

Conclusions.—Escalator-related foot injuries involving rubber clogs can result in severe crushing of the foot and even traumatic amputation. The broad toe-box design may give a false perception of the distance between the foot and the side of the escalator, whereas the 'softness' of these rubber clogs makes them vulnerable to crush by moving escalator steps. This is the first report in the literature describing escalator-related severe foot injuries in children who were wearing rubber clogs. Injuries sustained can be significant and permanent. The potential dangers of escalators and rubber clogs must not be underestimated.

Level of Evidence.—Level IV, Case Series.

▶ This report from Singapore is really scary since there is no reason to believe that a similar situation is not occurring in the United States. There is a fair amount of literature on escalator-related foot injuries. What is unique about this report from Singapore, however, is the linkage of such injuries to the wearing of rubber clogs by children. These rubber clogs have been on the market now for several years and clearly have evolved into a somewhat popular fashion accessory. This trendy footwear is comfortable and available in various colors and designs. The toe box at the front is perforated for ventilation, and a rubber hind strap that goes around the heel keeps the foot secured in the clog. The broad toe box design gives the appearance of an oversized footwear and, hence, a false perception of the distance between the foot and its surroundings. The softness of its material also makes it extremely pliable. As such, a rubber clog can be somewhat easily trapped into the edges of moving escalator steps and readily crushed by the steps once it has caught on to the metallic side panel. In recent years, rubber clogs have come under increased scrutiny owing to escalator accidents involving children. Various warnings have appeared about the hazards of wearing these and escalator injuries. The US Consumer Product Safety Commission reports that 77 escalator entrapment incidents were documented between 2006 and 2007. All but 2 involved soft-sided flexible rubber clogs.

The report from Singapore summarizes information on 17 children treated for escalator-related foot injuries between September 2006 and September 2008. The youngsters ranged in age from 2 to 9 years, and three-quarters of the children were wearing rubber clogs at the time of foot injury. Two-thirds of the children sustained severe foot injuries that required hospitalization for emergency surgery. A case of a 5-year old is illustrative of the problem. She had her left foot caught in an escalator. Her rubber clog was ripped into several parts (Fig 2). She sustained a complete amputation of her left great toe at the level of the base of the distal phalanx. The amputated toe was recovered, but the severity of the youngster's injury did not allow reattachment. The neurovascular bundle was completely crushed. She had to undergo disarticulation at the level of the interphalangeal joint. The wound eventually healed without complications.

In response to reports of escalator-related foot injuries owing to rubber clogs, Crocs, Inc, one of the principal manufacturers of these rubber clogs, launched the Escalator Safety Awareness Initiative. In this effort, Crocs uses tags on its

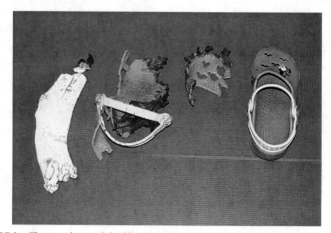

FIGURE 2.—The severely mangled rubber clog of a 5-year-old girl after being trapped in an escalator. (Reprinted from Leong Lim KB, Tey IK, Lokino ES, et al. Escalators, rubber clogs, and severe foot injuries in children. *J Pediatr Orthop*. 2010;30:414-419.)

shoes to provide its customers with escalator safety information. Although one of the future goals of this initiative is to push for changes in escalator safety code regulations regarding the design, installation, and maintenance, it also supports organizations that further the cause of safe escalator maintenance and use.

The data from this report are quite chilling. They are not a crock. The combination of childhood, Crocs, and escalators are a bad mix—a mix to be avoided.

J. A. Stockman III, MD

Prognostic Impact of Atypical Presentation in Pediatric Systemic Lupus Erythematosus: Results from a Multicenter Study

Taddio A, Rossetto E, Rosé CD, et al (Univ of Trieste, Italy; Thomas Jefferson Univ, Wilmington, DE; et al)
J Pediatr 156:972-977, 2010

Objectives.—The aim of the study is to assess the rate of atypical manifestations at onset in pediatric systemic lupus erythematosus (SLE) and to evaluate their effect on disease outcome.

Study Design.—This is a multicenter retrospective cohort study. A manifestation was considered atypical if it was not included in the American College Rheumatology classification criteria for SLE but was reported in literature as associated with SLE. Unfavorable outcome was considered presence of organ damage in the Systemic Lupus International Collaborative Clinics/American College of Rheumatology Damage Index at the last available evaluation.

Results.—One hundred patients were enrolled in the study; 24% presented atypical clinical features at onset. Univariate analysis showed a significant association of worse outcome variables with the presence of atypical manifestations at onset ($P = .004$), as well as renal involvement ($P = .027$). A multivariate logistic regression analysis showed that atypical manifestations at onset ($P = .018$), renal involvement at onset or during follow up ($P = .024$), and central nervous system disease involvement during follow up ($P = .021$) were independent predictors of poor prognosis.

Conclusions.—Our data support a relatively high rate of atypical onset in pediatric SLE. Presence of atypical manifestations at presentation and early kidney disease correlate with poor outcome. Similarly, during follow-up, kidney and central nervous system diseases are associated with worse outcome (Table 1).

▶ Most of us are familiar with the fact that autoimmune disorders can present in very atypical ways. This report from Italy and the Alfred I. duPont Hospital for Children in Delaware tells us just how atypically systemic lupus erythematosus (SLE) can present. Since SLE is a multisystem inflammatory autoimmune disease, its presentation can be very protean, with just 1 or 2 organ systems being the initial source of signs and symptoms. The multicenter retrospective cohort study of Taddio et al summarizes data from 100 patients with SLE (age range 3-18 years), followed up for 3 to 10 years. The investigators catalog atypical clinical features as those presenting with gastrointestinal involvement (abdominal pain, acute abdomen, intestinal perforation, intestinal bleeding, hemorrhagic or aseptic peritonitis, pseudo-obstruction, pancreatitis, hepatitis, and cholecystitis), cardiac involvement (myocarditis, acute valvular insufficiency), ocular involvement (retinal vasculitis, posterior uveitis), pulmonary involvement (acute and chronic lupus pneumonitis, pulmonary hemorrhage), endocrinopathy (hypoparathyroidism, primary hyperparathyroidism, hypothyroidism, parotiditis, sicca syndrome), neurologic involvement (chorea), and hemolytic uremic syndrome. One atypical manifestation of SLE was present in 24 patients, whereas 76 patients showed only classical manifestations fitting the usual classifying criteria for SLE by the American College of Rheumatology. The table shows the frequency of these atypical manifestations. Classical clinical manifestations included findings such as malar rash, photosensitivity, small-sized vessel leukocytoclastic vasculitis with intravascular thrombosis in deeper dermis, Raynaud phenomenon, arthritis/arthralgia, leukopenia, autoimmune hemolytic anemia, thrombocytopenia, fever, proteinuria, abnormal urinalysis, acute kidney failure, and nephrotic syndrome.

Thus in the pediatric population, about 1 in 4 patients with SLE may present with nonclassical clinical manifestations of the disease. When these nonclassical manifestations are isolated, the diagnosis may not easily be thought of. The authors of this report also tell us an important observation that atypical manifestations independently predict poorer outcome in patients with SLE.

In addition, the findings from this report underline the important finding that almost 10% of patients presenting with pediatric lupus will not have any classical clinical findings of lupus at all. Only later do the more typical findings

TABLE 1.—Atypical Manifestations at Onset in a Cohort of Patients with pSLE

	No. (%)
Gastrointestinal involvement	26 (67%)
Abdominal pain	6
Acute abdomen	7
Intestinal perforation	1
Intestinal bleeding	4
Hemorrhagic or aseptic peritonitis	—
Pseudoobstruction	—
Pancreatitis	1
Hepatitis	6
Cholecystitis	1
Cardiac involvement	3 (8%)
Myocarditis	1
Acute valvular insufficiency	2
Ocular involvement	2 (5%)
Retinal vasculitis	2
Posterior uveitis	—
Pulmonary involvement	2 (5%)
Acute or chronic lupus pneumonitis	1
Pulmonary hemorrhage	1
Endocrinopathy	6 (15%)
Hypoparathyroidism	—
Primary hyperparathyroidism	—
Hypothyroidism	—
Parotitis	1
Sicca syndrome	5
Neurologic involvement (Chorea)	—
HUS	—

appear in most of these patients. The bottom line is that we pediatricians should consider SLE in any patient presenting with fever and unexplained organ involvement even if the patient otherwise does not fit the American College of Rheumatology's classification criteria for SLE.

This commentary closes with an update on the first lupus drug approved in the last 50 years. In early March 2011, the US Food and Drug Administration (FDA) gave the green light to a new treatment for lupus. The therapy, called belimumab and marketed as Benlysta, is one of the first to be developed based on human genome research. It is far from perfect: the FDA estimated that about 11 people need to get the monoclonal antibody for one to benefit. Human Genome Sciences developed belimumab after it discovered a new protein in 1996 called BLyS, which helps to regulate B cells. When BLyS levels rise in lupus patients, the disease often worsens. More than 2 dozen lupus patients and advocates testified at a November 2010 FDA advisory meeting to discuss the therapy, pleading for approval. A phase III trial of the drug that included some older teenagers was recently reported and showed therapeutic advantages with modest toxicity.[1]

J. A. Stockman III, MD

Reference

1. Navarra S, Guzmán RM, Gallacher A. Efficacy and safety of belimumab in patients with active systemic lupus erythematosus: a randomized, placebo-controlled phase III trial. *Lancet.* 2011;377:721-731.

Familial Mediterranean Fever in the First Two Years of Life: A Unique Phenotype of Disease in Evolution

Padeh S, Livneh A, Pras E, et al (Edmond & Lily Safra Children's Hosp, Tel Hashomer, Israel; Sheba Med Ctr, Tel Hashomer, Israel)
J Pediatr 156:985-989, 2010

Objective.—To characterize the clinical and genetic features of familial Mediterranean fever (FMF).

Study Design.—Clinical presentation and MEditerranean FeVer mutation type of all patients with FMF, who first manifested the disease at ≤2 years of age were analyzed and compared with patients who first presented with FMF between 2 and 16 years.

Results.—Of 814 patients with FMF, in 254 patients (31.2%) the first FMF attack was at ≤2 years of age, with a mean age at onset of 1.1 ± 0.8 years. They were compared with 242 patients who presented with their first manifestation of FMF at 2 to 16 years. The clinical manifestations of FMF were comparable in the 2 patient groups, but the delay of diagnosis was longer in patients with early presentation (3.2 ± 3.2 years vs. 1.9 ± 2.7 years in the group with onset at 2-16 years, $P < .001$). A subgroup of patients (60/254), who were diagnosed at ≤2 years had the highest rate of attacks of fever alone as their sole manifestation (40.0% vs 8.4%, $P < .05$), and less peritonitis (45% vs 86.1%, $P < .05$) and pleuritis (3.4% vs 32.9%, $P < .05$). Most of these patients were homozygous for the *M694V* mutation and were of North African (Sephardic Jewish) extraction.

Conclusion.—In early life, FMF often begins with an atypical presentation, characterized by attacks of fever alone, and its diagnosis and initiation of treatment is therefore significantly delayed.

▶ Familial Mediterranean fever (FMF), while not common, is not rare in its presentation in children. Painful febrile episodes, the hallmark of the disease, are in most cases accompanied by signs of peritonitis, pleuritis, or acute synovitis, mainly in the lower extremities. Attacks of fever alone or with headache and general malaise may also occur. Over the course of the illness, a patient may experience several forms of attack. Symptoms related to FMF are often noted only when children become more verbal, usually after 2 years of age. In fact, the literature on FMF in patients presenting younger than 2 years of age is extremely limited, making most of us unaware of exactly how this disorder could present in very early childhood. The study by Padeh et al helps us all learn quite a bit about how the disease presents in this very young age group, presenting data from the Sheba Medical Center in Tel Aviv.

At the Sheba Medical Center in Israel, more than 800 patients with FMF have been diagnosed since early 2000. The medical center keeps an extremely detailed computerized database on all of its patients. One-third of the patients clearly had symptoms before 2 years of age. In those presenting before 2 years of age, fever as a sole manifestation of FMF was highly predominant when compared with older age patients. The younger patients had a much lower rate of abdominal attacks, pleuritis, and arthritis. Elevation of acute phase reactants during attacks was similar in all age groups.

There were other differences in the presentation of patients presenting at less than 2 years of age. Most predominantly was the observation that the rate of patients homozygous for the M694V mutation was significantly higher. All patients, regardless of age, had similar responses to colchicine prophylaxis with resolution or reduction in the number or intensity of the attacks. It also took just about the same amount of colchicine (when calculated based on body weight) to control the attacks, regardless of age. Colchicine was well tolerated by all patients.

For those in pediatric practice in the United States, most of us know that recurrent fever of undetermined origin at any age should lead one to suspect FMF in the differential diagnosis. This is an autosomal recessive disease, mainly affecting Jews, Armenians, Turks, Arabs, and other ethnic groups living around the Mediterranean basin, such as Druze, Greeks, and Italians. Given the melting pot aspect of our country, all of these populations are reflected on our shores. The FMF gene (*MEFV*) was identified almost 20 years ago along with its product, pyrin/marenostrin. As of now, more than 50 *MEFV* mutations have been described, and more are being described all the time. The diagnosis, however, is still largely clinically based and no other routine laboratory finding is disease specific. You may recall that this editor and his family for more than a decade enjoyed the presence of Riley, a female Sharpei. Riley, beginning at 15 weeks of age, started to experience periodic episodes of painful joints, swelling of the face and abdomen, and fever. After several episodes, a very astute veterinary canine internal medicine resident at the veterinary school of North Carolina State University made the correct diagnosis: familial Sharpei fever, which had just then been described as the animal model of FMF in humans. With careful monitoring and the use of colchicine, Riley far outlived the normal natural history of this disease. The natural course of FMF in both humans and Sharpeis is death from amyloidosis after varying periods of time.

This commentary closes with an observation having to do with physical activity. The musculoskeletal topic often contains information about injuries and other morbidities associated with physical activity. A recent report tells us about the association of episodic physical activity and sexual activity with the triggering of acute cardiac events. In a systematic review and meta-analysis of the literature, Dahabreh et al observed that physical activity increases the risk of sudden cardiac death by almost 5-fold.[1] The same was true of sexual activity. It should be noted, however, that if one engages in regular physical activity, this added risk is much, much less. The same may not be true for sexual activity. If there is a bottom line here it is that if one does not engage in regular physical activity, it might be better to engage in none at all, or so says one who believes that one is born with a fixed number of heart beats and that these should not be wasted on exercise.

J. A. Stockman III, MD

Reference

1. Dahabreh IJ, Paulus JK. Association of episodic physical activity and sexual activity with triggering of acute cardiac events. *JAMA*. 2011;305:1225-1233.

13 Neurology and Psychiatry

United States Head Circumference Growth Reference Charts: Birth to 21 Years

Rollins JD, Collins JS, Holden KR (Greenwood Genetic Ctr, SC)

J Pediatr 156:907-913, 2010

Objective.—To produce a more reliable, continuous set of occipito-frontal head circumference (OFC) growth reference charts for males and females from birth to adulthood in the United States.

Study Design.—After investigating the strengths and shortcomings of previous reports, we combined the most recent statistically reliable reports of OFC growth reference data into a locally weighted regression analysis to estimate percentile curves. We used cross-sectional prospective local pediatric data to validate our results.

Results.—We present new age- and sex-appropriate US OFC growth charts from birth to adulthood that include 3rd and 97th percentile cutoff values. Our local pediatric data validate that our new proposed OFC growth charts' assessment of attained OFC growth is comparable with previous references.

Conclusions.—We have eliminated disagreements between multiple current references by unifying previously reported US OFC data into a single set of smoothed male and female growth reference charts from birth to adulthood. This will reduce confusion or errors in interpretation of normal versus abnormal measurements currently encountered by primary care clinicians and subspecialists when using OFC growth charts for the US pediatric population.

▶ This report begins with a reminder that there are more than 500 conditions that manifest themselves with either microcephaly or macrocephaly. The issue, however, is what constitutes either of these. Currently the Centers for Disease Control (CDC) Occipitofrontal Circumference (OFC) growth charts are the most accepted and most reliable OFC reference to date. Unfortunately, these charts only address the age range from birth to 36 months. The most recent OFC growth charts from the CDC became available in 2000.[1] Traditionally, when a youngster outgrows the CDC charts, the health care provider must turn to other published OFC charts. The most recent normative OFC growth charts for children up to age 18 years were published in 1987.[2] In 2007, the

347

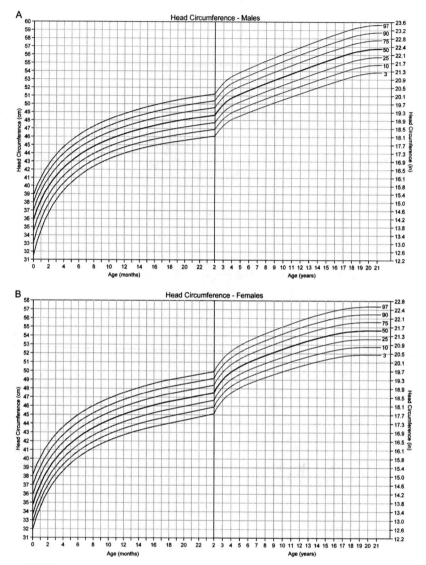

FIGURE 4.—Proposed OFC growth curves. A, Males. B, Females. (Reprinted from Journal of Pediatrics, Rollins JD, Collins JS, Holden KR. United States head circumference growth reference charts: birth to 21 years. *J Pediatr.* 2010;156:907-913. Copyright 2010 with permission from Elsevier.)

World Health Organization released OFC growth charts intended for international use. The latter charts are based on measurements of healthy children living under conditions likely to favor the achievement of full genetic growth potential. The youngsters measured also had careful histories taken to avoid inclusion of subjects exposed to maternal smoking. Other environmental factors were also standardized such as breast-feeding. Generally speaking, most individuals define microcephaly as −2 standard deviations (SDs) from the mean and macrocephaly as +2 SDs from the mean. The 3rd and 97th percentiles are ±1.88 SDs.

What Rollins et al have done is to reconcile previous work from multiple sources to create a set of unified OFC growth reference charts defined by the 3rd and 97th percentile for use by those responsible for pediatric care and clinical research in the United States. These curves take the best data from a variety of different sources and blend them together. By drawing on the strengths of multiple older OFC studies of various age ranges, the authors suggest that the new OFC growth reference charts presented in the figure appear to be more useful in the US clinical setting than any currently available chart. They could allow monitoring of OFC across all pediatric ages eliminating the confusion associated with switching references as a child grows (Fig 4).

While on the topic of microcephaly, an interesting report appeared recently in the neurology literature: a report, while having a distasteful title, "Pinheads," still provides very useful, interesting, and historical insights into how society once viewed medical disorders and labeled some individuals as freakish.[3] Unfortunately, the circus sideshow was a smorgasbord of human performers, shrewdly designed to entertain the middle class public and to exploit the attitudes of the time. Under the vernacular of "pinheads," people with microcephaly and mental retardation were displayed as "freaks." The report of Mateen et al pulled its original materials from the Ringling Brothers Circus Museum archives and Harvard Theater Collection, including sideshow banners, circus programs, song lyrics, and performance photographs in addition to contemporary newspaper articles, major medical journal publications and other secondary sources regarding microcephaly in the 19th and early 20th century circuses. Individuals with microcephaly were exhibited as "pinheads," portrayed as "missing links" or children from lost civilizations. These exhibitions eventually declined because of protective laws passed in part due to American circus "freak shows."

J. A. Stockman III, MD

References

1. Kuczmarski RJ, Ogden CL, Grummer-Strawn LM, et al. CDC growth charts: United States. *Adv Data.* 2000;314:1-27.
2. Roche AF, Mukherjee D, Guo S, Moore WM. Head circumference reference data: birth to 18 years. *Pediatrics.* 1987;79:706-712.
3. Mateen FJ, Boes CJ. "Pinheads": The exhibition of neurologic disorders at "The Greatest Show on Earth." *Neurol.* 2010;75:2028-2032.

Postnatal-Onset Microcephaly: Pathogenesis, Patterns of Growth, and Prediction of Outcome

Rosman NP, Tarquinio DC, Datseris M, et al (Boston Univ School of Medicine, MA; Albert Einstein College of Medicine at Long Island Jewish Med Ctr, Glen Oaks, NY; et al)

Pediatrics 127:665-671, 2011

Objective.—Although children with postnatal-onset microcephaly (POM) generally have poor development, we speculated that better somatic growth would predict better development in these children.

Patients and Methods.—We followed 57 children with POM for an average of 4.2 years (13 encephaloclastic, 14 dysgenetic, 6 with Rett syndrome, 24 idiopathic) and calculated the developmental quotient (DQ) at each visit (DQ >0.70 was considered normal). SD scores (SDS) for measurements were analyzed using a repeated measures mixed-effects model to assess effect of weight, height, head circumference (HC), and age on DQ. Pearson's correlation was used to examine the independent influence of each variable on final DQ.

Results.—Forty-four children (77%) had a low DQ (mean: 0.33), but 13 (23%) had a normal DQ (mean: 0.93), including 10 idiopathic and 3 encephaloclastic. Mean HC fell below -2 SDS in all before 1 year (destructive at 3.3 months, idiopathic low-DQ at 7.5 months, dysgenetic at 8.5 months, Rett syndrome at 11 months, and idiopathic normal-DQ at 11.5 months). Mean weights and heights both fell below -2 SDS for all low-DQ groups but remained normal in both normal-DQ groups. Weight, height, and HC were independent predictors of DQ ($P < .0001$). Final DQ correlated with weight ($r = 0.27$), height ($r = 0.41$), and HC ($r = 0.13$).

Conclusions.—Most children with POM have poor later development. Whatever the cause of POM, persons in whom postnatal body growth (weight, height, HC) is better sustained have more favorable development, and in one-quarter of such persons (mostly idiopathic POM), final DQ is normal (Table 1).

▶ There is virtually nothing written in the literature about postnatal-onset microcephaly. This is the importance of the report abstracted that elucidates the natural history of postnatal-onset microcephaly and tells us whether somatic growth can predict developmental outcome in these children. It is clear that although most youngsters with this problem will have a low developmental quotient, about 1 in 5 children will have a normal IQ. Table 1 illustrates the various causes of acquired microcephaly and its prognosis. The best prognosis is seen in those whose microcephaly is idiopathic. Three-fourths of those with normal development fell into this category.

On a related topic, recent literature tells us about how successful or not repositioning is with respect to the management of babies with asymmetrical heads (plagiocephaly). Such infants are conventionally treated with "active repositioning" or by wearing orthotic helmets, but the evidence to date has not pointed to either of these methods as being superior. An analysis of 3-dimensional surface

TABLE 1.—Fifty-seven Cases of Acquired Microcephaly: Pathogenesis, Somatic Growth, and Prognosis

	Encephaloclastic Low DQ (N=10)	Encephaloclastic Normal DQ (N=3)	Encephaloclastic Combined (N=13)	Dysgenetic Low DQ (N=14)	Rett Syndrome Low DQ (N=6)	Idiopathic Low DQ (N=14)	Idiopathic Normal DQ (N=10)	Idiopathic Combined (N=24)	Combined Low DQ (N=44)	Combined Normal DQ (N=13)	Total (N=57)
Birth weight percentile	57 (±29)	24 (±1.3)	51 (±31)	27 (±30)	57 (±39)	38 (±39)	43 (±30)	40 (±35)	42 (±39)	39 (±29)	41 (±37)
Birth height percentile	52 (±27)	22[a]	49 (±28)	7 (±34)	63 (±28)	51 (±31)	65 (±12)	57 (±24)	45 (±37)	59 (±18)	48 (±34)
Birth head circumference percentile	47 (±36)	23 (±34)	41 (±37)	38 (±47)	53 (±35)	35 (±28)	35 (±26)	35 (±27)	41 (±38)	32 (±28)	39 (±37)
Final weight percentile	3 (±35)	7 (±11)	4 (±31)	1 (±31)	1 (±0.04)	7 (±27)	12 (±32)	9 (±29)	1 (±33)	11 (±27)	2 (±38)
Final height percentile	6 (±38)	12 (±6)	7 (±34)	1 (±43)	2 (±37)	12 (±37)	41(±34)	25 (±42)	2 (±54)	35 (±35)	6 (±62)
Final head circumference percentile	1 (±0.5)	1 (±4)	1 (±1)	1 (±2)	1 (±0.4)	1 (±1)	1 (±2)	1 (±1)	1 (±1)	1 (±2)	1 (±2)
Final DQ	0.38 (±0.18)	0.78 (±0.08)	0.47 (±0.24)	0.32 (±0.17)	0.15 (±0.16)	0.39 (±0.17)	0.98 (±0.18)	0.64 (±0.34)	0.33 (±0.18)	0.93 (±0.18)	0.47 (±0.31)

All values reported as mean (± SD).
[a]Only 1 value present in this category.

scans of the whole head in 70 infants, using stereophotogrammetric imaging technology has shown that helmeting produces a greater reduction in asymmetry than active repositioning, most obviously in the occiput region. Whether this difference has any clinical significance is not yet known.[1]

J. A. Stockman III, MD

Reference

1. Lipira AB, Gordon S, Darvann PA. Helmet versus active repositioning for plagiocephaly: a 3-dimensional analysis. *Pediatrics.* 2010;126:e936-e945. Epub 2010 Sep 13.

Childhood Predictors of Use and Costs of Antidepressant Medication by Age 24 Years: Findings from the Finnish Nationwide 1981 Birth Cohort Study

Gyllenberg D, Sourander A, Niemelä S, et al (Univ of Helsinki and Helsinki Univ Hosp, Finland; Univ of Turku and Turku Univ Hosp, Finland; et al)
J Am Acad Child Adolesc Psychiatry 50:406-415, 2011

Objective.—Prior studies on antidepressant use in late adolescence and young adulthood have been cross-sectional, and prospective associations with childhood psychiatric problems have not been examined. The objective was to study the association between childhood problems and lifetime prevalence and costs of antidepressant medication by age 24 years.

Method.—A total of 5,547 subjects from a nation-wide birth cohort were linked to the National Prescription Register. Information about parent- and teacher-reported conduct, hyperkinetic and emotional symptoms, and self-reported depressive symptoms was gathered at age 8 years. The main outcome measure was national register-based lifetime information about purchases of antidepressants between ages 8 and 24 years. In addition, antidepressant costs were analyzed using a Heckman maximum likelihood model.

Results.—In all, 8.8% of males and 13.8% of females had used antidepressants between age 13 and 24 years. Among males, conduct problems independently predicted later antidepressant use. In both genders, self-reported depressive symptoms and living in other than a family with two biological parent at age 8 years independently predicted later antidepressant use. Significant gender interactions were found for conduct and hyperkinetic problems, indicating that more males who had these problems at age 8 have used antidepressants compared with females with the same problems.

Conclusions.—Childhood psychopathology predicts use of antidepressants, but the type of childhood psychopathology predicting antidepressant use is different among males and females.

▶ This report provides extraordinarily valuable information about the pervasive use of antidepressive medication by young people. Historical data show that between 1996 and 2005 in the United States, the percentage of persons aged

18 to 34 years who were treated with antidepressant medication during the course of a 1-year period increased from 4% to 7%.[1] Selective serotonin reuptake inhibitors, particularly fluoxetine, became popular in the late 1980s. Since then, new antidepressant medications have been associated with fewer side effects and lower toxicity in overdose. This reduced side effect rate has probably contributed to the increased use of antidepressants along with the publication of clinical guidelines supporting their use for a variety of conditions well beyond depression, including panic disorder, social phobia, and posttraumatic stress disorder. Additionally, there is wide use of off-label prescription of antidepressants for children and adolescents given the fact that most guidelines were developed for adults. Special attention has been drawn to the possibility of an elevated risk of suicidal behavior in teens. This has resulted in the US Food and Drug Administration marking antidepressant labels with a black box warning, in place since 2004.

Gyllenberg et al have updated us with information from a study describing antidepressant use between the ages of 13 and 24 years. They used information obtained from a registry first established in 1994. The aim of their study was to determine what kind of childhood psychopathology and family characteristics predict the later use of antidepressants. They also attempted to predict the lifetime cost of antidepressants. The data from this report represent the first population-based study examining predictive associations between childhood psychopathology and lifetime antidepressant use through adulthood. We see in this report data that among children younger than 15 years, the use of antidepressants is much higher in the United States than elsewhere. In fact, the use here on our shores is several times higher than in Europe.

We learn from this report that between the ages of 13 and 24 years, almost 10% of males and almost 14% of females are using antidepressants. Boys in particular with conduct disorders and boys and girls from homes with other than 2 biological parents are at significantly increased risk for using antidepressants. It is also clear that, for whatever reason, pharmaceutical companies manufacturing these drugs do financially better in the United States than elsewhere in the world.

J. A. Stockman III, MD

Reference

1. Olfson M, Marcus SC. National patterns in antidepressant medication treatment. *Arch Gen Psychiatr.* 2009;66:848-856.

Out-of-Hospital Hypertonic Resuscitation Following Severe Traumatic Brain Injury: A Randomized Controlled Trial

Bulger EM, for the ROC Investigators (Univ of Washington, Seattle; et al)
JAMA 304:1455-1464, 2010

Context.—Hypertonic fluids restore cerebral perfusion with reduced cerebral edema and modulate inflammatory response to reduce subsequent neuronal injury and thus have potential benefit in resuscitation of patients with traumatic brain injury (TBI).

Objective.—To determine whether out-of-hospital administration of hypertonic fluids improves neurologic outcome following severe TBI.

Design, Setting, and Participants.—Multicenter, double-blind, randomized, placebo-controlled clinical trial involving 114 North American emergency medical services agencies within the Resuscitation Outcomes Consortium, conducted between May 2006 and May 2009 among patients 15 years or older with blunt trauma and a prehospital Glasgow Coma Scale score of 8 or less who did not meet criteria for hypovolemic shock. Planned enrollment was 2122 patients.

Intervention.—A single 250-mL bolus of 7.5% saline/6% dextran 70 (hypertonic saline/dextran), 7.5% saline (hypertonic saline), or 0.9% saline (normal saline) initiated in the out-of-hospital setting.

Main Outcome Measure.—Six-month neurologic outcome based on the Extended Glasgow Outcome Scale (GOSE) (dichotomized as >4 or ≤4).

Results.—The study was terminated by the data and safety monitoring board after randomization of 1331 patients, having met prespecified futility criteria. Among the 1282 patients enrolled, 6-month outcomes data were available for 1087 (85%). Baseline characteristics of the groups were equivalent. There was no difference in 6-month neurologic outcome among groups with regard to proportions of patients with severe TBI (GOSE ≤4) (hypertonic saline/dextran vs normal saline: 53.7% vs 51.5%; difference, 2.2% [95% CI, −4.5% to 9.0%]; hypertonic saline vs normal saline: 54.3% vs 51.5%; difference, 2.9% [95% CI, −4.0% to 9.7%]; $P = .67$). There were no statistically significant differences in distribution of GOSE category or Disability Rating Score by treatment group. Survival at 28 days was 74.3% with hypertonic saline/dextran, 75.7% with hypertonic saline, and 75.1% with normal saline ($P = .88$).

Conclusion.—Among patients with severe TBI not in hypovolemic shock, initial resuscitation with either hypertonic saline or hypertonic saline/dextran, compared with normal saline, did not result in superior 6-month neurologic outcome or survival.

Trial Registration.—clinicaltrials.gov Identifier: NCT00316004.

▶ A lot is changing these days when it comes to resuscitation techniques. This report deals with some updated information about how those who have suffered severe traumatic brain injury might best be supported when first receiving medical attention. Often those who have had severe trauma to the head are hemodynamically stable, that is, not in hypovolemic shock, but show clear-cut evidence of significant brain injury when their Glasgow Coma Scale (GCS) score is measured. In such patients, the primary concern is not to allow anything to happen that might further compromise the long-term outcome of a patient by maneuvers that increase intracranial pressure (ICP). Indeed, current therapy following severe traumatic brain injury is focused on minimizing secondary injury by supporting systemic profusion and reducing ICP. Intravenous fluid resuscitation generally begins in the out-of-hospital setting; however, therapy for the management of cerebral edema is often delayed until after hospital arrival. If too much standard fluid is given in the field, it can only lead to further problems with increased ICP. Hypertonic fluids have been shown to decrease ICP and improve cerebral profusion in animal models and in patients with severe traumatic brain injury. Hypertonic saline has also been shown to have beneficial vasoregulatory, immunomodulatory, and neurochemical effects on the injured brain. Previous trials have suggested that early administration of hypertonic fluids to patients with severe traumatic brain injury might improve survival, but no large definitive trials have been reported, thus the value of the information provided by Bulger et al.

What these investigators have done is to include in an investigation of those individuals with traumatic brain injury as a result of blunt force trauma who were aged 15 years or older and who had a GCS of 8 or less. These individuals entered the protocol only if they did not have evidence of hemorrhagic shock. Subjects fitting the criteria received a single 250-mL bolus of 7.5% saline/6% dextran 70 (hypertonic saline/dextran), 7.5% saline (hypertonic saline), or 0.9% saline (normal saline) initiated in the out-of-hospital setting. The 6-month neurologic outcome was the end point of the study.

This study is the largest randomized trial of hypertonic resuscitation following traumatic brain injury. Unfortunately, the investigators were unable to demonstrate any improvement in 6-month neurologic outcome or survival in this patient population. This well-done study does not support a number of smaller studies that have reached a different conclusion. The authors hypothesize that starting hyperosmolar therapy in the out-of-hospital setting would reduce the subsequent sequelae leading to secondary brain injury. The lack of effect observed in this study may in fact be attributable to the need for more and more prolonged course of hyperosmolarity continuing into the early hospital period or the dilutional effects of crystalloid therapy, which did not differ after initial treatment.

The bottom line here is that in this randomized controlled trial, the investigators were unable to demonstrate any improvement in 6-month neurologic outcomes or survival for brain traumatized patients with presumed severe injury (out-of-hospital GCS ≤ 8) without evidence of hypovolemic shock who received a single bolus of hypertonic fluids compared with normal saline in the out-of-hospital setting. The data from this report do not preclude any benefit from hypertonic saline were it to have been administered differently, but at the present time there appears to be no compelling reason to adopt a practice of hypertonic fluid resuscitation for traumatic brain injury in such circumstances. Please note that this report did include adolescents, so the data most likely apply to this spectrum of the age group of children.

J. A. Stockman III, MD

Pediatric Concussions in United States Emergency Departments in the Years 2002 to 2006
Meehan WP III, Mannix R (Children's Hosp Boston, MA)
J Pediatr 157:889-893, 2010

Objectives.—To estimate the incidence and demographics of concussions in children coming to emergency departments (EDs) in the United States and describe the rates of neuroimaging and follow-up instructions in these patients.

Study Design.—This is a cross-sectional study of children 0 to 19 years old diagnosed with concussion from the National Hospital Ambulatory Medical Care Survey. National Hospital Ambulatory Medical Care Survey collects data on approximately 25 000 visits annually to 600 randomly selected hospital emergency and outpatient departments. We examined visits to United States emergency departments between 2002 and 2006. Simple descriptive statistics were used.

Results.—Of the 50 835 pediatric visits in the 5-year sample, 230 observations, representing 144 000 visits annually, were for concussions. Sixty-nine percent of concussion visits were by males. Thirty percent were sports-related. Sixty-nine percent of patients diagnosed with a concussion had head imaging. Twenty-eight percent of patients were discharged without specific instructions to follow-up with an outpatient provider for further treatment.

Conclusions.—Approximately 144 000 pediatric patients present to emergency departments each year with a concussion. Most of these patients undergo computed tomography of the head, and nearly one-third are discharged without specific instructions to follow-up with an outpatient provider for further treatment.

▶ Although most health care providers view concussions as evidence of a brain injury, the public at large generally does not quite think this way. A concussion is defined as "...a complex pathophysiological process involving the brain, induced by traumatic biomechanical forces.[1]" Unfortunately, the study of the epidemiology of concussion is often confused by a muddling of the terms concussion and mild traumatic brain injury. Meehan et al tell us about concussions in the United States based on data from the National Hospital Ambulatory Medical Care Survey. The data from the report by Meehan represent information on 50 835 pediatric visits to emergency rooms (ERs) for diagnosis and management of concussions.

What we learn from this report is that about 1 of every 200 patients seen in a pediatric ER is diagnosed with a concussion. This translates to about 144 000 visits annually. Boys, as might be expected, present more frequently than girls. In most instances, a CT scan is used to rule out structural brain injury. Given all the data appearing recently about the risks associated with CT radiation, one wonders whether we should be relying so heavily on such imaging, although most ER physicians believe that it is better to be safe than sorry and obtain a CT scan.

This report also tells us that all too often there is not time in the ER to explain all the things that should be taken into account during the recovery period from a concussion, including cognitive rest as well as physical rest and the risks of cognitive effects, impact on academic performance, and risk of recurrent injury. Most studies suggest that even with adequate instructions regarding follow-up, compliance is poor.

Fortunately, we are paying a great deal more attention to the short- and long-term consequences of children experiencing concussions. The authors of this report run a Sports Concussion Clinic at the Children' Hospital, Boston. The more we learn about concussion in children, the more we see that a simple knock on the head may not be all that simple in the long run. Careful follow-up with adequate recuperation is needed. Rapid reentry on the playing field is something to be very wary of.

Even in professional football we are hearing a great deal more about warnings of the long-term consequences of concussions. In late July 2010, for example, the National Football League (NFL) introduced a new poster to be hung in league locker rooms, warning players of possible long-term health effects of concussions. Each year, the poster reminds us that more than 1.5 million Americans sustain mild traumatic brain injuries with no loss of consciousness and no need for hospitalization; an equal number sustain injuries sufficient to impair consciousness, but insufficiently severe to necessitate hospitalization. It is the latter injury that is the very heart of the concern these days, particularly if such injuries are repeated. In professional sports where repetitive head injuries occur, such as boxing, cognitive decline may begin years after retirement from the game. Dementia pugilistica (punch drunk syndrome) is not something isolated to boxers. Those on any playing field sustaining repetitive head injury can experience this problem.[2]

J. A. Stockman III, MD

References

1. Callahan JM. Pediatric concussions in United States emergency departments: the tip of the iceberg. *J Pediatr.* 2010;157:873-875.
2. DeKosky ST, Ikonomovic MD, Gandy S. Traumatic brain injury—football, warfare, and long-term effects. *N Engl J Med.* 2010;363:1293-1296.

Decompressive Craniectomy in Diffuse Traumatic Brain Injury

Cooper DJ, for the DECRA Trial Investigators and the Australian and New Zealand Intensive Care Society Clinical Trials Group (Alfred Hosp, Melbourne, Victoria, Australia; et al)
N Engl J Med 364:1493-1502, 2011

Background.—It is unclear whether decompressive craniectomy improves the functional outcome in patients with severe traumatic brain injury and refractory raised intracranial pressure.

Methods.—From December 2002 through April 2010, we randomly assigned 155 adults with severe diffuse traumatic brain injury and intracranial hypertension that was refractory to first-tier therapies to undergo either bifrontotemporoparietal decompressive craniectomy or standard care. The original primary outcome was an unfavorable outcome (a composite of death, vegetative state, or severe disability), as evaluated on the Extended Glasgow Outcome Scale 6 months after the injury. The final primary outcome was the score on the Extended Glasgow Outcome Scale at 6 months.

Results.—Patients in the craniectomy group, as compared with those in the standard-care group, had less time with intracranial pressures above the treatment threshold (P<0.001), fewer interventions for increased intracranial pressure (P<0.02 for all comparisons), and fewer days in the intensive care unit (ICU) (P<0.001). However, patients undergoing craniectomy had worse scores on the Extended Glasgow Outcome Scale than those receiving standard care (odds ratio for a worse score in the craniectomy group, 1.84; 95% confidence interval [CI], 1.05 to 3.24; P = 0.03) and a greater risk of an unfavorable outcome (odds ratio, 2.21; 95% CI, 1.14 to 4.26; P = 0.02). Rates of death at 6 months were similar in the craniectomy group (19%) and the standard-care group (18%).

Conclusions.—In adults with severe diffuse traumatic brain injury and refractory intracranial hypertension, early bifrontotemporoparietal decompressive craniectomy decreased intracranial pressure and the length of stay in the ICU but was associated with more unfavorable outcomes. (Funded by the National Health and Medical Research Council of Australia and others; DECRA Australian Clinical Trials Registry number, ACTRN012605000009617.)

▶ This report did include teenagers who had suffered traumatic brain injuries, and therefore it is important for all of us to be familiar with the results of this study by Cooper et al. The report begins with a number of statistics about traumatic brain injury. It is noted that those with severe traumatic brain injury have a 60% likelihood of either dying or surviving with severe disability. In the United States, the annual burden of traumatic brain injury is more than $60 billion. Management of increased intracranial pressure associated with traumatic brain injury usually begins with pharmacologic agents. However, many patients with severe traumatic brain injury have raised intracranial pressure that is refractory to first-tier therapies. In such cases, surgical decompressive craniectomy is increasingly being performed to control intracranial pressure. To date, the data on the success of the latter approach have been spotty, thus the value of the information provided from the multicenter, randomized, controlled, Decompressive Craniectomy (DECRA) trial as summarized by Cooper et al.

The DECRA trial examined the efficacy of bifrontotemporoparietal decompressive craniectomy in adults younger than 60 years with traumatic brain injury in whom medical management had not maintained intracranial pressures below accepted targets. In this study, patients were randomly assigned to either undergo bifrontotemporoparietal decompressive craniectomy or stay on standard therapy. The results of this study show that in the craniectomy group, there was less time with intracranial pressures above treatment threshold levels. Patient stay in the intensive care unit (ICU) was lessened as well, but unfortunately the rates of death at 6 months were similar in the craniectomy group and the standard care group. Patients undergoing craniectomy also had worse scores on the Extended Glasgow Outcome Scale than those receiving standard care. The findings of this report differ from those of most nonrandomized studies of decompressive craniectomy. The investigators had speculated prior to the start of their study that in patients with severe traumatic brain injury, decompressive craniectomy would decrease intracranial pressure, improve functional outcomes, and decrease the number of survivors having severe disability. Unfortunately, despite the positive clinical signs in the ICU, decompressive craniectomy instead increased the likelihood of a poor outcome.

You can be absolutely certain that this report is receiving a great deal of attention and critical evaluation. It is also safe to say that many will not be influenced by the results of this study, given the desperate nature of some of these brain-injured patients. There is no substitute, however, for good data from properly designed randomized studies. An editorial that accompanied this report noted that it is important that craniectomy not be simply abandoned on the basis of the results of the study by Cooper et al. Rather, it is suggested that care providers must think more carefully about the risks and benefits of decompressive craniectomy before performing the procedure and must work to define the appropriate clinical setting for the procedure.[1] This editorial closes with the words of Seneca the Younger, *Errare humanum est, perseverare autem diabolicum* (to err is human, but to persist [in error] is diabolical). Enough said on this topic.

J. A. Stockman III, MD

Reference

1. Servadei F. Clinical value of decompressive craniectomy. *N Engl J Med.* 2011;364: 1558-1559.

"Traumatic Tap" Proportion in Pediatric Lumbar Puncture
Pappano D (East Tennessee Children's Hosp, Knoxville)
Pediatr Emerg Care 26:487-489, 2010

Objectives.—To determine the frequency of "traumatic" or "bloody" tap when pediatric lumbar puncture is performed by a physician who has completed training and performs the procedure frequently.

Methods.—The author identified 100 sequential patients presenting to a pediatric emergency department requiring lumbar puncture for clinical indications. Demographic information, cerebrospinal cell counts, and other relevant data were later obtained by retrospective chart review. Cell count results were categorized according to several previously used criteria: greater than 400, greater than 1000, and greater than 10,000/unsuccessful.

Results.—One procedure yielded only a small amount of bloody fluid on which no cell count was performed. The remaining 99 procedures yielded red blood cell counts less than 1000.

Conclusions.—The proportion of bloody or traumatic results from pediatric lumbar puncture reported from pediatric training centers is typically in the 20% to 30% range. This represents an overestimation of a more ideal proportion possible when the procedure is performed by a physician who has completed training and performs the procedure frequently.

▶ This is an interesting little report. It is fairly rare that journals will publish a series of outcomes undertaken by a single physician performing a single procedure, but that is what we see in this report. The author of the report completed his residency in 1995. This residency was followed by a 3-year pediatric emergency medicine fellowship and a 1-year pediatric neurology fellowship. The report tells us of this individual's outcomes in performing 100 consecutive lumbar punctures. Before this series of lumbar punctures was undertaken, this physician had performed somewhere between 250 and 300 lumbar punctures. The intent of the study was to tell us about the frequency of a seasoned doctor's traumatic taps.

Of the 100 lumbar punctures reported on, in 3 cases the indication for the lumbar puncture was to check for increased intracranial pressure. In the remaining 97, the indication was to rule in or rule out central nervous system infection. Most procedures (72%) were successful on the first attempt. One-third of the procedures resulted in no red blood cells in the cerebrospinal fluid (CSF). Seventy-one percent of procedures had fewer than 10 red blood cells. Lumbar puncture was unsuccessful in 1 patient. Organisms were isolated from CSF by bacterial culture in 2 cases and by viral culture in 3 cases.

Everyone knows that a traumatic tap or bloody contamination of CSF with circulating blood is a fairly common occurrence. In some cases, when there is a great deal of blood present, it is difficult to tell whether CSF has been obtained at all. Most of us are familiar with how to correct the white blood cell (WBC) count for the amount of red blood cells present. One can expect an elevation in the CSF WBC count by 1 WBC for every 1 to 1000 red blood cells. Traumatic taps with red blood cell counts less than 1000 usually do not cloud the clinical picture, whereas red blood cell counts greater than 10 000 are likely to introduce ambiguity in interpreting the WBC results.

Dr Pappano has set a benchmark for us. Because this is the only report that I am familiar with where a single physician has actually monitored his/her success rate for the performance of lumbar puncture, the data are enterable into the Guinness Records. Anyone want to challenge Dr Pappano?

J. A. Stockman III, MD

A clinical prediction rule for ambulation outcomes after traumatic spinal cord injury: a longitudinal cohort study
van Middendorp JJ, for the EM-SCI Study Group (Radboud Univ Nijmegen Med Centre, Netherlands; et al)
Lancet 377:1004-1010, 2011

Background.—Traumatic spinal cord injury is a serious disorder in which early prediction of ambulation is important to counsel patients and to plan rehabilitation. We developed a reliable, validated prediction rule to assess a patient's chances of walking independently after such injury.

Methods.—We undertook a longitudinal cohort study of adult patients with traumatic spinal cord injury, with early (within the first 15 days after injury) and late (1-year follow-up) clinical examinations, who were admitted to one of 19 European centres between July, 2001, and June, 2008. A clinical prediction rule based on age and neurological variables was derived from the international standards for neurological classification of spinal cord injury with a multivariate logistic regression model. Primary outcome measure 1 year after injury was independent indoor walking based on the Spinal Cord Independence Measure. Model performances were quantified with respect to discrimination (area under receiver-operating-characteristics curve [AUC]). Temporal validation was done in a second group of patients from July, 2008, to December, 2009.

Findings.—Of 1442 patients with spinal cord injury, 492 had available outcome measures. A combination of age (<65 *vs* ≥65 years), motor scores of the quadriceps femoris (L3), gastrocsoleus (S1) muscles, and light touch sensation of dermatomes L3 and S1 showed excellent discrimination in distinguishing independent walkers from dependent walkers and non-walkers (AUC 0·956, 95% CI 0·936−0·976, p<0·0001). Temporal validation in 99 patients confirmed excellent discriminating ability of the prediction rule (AUC 0·967, 0·939−0·995, p<0·0001).

Interpretation.—Our prediction rule, including age and four neurological tests, can give an early prognosis of an individual's ability to walk after traumatic spinal cord injury, which can be used to set rehabilitation goals and might improve the ability to stratify patients in interventional trials.

▶ This report from the Netherlands, Switzerland, and the United States about traumatic spinal cord injuries was largely based on adults with this problem, but the study did include teenagers as well, thus the inclusion of this report here. Prognostic indicators of neurological recovery and ambulation have been extensively studied over the last 50 years, but the report of Middendorp et al does add valuable new information to what we already know. These investigators have developed a validated prediction rule to assess a patient's chances of walking independently after traumatic spinal cord injury. They derive data from a large multicenter study of more than 1400 patients with a spinal cord injury. The information is important because a reliable prognosis of the patient's potential functional outcome is essential for counseling and to design a personalized rehabilitation program. To date, no reliable prediction rule for the ability to walk independently after a traumatic spinal cord injury has been available. On the basis of age and 4 clinical neurological parameters, a patient's long-term probability of walking independently after injury can now be calculated more accurately than with previous grading systems. You will need to read this report in some detail to understand how the new grading system is undertaken as part of the evaluation of newly injured patients.

While on the topic of neurological impairment, a new device has been described that lets the disabled move and communicate using their nose. Researchers have invented a device that allows the paralyzed to write, surf the web, and steer an electric wheelchair—all by sniffing. Sniffing is controlled in part by cranial nerves in the soft palate. Because these nerves emerge directly from the brain, as opposed to the spinal cord, they remain in tact for many severely paralyzed individuals. They also control the ability to blink, sip, and puff. Scientists have devised a sniff controller that uses a small plastic tube that fits into the nose. It measures pressure, translating variations in intensity, and frequency of sniffing into commands for a computer or wheelchair. Thirteen of 15 disabled individuals successfully used the technology to learn to write messages or surf the web. In addition to these capabilities, 1 individual was able to maneuver his wheelchair. The 15th volunteer made no progress with the technology.[1]

J. A. Stockman III, MD

Reference

1. Jabr F. The power of sniff: A new device lets the disabled move and communicate with their noses. *Scientific American*. September 2010:24.

Botulinumtoxin A treatment in toddlers with cerebral palsy
Tedroff K, Löwing K, Haglund-Åkerlind Y, et al (Astrid Lindgren Children's Hosp, Stockholm, Sweden)
Acta Paediatr 99:1156-1162, 2010

Aims.—In this study the aim was to evaluate the effect of botulinum toxin A (BoNT-A) treatment on muscle tone, contracture development and gait pattern in young children with cerebral palsy (CP).
Method.—Fifteen children with spastic CP (mean age = 16 months) were included in a randomized control study. All received a daily stretching programme and children in the BoNT-A group additionally received two injections, 6 months apart in the gastrocnemius muscle. Outcomes were assessed at baseline, and after 1 and 3.5 years. A 3D gait-analysis was performed at 5 years of age.
Results.—Plantarflexor muscle tone in the BoNT-A group was significantly reduced after 3.5 years, while the muscle tone at the ankle and knee in the control group remained unchanged. The change-score in knee-flexion muscle tone between the groups was significantly different after 3.5 years. The knee joint ROM was significantly increased at 1 year in the BoNT-A group but reduced at the knee and ankle joints in the control group after 3.5 years. No group differences were found for gait analysis, GMFM-66 or PEDI.
Conclusion.—Early treatment of BoNT-A in children with spastic CP may decrease muscle tone and decelerate contracture development after 3.5 years. The effect on gait development remains inconclusive.

▶ It has been almost 20 years since the first descriptions of the use of botulinum toxin A (BoNT-A) as a part of the management of children with cerebral palsy. What was initially heralded with great fanfare has not turned out to be a magic bullet for many of these youngsters. While initially producing improvement in spasticity, all too many children with cerebral palsy still would develop contractures over time. Tedroff et al have further evaluated this problem by following the long-term effects (3.5 years) after a year of repeated BoNT-A injections in addition to daily stretching programs, and compared these with the outcomes with stretching programs alone in young children (1 to 2 years old) with cerebral palsy. The investigators were particularly interested in following the effect on contracture and gait development. The study is one of the first to report the effect of BoNT-A in toddlers (less than 24 months old) with cerebral palsy.

In this report, toddlers with cerebral palsy received BoNT-A injections in the gastrocnemius muscle during a period when locomotion develops from crawling to independent walking. The results of this study suggest that early BoNT-A treatment during year one in toddlers with cerebral palsy does reduce the muscle tone and arrest the progress of contractures compared with a control group. The long-term effect, however, is much less clear, but the treatment might decelerate the expected increase in muscle tone and temporarily delay the development of contracture. Clearly more studies are needed before any clinical recommendation can be made in this young age group with respect to the true long-term benefits of the use of BoNT-A.

While on the topic of BoNT-A, it now is being used as part of the treatment of chronic cough in adults. Recently reported was the use of BoNT-A to decrease laryngeal hypertonicity in subjects with chronic cough.[1] It should be noted that this agent is very effective in producing aphonia when injected intralingually as administered to mother-in-laws who talk too much.

J. A. Stockman III, MD

Reference

1. Chu MW, Lieser JD, Sinacori JT. Use of botulinum toxin type A for chronic cough: a neuropathic model. *Arch Otolaryngol Head Neck Surg*. 2010;136:447-452.

The epidemiology of progressive intellectual and neurological deterioration in childhood
Verity C, Winstone AM, Stellitano L, et al (Addenbrooke's Hosp, Cambridge, UK; et al)
Arch Dis Child 95:361-364, 2010

Objective.—To study the epidemiology of diseases that cause progressive intellectual and neurological deterioration (PIND) in UK children.

Design.—Since May 1997, the authors have performed active surveillance to search for variant Creutzfeldt–Jakob Disease (vCJD) among the many diseases that cause neurological deterioration in children, using the monthly surveillance card sent to all UK consultant paediatricians by the British Paediatric Surveillance Unit. The authors obtain clinical details from reporting paediatricians by questionnaire or site visit, and an Expert Group then independently classifies the cases.

Results.—After 12 years, 2636 patients less than 16 years old with suspected PIND had been reported, of whom 1114 had a confirmed diagnosis to explain their deterioration: in these children, there were 147 different diseases. These were the six commonest diagnostic groups: leukoencephalopathies (183 cases), neuronal ceroid lipofuscinoses (141 cases), mitochondrial diseases (122 cases), mucopolysaccharidoses (102 cases), gangliosidoses (100 cases) and peroxisomal disorders (69 cases). Relatively large numbers of PIND children were reported from parts of the UK where there are high rates of consanguinity. Only six children with vCJD (four definite, two probable) had been identified.

Conclusions.—Although this study does not ascertain all UK cases, it provides a novel insight into the epidemiology of the neurodegenerative diseases that cause PIND in children. It is reassuring that in general these children are carefully investigated and that active surveillance has found only six children with vCJD. However, there is concern that more childhood vCJD cases may appear, possibly with a different genotype from those identified so far.

▶ It was about 15 years ago that Will et al first reported 10 cases of a new variant of Creutzfeldt-Jakob disease (vCJD).[1] As time has passed, it has become clear that vCJD has an earlier onset than sporadic CJD and has a novel neuropathological phenotype. Since 1996, in Great Britain, the National Creutzfeldt-Jakob Disease Surveillance Unit in Edinburgh has performed surveillance for vCJD. By early 2010, the definite and probable cases of vCJD had numbered 170. Of these, 166 patients were dead and 4 were still alive.[2]

The British Pediatric Surveillance Unit (BPSU) sends a monthly surveillance card listing the conditions currently under surveillance in Great Britain to all consultant pediatricians in the United Kingdom. They are asked to return this card reporting all cases seen under surveillance in the previous month. Currently, somewhere between 2800 and 2900 cards are sent monthly, and over 90% of these cards are returned. Data from the BPSU provide a rich source of information about the incidence of progressive intellectual and neurologic deterioration (PIND) in childhood. Cases of vCJD are included within the PIND surveillance. Thus, the BPSU provides a rich database of all the causes of PIND. The case definition for PIND may be seen in Table 1. After 12 years of active surveillance, 2636 cases of suspected PIND had been reported. Just 6 cases of vCJD were found among these cases. The youngest case reported was of a girl aged 12 years and the oldest was of a boy aged 15 years. The last child to develop symptoms did so in 2000. All reported youngsters with vCJD had died. Of the other children who met the PIND case definition, 1114 children had an underlying diagnosis that explained the deterioration. If all the specific diagnostic variants were counted separately, there were 147 known neurodegenerative conditions that were identified with PIND, which illustrates the complexity of classifying such children. The 30 most commonly identified diseases are shown in Table 2. Fig 2 shows the aggregate diagnostic grouping of the 6 largest groups causing PIND. Obviously, a number of children

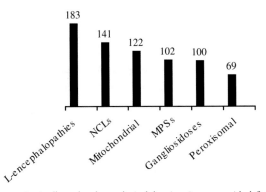

FIGURE 2.—Progressive intellectual and neurological deterioration cases with definite diagnoses: the six most commonly reported disease groups. L-encephalopathies, leukoencephalopathies; NCLs, neuronal ceroid lipofuscinoses; Mitochondrial, mitochondrial diseases; MPSs, mucopolysaccharidoses; Peroxisomal, peroxisomal disorders. (Reprinted from Verity C, Winstone AM, Stellitano L, et al. The epidemiology of progressive intellectual and neurological deterioration in childhood. *Arch Dis Child.* 2010;95:361-364, with permission from the BMJ Publishing Group Ltd.)

TABLE 1.—Case Definition—Progressive Intellectual and Neurological Deterioration

Any child (under 16 years of age at onset of symptoms) who fulfils *all* of the following three criteria:
▶ Progressive deterioration for more than 3 months
with
▶ Loss of already attained intellectual or developmental abilities
and
▶ Development of abnormal neurological signs.
Excluding:
　Static intellectual loss—for example, after encephalitis, head injury or near drowning.
Including:
　Children who meet the case definition, even if specific neurological diagnoses have been made
　Metabolic disorders leading to neurological deterioration
　Seizure disorders if associated with progressive deterioration
　Children who have been diagnosed as having neurodegenerative disorders who have not yet
　　developed symptoms
Reporting restricted to cases seen in the last month but including those whose condition began earlier (ie, including 'old cases' of children in follow-up if seen in that month).

with PIND had deteriorated or died without a diagnosis. Review of these cases seemed to exclude vCJD as a potential cause of the PIND.

The authors of this report are careful to warn that the data derived from BPSU do not allow a means of accurately determining the incidence or prevalence rates of certain neurodegenerative diseases. This is because of underreporting of cases for various reasons. Also, some diseases do not always progress over time. A classic example is Rett syndrome, in which patients may deteriorate but only to a plateau. Despite these caveats, this report from Great Britain has yielded valuable information about the clinical presentation and mode of diagnosis of many of the diseases that cause PIND.

While on the topic of progressive intellectual and neurologic deterioration, it appears that walking for 40 minutes 3 times per week actually has the opposite

TABLE 2.—Thirty Most Commonly Reported Confirmed Diagnoses

Condition	No of Cases
NCL late infantile	73
Mucopolysaccharidosis IIIA (San Filippo)	69
Rett syndrome	60
Metachromatic leukodystrophy	59
Adrenoleukodystrophy	56
NCL juvenile	44
GM2 gangliosidosis type 1 (Tay–Sachs)	41
Niemann–Pick Type C	38
Krabbe disease	33
GM2 gangliosidosis type 2 (Sandhoff)	33
GM1 gangliosidosis	23
Huntington disease	22
NCL infantile	22
PKAN/NBIA*	21
Pelizaeus–Merzbacher disease	17
Leigh syndrome	17
NARP (including NARP/MILS)	17
Menkes disease	16
Mucopolysaccharidosis IIA (Hunter disease)	15
Cockayne disease	15
Canavan disease	13
Neuroaxonal dystrophy	12
Vanishing white matter disease	11
Aicardi–Goutieres syndrome	10
Alexander disease	10
Glutaric aciduria type 1	10
Molybdenum cofactor deficiency	10
Ataxia telangiectasia	9
Subacute sclerosing panencephalitis	9
Rasmussen syndrome	8

NARP, neuropathy ataxia retinitis pigmentosa; NARP/MILS, NARP/maternally inherited Leigh syndrome; NCL, neuronal ceroid-lipofuscinosis.
*PKAN (pantothenate kinase-associated neurodegeneration) also known as NBIA (neurodegeneration with brain iron accumulation), previously Hallevorden–Spatz disease.

effect, increasing brain volume and memory. A randomized study recently reported that 60 healthy older adults who participated in aerobic training for a year increased their hippocampal volume by 2%, whereas a control group had 1.4% loss of volume, consistent with normal aging. The 2% increase reversed the usual age-related loss in volume by 1 to 2 years, and it led to improvement in spacial memory. Aerobic exercise may boost levels of brain-derived neurotrophic factor. Win 1 for exercise for the elderly![3]

J. A. Stockman III, MD

References

1. Will RG, Ironside JW, Zeidler M, et al. A new variant of Creutzfeldt-Jakob disease in the UK. *Lancet.* 1996;347:921-925.
2. The National CJD Surveillance Unit. Creutzfeldt-Jakob disease statistics. http://www.jcd.ac.uk. Accessed June 30, 2010.
3. Erickson KI, Voss MW, Prakash RS, et al. Exercise training increases size of hippocampus and improves memory. *Proc Natl Acad Sci U S A.* 2011;108:3017-3022. Epub 2011 Jan 31.

Streptococcal Upper Respiratory Tract Infections and Exacerbations of Tic and Obsessive-Compulsive Symptoms: A Prospective Longitudinal Study

Leckman JF, King RA, Gilbert DL, et al (Yale Univ School of Medicine, New Haven, CT; Univ of Cincinnati, OH; et al)
J Am Acad Child Adolesc Psychiatry 50:108-118, 2011

Objective.—The objective of this blinded, prospective, longitudinal study was to determine whether new group A β hemolytic streptococcal (GABHS) infections are temporally associated with exacerbations of tic or obsessive-compulsive (OC) symptoms in children who met published criteria for pediatric autoimmune neuropsychiatric disorders associated with streptococcal infections (PANDAS). A group of children with Tourette syndrome and/or OC disorder without a PANDAS history served as the comparison (non-PANDAS) group.

Method.—Consecutive clinical ratings of tic and OC symptom severity were obtained for 31 PANDAS subjects and 53 non-PANDAS subjects. Clinical symptoms and laboratory values (throat cultures and streptococcal antibody titers) were evaluated at regular intervals during a 25-month period. Additional testing occurred at the time of any tic or OC symptom exacerbation. New GABHS infections were established by throat swab cultures and/ or recent significant rise in streptococcal antibodies. Laboratory personnel were blinded to case or control status, clinical (exacerbation or not) condition, and clinical evaluators were blinded to the laboratory results.

Results.—No group differences were observed in the number of clinical exacerbations or the number of newly diagnosed GABHS infections. On only six occasions of a total of 51 (12%), a newly diagnosed GABHS infection was followed, within 2 months, by an exacerbation of tic and/or OC symptoms. In every instance, this association occurred in the non-PANDAS group.

Conclusions.—This study provides no evidence for a temporal association between GABHS infections and tic/OC symptom exacerbations in children who meet the published PANDAS diagnostic criteria.

▶ It was back in 1998 that Swedo et al in a psychiatry journal described the disorder that now goes by the acronym PANDAS (pediatric autoimmune neuropsychiatric disorders associated with streptococcal infections).[1] Subsequent clinical and laboratory-based studies have failed to uniformly provide support for the existence of PANDAS. A major shortcoming of the PANDAS hypothesis has been the very small number of adequately designed prospective studies examining any temporal relation between antecedent bona fide group A β hemolytic streptococci (GABHS) infection and the onset of exacerbations of tic and obsessive-compulsive (OC) symptoms. Leckman et al have conducted an intensive, blinded clinical and laboratory prospective cohort study that included PANDAS and non-PANDAS comparison subjects. The hypothesis was that if PANDAS is a unique clinical entity, then PANDAS cases would have more clinical exacerbations temporally linked to antecedent GABHS infections than non-PANDAS comparison subjects.

The results of this study of children who met established published diagnostic criteria for PANDAS showed there was no temporal association between clinical exacerbations and antecedent GABHS infections documented by microbiologic and/or immunologic criteria. These findings support those from earlier prospective blinded, case-controlled studies in which more than 75% of clinical exacerbations were not temporally related to infections.[2] Taken together, the implication from these independent studies is that there is no convincing evidence for an ongoing causal association between GABHS and tic/OC exacerbations in children who met the published PANDAS diagnostic criteria.

It should be noted that although GABHS infections have been postulated as the main initial autoimmune response—inciting event contributing to the sudden onset of severe neuropsychiatric symptoms, it is well documented that sudden OC and tic symptom onset or worsening can be triggered by other infectious agents (eg, herpes simplex virus, varicella zoster virus, human immunodeficiency virus, *Borrelia burgdorferi*, *Mycoplasma pneumoniae*, sinusitis, and the common cold).

The authors of this report say the most important conclusion of their study is that children who meet the published criteria for PANDAS, particularly those whose exacerbations limited to just tics or OC symptoms, typically do not require the performance of throat cultures in the absence of symptoms of pharyngitis and that there is no convincing rationale for the use of prophylactic antibiotics in such circumstances. Needless to say debate will continue in this regard. As an aside, if you want to read an extraordinarily up-to-date review of streptococcal pharyngitis, see the clinical practice review by Wessels.[3]

This commentary closes with a reading recommendation. For any interested in medical disorders in historical figures, a book recently appeared that talked about neurologic disorders in famous artists.[4] You will learn that the great composer Wolfgang Amadeus Mozart (1756-1791) most likely had obsessive compulsive disorder associated with Tourette syndrome, which manifested itself in early childhood but came into full force in adolescence. A detailed analysis of Mozart's letters has demonstrated an abundance of coprolalia, mostly scatological expressions and sexual insinuations, which are typical for this clinical entity. It should also be noted that the Hungarian composer, Bela Bartock (1881-1945) most likely had mild autism. Enjoy this book, if you can find it. You will acquire knowledge about Marcel Proust, Gustave Flaubert, Fyodor Dostoyevsky, Andy Warhol, Robert Schumann, and others. To read a review of the book, see the excellent piece by Carl Lyndgren.[5]

J. A. Stockman III, MD

References

1. Swedo SE, Leonard HL, Garvey M, et al. Pediatric autoimmune neuropsychiatric disorders associated with streptococcal infections: clinical description of the first 50 cases. *Am J Psychiatry.* 1998;155:264-271.
2. Kurlan R, Johnson D, Kaplan EL; and the Tourette Syndrome Study Group. Streptococcal infection and exacerbations of childhood tics and obsessive-compulsive symptoms: a prospective blinded cohort study. *Pediatrics.* 2008;121:1188-1197.
3. Wessels MR, Clinical practice. Streptococcal pharyngitis. *N Engl J Med.* 2011; 364:648-655.

4. Bogousslavsky J, Boller F, eds. *Neurologic disorders and famous artists (frontiers of neurology and neuroscience)*. Carger, Basel: S Karger Pub; 2005.
5. Lyndgren C. Neurologic disorders in famous artists. *Acta Paediatr.* 2011;100: 628-629.

L-Histidine Decarboxylase and Tourette's Syndrome

Ercan-Sencicek AG, Stillman AA, Ghosh AK, et al (Yale Univ School of Medicine, New Haven, CT; Weill Med College of Cornell Univ, NY; et al)

N Engl J Med 362:1901-1908, 2010

Tourette's syndrome is a common developmental neuropsychiatric disorder characterized by chronic motor and vocal tics. Despite a strong genetic contribution, inheritance is complex, and risk alleles have proven difficult to identify. Here, we describe an analysis of linkage in a two-generation pedigree leading to the identification of a rare functional mutation in the *HDC* gene encoding L-histidine decarboxylase, the rate-limiting enzyme in histamine biosynthesis. Our findings, together with previously published data from model systems, point to a role for histaminergic neurotransmission in the mechanism and modulation of Tourette's syndrome and tics.

▶ As noted in other related commentaries, there are a number of treatments available to help manage patients with Tourette syndrome. Current therapies include the use of medications such as haloperidol and behavioral therapies, including habit reversal training and self-hypnosis. No current therapy, of course, gets at the heart of the problem of what causes Tourette syndrome, which has largely remained a mystery. The molecular underpinnings of the disorder have remained uncertain, although there is evidence to suggest involvement of dopaminergic neurotransmission and abnormalities involving the cortical-striatal-thalamic-cortical circuitry. Until the pathophysiology is clearly known, no treatment is likely to be totally effective, thus the importance of this report, which looks at the potential genetic origins of the disorder.

It has been understood for some time that there is a large genetic contribution to Tourette syndrome. Rare functional variants in the neuronal transmembrane molecule SLITRK1 (the SLIT and NTRK-like family, member 1 protein) have been associated with Tourette syndrome. Unfortunately, mutations were found in only a small proportion of affected persons, and little is known about how the proteins produced by these genes contribute to Tourette syndrome. What these authors from the United States and the Netherlands have done is to describe an analysis of linkage in a 2-generation pedigree that led to the identification of a functional mutation in the *HDC* gene encoding L-histidine decarboxylase. The latter enzyme is the rate-limiting enzyme in histamine biosynthesis. This family appears to carry a Mendelian form of the syndrome. Eighty individuals over 2 generations have been affected. It seems extremely unlikely that chance alone would have accounted for the clinical and laboratory findings.

The importance of this article is that it describes very clearly a link between histaminergic neurotransmission and tics, findings anchored on genetics. Several compounds are now under investigation that would target the presynaptic autoreceptor, H3 receptor. These findings suggest an approach to treatment that may prove effective not just to these fairly rare 8 patients but to others with Tourette syndrome. The importance of this report cannot be underestimated. Rarely do you see a description of 8 patients appearing in the *New England Journal of Medicine*, unless the report is having some significant gravitas.

J. A. Stockman III, MD

Behavior Therapy for Children With Tourette Disorder: A Randomized Controlled Trial

Piacentini J, Woods DW, Scahill L, et al (Univ of California at Los Angeles; Univ of Wisconsin—Milwaukee; Yale Child Study Ctr, New Haven, CT; et al)
JAMA 303:1929-1937, 2010

Context.—Tourette disorder is a chronic and typically impairing childhood-onset neurologic condition. Antipsychotic medications, the first-line treatments for moderate to severe tics, are often associated with adverse effects. Behavioral interventions, although promising, have not been evaluated in large-scale controlled trials.

Objective.—To determine the efficacy of a comprehensive behavioral intervention for reducing tic severity in children and adolescents.

Design, Setting, and Participants.—Randomized, observer-blind, controlled trial of 126 children recruited from December 2004 through May 2007 and aged 9 through 17 years, with impairing Tourette or chronic tic disorder as a primary diagnosis, randomly assigned to 8 sessions during 10 weeks of behavior therapy (n = 61) or a control treatment consisting of supportive therapy and education (n = 65). Responders received 3 monthly booster treatment sessions and were reassessed at 3 and 6 months following treatment.

Intervention.—Comprehensive behavioral intervention.

Main Outcome Measures.—Yale Global Tic Severity Scale (range 0-50, score > 15 indicating clinically significant tics) and Clinical Global Impressions—Improvement Scale (range 1 [very much improved] to 8 [very much worse]).

Results.—Behavioral intervention led to a significantly greater decrease on the Yale Global Tic Severity Scale (24.7 [95% confidence interval {CI}, 23.1-26.3] to 17.1 [95% CI, 15.1-19.1]) from baseline to end point compared with the control treatment (24.6 [95% CI, 23.2-26.0] to 21.1 [95% CI, 19.2-23.0]) ($P < .001$; difference between groups, 4.1; 95% CI, 2.0-6.2) (effect size = 0.68). Significantly more children receiving behavioral intervention compared with those in the control group were rated as being very much improved or much improved on the Clinical Global

Impressions—Improvement scale (52.5% vs 18.5%, respectively; *P*< .001; number needed to treat = 3). Attrition was low (12/126, or 9.5%); tic worsening was reported by 4% of children (5/126). Treatment gains were durable, with 87% of available responders to behavior therapy exhibiting continued benefit 6 months following treatment.

Conclusion.—A comprehensive behavioral intervention, compared with supportive therapy and education, resulted in greater improvement in symptom severity among children with Tourette and chronic tic disorder.

Trial Registration.—clinicaltrials.gov Identifier: NCT00218777.

▶ There has been a great deal written about the nonpharmacologic treatment of Tourette disorder. Those affected with Tourette disorder usually begin with tics in childhood with the severity of the entity peaking in early adolescence, often declining in young adulthood. The tics are commonly preceded by premonitory urges or sensations that are experienced as noxious and relieved on the completion of the tic. While not a common disorder, it is not rare, with an estimated 6 per 1000 children affected.

A wide variety of medications have been used to treat Tourette disorder, including haloperidol, pimozide, and risperidone. These drugs rarely eliminate tics altogether and frequently are associated with unacceptable sedation, weight gain, dulling of affect, and sometimes also elicit adverse motor effects. There have been relatively few good studies documenting the long-term effectiveness of drug therapy. Because of the less than successful use of medication, many have offered these youngsters behavioral intervention, usually in the form of habit reversal training. Habit reversal acknowledges the neurologic basis of tics but proposes that situational factors, including the reaction of others to the tics as well as the internal experience of premonitory urges, play an important and ongoing role in the expression of tics. The results of the trial reported by Piacentini et al give affected individuals and their family some good news about the outcomes of a comprehensive behavioral intervention program. This randomized, observer-blinded, controlled trial of 126 children showed a significant decrease in the number of tics in children treated with behavioral intervention.

An important aspect of any treatment for Tourette disorder is whether the effect of treatment is durable. In the randomized controlled trial reported, the behavioral therapy was habit reversal training. This involves making the individual aware of the tics and competing responses that need to be addressed. Awareness training entails self-monitoring of current tics, focusing on the prodrome urge or other early signs that a tic is about to occur. Competing-response training involves engagement in a voluntary behavior physically incompatible with the tic, contingent on the premonitory urge or other signs of impeding tic occurrence. Competing-response training is distinct from deliberate tic suppression in that it teaches the patient to initiate a voluntary behavior to manage the premonitory urge and disrupt the negative reinforcement cycle rather than simply suppressing the tic. Although the study design did not include evaluation of all children for great lengths of time posttreatment, the findings did provide preliminary support for the durability of response to behavioral intervention.

Most individuals conceptualize Tourette disorder as a neurotransmitter-based neurologic disorder. This theory is probably correct, but acknowledging that behavioral and learning processes play a role in tic severity does open another avenue of treatment beyond haloperidol, the drug therapy of choice now for over 40 years.

J. A. Stockman III, MD

Nonpharmacological Treatment of Tics in Tourette Syndrome Adding Videotape Training to Self-Hypnosis

Lazarus JE, Klein SK (Univ Hosps Case Med Ctr, Cleveland, OH)
J Dev Behav Pediatr 31:498-504, 2010

Objective.—This case series examines the practicality of using a standardized method of training children in self-hypnosis (SH) methods to explore its efficiency and short-term efficacy in treating tics in patients with Tourette syndrome.

Methods.—The files of 37 children and adolescents with Tourette syndrome referred for SH training were reviewed, yielding 33 patients for analysis. As part of a protocol for SH training, all viewed a videotape series of a boy undergoing SH training for tic control. Improvement in tic control was abstracted from subjective patient report.

Results.—Seventy-nine percent of the patients trained in this technique experienced short-term clinical response, defined as control over the average 6-week follow-up period. Of the responders, 46% achieved tic control with SH after only 2 sessions and 96% after 3 visits. One patient required 4 visits.

Conclusions.—Instruction in SH, aided by the use of videotape training, augments a protocol and probably shortens the time of training in this technique. If SH is made more accessible in this way, it will be a valuable addition to multi-disciplinary management of tic disorders in Tourette syndrome.

▶ Self-hypnosis represents another form of nonpharmacologic treatment for tics in Tourette syndrome. Self-hypnosis is one of a number of self-regulation techniques that have been used to treat unwanted behaviors. Other therapies have included biofeedback training, self-monitoring, relaxation training, massed negative practice, contingency management, and habit reversal. The latter form of behavioral modification is noted in the previous commentary. Self-hypnosis has been used to treat migraine headaches, warts, primary nocturnal enuresis, various habits, such as nailbiting, hair pulling, thumb sucking, scratching, picking, and itching, and also has been used in the management of the side effects of chemotherapy, pain management, insomnia, and asthma.

Managing tics in patients with Tourette syndrome with nonpharmacologic therapy including behavioral therapy has been around for almost 50 years. Such therapies are frequently used since medications, usually haloperidol, can be associated with less-than-pleasant side effects. Medication therapy is often ineffective as well. Habit reversal is the most commonly used nonpharmacologic therapy. Self-hypnosis has also been reported but using poorly identified protocols with less than standardized methodologies and experimental design. What Lazarus et al have done is to attempt to apply rigor to investigating self-hypnosis as a treatment of tics in patients with Tourette syndrome. They also used videotaped training to enhance the efficacy of self-hypnosis.

You should read this report in detail to see exactly how these investigators used self-hypnosis and videotaped training to control tics. In this series of 33 patients undergoing self-hypnosis, 12 experienced a dramatic response in tic control after only 2 visits, 13 after 3 visits, and 1 after 4 visits. Compared with medical management with drugs, self-hypnosis appears to be safe and free of side effects. Unfortunately, we do not have good data on truly long-term follow-up with self-hypnosis. Although the visits are fairly lengthy to teach self-hypnosis (90 minutes each), it seems well worth 2 or 3 (and perhaps 4) tries at it. Just reading this article made this editor more relaxed.

J. A. Stockman III, MD

Long-Term Mortality in Childhood-Onset Epilepsy

Sillanpää M, Shinnar S (Univ of Turku and Turku Univ Hosp, Finland; Albert Einstein College of Medicine, Bronx, NY)
N Engl J Med 363:2522-2529, 2010

Background.—There are few studies on long-term mortality in prospectively followed, well-characterized cohorts of children with epilepsy. We report on long-term mortality in a Finnish cohort of subjects with a diagnosis of epilepsy in childhood.

Methods.—We assessed seizure outcomes and mortality in a population-based cohort of 245 children with a diagnosis of epilepsy in 1964; this cohort was prospectively followed for 40 years. Rates of sudden, unexplained death were estimated. The very high autopsy rate in the cohort allowed for a specific diagnosis in almost all subjects.

Results.—Sixty subjects died (24%); this rate is three times as high as the expected age-and sex-adjusted mortality in the general population. The subjects who died included 51 of 107 subjects (48%) who were not in 5-year terminal remission (i.e., ≥5 years seizure-free at the time of death or last follow-up). A remote symptomatic cause of epilepsy (i.e., a major neurologic impairment or insult) was also associated with an increased risk of death as compared with an idiopathic or cryptogenic cause (37% vs. 12%, P<0.001). Of the 60 deaths, 33 (55%) were related to epilepsy, including sudden, unexplained death in 18 subjects (30%), definite or probable seizure in 9 (15%), and accidental drowning in 6 (10%). The deaths that were not related to epilepsy occurred primarily in subjects with remote symptomatic epilepsy. The cumulative risk of sudden, unexplained death was 7% at 40 years overall and 12% in an analysis that was limited to subjects who were not in long-term remission and not receiving medication.

Among subjects with idiopathic or cryptogenic epilepsy, there were no sudden, unexplained deaths in subjects younger than 14 years of age.

Conclusions.—Childhood-onset epilepsy was associated with a substantial risk of epilepsy-related death, including sudden, unexplained death. The risk was especially high among children who were not in remission. (Funded by the Finnish Epilepsy Research Foundation.)

▶ This is one of the most important reports in recent times in the field of child neurology. Few investigations have studied the long-term outcomes, including mortality, of children with seizures. At best, in pediatric series, the follow-up has been 5 to 10 years. Accurate autopsy data in those who are known to have seizures and die have rarely been reported.

What Sillanpää and Shinnar have done is present mortality data on 245 individuals who had epilepsy onset in childhood and were followed for a minimum of 40 years. The diagnosis of epilepsy was made before 16 years of age. The diagnosis was defined as having 2 unprovoked seizures. All were carefully followed for decades. During this period, there were 60 deaths. Autopsy rates were high at 70%. Virtually all the autopsies included toxicologic screening. Of the patients who did not have autopsy, the cause of death was clearly defined and unrelated to epilepsy except in a single individual who died after a documented epileptic seizure.

The data from Finland clearly show an increased risk of death associated with child-onset epilepsy, a risk that was substantial and persisted into adulthood. The most important significant factor for death from any cause as well as for epilepsy-related deaths specifically was the absence of a 5-year remission from seizures. By definition, epilepsy-related deaths occurred exclusively in subjects who were not in a 5-year remission. It was somewhat surprising that other factors known to be associated with increased mortality among patients with epilepsy did not emerge as significant risk factors. For example, severe cognitive impairment, frequently associated with epilepsy, was not a marker for early death in and of itself. Overall, some 9% of those diagnosed with epilepsy in childhood experienced sudden unexplained death, but this percentage included all those in the study, not just those who were not in remission for periods of 5 years before they died. Unexplained death occurred generally between 20 and 40 years of age and then again after 50 years of age. While the data from this report do not provide support for aggressive treatment to prevent sudden unexplained death in patients with epilepsy, it would seem to make sense that whatever one can do to modify the risk of sudden unexplained death by keeping patients seizure free would be reasonable.

As an aside, there are some interesting data from Great Britain about whether it is safe to drive after one experiences a first seizure. Currently, in Great Britain, patients who have had a single unprovoked seizure (whether they are taking antiepileptic drugs or not) are banned from driving for 6 months. The law applies to patients who have no clinical factors or investigation results that suggest an unacceptably high risk of a further seizure (20% or greater in the next 12 months), but the law does not specify what these various factors might be. Legislation is based on recommendations of the Driving in Vehicle

Licensing Agency's Neurology Panel that individuals should be barred from driving who have an estimated risk of an epileptic seizure or any other kind of sudden unexpected attack of more than 20% in any given year (or more than 2% for a heavy goods vehicle license, such as a trucker). Laws began to be put into place in this regard in the 1930s after a seizure of a man at the wheel of an automobile that caused him to drive into a crowd watching the changing of the guard at Buckingham Palace, killing an onlooker. This resulted in epilepsy being the first medical condition to be declared an absolute bar to driving. This draconian rule was relaxed in the 1960s. In the United States, guidelines with respect to restriction of driving privileges vary enormously among the various states and territories.

J. A. Stockman III, MD

Course and outcome of childhood epilepsy: A 15-year follow-up of the Dutch Study of Epilepsy in Childhood

Geerts A, Arts WF, Stroink H, et al (Erasmus MC, Rotterdam, The Netherlands; Erasmus MC-Sophia Children's Hosp, Rotterdam, The Netherlands; Canisius-Wilhelmina Hosp, Nijmegen, The Netherlands; et al)
Epilepsia 51:1189-1197, 2010

Purpose.—To study the course and outcome of childhood-onset epilepsy during 15-year follow-up (FU).

Methods.—We extended FU in 413 of 494 children with new-onset epilepsy recruited in a previously described prospective hospital-based study by questionnaire.

Results.—Mean FU was 14.8 years (range 11.6–17.5 years). Five-year terminal remission (TR) was reached by 71% of the cohort. Course during FU was favorable in 50%, improving in 29%, and poor or deteriorating in 16%. Mean duration of seizure activity was 6.0 years (range 0–21.5 years), strongly depending on etiology and epilepsy type. Duration was <1 year in 25% of the cohort and exceeded 12 years in another 25%. Antiepileptic drugs (AEDs) were used by 86% during a mean of 7.4 years: one-third had their last seizure within 1 year of treatment, and onethird continued treatment at the end, although some had a 5-year TR. At last contact, 9% of the cohort was intractable. In multivariate analysis, predictors were non-idiopathic etiology, febrile seizures, no 3-month remission, and early intractability. Eighteen patients died; 17 had remote symptomatic etiology. Standardized mortality ratio for remote symptomatic etiology was 31.6 [95% confidence interval (CI) 18.4–50.6], versus 0.8 [95% CI 0.02–4.2] for idiopathic/cryptogenic etiology.

Discussion.—In most children with newly diagnosed epilepsy, the long-term prognosis of epilepsy is favorable, and in particular, patients with idiopathic etiology will eventually reach remission. In contrast, epilepsy remains active in ~30% and becomes intractable in ~10%. AEDs probably do not influence epilepsy course; they merely suppress seizures.

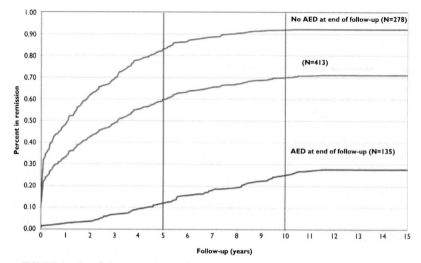

FIGURE 2.—Cumulative proportion reaching a 5-year terminal remission (TR$_E$) during follow-up. AED, antiepileptic drug. (Reprinted from Geerts A, Arts WF, Stroink H, et al. Course and outcome of childhood epilepsy: a 15-year follow-up of the dutch study of epilepsy in childhood. *Epilepsia.* 2010;51: 1189-1197. John Wiley and Sons [www.interscience.wiley.com].)

Mortality is significantly higher only in those with remote symptomatic etiology (Fig 2).

▶ This is an important report. The investigators have followed newly diagnosed children with childhood epilepsy for 15 years and now tell us how well these youngsters are doing. More than 400 children diagnosed with epilepsy are included in this follow-up study. All the youngsters enrolled in this study had at least 2 unprovoked epileptic seizures or 1 unprovoked status epilepticus episode before enrollment. The etiology of the seizure disorder had to be idiopathic to be included in this report. Some children did show evidence of mental retardation (IQ < 70). As can be seen in Fig 2, the long-term outlook for most children is excellent with 71% of youngsters being in remission for at least 5 years. Unfortunately, 8.5% of the population followed continued to have intractable seizures even as long as 15 years from the time of diagnosis (Fig 2). During the period of follow-up, the course of epilepsy was found to be variable in many patients with periods of remission interchanging with periods of seizures. Eighteen of 413 patients died. All but one of these had persistent seizure activity over the years.

This commentary closes with a challenge to your diagnostic prowess. See how you would handle the following case in terms of making a diagnosis. The 36-year-old nursing instructor is referred to the neurology service. Since this individual was 17 years of age, within a minute of starting to read, he would have perioral twitching and an abnormal tongue sensation. These symptoms occurred while reading silently or aloud, and were not specific to content or language. The symptoms were not obvious to others, but if he read aloud he stuttered. He experienced similar symptoms while teaching, speaking, or discussing subject matter, but never while singing hymns or during casual conversation. A year after the onset of symptoms, he experienced jerks of his right arm while writing which meant he could not write beyond a few lines. These symptoms affected his job and social life, forcing him to quit his occupation. Psychiatric consultation was of no help.

Your diagnosis? If you diagnosed this patient as having a classic description of primary reading epilepsy, you would be right. Primary reading epilepsy is one of the important types of complex reflex epilepsies, usually beginning in adolescence. The exact incidence and prevalence of this form of epilepsy are unknown. Patients report jaw jerking or movements of the orofacial muscles, which appear as stuttering mostly after reading for some time. These represent partial seizures or localized myoclonus. If reading is continued, a generalized seizure can ensue. Seizures can also be precipitated by argumentative conversation, writing, calculating, copying figures, or playing piano, chess, card games, or crossword puzzles. Most patients learn to avoid an attack of generalized seizure by recognizing the orofacial symptoms and stopping reading. Broad spectrum antiepileptic drugs such as sodium valproate or levetiracetam can raise the threshold for seizure precipitation. The nursing instructor described was documented to have this problem by means of monitoring with a continuous video-electroencephalogram. To read more about this problem, see the case report by Baheti et al.[1]

J. A. Stockman III, MD

Reference

1. Baheti NN, Cherian A, Menon R, Radhakrishnan A. The nursing instructor's speech. *Lancet*. 2011;377:1210.

Patterns of Nonadherence to Antiepileptic Drug Therapy in Children With Newly Diagnosed Epilepsy
Modi AC, Rausch JR, Glauser TA (Cincinnati Children's Hosp Med Ctr, OH)
JAMA 305:1669-1676, 2011

Context.—Because of epilepsy's common occurrence, the narrow therapeutic and safety margins of antiepileptic medications, and the recognized complications of medication nonadherence in adults with epilepsy, identifying the rates, patterns, and predictors of nonadherence in children with epilepsy is imperative. The onset and evolution of antiepileptic drug nonadherence in children with newly diagnosed epilepsy remains unknown.

Objectives.—To identify and characterize trajectories of adherence in children with newly diagnosed epilepsy over the first 6 months of therapy and to determine sociodemographic and epilepsy-specific predictors of adherence trajectories.

Design, Setting, and Patients.—Prospective, longitudinal observational study of antiepileptic drug adherence in a consecutive cohort of 124 children (2-12 years old) with newly diagnosed epilepsy at Cincinnati

Children's Hospital Medical Center. Patients were recruited from April 2006 through March 2009, and final data collection occurred in September 2009.

Main Outcome Measure.—Objective adherence measured using electronic monitors.

Results.—Fifty-eight percent of children with newly diagnosed epilepsy demonstrated persistent nonadherence during the first 6 months of therapy. Group-based trajectory models identified 5 differential adherence patterns (Bayesian information criterion$=-23611.8$): severe early nonadherence (13%; 95% confidence interval [CI], 8%-20%), severe delayed nonadherence (7%; 95% CI, 3%-12%), moderate nonadherence (13%; 95% CI, 8%-20%), mild nonadherence (26%; 95% CI, 19%-34%), and near-perfect adherence (42%; 95% CI, 33%-50%). The adherence pattern of most patients was established by the first month of therapy. Socioeconomic status was the sole predictor of adherence trajectory group status ($x^2_4 = 19.3$ [n = 115]; $P < .001$; partial $r^2 = 0.25$), with lower socioeconomic status associated with higher nonadherence.

Conclusion.—Five trajectory patterns were identified that captured the spectrum of nonadherence to antiepileptic drugs among children with newly diagnosed epilepsy; the patterns were significantly associated with socioeconomic status.

▶ In adults, it is well known that noncompliance with epilepsy therapy is associated with increased morbidity, in the form of continued seizures, elevated mortality, and greater health care costs. It remains uncertain whether this similar set of circumstances occurs among our youth with epilepsy because the situation is substantially different because parents and others are involved with compliance.

Modi et al have attempted to identify those factors associated with adherence to drug therapy in newly diagnosed children with a seizure disorder. The children followed were at the new-onset seizure clinic at Cincinnati Children's Hospital Medical Center. The youngsters ranged in age from 2 to 12 years. To enter the study, the children could not have findings of significant developmental disorders or comorbid chronic diseases requiring daily medication. Compliance with seizure medications evaluated using the Medication Event Monitoring Systems TrackCap (Aardex Group, Sion, Switzerland). The latter involves an electronic monitoring system that measures the dosing histories of patients prescribed oral medications. The cap on the medication bottle contains a microelectronic circuit to register the dates and times the bottle is opened and closed. The device stores the times and dates for up to 3518 events for a period as long as 36 months. The data are downloadable to a Windows-based computer.

The report of Modi et al shows that almost 60% of newly diagnosed pediatric patients with seizure disorders were nonadherent in the first 6 months postdiagnosis. You will have to read this report in some detail to look at the statistical model used, but nonadherence was definitely a problem. Socioeconomic status was the only significant predictor of nonadherence, and the authors believe that it can help identify patients at the greatest risk of not taking medication. The authors also concluded that because this is such a common problem, clinicians should consider routinely assessing adherence to antiepileptic drug therapy in all children with epilepsy.

The severe early nonadherent subset of children who took between a quarter and one-half of their antiepileptic drug doses in the first month of therapy and then became completely nonadherent over some time suggests a volitional non-adherence, wherein parents may have actively decided that their children should not take antiepileptic drugs. This may be a denial that the child has epilepsy, the belief that being seizure free means the child is over their problem, or perhaps concern about the risks of antiepileptic drugs outweighing the risk of seizures.

It should be noted that the authors did not examine the effect of adherence on health outcomes, including frequency of seizures and health-related quality of life. It was noted that 6 months of therapy is too short to rigorously determine the efficacy of antiepileptic drug therapy in a group of children with a variety of seizure types. Nonetheless, the rate of nonadherence over the course of the first 6 months of therapy is concerning and suggests a need for intervention studies that aim to optimize adherence early in the course of treatment. To read more about epilepsy, see the Patient Page in the April 27, 2011, issue of the *Journal of the American Medical Association.*[1]

J. A. Stockman III, MD

Reference

1. Parmet S, Lynm C, Golub RM. JAMA patient page. Epilepsy. *JAMA*. 2011;305: 1722.

Suicide-Related Events in Patients Treated with Antiepileptic Drugs

Arana A, Wentworth CE, Ayuso-Mateos JL, et al (Risk MR Pharmacovigilance Services, Zaragoza, Spain; Risk MR, Bridgewater, NJ; Universidad Autónoma de Madrid, Spain)

N Engl J Med 363:542-551, 2010

Background.—A previous meta-analysis of data from clinical trials showed an association between antiepileptic drugs and suicidality (suicidal ideation, behavior, or both). We used observational data to examine the association between the use or nonuse of antiepileptic drugs and suicide-related events (attempted suicides and completed suicides) in patients with epilepsy, depression, or bipolar disorder.

Methods.—We used data collected as part of the clinical care of patients who were representative of the general population in the United Kingdom to identify patients with epilepsy, depression, or bipolar disorder and to determine whether they received antiepileptic drugs. We estimated the incidence rate of suicide-related events and used logistic regression to compute odds ratios, controlling for confounding factors.

Results.—In a cohort of 5,130,795 patients, the incidence of suicide-related events per 100,000 person-years was 15.0 (95% confidence interval [CI], 14.6 to 15.5) among patients without epilepsy, depression, bipolar disorder, or antiepileptic-drug treatment, 38.2 (95% CI, 26.3 to 53.7) among patients with epilepsy who did not receive antiepileptic drugs, and 48.2 (95% CI, 39.4 to 58.5) among patients with epilepsy who received antiepileptic drugs. In adjusted analyses, the use of antiepileptic drugs was not associated with an increased risk of suicide-related events among patients with epilepsy (odds ratio, 0.59; 95% CI, 0.35 to 0.98) or bipolar disorder (1.13; 95% CI, 0.35 to 3.61) but was significantly associated with an increased risk among patients with depression (1.65; 95% CI, 1.24 to 2.19) and those who did not have epilepsy, depression, or bipolar disorder (2.57; 95% CI, 1.78 to 3.71).

Conclusions.—The current use of antiepileptic drugs was not associated with an increased risk of suicide-related events among patients with epilepsy, but it was associated with an increased risk of such events among patients with depression and among those who did not have epilepsy, depression, or bipolar disorder.

▶ It was in early 2008 that the Food and Drug Administration (FDA) first issued a safety warning on the risk of suicide associated with antiepileptic drugs. This warning cataloged the findings of a meta-analysis of placebo-controlled clinical trials of 11 antiepileptic drugs. This meta-analysis showed a risk of the development of suicidality (primarily suicidal behavior or ideation) that was twice as high among patients who received antiseizure drugs as among patients who had received a placebo. Such a risk began soon after the start of antiseizure medications and was elevated regardless of the type of antiepileptic drug used or the indication for the drug.

What Arana et al have done was attempt to reexamine this problem dealing with the several limitations that existed in the FDA's report, such as the lack of systematic or standardized language to define suicidal ideation and behavior across the clinical trials. Specifically, the investigators examined the association between antiseizure drugs and suicide-related events defined as suicide attempts and completed suicides, using data collected as part of a clinical practice in the United Kingdom. The study itself was designed by investigators in Spain. Specifically, the investigation used the Health Improvement Network database information representative of the general population of the United Kingdom that includes more than 6.7 million patients. It should be noted that a large portion of the population included categories of patients younger than 20 years and patients in young adulthood (20-34 years of age) and thus the study most likely does apply to the older pediatric population.

The findings from the United Kingdom note a crude incidence of suicide-related events of 38.2 per 100 000 person-years among patients with epilepsy who did not receive antiepileptic drugs, and the incidence was slightly higher (48.2 per 100 000 person-years) among patients with epilepsy who received antiepileptic drugs. The most likely explanation for the difference between the unadjusted and adjusted findings is that patients who received antiepileptic drugs were older and had more coexisting conditions and risk factors than those who did not receive antiepileptic drugs. The risk of suicide-related events was increased among patients who received antiepileptic drugs for indications other than epilepsy, bipolar disorder, or depression (odds ratio, 2.57; 95% confidence interval, 1.78-3.71). It was not possible to be certain about the indications for the use of antiepileptic drugs among these patients, but it is likely that for some patients, the indications were pain related (eg, herpes zoster). Pain itself, particularly chronic pain, has been associated with an increased risk of suicide. In patients with depression, the risk was also higher among current users of antiepileptic drugs than among nonusers. Although a causal role of antiepileptic drugs is possible, it is also possible that the use of antiepileptic drugs in these patients is a marker of severe depression or the presence of another condition that may be associated with an increased risk of suicide-related events.

In general, the results from the United Kingdom do not strongly confirm the findings previously reported by the FDA. The FDA study was a meta-analysis of data from placebo-controlled clinical trials of the use of antiepileptic drugs across a number of indications for up to 24 weeks. Among the 142 cases of suicide-related events included in the FDA analysis, 4 (2.8%) were completed suicides and 38 (26.8%) were suicide attempts. The British study focused on these "harder" end points that are of greatest clinical concern and involved a longer mean follow-up of 6.2 years. Unlike the FDA report, the results from England suggest that in patients with epilepsy, the use of antiepileptic drugs is not associated with a marked increased risk of suicide attempts or completed suicide. The results were similar for patients with bipolar disorder, not finding a significant effect of antiepileptic drugs on suicide-related events among patients with this condition, which itself is associated with a high risk of suicide.

The bottom line is that the findings from this report do not provide support for a strong association between antiepileptic drugs and suicide-related events among patients receiving antiepileptic drugs for epilepsy. However, an association was observed between the current use of antiepileptic drug and suicide-related events among patients with depression and among patients who did not have epilepsy, depression, or bipolar disorder. Whether the findings from this report can be totally translated to the United States is something to be debated. Chances are the data, however, are correct and do apply to the older childhood population here.

J. A. Stockman III, MD

Screening, Triage, and Referral of Patients Who Report Suicidal Thought During a Primary Care Visit
Gardner W, Klima J, Chisolm D, et al (Ohio State Univ, Columbus; Nationwide Children's Hosp, Columbus, OH)
Pediatrics 125:945-952, 2010

Objective.—Suicidal youths are rarely identified in primary care settings. We describe here a care process that includes a computerized screen, colocated social workers, and a coordinated suicide-prevention team at a specialty mental health unit.

Patients and Methods.—Patients were 1547 youths aged 11 to 20 years seen in an urban primary care system during 2005 and 2006. We performed an observational study of services provided to youths who screened positive for suicidal ideation on a computerized behavioral health screen during visits to pediatric primary care clinics. Data included clinical records, provider notes, and patients' responses to the screen.

Results.—A total of 209 (14%) youths reported suicidal thought in the previous month. Suicidal thought was more common among girls, younger youths, substance users, depressed youths, youths who carried weapons, and those who had been in fights; 87% reported at least 1 other serious behavioral health problem. Social workers were able to triage 205 (98%) youths. Triage occurred on the visit day for 193 youths (94%). Mental health evaluations were recommended for 152 (74%) of the triaged youths. Of the 109 subjects referred to a clinic with records accessible for review, 71 (65%) received a mental health service within 6 months.

Conclusions.—Pediatric primary care is a feasible setting in which to screen for suicidal youths and link them with mental health services. Youths who visit primary care clinics are willing to disclose suicidal ideation on a computerized screen. Youths who screen positive for suicide have many associated behavioral health needs. The use of information technology, colocated physician extenders, and a coordinated team on the mental health side can facilitate rapid, personal contact between the family and mental health service providers, and has the potential to overcome barriers to care for youths with suicidal ideation in the primary care setting.

▶ It is a sad fact that adolescents who have suicidal ideation are rarely identified in a primary care setting. This is despite the fact that suicide is the third leading cause of death for persons aged 10 to 19 years in the United States. Some 11% of all deaths in teens are the result of suicide. Most studies suggest that 1 in 7 high school students report having had considered suicide within the previous year. Given the fact that most insured teenagers and even most uninsured teenagers are seen annually in primary care settings, there is a heavy responsibility to consider as part of our triage the potential for a teen to do serious harm to herself or himself. Screening alone, however, is hardly enough. It is useful only if followed by effective care.

The report of Gardner et al from Columbus, Ohio, describes a primary care screening, triage, and referral process for youth with suicidal ideation. The investigators examined factors that might explain which at-risk youth receive mental health services. The investigators basically asked 4 questions: (1) Will adolescents report suicidal thought, knowing that a physician will read their answers? (2) What are the characteristics of patients who report suicidal thought? (3) If an adolescent discloses suicidal thoughts on a primary care screen, how often will that youth later receive a mental health service (not including the screening and triage process at the beginning)? and (4) Does a positive mental health screen predict subsequent suicidal ideation or behavior?

The data from this report clearly document that teens will disclose suicidal thoughts when screened in primary care, even when they know that the care provider will see the answer. Consistent with the literature, nearly 1 in 6 patients who visited a primary care office in Ohio reported suicidal thoughts in the previous month when asked the question on a computerized survey. This rate is quite comparable with results from anonymous surveys. Such thoughts, as one might anticipate, were most common among teens who were clinically depressed. Importantly, 6 of 7 youths who answered yes to the question about suicidal thoughts, also acknowledged substance abuse, carrying weapons, participation in violence, or depression. A positive suicidal thought screen result does identify a youth at risk, and it should be followed by a comprehensive behavioral health evaluation, ideally one done by a skilled social worker during the primary care visit, obviating the need for a referral to a mental health specialist for this purpose. Automatically making a referral, unfortunately, has the effect of making the assessment and subsequent linkage with intervention less likely than if mental health services were integrated in the primary care setting.

When the investigators asked what youth factors were associated with a patient receiving a referral, they found that black youths were less likely to be referred to specialty mental health services. It is unfortunate, but there is no information in this report to tell us whether this was because the providers were less likely to recommend a mental health referral to the family or because black families were more likely to refuse the offer.

The interesting aspect of this report is that the youths included in the study provided answers using a computerized screen administered while they waited for an office visit. The responses were very quickly reviewed before being seen, and based on the responses, the appropriate teams could be organized right then and there as the visit was underway. We should be grateful to these investigators from the Departments of Pediatrics and Psychiatry at Ohio State University/Nationwide Children's Hospital for showing us how all this can be done to the benefit of the teens that we are committed to serving.

J. A. Stockman III, MD

Comparative Safety of Antidepressant Agents for Children and Adolescents Regarding Suicidal Acts
Schneeweiss S, Patrick AR, Solomon DH, et al (Harvard Med School, Boston, MA; et al)
Pediatrics 125:876-888, 2010

Objective.—The objective of this study was to assess the risk of suicide attempts and suicides after initiation of antidepressant medication use by children and adolescents, for individual agents.

Methods.—We conducted a 9-year cohort study by using population-wide data from British Columbia. We identified new users of antidepressants who were 10 to 18 years of age with a recorded diagnosis of depression. Study outcomes were hospitalization attributable to intentional self-harm and suicide death.

Results.—Of 20 906 children who initiated antidepressant therapy, 16 774 (80%) had no previous antidepressant use. During the first year of use, we observed 266 attempted and 3 completed suicides, which yielded an event rate of 27.04 suicidal acts per 1000 person-years (95% confidence interval [CI]: 23.9—30.5 suicidal acts per 1000 person-years). There were no meaningful differences in the rate ratios (RRs) comparing fluoxetine with citalopram (RR: 0.97 [95% CI: 0.54—1.76]), fluvoxamine (RR: 1.05 [95% CI: 0.46—2.43]), paroxetine (RR: 0.80 [95% CI: 0.47—1.37]), and sertraline (RR: 1.02 [95% CI: 0.56—1.84]). Tricyclic agents showed risks similar to those of selective serotonin reuptake inhibitors (RR: 0.92 [95% CI: 0.43—2.00]).

Conclusion.—Our finding of equal event rates among antidepressant agents supports the decision of the Food and Drug Administration to include all antidepressants in the black box warning regarding potentially increased suicidality risk for children and adolescents beginning use of antidepressants.

▶ It has been about 8 years now since the US Food and Drug Administration (FDA) first issued the advisory that antidepressants might be associated with an increased risk of suicidal thoughts and behavior in children and adolescents. The data that prompted these warnings were based on a meta-analysis of all the then-available randomized trials of antidepressants in this age group, in which patients assigned randomly to receive antidepressants had nearly twice the rate of suicidal ideation or behavior, compared with those who received placebo. Unfortunately, the original interpretation of these findings was very cautionary and limited by a number of factors, including the brief duration of the trials that were included in the meta-analysis, few actual suicide attempts, and almost no completed suicides. The studies were also severely limited in their ability to compare suicide risk across individual antidepressant agents. This leaves practitioners with little or no advice with respect to guidance on treatment decisions.

The authors of this report from the Harvard Medical School, the University of British Columbia, and the National Institute of Mental Health provide us with important information about whether the risk of suicidal thoughts, and the possibility of suicide itself, applies equally to all antidepressant classes and duration of use or whether there are particular treatment regimens with safety advantages that might be prescribed in preference to others in the pediatric and adolescent age population. With the information from a 9-year cohort study using population-wide data from British Columbia, the investigators analyzed data from new users of antidepressants who were 10 to 18 years of age. More than 20 000 children were found who had initiated antidepressant therapy, 80% of whom had no previous antidepressant use. It was in the latter group of children that a detailed analysis was undertaken. The bottom line was very clear. There were no meaningful differences in attempted or completed suicides when comparing fluoxetine with citalopram, fluvoxamine, paroxetine, or sertraline. More broadly speaking, tricyclic antidepressants were no different in terms of untoward outcomes in comparison with selective serotonin reuptake inhibitors.

The data from this report are consistent with the findings of several other observational studies of much smaller size that have reported small or no differences in the rates of suicide and suicide attempts between antidepressant classes. This report, however, because of its enormous sample size, has the greatest power to detect a difference in suicidal act rates among the various drugs that are used to treat depression. This report therefore will be the gold standard against which all subsequent reports will be judged. The analysis, in fact, goes a long way to support the decision of the FDA to include all antidepressants in the black box warning regarding increased suicidality risk in children and adolescents. This allows clinicians to make a decision to initiate pharmacotherapy solely on the basis of likely efficacy and less so on the basis of safety. All involved with the care of children starting on antidepressants must be vigilant in monitoring children and adolescents for worsening of suicidal ideation.

J. A. Stockman III, MD

Lifetime Prevalence of Mental Disorders in U.S. Adolescents: Results from the National Comorbidity Survey Replication—Adolescent Supplement (NCS-A)

Merikangas KR, He J-P, Burstein M, et al (Natl Inst of Mental Health, Bethesda, MD; et al)

J Am Acad Child Adolesc Psychiatry 49:980-989, 2010

Objective.—To present estimates of the lifetime prevalence of *DSM-IV* mental disorders with and without severe impairment, their comorbidity across broad classes of disorder, and their sociodemographic correlates.

Method.—The National Comorbidity Survey—Adolescent Supplement NCS-A is a nationally representative face-to-face survey of 10,123 adolescents aged 13 to 18 years in the continental United States. *DSM-IV* mental disorders were assessed using a modified version of the fully structured World Health Organization Composite International Diagnostic Interview.

Results.—Anxiety disorders were the most common condition (31.9%), followed by behavior disorders (19.1%), mood disorders (14.3%), and substance use disorders (11.4%), with approximately 40% of participants with one class of disorder also meeting criteria for another class of lifetime disorder. The overall prevalence of disorders with severe impairment and/or distress was 22.2% (11.2% with mood disorders, 8.3% with anxiety disorders, and 9.6% behavior disorders). The median age of onset for disorder classes was earliest for anxiety (6 years), followed by 11 years for behavior, 13 years for mood, and 15 years for substance use disorders.

Conclusions.—These findings provide the first prevalence data on a broad range of mental disorders in a nationally representative sample

TABLE 2.—Lifetime Prevalence of DSM-IV Disorders by Sex and Age Group and Severe Impairment in the National Comorbidity Survey—Adolescent Supplement (NCS-A)

DSM-IV Disorder	Sex				Age						DSM-IV Disorder		Adolescents with Severe Impairment	
	Female		Male		13-14 y		15-16 y		17-18 y		Total			
	%	SE	%	SE	%	SE	%	SE	%	SE	%	SE	%	SE
Mood disorders														
Major depressive disorder or dysthymia	15.9	1.3	7.7	0.8	8.4	1.3	12.6	1.3	15.4	1.4	11.7	0.9	8.7	0.8
Bipolar I or II	3.3	0.4	2.6	0.3	1.9	0.3	3.1	0.3	4.3	0.7	2.9	0.3	2.6	0.2
Any mood disorder	18.3	1.4	10.5	1.1	10.5	1.3	15.5	1.4	18.1	1.6	14.3	1.0	11.2	1.0
Anxiety disorders														
Agoraphobia	3.4	0.4	1.4	0.3	2.5	0.4	2.5	0.4	2.0	0.5	2.4	0.2	—	—
Generalized anxiety disorder	3.0	0.6	1.5	0.3	1.0	0.3	2.8	0.6	3.0	0.5	2.2	0.3	0.9	0.2
Social phobia	11.2	0.7	7.0	0.5	7.7	0.6	9.7	0.7	10.1	1.0	9.1	0.4	1.3	0.2
Specific phobia	22.1	1.1	16.7	0.9	21.6	1.6	18.3	1.0	17.7	1.3	19.3	0.8	0.6	0.1
Panic disorder	2.6	0.3	2.0	0.3	1.8	0.4	2.3	0.3	3.3	0.7	2.3	0.2	—	—
Post-traumatic stress disorder	8.0	0.7	2.3	0.4	3.7	0.5	5.1	0.5	7.0	0.8	5.0	0.3	1.5	0.2
Separation anxiety disorder	9.0	0.6	6.3	0.5	7.8	0.6	8.0	0.7	6.7	0.8	7.6	0.3	0.6	0.1
Any anxiety disorder	38.0	1.4	26.1	0.8	31.4	1.9	32.1	1.0	32.3	1.7	31.9	0.8	8.3	0.4
Behavior disorders														
Attention deficit hyperactivity disorder	4.2	0.5	13.0	1.0	8.8	0.9	8.6	0.8	9.0	1.1	8.7	0.6	4.2	0.4
Oppositional defiant disorder	11.3	0.9	13.9	1.2	12.0	1.2	12.6	1.3	13.6	1.4	12.6	0.9	6.5	0.7
Conduct disorder	5.8	1.1	7.9	1.2	4.4	1.2	7.5	1.2	9.6	1.3	6.8	0.9	2.2	0.4
Any behavior disorder	15.5	1.2	23.5	1.6	18.2	1.5	19.5	1.7	21.9	1.8	19.6	1.2	9.6	0.8
Substance use disorders														
Alcohol abuse/dependence	5.8	0.5	7.0	0.6	1.3	0.3	6.5	0.6	14.5	1.2	6.4	0.4	—	—
Drug abuse/dependence	8.0	0.8	9.8	0.8	3.4	0.6	9.7	0.9	16.3	1.5	8.9	0.7	—	—
Any substance use disorder	10.2	0.9	12.5	0.8	3.7	0.6	12.2	0.9	22.3	1.6	11.4	0.7	—	—
Other														
Eating disorders	3.8	0.4	1.5	0.3	2.4	0.4	2.8	0.3	3.0	0.4	2.7	0.2	—	—
Any class[a]	51.0	1.4	48.1	1.6	45.3	2.1	49.3	1.9	56.7	2.7	49.5	1.2	22.2[b]	1.0
1 class	30.3	1.3	30.3	1.3	31.2	1.8	29.4	1.4	30.4	2.3	30.3	0.9	16.2	0.6
2 classes	12.6	0.9	12.1	1.2	9.2	1.0	13.0	1.3	16.5	1.7	12.4	0.9	5.2	0.7
3 or 4 classes	8.1	1.1	5.7	0.6	5.0	1.1	6.9	0.9	9.9	1.3	6.9	0.7	0.8	0.2

Note:
[a]Excludes eating disorders.
[b]Excluding substance use disorders [with substance use disorders: any class = 27.6 (1.0); 1 class = 18.1 (0.7); 2 classes = 6.7 (0.5); 3 or 4 classes = 2.9 (0.6)].

of U.S. adolescents. Approximately one in every four to five youth in the U.S. meets criteria for a mental disorder with severe impairment across their lifetime. The likelihood that common mental disorders in adults first emerge in childhood and adolescence highlights the need for a transition from the common focus on treatment of U.S. youth to that of prevention and early intervention.

▶ Most surveys performed in the United States suggest that about 1 of every 3 to 4 children will experience a mental disorder and that about 1 in 10 will have a serious emotional disturbance. Unfortunately, there have been a lack of empirical data on the prevalence and distribution of a wide range of *Diagnostic and Statistical Manual of Mental Disorders (Fourth Edition)* (*DSM-IV*) mental disorders from a nationally representative sample of children or adolescents. Without accurate information, it is difficult to establish resource allocation priorities for prevention, treatment, and research. The report of Merikangas et al provides information from the National Comorbidity Survey. This is a nationally representative face-to-face survey of more than 10 000 adolescents aged 13 to 18 years within the continental United States. The findings from this report provide the first lifetime prevalence data on a broad range of mental disorders in a truly nationally representative sample of US adolescents. Almost half of the sample (49.5%) had at least one class of disorder, and approximately a quarter (27.6%) had severe impairment. A mood disorder was present in 14.3% with a nearly 2-fold increase in prevalence from the age group of 13 to 14 years to 17 to 18 years. Nearly one-third of adolescents met the criteria for an anxiety disorder (31.9%). In addition to these findings, 11.3% of adolescents met the criteria for a substance use disorder. An interesting finding was that those adolescents whose parents had not graduated from college were at significant increased risk for all disorder classes.

Among the specific findings of this report was the documentation of the prevalence of attention deficit hyperactivity disorder at 8.7%, with 3 times as many males being affected with this condition as females. The prevalence of severe attention deficit hyperactivity disorder was 4.2%. Some 12.6% of the sample manifested oppositional defiant disorder (6.5% for severe cases), and 6.8% met criteria for conduct disorder (2.2% for severe cases). Table 2 provides detailed information on the lifetime prevalence of *DSM-IV* disorders by sex and age.

The conclusions of this report are fairly straightforward. Adolescence, for many, is a rough ride. The public health importance of these findings cannot be underestimated.

J. A. Stockman III, MD

Association of suicide attempts with acne and treatment with isotretinoin: retrospective Swedish cohort study

Sundström A, Alfredsson L, Sjölin-Forsberg G, et al (Karolinska Univ Hosp, Stockholm, Sweden; Karolinska Inst, Stockholm, Sweden; Med Products Agency, Uppsala, Sweden)

BMJ 341:c5812, 2010

Objective.—To assess the risk of attempted suicide before, during, and after treatment with isotretinoin for severe acne.

Design.—Retrospective cohort study linking a named patient register of isotretinoin users (1980-9) to hospital discharge and cause of death registers (1980-2001).

Setting.—Sweden, 1980-2001.

Population.—5756 patients aged 15 to 49 years prescribed isotretinoin for severe acne observed for 17 197 person years before, 2905 person years during, and 87 120 person years after treatment.

Main Outcome Measures.—Standardised incidence ratio (observed number divided by expected number of suicide attempts standardised by sex, age, and calendar year), calculated up to three years before, during, and up to 15 years after end of treatment.

Results.—128 patients were admitted to hospital for attempted suicide. During the year before treatment, the standardised incidence ratio for attempted suicide was raised: 1.57 (95% confidence interval 0.86 to 2.63) for all (including repeat) attempts and 1.36 (0.65 to 2.50) counting only first attempts. The standardised incidence ratio during and up to six months after treatment was 1.78 (1.04 to 2.85) for all attempts and 1.93 (1.08 to 3.18) for first attempts. Three years after treatment stopped, the observed number of attempts was close to the expected number and remained so during the 15 years of follow-up: standardised incidence ratio 1.04 (0.74 to 1.43) for all attempts and 0.97 (0.64 to 1.40) for first attempts. Twelve (38%) of 32 patients who made their first suicide attempt before treatment made a new attempt or committed suicide thereafter. In contrast, 10 (71%) of the 14 who made their first suicide attempt within six months after treatment stopped made a new attempt or committed suicide during follow-up (two sample test of proportions, P=0.034). The number needed to harm was 2300 new six month treatments per year for one additional first suicide attempt to occur and 5000 per year for one additional repeat attempt.

Conclusions.—An increased risk of attempted suicide was apparent up to six months after the end of treatment with isotretinoin, which motivates a close monitoring of patients for suicidal behaviour for up to a year after treatment has ended. However, the risk of attempted suicide was already rising before treatment, so an additional risk due to the isotretinoin treatment cannot be established. As patients with a history of suicide attempts before treatment made new attempts to a lesser extent than did patients who started such behaviour in connection with treatment, patients with severe acne should not automatically have isotretinoin treatment withheld because of a history of attempted suicide.

▶ Sundström et al have assessed the association between isotretinoin use and attempted suicide. We all know that isotretinoin is effective for severe nodulo-cystic or treatment-resistant acne, but its use remains controversial. Isotretinoin is associated with considerable mucocutaneous side effects, a high risk of tera-togenicity, and other adverse effects. There have also been rumblings about an association with depression and suicide. These concerns were initially prompt-ed by case reports and case series. Although a causative association is biolog-ically possible, epidemiological studies have generally failed to find one. Small studies performed to date have observed no increase in depression, attempted suicide, or suicide in people with acne who used isotretinoin compared with those who used antibiotics and no changes in these outcomes before and after treatment with isotretinoin.[1] In addition, a study of Finnish military conscripts shows that isotretinoin was not associated with an increased suicidal ideation.[2] With regard to depression, a retrospective analysis performed here in the United States of isotretinoin and antidepressant prescriptions found no association but a Canadian analysis of prescriptions and hospital admissions did find a significant association.[3,4]

It was against this background of uncertainty that Sundström et al undertook their retrospective cohort study of suicide attempts up to 3 years before treat-ment, during treatment, and up to 15 years after treatment with isotretinoin. The authors found an increased risk of suicide attempts in those taking isotre-tinoin and that this risk peaks in the months after the start of treatment. Using standardized incidence ratios (observed number divided by expected number of suicide attempts standardized by gender, age, and calendar year) for attempted suicide, they found a significantly increased risk during and 6 months after the end of treatment for the first attempt (standardized incident ratio, 1.93; 95% confidence interval, 1.08-3.18) and for all attempts (standardized incident ratio, 1.78; 95% confidence interval, 1.04-2.85).

The real issue with reports such as that of Sundström et al is whether acne alone may be what causes an increased risk of attempted suicide. It is possible that the increased risk of attempted suicide during treatment might be acne related rather than treatment related. Isotretinoin is often associated with an initial worsening of the acne. Is it possible that those who have high expecta-tions of benefits from treatment that are not met react to it in a negative way with a resultant depression? These are the types of issues that are not addressed in the report by Sundström et al.

Because there are so many unanswered questions, it seems reasonable that during and after treatment with isotretinoin (perhaps, especially, unsuccessful treatment), patients should be carefully monitored for depression and suicidal thoughts. The issue of who would do this monitoring needs to be worked out. Last, all care providers should be aware of the influence of YouTube. YouTube and other video-sharing Web sites may propagate the risk of nonsui-cidal self-injury in young people. Using YouTube's own search engine and keywords "self-injury" and "self-harm," the 100 most viewed video clips were examined involving both live individuals and those that depicted photographs or other images. The top 100 have been viewed over 2 million times, and 80% were accessible to the general audience. Explicit imagery of self-harm was common in these videos.[5]

J. A. Stockman III, MD

References

1. Jick SM, Kremers HM, Vasilakis-Ecaramozza C. Isotretinoin use and risk of depression, psychotic symptoms, suicide and attempted suicide. *Arch Dermatol.* 2000;136:1231-1236.
2. Rehn LM, Meririnne E, Höök-Nikanne J, Isometsä E, Henriksson M. Depressive symptoms and suicidal ideation among isotretinoin treatment: a 12-week followup study of male Finnish military conscripts. *J Eur Acad Dermatol Venereol.* 2009;23: 1294-1297.
3. Hersom K, Neary NP, Levaux HP, Klaskala W, Strauss JS. Isotretinoin and antidepressant pharmacotherapy: a prescription sequence symmetry analysis. *J Am Acad Dermatol.* 2003;49:424-432.
4. Azoulay L, Blais L, Koren G, LeLorier J, Bérard A. Isotretinoin and the risk of depression in patients with acne vulgaris: a case-crossover study. *J Clin Psychiatry.* 2008;69:526-532.
5. Lewis SP, Heath NL, St Denis JM, Noble R. The scope of nonsuicidal self-injury in YouTube. *Pediatrics.* 2011;127:e552-e557. Epub 2011 Feb 21.

Depression, Stigma, and Suicidal Ideation in Medical Students
Schwenk TL, Davis L, Wimsatt LA (Univ of Michigan, Ann Arbor)
JAMA 304:1181-1190, 2010

Context.—There is a concerning prevalence of depression and suicidal ideation among medical students, a group that may experience poor mental health care due to stigmatization.

Objective.—To characterize the perceptions of depressed and nondepressed medical students regarding stigma associated with depression.

Design, Setting, and Participants.—Cross-sectional Web-based survey conducted in September-November 2009 among all students enrolled at the University of Michigan Medical School (N = 769).

Main Outcome Measures.—Prevalence of self-reported moderate to severe depression and suicidal ideation and the association of stigma perceptions with clinical and demographic variables.

Results.—Survey response rate was 65.7% (505 of 769). Prevalence of moderate to severe depression was 14.3% (95% confidence interval [CI], 11.3%-17.3%). Women were more likely than men to have moderate to severe depression (18.0% vs 9.0%; 95% CI for difference, −14.8% to −3.1%; $P = .001$). Third- and fourth-year students were more likely than first- and second-year students to report suicidal ideation (7.9% vs 1.4%; 95% CI for difference, 2.7%-10.3%; $P = .001$). Students with moderate to severe depression, compared with no to minimal depression, more frequently agreed that "if I were depressed, fellow medical students would respect my opinions less" (56.0% vs 23.7%; 95% CI for difference,

17.3%-47.3%; $P < .001$), and that faculty members would view them as being unable to handle their responsibilities (83.1% vs 55.1%; 95% CI for difference, 16.1%-39.8%; $P < .001$). Men agreed more commonly than women that depressed students could endanger patients (36.3% vs 20.1%; 95% CI for difference, 6.1%-26.3%; $P = .002$). First- and second-year students more frequently agreed than third- and fourth-year students that seeking help for depression would make them feel less intelligent (34.1% vs 22.9%; 95% CI for difference, 2.3%-20.1%; $P < .01$).

Conclusions.—Depressed medical students more frequently endorsed several depression stigma attitudes than nondepressed students. Stigma perceptions also differed by sex and class year.

▶ There is no question that the life of a medical student is not always an easy one. Medical students experience much higher degrees of depression, burnout, and mental illness than their peers in the overall population. On careful examination, one can see that medical students have a significantly higher risk of suicidal ideation and suicide, higher rates of burnout, and a lower quality of life than their age-matched peers. It is sad to say, but medical students are less likely than the general population to receive appropriate treatment of these psychological issues despite seemingly better access to care. In part, this relates to the stigma associated with depression and the use of health care services. One study has identified stigma as an explicit barrier to the use of mental health services by a significant proportion of first- and second-year medical students who were experiencing depression.[1] As many as a quarter of medical students fear that documentation in their academic record that they were receiving mental health services would be a barrier to their future success, making them less competitive for residency position. All too often this leads to antidepressant self-prescription or other potentially harmful methods of coping such as excessive alcohol consumption.

In a cross-sectional study with 505 medical student participants at the University of Michigan, Schwenk et al have found that 14% expressed symptoms consistent with moderate to severe depression. Symptoms of anxiety disorders, including acute and posttraumatic stress associated with clinical training activities, may in fact be more common than mood disorders among medical students. Depressed students were more likely to seriously consider suicide, think about dropping out of school, and express greater sensitivities to the stigma associated with being recognized as depressed by peers, teachers, and clinical caregivers. This report is also consistent with other literature on the personal health concerns of medical students, their perceptions of academic vulnerability, and barriers to appropriate care.

In a commentary that accompanied the report of Schwenk et al, Laura Weiss Roberts suggests that the report by Schwenk et al issues a clear invitation to intervene with depressed and at-risk students, particularly during the transition between the second and third years of medical school when suicidal thoughts and the wish to leave medical training seem to be greatest.[2] Needless to say, everything we can do to destigmatize mental health issues among medical students would go a long way to helping our progeny face these early rigors of medicine better.

To read more about loneliness, a major contributory factor to depression in medical students and others with depression, see the excellent review of this topic by Miller.[3] You will see reference to new research that suggests chronic loneliness is associated with changes in the cardiovascular, immune, and nervous systems.

J. A. Stockman III, MD

References

1. Givens JL, Tjia J. Depressed medical students' use of mental health services and barriers to use. *Acad Med.* 2002;77:918-921.
2. Roberts LW. Understanding depression and distress among medical students. *JAMA.* 2010;304:1231-1232.
3. Miller G. Social neuroscience. Why loneliness is hazardous to your health. *Science.* 2011;331:138-140.

Effect of a barrier at Bloor Street Viaduct on suicide rates in Toronto: natural experiment

Sinyor M, Levitt AJ (Univ of Toronto, Ontario, Canada; Sunnybrook Health Sciences Centre and Women's College Hosp, Toronto, Ontario, Canada)
BMJ 341:c2884, 2010

Objective.—To determine whether rates of suicide changed in Toronto after a barrier was erected at Bloor Street Viaduct, the bridge with the world's second highest annual rate of suicide by jumping after Golden Gate Bridge in San Francisco.

Design.—Natural experiment.

Setting.—City of Toronto and province of Ontario, Canada; records at the chief coroner's office of Ontario 1993-2001 (nine years before the barrier) and July 2003-June 2007 (four years after the barrier).

Participants.—14 789 people who completed suicide in the city of Toronto and in Ontario.

Main Outcome Measure.—Changes in yearly rates of suicide by jumping at Bloor Street Viaduct, other bridges, and buildings, and by other means.

Results.—Yearly rates of suicide by jumping in Toronto remained unchanged between the periods before and after the construction of a barrier at Bloor Street Viaduct (56.4 v 56.6, P=0.95). A mean of 9.3 suicides occurred annually at Bloor Street Viaduct before the barrier and none after the barrier (P<0.01). Yearly rates of suicide by jumping from other bridges and buildings were higher in the period after the barrier although only significant for other bridges (other bridges: 8.7 v 14.2, P=0.01; buildings: 38.5 v 42.7, P=0.32).

Conclusions.—Although the barrier prevented suicides at Bloor Street Viaduct, the rate of suicide by jumping in Toronto remained unchanged.

This lack of change might have been due to a reciprocal increase in suicides from other bridges and buildings. This finding suggests that Bloor Street Viaduct may not have been a uniquely attractive location for suicide and that barriers on bridges may not alter absolute rates of suicide by jumping when comparable bridges are nearby.

▶ Worldwide, suicide is the 13th leading cause of death, and attempted suicide is a major cause of injury. Statistically speaking, suicide is an even more common cause of death in the older pediatric population. This report by Sinyor et al is an interesting one because it takes a fairly direct approach to the prevention of suicide. One of the few approaches with a strong evidence base in the prevention of suicide is the attempt to limit access to methods that are highly lethal and commonly used in suicide acts.[1] The rationale for such an approach is based on 4 observations: suicide attempts are often impulsive, crises are often fleeting, prognosis is good after a nonfatal attempt, and acts are more likely to be fatal when highly fatal methods are used. You may have noted that one attempt to limit exposure to highly lethal methods is the placing of barriers on bridges and other common sites from which suicide attempted. This seems a sensible approach. Jumping is highly lethal, and deaths are often very public, leading to media reporting and possible contagion.

In the report of Sinyor et al, we see a description of the apparent failure of the Bloor Street Viaduct barrier in Toronto to reduce suicide by jumping. Such barriers decrease or eliminate suicides at bridges commonly used for suicide, but it has been unclear whether such barriers actually prevent suicides overall. Will people simply substitute one bridge for another as a means of suicide? Sinyor et al accessed the yearly rates of suicide by jumping at the Bloor Street Viaduct from 1993 to 2001 (9 years before the barrier) and from July 2003 to June 2007 (4 years after the barrier). The barrier itself prevented all suicides from the bridge; deaths fell from 9.3 a year to 0. Unfortunately, preventing suicides at the most common site of suicides had no effect on overall rates of suicide by jumping in the region as a whole. There was a compensatory increase in suicides from other bridges.

So what do we learn from what has happened in Toronto? There are several notes of caution about abandoning barrier construction on suicide bridges. Firstly, the relatively small number of suicides from the Bloor Street Viaduct (9.3 per year before the barrier; < 4% of suicides in Toronto) make it impossible to draw any conclusions about the net effect of the barrier on suicide deaths overall. Secondly, suicides from other bridges may have been increasing in the years before the barrier was erected. Thus, the rise in suicides from other bridges may have resulted from an increase in the popularity of bridge jumping rather than substitution. Thirdly, other studies of bridge barriers have been more favorable. For example, barriers on the Clifton Suspension Bridge in the United Kingdom led to a halving of deaths from the bridge and a reduction in overall suicides by jumping in the area by men (90% of those who jumped from the Clifton Suspension Bridge before the barriers were put in place were men). Lastly, as the authors point out in their report, people who jumped from bridges, such as the Bloor Street Viaduct, that span hard surfaces (rather than water) and do not have the iconic status or esthetic distinction of the Golden Gate may differ from those who jump from iconic sites. Moreover, jumpers may be less impulsive than people who use other common suicide methods. There are ample data to show that jumpers are less likely to have same-day crises, such as interpersonal conflicts on the day of suicide than people who use methods other than jumping (most of whom die in their homes); this suggests that restricting access to highly lethal household methods may, on average, be more effective. Suicide barriers do reduce the number of people who witness gruesome public suicides and the press that goes with it. The latter may trigger other additional suicide deaths.

The study of Sinyor et al reminds us that means restrictions may not work everywhere when it comes to prevention of suicide. The most common methods of suicide are perhaps amenable to modulation, such as handgun use and limitation of certain forms of toxins. When and where restriction work, this approach may save more lives than other suicide prevention strategies, especially in teens and young adults who tend to act impulsively.

In conclusion, we offer a little-known fact: while most suicides occur in the home, many occur in public places, including national parks. The Centers for Disease Control and the National Park Service recently analyzed reports of suicides (suicides and attempted suicides) occurring in national parks during the period 2003 to 2007. During this 7-year span, 84 national parks reported 286 suicide events, an average of 41 events per year. Of these 286 events, 68% were fatal. The 2 most commonly used methods of suicide were firearms and falls. Consistent with national patterns, 83% of suicides were among males. The 2 parks with the highest number of suicides and attempted suicides were the Blue Ridge Parkway in North Carolina and Virginia and the Grand Canyon National Park in Arizona, each with 21 suicides or attempted suicides.[2]

J. A. Stockman III, MD

References

1. Mann JJ, Apter A, Bertolote J, et al. Suicide prevention strategies: a systematic review. *JAMA.* 2005;294:2064-2074.
2. Newman S, Akre E, Bossarte R, Mack K, Crosby A. Suicides in national parks—United States, 2003-2009. *MMWR.* 2010;59:1546-1549.

14 Newborn

Perinatal Regionalization for Very Low-Birth-Weight and Very Preterm Infants: A Meta-Analysis

Lasswell SM, Barfield WD, Rochat RW, et al (Natl Ctr for Chronic Disease Prevention and Health Promotion, Atlanta, GA; Emory Univ, Atlanta, GA; et al)
JAMA 304:992-1000, 2010

Context.—For more than 30 years, guidelines for perinatal regionalization have recommended that very low-birth-weight (VLBW) infants be born at highly specialized hospitals, most commonly designated as level III hospitals. Despite these recommendations, some regions continue to have large percentages of VLBW infants born in lower-level hospitals.

Objective.—To evaluate published data on associations between hospital level at birth and neonatal or predischarge mortality for VLBW and very preterm (VPT) infants.

Data Sources.—Systematic search of published literature (1976–May 2010) in MEDLINE, CINAHL, EMBASE, and PubMed databases and manual searches of reference lists.

Study Selection and Data Extraction.—Forty-one publications met a priori inclusion criteria (randomized controlled trial, cohort, and case-control studies measuring neonatal or predischarge mortality among live-born infants ≤1500 g or ≤32 weeks' gestation delivered at a level III vs lower-level facility). Paired reviewers independently assessed publications for inclusion and extracted data using standardized forms. Discrepancies were decided by a third reviewer. Publications were reviewed for quality by 3 authors based on 2 content areas: adjustment for confounding and description of hospital levels. We calculated weighted, combined odds ratios (ORs) using a random-effects model and comparative unadjusted pooled mortality rates.

Data Synthesis.—We observed increased odds of death for VLBW infants (38% vs 23%; adjusted OR, 1.62; 95% confidence interval [CI], 1.44-1.83) and VPT infants (15% vs 17%; adjusted OR, 1.55; 95% CI, 1.21-1.98) born outside of level III hospitals. Consistent results were obtained when restricted to higher-quality evidence (mortality in VLBW infants, 36% vs 21%; adjusted OR, 1.60; 95% CI, 1.33-1.92 and in VPT infants, 7% vs 12%; adjusted OR, 1.42; 95% CI, 1.06-1.88) and infants weighing less than 1000 g (59% vs 32%; adjusted OR, 1.80; 95% CI, 1.31-2.46). No significant differences were found through subgroup analysis of study characteristics. Meta-regression by year of publication did not reveal a change over time (slope, 0.00; $P=.87$).

395

Conclusion.—For VLBW and VPT infants, birth outside of a level III hospital is significantly associated with increased likelihood of neonatal or predischarge death.

▶ It should come as no surprise that for very low birth weight (VLBW) and very preterm (VPT) infants being born outside of a level III hospital is likely to be associated with not doing well. Almost 40 years ago, the Committee on Perinatal Health and the March of Dimes issued a statement *Toward Improving the Outcome of Pregnancy*, which outlined a model for the regionalization of perinatal services to be implemented throughout the United States.[1] Within regions, hospitals were classified as: level I, providing basic uncomplicated neonatal care; level II, able to care for moderately ill infants; and level III, equipped to handle serious neonatal illnesses and abnormalities including VLBW (<1500 g). Largely on a voluntary basis, most areas of the country regionalized around these characterizations, but by the late 1980s, there appeared to be some weakening in the regional systems. This led to a reissuing by the March of Dimes of a second document underscoring the importance of perinatal regionalization. Despite renewed efforts, deregionalization has continued over the last 15 years or so, resulting in an increase in VLBW infants being born outside of level III hospitals, as well as a proliferation of small neonatal intensive care units competing for market share in the same region. Data from the Federal Maternal and Child Health Bureau show slow progress toward the goal of 90% of VLBW infants in each state being born in level III centers. In 2008, for example, only 5 states had reached 90% level, while 10 states are below 70%.[2]

The report of Lasswell et al provides information from a meta-analysis of more than 30 years of published data on the relationship between hospital level at birth and neonatal mortality and predischarge mortality for VLBW and VPT infants. As can be seen in the abstract, there is a significantly increased odds of death for VLBW infants and VPT infants born outside level III hospitals. The authors of this report remind us that although they represent less than 2% of US births, 55% of infant deaths occur among VLBW infants and that strengthening perinatal regionalization systems in states with high percentages of VLBW and VPT infants born outside of level III centers could potentially save thousands of infant lives each year.

Also clear from these data is that everyone is doing a better job of saving small babies, no matter where they are born. Much has changed in the field of neonatology since the introduction of perinatal regionalization. The introduction of surfactant therapy in the late 1980s and antenatal steroids in the mid-1990s has improved outcomes for VLBW infants. Also, the supply of neonatologists has increased as has the analytic epidemiologic capacity to determine best outcomes. These improvement factors having been noted, it is still far better to be born in a level III hospital capable of a full range of services when you are a tiny baby.

This commentary closes with a fast fact related to birth rates in the United States. Provisional data from the US National Center for Health Statistics show that the national number of births was 4 136 000 in 2009, a fall of 2.6% from 2008. The fertility rate (live births per 1000 women aged 15 to 44) fell from 68.4 in 2008 to 66.8 in 2009. Births fell in all age groups except women aged 40 years or older.[3]

J. A. Stockman III, MD

References

1. Committee on Perinatal Health. *Toward Improving the Outcome of Pregnancy: Recommendations for the Regional Development of Maternal and Perinatal Health Services.* White Plains, NY: March of Dimes National Foundation; 1976.
2. US Department of Health and Human Services. Health Resources and Services Administration. Maternal and Child Health Bureau: Multi-year report, performance measure No.1. https://perfdata.hrsa.gov/mchb/TVISReports/MeasurementData/standardnationalmeasureindicatorsearch.aspx?measuretype+performance&year type=mostrecent. Accessed January 15, 2009.
3. Editorial comment. US births fell during recession. *BMJ.* 2010;341:c4771.

Time of birth and risk of neonatal death at term: retrospective cohort study
Pasupathy D, Wood AM, Pell JP, et al (Univ of Cambridge, UK; Univ of Glasgow, Scotland, UK; et al)
BMJ 341:c3498, 2010

Objective.—To determine the effect of time and day of birth on the risk of neonatal death at term.

Design.—Population based retrospective cohort study.

Setting.—Data from the linked Scottish morbidity records, Stillbirth and Infant Death Survey, and birth certificate database of live births in Scotland, 1985-2004.

Subjects.—Liveborn term singletons with cephalic presentation. Perinatal deaths from congenital anomalies excluded. Final sample comprised 1 039 560 live births.

Main Outcome Measure.—All neonatal deaths (in the first four weeks of life) unrelated to congenital abnormality, plus a subgroup of deaths ascribed to intrapartum anoxia.

Results.—The risk of neonatal death was 4.2 per 10 000 during the normal working week (Monday to Friday, 0900-1700) and 5.6 per 10 000 at all other times (out of hours) (unadjusted odds ratio 1.3, 95% confidence interval 1.1 to 1.6). Adjustment for maternal characteristics had no material effect. The higher rate of death out of hours was because of an increased risk of death ascribed to intrapartum anoxia (adjusted odds ratio 1.7, 1.2 to 2.3). Though exclusion of elective caesarean deliveries attenuated the association between death ascribed to anoxia and delivery out of hours, a significant association persisted (adjusted odds ratio 1.5, 1.1 to 2.0). The attributable fraction of neonatal deaths ascribed to intrapartum anoxia associated with delivery out of hours was 26% (95% confidence interval 5% to 42%).

Conclusions.—Delivering an infant outside the normal working week was associated with an increased risk of neonatal death at term ascribed to intrapartum anoxia.

▶ Everyone knows that delivery rooms operate 24 hours a day. The study of Pasupathy et al from Great Britain suggests that having a baby may not be consistently safe around the clock. In a retrospective study, these investigators looked at whether the risk of neonatal death varied according to time and day of birth among just over 1 million term babies born in Scotland between 1985 and 2004. After adjusting for several possible confounders, the investigators found that babies born outside of the hours 9:00 AM to 5:00 PM, Monday through Friday, were more likely to die around the time of birth than those born during normal working hours. Out-of-hours deliveries were responsible for an additional 1 to 2 extra deaths per 10 000 live births, with anoxia being the main cause of mortality.

Although this study from Scotland was unable to determine the cause of the small but significant difference in neonatal mortality related to the time of birth, it does raise concerns that staff issues are at the heart of the problem. Twenty-four–hour safety in labor and delivery areas of hospitals is a hot topic outside the United Kingdom as well. The Netherlands, for example, lags behind in the steady decrease in perinatal mortality in Western countries, and in 2008 the Netherlands' Health Minister installed a steering committee on pregnancy and birth to come up with a solution. One of the recommendations of their report that came out in December 2009 was that gynecologists and paramedics should be available for obstetric and perinatal care 24 hours a day, 7 days a week. If they are on call they must be able to reach the hospital within 15 minutes, according to the guidelines.

It should be noted that one of the concerns in Great Britain is the fact that trainees now have much less in the way of hands-on experience. In an editorial that accompanied the report of Pasupathy et al, it was noted that provision of more rested, but generally less experienced, doctors does not result in improved quality of care. Surgeons in the European Union claim that European Working Time Directives in fact put patients' lives at risk.[1] The European Working Time Directives resulted in a 48-hour working week for trainees with the consequence that many junior doctors are working more frequent, albeit shorter, on-call shifts, with more handovers between shifts. Such systems reduce patient care continuity and increase the risk of adverse events during handovers. An investigation was undertaken in Europe looking at the frequency and quality of handovers of out-of-hours urology admissions more than 2 months in 2009.[1] Seventy-three patients were admitted between 5:00 PM and 8:00 AM. Twenty patients had their cases handed over orally or in writing, but 53 patients had no handover at all. In only 7 of the 20 cases handed over were essential details given and clinical urgency indicated. Only 27% of out-of-hour admissions were adequately handed over the following morning. As a result, patients were missed on ward rounds, delaying appropriate treatment and investigation. While no critical incidents resulted in long-term harm, several near misses occurred. Needless to say, residents in the United States are not down to a 48-hour working week, but at the current trajectory, we should be there sometime in the not-too-distant future if things do not change.

This commentary closes with an observation about birth rates unrelated to time of the day but rather, to the country of origin. It appears that the one-child policy in China is now producing aberrations that are likely to seriously challenge that country's economy and social fabric. The one-child policy has created a generation in which men seriously outnumber women and has slowed population growth dramatically, resulting in a rapidly aging population, a shrinking labor force, and a skewed sex ratio at birth. The policy is now 30 years old and some have said that it has run its course. Interestingly, when the policy was instituted on September 25, 1980, the intervention was not meant to last forever. The Communist party and the Communist youth league foresaw it lasting a span of 1 generation. To see some interesting statistics on how fast things can go off course within a society demographics-wise, see the interesting commentary on this topic by Hvistendahl.[2]

J. A. Stockman III, MD

References

1. Manjunath A, Srirangam SJ. Risks of working time directive. Shorter shifts and more frequent handover. *BMJ*. 2010;341:c4858.
2. Hvistendahl M. Demography. Has China outgrown the one-child policy? *Science*. 2011;329:1458-1461.

Respiratory Morbidity in Late Preterm Births

The Consortium on Safe Labor (Univ of Illinois at Chicago; Natl Inst of Child Health and Human Development, Bethesda, MD; Cedars-Sinai Med Ctr, Los Angeles, CA; et al)
JAMA 304:419-425, 2010

Context.—Late preterm births (34 0/7 – 36 6/7 weeks) account for an increasing proportion of prematurity-associated short-term morbidities, particularly respiratory, that require specialized care and prolonged neonatal hospital stays.

Objective.—To assess short-term respiratory morbidity in late preterm births compared with term births in a contemporary cohort of deliveries in the United States.

Design, Setting, and Participants.—Retrospective collection of electronic data from 12 institutions (19 hospitals) across the United States on 233 844 deliveries between 2002 and 2008. Charts were abstracted for all neonates with respiratory compromise admitted to a neonatal intensive care unit (NICU), and late preterm births were compared with term births in regard to resuscitation, respiratory support, and respiratory diagnoses. A multivariate logistic regression analysis compared infants at each gestational week, controlling for factors that influence respiratory outcomes.

Main Outcome Measures.—Respiratory distress syndrome, transient tachypnea of the newborn, pneumonia, respiratory failure, and standard and oscillatory ventilator support.

Results.—Of 19 334 late preterm births, 7055 (36.5%) were admitted to a NICU and 2032 had respiratory compromise. Of 165 993 term infants, 11 980 (7.2%) were admitted to a NICU, 1874 with respiratory morbidity. The incidence of respiratory distress syndrome was 10.5% (390/3700) for infants born at 34 weeks' gestation vs 0.3% (140/41 764) at 38 weeks. Similarly, incidence of transient tachypnea of the newborn was 6.4% (n = 236) for those born at 34 weeks vs 0.4% (n = 155) at 38 weeks, pneumonia was 1.5% (n = 55) vs 0.1% (n = 62), and respiratory failure was 1.6% (n = 61) vs 0.2% (n = 63). Standard and oscillatory ventilator support had similar patterns. Odds of respiratory distress syndrome decreased with each advancing week of gestation until 38 weeks compared with 39 to 40 weeks (adjusted odds ratio [OR] at 34 weeks, 40.1; 95% confidence interval [CI], 32.0-50.3 and at 38 weeks, 1.1; 95% CI, 0.9-1.4). At 37 weeks, odds of respiratory distress syndrome were greater than at 39 to 40 weeks (adjusted OR, 3.1; 95% CI, 2.5-3.7), but the odds at 38 weeks did not differ from 39 to 40 weeks. Similar patterns were noted for transient tachypnea of the newborn (adjusted OR at 34 weeks, 14.7; 95% CI, 11.7-18.4 and at 38 weeks, 1.0; 95% CI, 0.8-1.2), pneumonia (adjusted OR at 34 weeks, 7.6; 95% CI, 5.2-11.2 and at 38 weeks, 0.9; 95% CI, 0.6-1.2), and respiratory failure (adjusted OR at 34 weeks, 10.5; 95% CI, 6.9-16.1 and at 38 weeks, 1.4; 95% CI, 1.0-1.9).

Conclusion.—In a contemporary cohort, late preterm birth, compared with term delivery, was associated with increased risk of respiratory distress syndrome and other respiratory morbidity.

▶ This report telling us about the current status of respiratory morbidity in late preterm infants is full of important facts. Three-quarters of all preterm births here occur between 34 and 37 weeks' gestation, the definition of late preterm birth. These account for 9.1% of all deliveries in our country. There is ample evidence over time that such late preterm births are associated with significant morbidity, especially respiratory distress syndrome (RDS). However, most of the data documenting these morbidities are quite old, thus the importance of this report from the Consortium on Safe Labor summarizing modern data from nationwide cohorts of deliveries. The data analyzed were largely related to deliveries occurring between 2005 and 2007. Late preterm births were defined as delivery between 34 0/7 and 36 6/7 weeks' gestation, while term birth was defined as 37 0/7 to 40 6/7 weeks' gestation. Gestational age was determined by best obstetric estimate, in most cases, by last menstrual period with a confirmatory sonogram.

The data of the consortium were derived from an analysis of 228 666 women who delivered 233 844 infants at 12 obstetrical centers. Late preterm births averaged 9.1% with 78.6% of deliveries occurring at term. Infants delivered at 34 weeks required more oxygen supplementation (8.3%), delivery of oxygen by bag and mask (4.0%), intubation (2.9%), and chest compression (0.2%) in the delivery room than infants born at each successive week of gestational age until 39 weeks (oxygen supplementation [0.30%], bag and mask [0.12%], intubation [0.10%], and chest compressions [0.03%]). With the exception of intubation for meconium, level of resuscitation required in the delivery room and neonatal intensive care unit (NICU) respiratory support decreased significantly with each advancing week gestation until 39 weeks. RDS/hyaline membrane disease was the most common respiratory morbidity occurring in 10.5% of 34-week deliveries, decreasing with gestational age to 0.35% at 40 weeks. Transient tachypnea of the newborn was the second most common morbidity in 6.4% at 34 weeks, reaching a low of 0.3% at 39 weeks. Also decreasing from 34 weeks were pneumonia (from 1.5% to 0.1% at 39 weeks); persistent apnea and bradycardia (from 1.6% to 0.02%); pulmonary hypertension (from 0.5% to 0.06%); pneumothorax (from 0.8% to 0.07%); and overall respiratory failure (from 1.6% to 0.09%). If you run the numbers, the odds ratio for having RDS is 40-fold greater at 34 weeks than at 39 weeks. The odds of needing surfactant administration decreases from 7.4% to 0.2% in these same age ranges.

The report of the consortium is the largest investigation to date of respiratory morbidity in late preterm infants using modern medical electronic data accumulation and controlling for multiple factors. There is nothing more powerful than solid data when it comes to information such as this. Needless to say, it is best for babies to stay inside a mother's womb until term. Even at 37 weeks, however, the odds of RDS are still 3-fold greater than at 39 or 40 weeks.

Please do not think that the information provided from this report is entirely complete. The report's retrospective design precludes collection of information not supplied in the electronic medical record or the NICU chart. For example, it is quite certain that the authors would have preferred to include information on the effect of administration of steroids for fetal lung maturity on neonates, but these data were not in a discrete field in the medical records. More than a third of late preterm births and a third of term births did not have information on whether mothers had received steroids to improve fetal lung maturity. Another potential weakness of the report, one not easily overcome, was the inability to corroborate gestational age.

The conclusion of this report is obviously straightforward and that is that clinicians should do the most to prevent even late preterm birth. Improved pregnancy dating through early ultrasound confirmation of estimated due dates may help prevent neonatal morbidity associated with erroneous early delivery of a neonate.

While on the topic of a safe pregnancy, the penultimate in safe pregnancy and delivery is seen among the mongooses. Four times a year, a female mongoose gives birth to her pups on the exact same night as more than half the other females in her group. The small carnivores are not planning a massive birthday celebration. Rather they are trying to ensure the survival of their pups. Researchers have shown that mongoose litters born a day or two earlier than others are 30% more likely to be killed by adult female mongooses. These females do not want competition for their own offspring, so they kill the pups while their mothers are out foraging. But if the litters are born together, all of the moms are out foraging at the same time—so there is no one left behind to kill the babies. Similar scenarios in ancient human societies may explain why women's menstrual cycles often end up being in sync when they spend a lot of time together. To read more about this, see the commentary on this topic that appeared in *Science*.[1]

J. A. Stockman III, MD

Reference

1. Krishnaswamy DJ. ScienceShot: Why Mongoose Moms Synchronize Births. *Science.* http://news.sciencemag.org/sciencenow/2010/08/scienceshots-why-mongoose-moms-s.html. Published August 3, 2010. Accessed August 23, 2011.

Cerebral Palsy Among Term and Postterm Births
Moster D, Wilcox AJ, Vollset SE, et al (Univ of Bergen, Norway; Natl Insts of Health, Durham, NC)
JAMA 304:976-982, 2010

Context.—Although preterm delivery is a well-established risk factor for cerebral palsy (CP), preterm deliveries contribute only a minority of affected infants. There is little information on the relation of CP risk to gestational age in the term range, where most CP occurs.

Objective.—To determine whether timing of birth in the term and postterm period is associated with risk of CP.

Design, Setting, and Participants.—Population-based follow-up study using the Medical Birth Registry of Norway to identify 1 682 441 singleton children born in the years 1967-2001 with a gestational age of 37 through 44 weeks and no congenital anomalies. The cohort was followed up through 2005 by linkage to other national registries.

Main Outcome Measures.—Absolute and relative risk of CP for children surviving to at least 4 years of age.

Results.—Of the cohort of term and postterm children, 1938 were registered with CP in the National Insurance Scheme. Infants born at 40 weeks had the lowest risk of CP, with a prevalence of 0.99/1000 (95% confidence interval [CI], 0.90-1.08). Risk for CP was higher with earlier or later delivery, with a prevalence at 37 weeks of 1.91/1000 (95% CI, 1.58-2.25) and a relative risk (RR) of 1.9 (95% CI, 1.6-2.4), a prevalence at 38 weeks of 1.25/1000 (95% CI, 1.07-1.42) and an RR of 1.3 (95% CI, 1.1-1.6), a prevalence at 42 weeks of 1.36/1000 (95% CI, 1.19-1.53) and an RR of 1.4 (95% CI, 1.2-1.6), and a prevalence after 42 weeks of 1.44 (95% CI, 1.15-1.72) and an RR of 1.4 (95% CI, 1.1-1.8). These associations were even stronger in a subset with gestational age based on ultrasound measurements: at 37 weeks the prevalence was 1.17/1000 (95% CI, 0.30-2.04) and the relative risk was 3.7 (95% CI, 1.5-9.1). At 42 weeks the prevalence was 0.85/1000 (95% CI, 0.33-1.38) and the relative risk was 2.4 (95% CI, 1.1-5.3). Adjustment for infant sex, maternal age, and various socioeconomic measures had little effect.

Conclusion.—Compared with delivery at 40 weeks' gestation, delivery at 37 or 38 weeks or at 42 weeks or later was associated with an increased risk of CP.

▶ Everyone knows that there is no way to pinpoint the many instances of underlying causes of cerebral palsy. It is associated with complicated labor and delivery, but that and preterm birth aside, most cases had little apparent association with delivery care. One of the strongest predictors of cerebral palsy is preterm birth in and of itself. It has been estimated that three-fourths of all infants with cerebral palsy, however, are in fact born within 4 weeks of term.[1]

The report of Moster et al provides powerful additional information about the root origins of cerebral palsy based on data from the Medical Birth Registry of Norway. This registry has been in operation since 1967. All babies born in Norway are registered. The data from this registry confirm that the risk of cerebral palsy increases with increasing preterm delivery, but nonetheless, most cerebral palsy occurs among term deliveries. The actual risk of cerebral palsy is lowest at 40 weeks, with the highest risks occurring at 37 weeks and at 42 weeks or later. These data can be translated into the statistical observation that cerebral palsy risk has a very robust U-shaped association with gestational age. The lowest point in that U is at 40 weeks, and sharp flexions in the risk are seen on either side of 40 weeks (Fig 1 in the original article).

The authors of this report suggest 2 possible relationships between gestational age and the risk of cerebral palsy. One possible interpretation is that delivery too early or too late even within the limited range of term and postterm births increases the risk of cerebral palsy. However, an equally plausible interpretation is that fetuses predisposed to cerebral palsy have a disturbance in the timing of their delivery, which causes them to be more often delivered early or late. This apparently happens with other fetal conditions. For example, there is a U-shaped pattern in the risk of congenital anomalies. The most plausible explanation is reverse causation; malformed infants experience disruptions at the time of delivery, with increased chance of delivery either earlier or later than 40 weeks. Needless to say, the type of malformation tends to determine the specific relationship with gestational age. As an example, anencephalic fetuses have a tendency to be born postterm, while children with trisomy 18 generally are born preterm or postterm. Those with Down syndrome mostly are born early.

At least as far as cerebral palsy is concerned, weeks 37 and 38 of gestation seem to resemble weeks 40 and 42 of gestation leaving 39 to 41 weeks as the optimal time for delivery. If the time of delivery affects cerebral palsy risk, then intervention at 40 weeks might reduce the overall risk of this neurologic disorder, while elective surgery at 37 or 38 weeks might increase it. On the other hand, if you believe that infants prone to cerebral palsy are disrupted in their delivery times, the presence of cerebral palsy will remain unchanged regardless of the time of delivery. There is little way to address this conundrum because a definitive answer would require a randomized clinical trial of deliveries at various gestational ages, an impractical option. If cerebral palsy is analogous to congenital malformations in its distribution based on gestational age, then a change in time of delivery would have no influence on a child's underlying likelihood of having cerebral palsy. The bottom line is that until the biological mechanisms for these patterns of risk in term and postterm babies are better understood, it is better to deliver babies mandatorily within a week of term, if at all possible.

This commentary closes with a question related to neonatal/perinatal medicine. Is it better or worse, in general, to deliver in a squatting position? The answer to this query comes from a recent report showing that adoption of a third-stage delivery protocol in which the placenta was delivered in a squatting position within 5 minutes of giving birth results in a postpartum hemorrhage rate of under 1%.[2] Needless to say, it is likely that this intervention will apply only to some women in specific circumstances, not the typical delivery in a maternity ward delivery room.

J. A. Stockman III, MD

References

1. Moster D, Lie RT, Markestad T. Long term medical and social consequences of preterm birth. *N Engl J Med.* 2008;359:262-273.
2. Editorial comment. Postpartum hemorrhage post method of delivery. *BMJ.* 2010; 341:c5424.

A Randomized Trial of Prenatal versus Postnatal Repair of Myelomeningocele

Adzick NS, for the MOMS Investigators (Children's Hosp of Philadelphia, PA; et al)
N Engl J Med 364:993-1004, 2011

Background.—Prenatal repair of myelomeningocele, the most common form of spina bifida, may result in better neurologic function than repair deferred until after delivery. We compared outcomes of in utero repair with standard postnatal repair.

Methods.—We randomly assigned eligible women to undergo either prenatal surgery before 26 weeks of gestation or standard postnatal repair. One primary outcome was a composite of fetal or neonatal death or the need for placement of a cerebrospinal fluid shunt by the age of 12 months. Another primary outcome at 30 months was a composite of mental development and motor function.

Results.—The trial was stopped for efficacy of prenatal surgery after the recruitment of 183 of a planned 200 patients. This report is based on results in 158 patients whose children were evaluated at 12 months. The first primary outcome occurred in 68% of the infants in the prenatal-surgery group and in 98% of those in the postnatal-surgery group (relative risk, 0.70; 97.7% confidence interval [CI], 0.58 to 0.84; P<0.001). Actual rates of shunt placement were 40% in the prenatal-surgery group and 82% in the postnatal-surgery group (relative risk, 0.48; 97.7% CI, 0.36

to 0.64; P<0.001). Prenatal surgery also resulted in improvement in the composite score for mental development and motor function at 30 months (P = 0.007) and in improvement in several secondary outcomes, including hindbrain herniation by 12 months and ambulation by 30 months. However, prenatal surgery was associated with an increased risk of preterm delivery and uterine dehiscence at delivery.

Conclusions.—Prenatal surgery for myelomeningocele reduced the need for shunting and improved motor outcomes at 30 months but was associated with maternal and fetal risks. (Funded by the National Institutes of Health; ClinicalTrials.gov number, NCT00060606.)

▶ The concept of fetal surgery for management of myelomeningocele is not a new concept. Theoretically, earlier in utero repair would provide superior outcomes for the offspring than postnatal surgery. Despite the promise of fetal surgical procedures, repair of structural malformations in utero has not been shown to be better than postnatal repair at improving the outcome in randomized controlled trials for the management with fetal tracheal occlusion for congenital diaphragmatic hernia.[1] Studies done over the years of open fetal surgery to repair myelomeningocele reported serious maternal and fetal complications. These reports, however, were based on relatively small non-randomized patient populations.

Adzick et al report the results of the Management of Myelomeningocele Study (MOMS) that was designed to assess outcomes of prenatal surgery as compared with postnatal surgery. In the study, the researchers describe 158 pregnant women who had a fetus diagnosed with myelomeningocele. Half had been randomized to fetal surgery and the others to delayed procedure post-birth. The results show that 42% of children who had surgery in the womb were able to walk unassisted in 30 months compared with 21% of those who received surgery postnatally. There were no marked differences in mental development between the groups.

So what is the rub? Nearly four-fifths of babies who had surgery in utero were born prematurely, with 10 of 78 born before 30 weeks' gestation. In the postbirth surgical treatment group, just 15% were born prematurely. Specifically, the prenatal surgery group had higher rates of maternal and fetal complications, including spontaneous membrane rupture (46% in the prenatal surgery group vs 8% in the postnatal surgery group), oligohydramnios (21% vs 4%), and more overall complications related to the increased rate of prematurity. More than one-third of mothers in the prenatal surgery group showed dehiscence or a very thin uterine wall at the hysterotomy site.

In an editorial by Simpson and Green that accompanied this report, it was commented that the degree to which intrauterine repair will transform the outcomes of fetuses with myelomeningocele remains unclear.[2] It should be recognized that the outcomes after prenatal surgery are less than perfect in MOMS, but parents now have options to consider. It should also be recognized that all these surgeries were funneled to just 3 centers that presumably have acquired all the technical expertise to get high-quality outcomes, or at least the best high-quality outcomes. With the trial complete, it is difficult to say whether other centers in the United States are likely to be able to replicate these findings anytime soon. Nonetheless, the study by Adzick et al is a major step in the right direction. Hopefully, there will be less invasive methodologies designed that will minimize maternal and fetal complications.

J. A. Stockman III, MD

References

1. Harrison MR, Keller RL, Hawgood SB, et al. A randomized trial of fetal endoscopic tracheal occlusion for severe fetal congenital diaphragmatic hernia. *N Engl J Med.* 2003;349:1916-1924.
2. Simpson JL, Greene MF. Fetal surgery for myelomeningocele? *N Engl J Med.* 2011;364:1076-1077.

Continuous Glucose Monitoring in Newborn Babies at Risk of Hypoglycemia

Harris DL, Battin MR, Weston PJ, et al (Waikato District Health Board, Hamilton, New Zealand; Univ of Auckland, New Zealand)
J Pediatr 157:198-202, 2010

Objective.—To determine the usefulness of continuous glucose monitoring in babies at risk of neonatal hypoglycemia.

Study Design.—Babies ≥32 weeks old who were at risk of hypoglycemia and admitted to newborn intensive care received routine treatment, including intermittent blood glucose measurement using the glucose oxidase method, and blinded continuous interstitial glucose monitoring.

Results.—Continuous glucose monitoring was well tolerated in 102 infants. There was good agreement between blood and interstitial glucose concentrations (mean difference, 0.0 mmol/L; 95% CI, −1.1–1.1). Low glucose concentrations (<2.6 mmol/L) were detected in 32 babies (32%) with blood sampling and in 45 babies (44%) with continuous monitoring. There were 265 episodes of low interstitial glucose concentrations, 215 (81%) of which were not detected with blood glucose measurement. One hundred seven episodes in 34 babies lasted >30 minutes, 78 (73%) of which were not detected with blood glucose measurement.

Conclusion.—Continuous interstitial glucose monitoring detects many more episodes of low glucose concentrations than blood glucose measurement. The physiological significance of these previously undetected episodes is unknown.

▶ For some time now, continuous interstitial glucose monitoring has been used as a part of the management of diabetes mellitus, largely to monitor high blood glucose levels in diabetics. The techniques used are safe and reliable and certainly lead to improved metabolic control, minimizing periods of high and low blood sugars in those diabetics so monitored. There are also some data about continuous glucose monitoring being safe and reliable in extremely low birth weight infants, but there are few data about its use in larger newborns.[1] There are obvious benefits to such continuous monitoring in discovering recurrent episodes of low glucose concentration in any newborn. Presumably, such monitoring could determine when treatment is necessary and when treatment can be safely discontinued. Continuous glucose monitoring could also reduce the number of blood tests required in infants at risk for hypoglycemia.

In the report of Harris et al, more than 100 newborns of 32 weeks or greater gestation were monitored with interstitial glucose concentrations. The Continuous Glucose Monitor Sensor (CGMS System Gold, Medtronic, MiniMed, Northridge, California) was used for the continuous monitoring. The CGMS is made up of a platinum glucose oxidase—coated sensor, a cable, and a monitor that is similar in size to a pager. The sensor was placed into the lateral aspect of the baby's thigh with a trigger-loaded insertion device and is secured with clear adhesive dressing. The interstitial glucose concentration is converted into an electrical signal that is stored every 10 seconds. The monitor then averages the signal every 5 minutes, providing 288 interstitial glucose concentration data points per day. In this study, the interstitial glucose concentrations were not viewed in real time; rather, they were compared in retrospect with the blood glucose samples that were taken. Some 265 episodes of low interstitial glucose concentrations were observed, 81% of which were not detected with intermittent blood glucose measurement. Some 107 episodes in 34 babies lasted more than one-half hour, and 73% of these were not detected by blood glucose measurement.

It is fairly clear from this study that continuous interstitial glucose monitoring will detect more episodes of low glucose concentration than blood glucose measurement. The authors of this report warn us that the actual significance of such detectable episodes is unknown. In an editorial that accompanied this report, Hay and Rozance ask the question: "Do such observations support continuous glucose monitoring in neonates?"[2] These authors suggest that there is reason for caution. Currently, we have no knowledge of what to do with the information coming from data on continuous versus intermittent assessment of glucose concentrations, challenging us with new sets of problems related to low glucose concentrations. Basically, since there is no information about the clinical significance of these episodes, we do not have a clue as to what should be done about them. There is no way to incorporate continuous glucose monitoring into clinical practice without a critical assessment of the meaning of the findings; otherwise we could see many more infants being treated than might be necessary. It is also noted that there is considerable potential for interstitial glucose continuous monitoring to yield data that lawyers may use in lawsuits even though there is no substantiation that continuous monitoring is better than intermittent monitoring, at least at the present time. None of this means that we should not be aggressively moving toward interstitial monitoring— simply that we need to learn as quickly as possible how to use this important new tool.

This commentary closes with a brief unrelated observation regarding the effect of drinking caffeinated drinks while pregnant. The effect on the risk of preterm deliveries has been studied for the past several decades without any consistent results. A recent meta-analysis, however, of 32 relevant cohort and case-control studies since 1966 now reports no important association between caffeine intake during pregnancy and preterm delivery.[3] Caffeine restriction may still be sensible, though, to reduce the risk of low birth weight, which can occur with even low doses of caffeine.

J. A. Stockman III, MD

References

1. Beardsall K, Ogilvy-Stuart AL, Ahluwalia J, Thompson M, Dunger DB. The continuous glucose monitoring sensor in neonatal intensive care. *Arch Dis Child Fetal Neonatal Ed.* 2005;90:F307-F310.
2. Hay WW Jr, Rozance PJ. Continuous glucose monitoring for diagnosis and treatment of neonatal hypoglycemia. *J Pediatr.* 2010;157:180-182.
3. Maslova E, Bhattacharya S, Lin SW, Michels KB. Caffeine consumption during pregnancy and risk of preterm birth: a meta-analysis. *Am J Clin Nutr.* 2010;92: 1120-1132. Epub 2010 Sep 15.

Hour-Specific Bilirubin Nomogram in Infants With ABO Incompatibility and Direct Coombs-Positive Results

Schutzman DL, Sekhon R, Hundalani S (Albert Einstein Med Ctr, Philadelphia, PA)
Arch Pediatr Adolesc Med 164:1158-1164, 2010

Objective.—To determine the usefulness of the hour-specific Bhutani et al bilirubin nomogram when applied to infants with Coombs-positive test results.

Design.—Retrospective chart review.

Setting.—Term nursery and neonatal intensive care unit of a university-affiliated hospital.

Patients.—All infants with A+ or B+ blood type born in our center from September 1, 2006, through August 31, 2008, to mothers with O+ blood.

Outcomes.—Proportion of infants with Coombs-positive results from the nomogram zones who required phototherapy and comparison of the percentage of infants with Coombs-positive results in each zone with the percentage of those with Coombs-negative results in each zone.

Results.—A total of 240 infants with Coombs-positive and 460 with Coombs-negative results having a gestational age of 35 weeks or older were evaluated. Sensitivity and specificity of data for infants with direct Coombs-positive results in zone 4 (high risk; 74.2% and 97.1%) and those for infants in zones 3 (high-intermediate risk) and 4 combined (96.7% and 83.7%) compared favorably with the data from the Bhutani et al cohort, which had direct Coombs-negative results (54.0% and 96.2% for zone 4; 90.5% and 84.7% for zones 3 and 4 combined). The likelihood ratio for infants with direct Coombs-positive results in zone 4, 25.8 (95% confidence interval, 11.4-58.4), was twice that of the Bhutani et al cohort, 14.1 (11.0-18.1). The nomogram performed well in directing the timing of bilirubin level follow-up. All infants in zones 3 and 4 with Coombs-positive results were followed up after hospital discharge. None required an exchange transfusion or developed bilirubin encephalopathy.

Conclusions.—The Bhutani et al bilirubin nomogram reliably identified infants at gestational age of older than 35 weeks with direct Coombs-positive results who were at risk for significant hyperbilirubinemia and directed the timing of follow-up for these infants. This finding has direct clinical applicability to the health care professional practicing in the newborn nursery.

▶ Just about every newborn nursery on the planet now uses the Bhutani nomogram. It was in 1999 that Bhutani et al published their classic report showing the hour-specific bilirubin levels of an infant, relating this to the risk of needing treatment for hyperbilirubinemia. Nurseries now routinely chart bilirubin levels using the Bhutani nomogram (Fig in the original article). It should be noted, however, that this nomogram was developed in a way that excluded infants who had direct Coombs-positive test results. Technically speaking, the nomogram therefore has limited applicability, and the information provided relates just to infants with direct Coombs-negative test results. What Schutzman et al have done is to report how neonates that are direct Coombs positive plot out on the Bhutani nomogram as well as show what becomes of these neonates in terms of a need for management of hyperbilirubinemia.

The most significant information derived from this report is the positive predictive value (PPV) of the information provided by the Bhutani nomogram in direct Coombs-positive infants. In the cohort of infants in this report with direct Coombs-positive results, those who were placed in zone 4, the high-risk group, had a PPV of 79.3%, indicating an extremely high likelihood for the need of phototherapy. While the PPV of the infants in this report in zone 3 was just 20%, this result still reflects a substantial risk that requires close follow-up on discharge. Interestingly, gestational age added no significant effect on the ability of zone 4 to predict the need for phototherapy because the PPV was already so high.

One interesting observation in this report was that only 12.9% of direct Coombs-positive infants ultimately required phototherapy using the guidelines provided by the American Academy of Pediatrics Subcommittee on Hyperbilirubinemia.[1] This finding is significantly less than the reported incidence of a requirement for phototherapy in other series. It is important to recognize that this relatively low incidence of required phototherapy likely represents the difference among demographics of the patients in this study as opposed to those in other series. There are marked ethnic differences in the incidence of hyperbilirubinemia, at least partly related to genetic variability in the uridine diphosphate glucuronosyl transferase 1 promoter region. On ethnic differences alone, some infants will more rapidly metabolize bilirubin than others.

The message in this report is fairly clear: although the Bhutani nomogram was not specifically developed for infants with Coombs-positive results, the nomogram can be applied to these infants with a high degree of success in predicting which babies will need phototherapy. It is nice to see that the nomogram has proven to be very durable.[2]

J. A. Stockman III, MD

References

1. American Academy of Pediatrics Subcommittee on Hyperbilirubinemia. Management of hyperbilirubinemia in the newborn infant 35 or more weeks of gestation. *Pediatrics*. 2004;114:297-316.
2. Bhutani VK, Johnson L, Sivieri EM. Predictive ability of a predischarge hour-specific serum bilirubin for subsequent significant hyperbilirubinemia in healthy term and near term newborns. *Pediatrics*. 1999;103:6-14.

Neonatal non-hemolytic hyperbilirubinemia: a prevalence study of adult neuropsychiatric disability and cognitive function in 463 male Danish conscripts

Ebbesen F, Ehrenstein V, Traeger M, et al (Aarhus Univ Hosp, Aalborg, Denmark; Aarhus Univ Hosp, Denmark)
Arch Dis Child 95:583-587, 2010

Objective.—To examine whether neonatal nonhemolytic hyperbilirubinemia is associated with adult neuropsychiatric disability and cognitive function.

Methods.—The study included all men born as singletons ≥35 gestational weeks in two Danish counties from 1 January1977 to 31 December 1983 that registered at conscription in a Danish region. Their infant levels of hyperbilirubinemia was ascertained from hospital records. At conscription, the prevalence of neurologic conditions and performance on a standard group intelligence test (Boerge Prien test) was compared between men with and without neonatal non-hemolytic hyperbilirubinemia.

Results.—The study group consisted of 463 conscripts exposed to neonatal non-hemolytic hyperbilirubinemia and 12 718 unexposed conscripts. The median value of maximum serum bilirubin concentration was 256 μmol/l (range 105−482). Among the exposed, 5.6% were deemed unfit for military service due to a neurologic or a psychiatric condition, compared with 4.8% among the unexposed (prevalence ratio 1.18, 95% CI 0.81 to 1.73). Among men with Boerge Prien measurement, mean Boerge Prien test score among 391 exposed men was 42.4 points compared with 43.4 points among 11 248 unexposed men (mean difference 1.0 points, 95% CI 0.0 to 1.9). There was no association between level of hyperbilirubinemia and cognitive score. Adjusted prevalence ratio of obtaining a Boerge Prien test score in the lowest quartile was 1.04 (95% CI 0.87 to 1.23).

Conclusion.—The study found no evidence of an association between neonatal non-hemolytic hyperbilirubinemia and adult neurodevelopment and cognitive performance in male conscripts. Since cognitive performance was not associated with the severity of hyperbilirubinemia we ascribe the slightly lower cognitive scores among exposed to uncontrolled confounding.

▶ When in training, I was taught that nonhemolytic hyperbilirubinemia should not be as worrisome as hyperbilirubinemia due to hemolysis. These teachings, prevalent at the time, persist to this day but with very little substantiation. Because of this lack of substantiation, many take the conservative road and use exactly the same criteria to manage nonhemolytic hyperbilirubinemia as caused by Rh hemolytic disease, ABO incompatibility, and hereditary spherocytosis, the 3 most common causes of hemolytic hyperbilirubinemia in the neonatal period.

What Ebbesen et al have done is to explore the issue of neonatal nonhemolytic hyperbilirubinemia in much greater detail than has been true in the past by doing neuropsychiatric and cognitive assessments on those entering the military in Denmark. Everyone entering the military in Denmark has a medical record that goes all the way back to the neonatal period, and it was quite easy to determine whether these young military conscripts had evidence of neonatal hyperbilirubinemia and its cause.

Almost 500 Danish conscripts were evaluated along with controls. All had evidence of significant hyperbilirubinemia in the neonatal period. Excluded from the study were those who were born at a gestational age of less than 35 weeks, those who had maximum bilirubin levels beyond 14 days of age, and those who had hemolytic causes of the hyperbilirubinemia as demonstrated by Rh blood typing, ABO incompatibility, or the presence of hereditary spherocytosis. Infants who were profoundly anemic were excluded as were those who had documented hypothyroidism. Included in the study were those whose bilirubin levels were in excess of those requiring phototherapy or in excess of the levels set in Denmark for requiring exchange transfusion. The conclusions of the data from this report are clear. The investigators found no evidence of increased risk of psychiatric morbidity or worse cognitive performance among male conscripts exposed to periods of significant hyperbilirubinemia as neonates. It is hard to say whether this report alone will assuage those who treat all forms of hyperbilirubinemia the same when it comes to the criteria for phototherapy or exchange transfusion.

J. A. Stockman III, MD

Methaemoglobinaemia risk factors with inhaled nitric oxide therapy in newborn infants

Hamon I, Gauthier-Moulinier H, Grelet-Dessioux E, et al (Maternité Régionale Universitaire, Nancy, France; Hôpital Jeanne de Flandre, CHU Lille, France)
Acta Paediatr 99:1467-1473, 2010

Background.—Inhaled nitric oxide (iNO), commonly used for hypoxic neonates, may react with haemoglobin to form methaemoglobin (MetHb). MetHb monitoring during iNO therapy has been questioned since low doses of iNO are used.

Aim.—To evaluate the incidence of and identify risk factors associated with elevated MetHb in neonates treated with iNO.

Methods.—Neonates who were treated with iNO and had at least one MetHb measurement were included. Demographic characteristics and methods of iNO administration (dosage, duration) at the time of each MetHb measurement were analysed.

Results.—Four hundred and fifty-two MetHb measurements from 81 premature and 82 term and near-term infants were analysed. MetHb was above 5% in one-term infant, and between 2.5−5% in 16 infants. A higher maximum dose of iNO (22.7 vs 17.7 p.p.m.), but not gestational age, was a significant risk factor for elevated MetHb. Significantly higher oxygen levels (75.5% vs 51.7%) were associated with higher MetHb in term infants. Preterm infants had no risk for high MetHb when iNO was kept below 8 p.p.m. These data suggest the possibility of limiting blood withdrawal when low doses iNO are used.

Conclusion.—High MetHb is exceptional in neonates treated with low dose iNO. Associated risk factors are related to high iNO dose and the simultaneous use of high concentrations of oxygen.

▶ We are seeing more and more usage of inhaled nitric oxide (NO), largely used to improve oxygenation and reduce the need for extracorporeal membrane oxygenation in term or near-term hypoxic neonates. One of the side effects, however, of NO is that it has a high oxidative stress potential, at least in experimental studies. It does diffuse into the bloodstream and rapidly reacts with hemoglobin to form methemoglobin. Methemoglobin, of course, is hemoglobin in which the iron is carried in the ferric state. The oxygen-carrying capacities of hemoglobin depend on oxygen binding to ferrous iron at each of the 4 heme groups. Methemoglobin is unable to bind oxygen and transport it throughout the body. Methemoglobin concentrations greater than 10% will result in cyanosis. The body has a mechanism to convert methemoglobin back to oxyhemoglobin at a rate of about 2% to 3% a day.

The report of Hamon et al tells us about neonates who have been treated with inhaled NO. The investigators observed a 4.6% increase of methemoglobin concentrations greater than 2.5% in infants treated with inhaled NO. Only 1 term infant in the entire study exceeded a methemoglobin concentration of 5%, and no clinical consequences could be seen in any infant treated with NO. Five percent is considered by some to be the toxic threshold of methemoglobin. The conclusion is that if the appropriate doses of inhaled NO are used for near-term or term infants, toxic levels of methemoglobin should rarely occur. Nonetheless, it is possible for infants receiving NO therapy to be at risk, albeit quite low, for the development of a serious complication such as methemoglobinemia.

On a related subject, according to an independent consensus panel appointed by the National Institutes of Health (NIH), inhaled nitric oxide therapy should not be used routinely to treat newborns born before 34 weeks' gestation. Inhaled nitric oxide therapy has been approved by the US Food and Drug Administration for routine treatment of pulmonary hypertension in term or near-term infants. Based on this, some scientists have launched clinical trials of inhaled nitric oxide therapy on infants born before 34 weeks' gestation who have underdeveloped lungs, and some hospitals have begun using the treatment off-label in this population. Such off-label use in premature infants has been very controversial in part because its cost can exceed $3000 per day and some insurers have refused to cover it. The consensus panel has noted that clinical trials to date have not clearly demonstrated the effect of such therapy on pulmonary outcome, survival, and neurodevelopment. At the same time, the panel did note that this therapy may be beneficial in infants born before 34 weeks' gestation with pulmonary hypertension and lung hypoplasia, but these uses have not been adequately studied as of the NIH consensus panel report.[1]

J. A. Stockman III, MD

Reference

1. Kuehn BM. Consensus panel discourages routine use of nitric oxide in premature infants. *JAMA.* 2010;304:2466.

Inhaled nitric oxide for prevention of bronchopulmonary dysplasia in premature babies (EUNO): a randomised controlled trial
Mercier J-C, for the EUNO Study Group (Hôpital Robert Debré, Paris, France; et al)
Lancet 376:346-354, 2010

Background.—In animal models, inhaled nitric oxide improved gas exchange and lung structural development, but its use in premature infants at risk of developing bronchopulmonary dysplasia remains controversial. We therefore tested the hypothesis that inhaled nitric oxide at a low concentration, started early and maintained for an extended period in babies with mild respiratory failure, might reduce the incidence of bronchopulmonary dysplasia.

Methods.—800 preterm infants with a gestational age at birth of between 24 weeks and 28 weeks plus 6 days (inclusive), weighing at least 500 g, requiring surfactant or continuous positive airway pressure for respiratory distress syndrome within 24 h of birth were randomly assigned in a one-to-one ratio to inhaled nitric oxide (5 parts per million) or placebo gas (nitrogen gas) for a minimum of 7 days and a maximum of 21 days in a double-blind study done at 36 centres in nine countries in the European Union. Care providers and investigators were masked to the computer-generated treatment assignment. The primary outcome was survival without development of bronchopulmonary dysplasia at postmenstrual age 36 weeks. Analysis was by intention to treat. This study is registered with ClinicalTrials. gov, number NCT00551642.

Findings.—399 infants were assigned to inhaled nitric oxide, and 401 to placebo. 395 and 400, respectively, were analysed. Treatment with inhaled nitric oxide and placebo did not result in significant differences in survival of infants without development of bronchopulmonary dysplasia (258 [65%] of 395 *vs* 262 [66%] of 400, respectively; relative risk 1·05, 95% CI 0·78−1·43); in survival at 36 weeks' postmenstrual age (343 [86%] of 399 *vs* 359 [90%] of 401, respectively; 0·74, 0·48−1·15); and in development of bronchopulmonary dysplasia (81 [24%] of 339 *vs* 96 [27%] of 358, respectively; 0·83, 0·58−1·17).

Interpretation.—Early use of low-dose inhaled nitric oxide in very premature babies did not improve survival without bronchopulmonary dysplasia or brain injury, suggesting that such a preventive treatment strategy is unsuccessful.

▶ There are lots of reasons to think that nitric oxide (NO) might be helpful in the management/prevention of the long-term complications of bronchopulmonary dysplasia. NO does have a vasodilatory role in pulmonary hypertension in term infants. This has been documented. NO also shows positive effects in animal models of lung immaturity and lung injury including a reduction in lung inflammation, neutrophil infiltration into the lung, protection against oxidant lung injury, reversal of the effects of inhibition of vascular endothelial growth factor, and stimulation of angiogenesis and the maturation of alveoli.

The report of Mercier et al tells us about the use of NO in 800 patients. Unfortunately, the data from this report show that the early use of low-dose inhaled nitric acid in very premature babies does not improve survival. The information from this report illustrates how varying the findings have been from trials with NO. To date, some studies have shown benefit, others no benefit to NO use as part of the prevention of bronchopulmonary dysplasia.

In an editorial that accompanied this report, Sosenko and Bancalari asked the question: can the clinician, with the data available from 6 large-scale clinical trials, make an evidence-based decision about the use of inhaled NO in premature infants without bronchopulmonary dysplasia to improve their survival?[1] They replied that so far, the answer is no. While some infants seem to be improved with NO, more studies are clearly needed to define the optimal dose and duration and the target population in terms of maturity, severity of illness, race, and age at enrollment at which the infant would optimally and potentially be most responsive to the intervention provided by inhaled NO, if any.

Thus, it is that inhaled NO can and should be used for certain purposes such as to improve oxygenation and reduce the need for extracorporeal membrane oxygenation in term or near-term hypoxic neonates, but when it comes to the prevention of bronchopulmonary dysplasia, we have to wait for more evidence.

J. A. Stockman III, MD

Reference

1. Sosenko IRS, Bancalari E. NO for preterm infants at risk for bronchopulmonary dysplasia. *Lancet.* 2010;376:308-310.

Neonatal Abstinence Syndrome after Methadone or Buprenorphine Exposure

Jones HE, Kaltenbach K, Heil SH, et al (Johns Hopkins Univ School of Medicine, Baltimore, MD; Thomas Jefferson Univ, Philadelphia, PA; Univ of Vermont, Burlington; et al)

N Engl J Med 363:2320-2331, 2010

Background.—Methadone, a full mu-opioid agonist, is the recommended treatment for opioid dependence during pregnancy. However, prenatal exposure to methadone is associated with a neonatal abstinence syndrome (NAS) characterized by central nervous system hyperirritability and autonomic nervous system dysfunction, which often requires medication and extended hospitalization. Buprenorphine, a partial mu-opioid agonist, is an alternative treatment for opioid dependence but has not been extensively studied in pregnancy.

Methods.—We conducted a double-blind, double-dummy, flexible-dosing, randomized, controlled study in which buprenorphine and methadone were compared for use in the comprehensive care of 175 pregnant women with opioid dependency at eight international sites. Primary outcomes were the number of neonates requiring treatment for NAS, the peak NAS score, the total amount of morphine needed to treat NAS, the length of the hospital stay for neonates, and neonatal head circumference.

Results.—Treatment was discontinued by 16 of the 89 women in the methadone group (18%) and 28 of the 86 women in the buprenorphine group (33%). A comparison of the 131 neonates whose mothers were followed to the end of pregnancy according to treatment group (with 58 exposed to buprenorphine and 73 exposed to methadone) showed that the former group required significantly less morphine (mean dose, 1.1 mg vs. 10.4 mg; $P<0.0091$), had a significantly shorter hospital stay (10.0 days vs. 17.5 days, $P<0.0091$), and had a significantly shorter duration of treatment for the neonatal abstinence syndrome (4.1 days vs. 9.9 days, $P<0.003125$) (P values calculated in accordance with prespecified thresholds for significance). There were no significant differences between groups in other primary or secondary outcomes or in the rates of maternal or neonatal adverse events.

Conclusions.—These results are consistent with the use of buprenorphine as an acceptable treatment for opioid dependence in pregnant women. (Funded by the National Institute on Drug Abuse; ClinicalTrials.gov number, NCT00271219.)

▶ As is true of nonpregnant drug-using patients, methadone is used as part of a comprehensive approach to the care of pregnant women and does improve both maternal and neonatal outcomes in comparison with no treatment. Unfortunately, exposure to methadone in utero can result in a disorder known as neonatal abstinence syndrome. This syndrome is characterized by a newborn having irritability of the central nervous system and dysfunction in the autonomic nervous system affecting the gastrointestinal tract and respiratory systems. Untreated neonatal abstinence syndrome can cause serious problems, including diarrhea, feeding difficulties, weight loss, and seizures. Death has also been reported. For these reasons, care providers have been looking for an alternative to methadone to manage pregnant women addicted to opioids.

We see in this report that buprenorphine may be a useful alternative to the use of methadone in pregnancy. Buprenorphine is a partial μ-opioid agonist and a κ-opioid antagonist. It has been used to treat opioid dependence. Its intrinsic receptor efficacy results in a less-than-maximal opioid effect and a diminished risk of overdose, as compared with methadone. In nonpregnant adults, the effects of abrupt withdrawal of buprenorphine are minimal relative to the effects of withdrawal of a full μ-opioid agonist. Small studies have suggested that neonates exposed to buprenorphine might be less likely to require treatment of neonatal abstinence syndrome than those exposed to methadone. The study of Jones et al confirms this. Jones et al conducted a double-blind study comparing buprenorphine with methadone when used in 175 pregnant women. They looked at 5 primary neonatal outcome measures related to neonatal abstinence syndrome as well as length of hospital stay and head circumference. In terms of outcomes, the percentage of neonates requiring neonatal abstinence syndrome treatment did not differ significantly between the 2 treatment groups. There was also no difference in head circumference. There were, however, significant differences in the amount of morphine needed for the treatment of neonatal abstinence syndrome and the length of hospital stay in neonates. On average, neonates exposed to buprenorphine required 89% less morphine than did neonates exposed to methadone. These babies also required less time in the neonatal unit (10 days vs 17.5 days). The 2 medication groups did not differ significantly with respect to any serious maternal or neonatal adverse events.

This randomized double-blind trial documents that infants who had prenatal exposure to buprenorphine require significantly less morphine for the treatment of neonatal abstinence syndrome, a significantly shorter period of treatment of neonatal abstinence syndrome, and a significantly shorter hospital stay than do infants with prenatal exposure to methadone. Unfortunately, women who are taking buprenorphine are more likely to discontinue treatment during their pregnancies. Why this observation occurred is unexplained. The high rate of satisfaction with methadone affirms the important role it plays in the treatment of pregnant women who are highly dependent on opioids. Moreover, given the partial agonistic activity of buprenorphine and its ceiling effects of at maximal doses, it will not be the optimal treatment for all pregnant patients with dependency on opioids.

The bottom line here is that for many, buprenorphine is a suitable alternative methadone for the treatment of opioid dependency during pregnancy, at least from the infant's point of view. It would seem that a good recommendation would be to at least attempt to use this drug to manage a pregnancy unless a woman finds that buprenorphine is not a suitable alternative to methadone in controlling opioid dependency.

J. A. Stockman III, MD

Secondhand Smoke and Adverse Fetal Outcomes in Nonsmoking Pregnant Women: A Meta-analysis

Leonardi-Bee J, Britton J, Venn A (Univ of Nottingham, UK)
Pediatrics 127:734-741, 2011

Objective.—To determine the risk of adverse fetal outcomes of second-hand smoke exposure in nonsmoking pregnant women.

Methods.—This was a systematic review and meta-analysis in accordance with Meta-analysis of Observational Studies in Epidemiology (MOOSE) guidelines. We searched Medline and Embase (to March 2009) and reference lists for eligible studies; no language restrictions were imposed. Pooled odds ratios (ORs) with 95% confidence intervals (CIs) were estimated by using random-effect models. Our search was for epidemiologic studies of maternal exposure to secondhand smoke during pregnancy in nonsmoking pregnant women. The main outcome measures were spontaneous abortion, perinatal and neonatal death, stillbirth, and congenital malformations.

Results.—We identified 19 studies that assessed the effects of second-hand smoke exposure in nonsmoking pregnant women. We found no evidence of a statistically significant effect of secondhand smoke exposure on the risk of spontaneous abortion (OR: 1.17 [95% CI: 0.88–1.54]; 6 studies). However, secondhand smoke exposure significantly increased the risk of stillbirth (OR: 1.23 [95% CI: 1.09–1.38]; 4 studies) and congenital malformation (OR: 1.13 [95% CI: 1.01–1.26]; 7 studies), although none of the associations with specific congenital abnormalities were individually significant. Secondhand smoke exposure had no significant effect on perinatal or neonatal death.

Conclusions.—Pregnant women who are exposed to secondhand smoke are estimated to be 23% more likely to experience stillbirth and 13% more likely give birth to a child with a congenital malformation. Because the timing and mechanism of this effect is not clear, it is important to prevent secondhand smoke exposure in women before and during pregnancy.

▶ Everyone knows that drinking alcoholic beverages and smoking during pregnancy are not good for an unborn baby. There is not only an increased risk of fetal mortality and morbidity but also a risk for being born small for gestational age, particularly in infants born of actively smoking mothers. Birth weights of infants born to mothers who smoke during pregnancy average about 250 g less than those born to nonsmoking mothers.[1] What is not well known is whether secondhand smoke might cause some degree of similar difficulties. A recent systematic review and meta-analysis did report that secondhand smoke exposure in nonsmoking pregnant women would decrease birth weight by about 33 g and also would increase the risk of low birth weight.[2] The effect of maternal secondhand smoke exposure on other fetal outcomes including mortality and congenital malformation, however, has been less widely noted, thus the importance of the results of this study.

Leonardi-Bee et al report on results of a systematic review and meta-analysis of the world's literature in an attempt to quantify the effect of maternal second-hand smoke exposure during pregnancy on a range of adverse fetal outcomes, including spontaneous abortion, fetal death, stillbirth, and major malformations. After screening more than 4000 articles identified in a search engine, 19 studies were found to meet all the inclusion criteria to form a proper systematic review and meta-analysis. Secondhand smoke exposure during pregnancy increased the risk of stillbirth by 23% and congenital malformations by 13%. It had no significant effect on perinatal or neonatal death. The latter is not surprising given the fact that typical secondhand smoke exposure consists of only about 1% of typical active smoking exposure.

The authors of this report conclude that the effects of secondhand smoke on adverse fetal outcomes are likely to be the result of the impact of sidestream smoke, which is the primary component of secondhand smoke exposure and has been shown to be more harmful than mainstream smoke because it contains greater concentrations of toxins that are harmful to the fetus. It is speculated that the mechanism by which secondhand smoke exposure exerts its effects could be the mother's exposure to sidestream smoke during a particular period in pregnancy and/or during the preconception period or could be the direct effect of active smoking by the father on spermatogenesis, thereby inducing genotoxic effects.

The conclusions of this report provide confirmatory evidence that there are adverse effects in maternal secondhand smoke exposure during pregnancy on the health of the fetus. As an aside, Bandiera et al have recently shown data that among nonsmokers exposed to secondhand smoke, serum cotinine levels are potentially associated with symptoms of the *Diagnostic and Statistical Manual of Mental Disorders* (Fourth Edition) major depressive disorder, general anxiety disorder, attention deficit/hyperactivity disorder, and conduct disorder after adjusting for age, sex, race/ethnicity, poverty, migraine, asthma, hay fever, and maternal smoking during pregnancy.[3] These results are consistent with a growing body of research documenting an association between second-hand smoke exposure and mental health outcomes.

J. A. Stockman III, MD

References

1. Shah NR, Bracken MB. A systematic review and meta-analysis of prospective studies on the association between maternal cigarette smoking and preterm delivery. *Am J Obstet Gynecol.* 2000;182:465-472.
2. Leonardi-Bee J, Smyth A, Britton J, Coleman T. Environmental tobacco smoke and fetal health: systematic review and meta-analysis. *Arch Dis Child Fetal Neonatal Ed.* 2008;93:F351-F361.
3. Bandiera FC, Richardson AK, Lee DJ, et al. Secondhand smoke exposure and mental health among children and adolescents. *Arch Pediatr Adolesc Med.* 2011;165:332-338.

Effectiveness of antenatal corticosteroids in reducing respiratory disorders in late preterm infants: randomised clinical trial

Porto AMF, Coutinho IC, Correia JB, et al (Instituto de Medicina Integral Professor Fernando Figueira (IMIP), Recife, Pernambuco, Brazil)
BMJ 342:d1696, 2011

Objectives.—To determine the effectiveness of corticosteroids in reducing respiratory disorders in infants born at 34-36 weeks' gestation.
Design.—Randomised triple blind clinical trial.
Setting.—A large tertiary teaching hospital in northeast of Brazil.
Participants.—Women at 34-36 weeks of pregnancy at risk of imminent premature delivery.
Interventions.—Betamethasone 12 mg or placebo intramuscularly for two consecutive days.
Main Outcomes Measures.—Primary outcome was the incidence of respiratory disorders (respiratory distress syndrome and transient tachypnoea of the newborn). Secondary outcomes included the need for ventilatory support, neonatal morbidity, and duration of stay in hospital.
Results.—320 women were randomised, 163 of whom were assigned to the treatment group and 157 to the controls. Final analysis included 143 and 130 infants, respectively. The rate of respiratory distress syndrome was low (two (1.4%) in the corticosteroid group; one (0.8%) in the placebo group; P=0.54), while the rate of transient tachypnoea was high in both groups (34 (24%) v 29 (22%); P=0.77). There was no reduction in the risk of respiratory morbidity with corticosteroid use even after adjustment for subgroups of gestational age (34-34^{+6} weeks, 35-35^{+6} weeks, and $\geq$36 weeks). The adjusted risk of respiratory morbidity was 1.12 (95% confidence interval 0.74 to 1.70). The need for ventilatory support was around 20% in both groups. There was no difference in neonatal morbidity (88 (62%) v 93 (72%); P=0.08) or in the duration of stay in hospital between the two groups (5.12 v 5.22 days; P=0.87). Phototherapy for jaundice was required less often in babies whose mothers received corticosteroids (risk ratio 0.63, 0.44 to 0.91).
Conclusions.—Antenatal treatment with corticosteroids at 34-36 weeks of pregnancy does not reduce the incidence of respiratory disorders in newborn infants.
Trial Registration.—Clinical Trials NCT00675246.

▶ No one will argue, based on a substantial body of evidence, that antenatal corticosteroids safely reduce the incidence of neonatal respiratory disorders in infants born before 34 weeks' gestation. What comes in a slightly older gestational age group, however, has been a bit murkier. Currently, such intervention is not universally recommended. Subgroup analyses from meta-analyses have not yet answered the question as to whether corticosteroids might be of value after 34 weeks.

Porto et al from Brazil conducted a new randomized controlled trial to examine this issue. Pregnant women at risk of imminent premature delivery between 34 and 36 weeks were allocated to receive either 12-mg betamethasone or placebo intramuscularly for 2 consecutive days. The intervention was shown to have no different outcome with respect to the incidence of respiratory distress syndrome and transient tachypnea in the newborn.

In an editorial that accompanied this report, it was mentioned that the report of Porto et al, which has received a lot of attention, has some limitations. The study may not have been sufficiently powered to assess the differences in rates of respiratory distress syndrome, raising the possibility that the overall rates of this syndrome were too small to detect the effect of antenatal corticosteroids.[1] The commentary suggests that clinicians should not alter their current practice on the basis of this single possibly underpowered randomized controlled trial, but rather should await incorporation of these results into a systematic review of antenatal steroids, which is currently being updated.[2]

It will be interesting to see what further evidence evolves or doesn't evolve to tell us whether steroids are useful in more mature infants. Fetal lungs are assumed to have reached surfactant maturity by 34 weeks, and this is the reason so few studies have specifically looked at the efficacy of antenatal corticosteroids between 34 and 36 weeks of pregnancy. While there is not a uniform consensus about the application of steroids beyond 34 weeks, they are used in many places because, between 34 and 36 weeks, infants are still at risk of respiratory morbidity, mainly transient tachypnea of the newborn and respiratory distress syndrome.

J. A. Stockman III, MD

References

1. Roberts D. Antenatal corticosteroids in late preterm infants: limited evidence suggest no effect on respiratory disorders or other complications of prematurity. *BMJ.* 2011;342:833-834.
2. Roberts D, Dalziel S. Antenatal corticosteroids for accelerating fetal lung maturation for women at risk of preterm birth. *Cochrane Database Syst Rev.* 2006;(3). CD004454.

Hemolysis and Hyperbilirubinemia in Antiglobulin Positive, Direct ABO Blood Group Heterospecific Neonates
Kaplan M, Hammerman C, Vreman HJ, et al (Shaare Zedek Med Ctr, Jerusalem, Israel; Stanford Univ School of Medicine, CA)
J Pediatr 157:772-777, 2010

Objective.—We quantified hemolysis and determined the incidence of hyperbilirubinemia in neonates who were direct antiglobulin titer (DAT)-positive, ABO heterospecific, and compared variables among O-A and O-B subgroups.

Study Design.—Plasma total bilirubin (PTB) was determined before the neonates were discharged from the hospital and more frequently when clinically warranted, in neonates who were DAT positive with blood group A or B and with mothers who had blood group O. Heme catabolism (and therefore bilirubin production) was indexed by blood carboxyhemo-globin corrected for inspired carbon monoxide (COHbc). Hyperbilirubi-nemia was defined as any PTB concentration >95th percentile on the hour-of-life-specific bilirubin nomogram.

Results.—Of 164 neonates, 111 were O-A and 53 O-B. Overall, hyper-bilirubinemia developed in 85 neonates (51.8%), and it tended to be more prevalent in the O-B neonates than O-A neonates (62.3% versus 46.8%; $P = .053$). Hyperbilirubinemia developed in more O-B newborns than O-A newborns at <24 ours (93.9% versus 48.1%; $P < .0001$). COHbc values were globally higher than our previously published newborn values. Babies in whom hyperbilirubinemia developed had higher COHbc values than the already high values of babies who were non-hyperbilirubinemic, and O-B newborns tended to have higher values than their O-A counterparts.

Conclusions.—DAT-positive, ABO heterospecificity is associated with increased hemolysis and a high incidence of neonatal hyperbilirubinemia. O-B heterospecificity tends to confer even higher risk than O-A counterparts.

▶ One would have thought that after decades of the acquisition of knowledge regarding hyperbilirubinemia, we would have perfected, or at least come to near perfection, our knowledge about the role of ABO incompatibility and the risk of significant hyperbilirubinemia. Apparently we have not come close to the mark as yet because the information provided in the report of Kaplan et al continues to add significant and important new knowledge on this topic.

For some, the term heterospecific blood grouping is relatively new. When it comes to ABO blood grouping, all the term means is that the mother is of blood group O and the newborn is of blood group A or B. Obviously in such circumstances, if the direct antiglobulin titer (DAT) is positive, there is an increased risk of the development of hyperbilirubinemia. The experience of anyone in practice, however, is that there seems to be little predictability when it comes to who will and will not develop hyperbilirubinemia in the circum-stances of a positive DAT and ABO blood group heterospecific specificity. Now we see exactly how common, or uncommon, newborn blood group heter-ospecificity truly is. At the Shaare Zedek Medical Center in Jerusalem, 21% of newborns are of blood group A or B and are born to blood group O mothers. Some 15% of the latter newborns are DAP positive, and of these, 52% develop hyperbilirubinemia. Elevated carboxyhemoglobin concentrations confirmed the hemolytic nature of DAT-positive ABO heterospecificity in this population. Indeed, the percentage of hyperbilirubinemic neonates increases with increasing carboxyhemoglobin concentration values. Greater degrees of hemolysis and hyperbilirubinemia were noted when a baby with blood group B was born of a blood group O mother in comparison with a baby born with blood group A of a blood group O mother. Also in the O-B circumstance, hyperbilirubinemia occurred earlier and more often in the first 24 hours of life. No baby in this series developed kernicterus. A number of babies, however, did require intervention in the form of phototherapy. The apparent mild nature of the disease should not cause complacency for ABO hemolytic disease because there are reports in the literature of severe hyperbilirubinemia and kernicterus in such circumstances.

J. A. Stockman III, MD

Nasal continuous positive airway pressure (CPAP) versus bi-level nasal CPAP in preterm babies with respiratory distress syndrome: a randomised control trial

Lista G, Castoldi F, Fontana P, et al (Children's Hosp, Via Castelvetro, Milan, Italy; et al)

Arch Dis Child Fetal Neonatal Ed 95:F85-F89, 2010

Objective.—To evaluate the clinical course, respiratory outcomes and markers of inflammation in preterm infants with moderate respiratory distress syndrome (RDS) assigned from birth to nasal continuous positive airway pressure (NCPAP) or bi-level NCPAP.

Methods.—A total of 40 infants with a gestational age (GA) of 28–34 weeks (<35 weeks' GA), affected by moderate RDS, were considered eligible and were randomised to NCPAP (group A; n = 20, CPAP level = 6 cm H_2O) or to bi-level NCPAP (group B; n = 20, lower CPAP level = 4.5 cm H_2O, higher CPAP level = 8 cm H_2O), provided with variable flow devices. Inflammatory response was the primary outcome; serum cytokines were measured on days 1 and 7 of life. Length of ventilation, oxygen dependency, need for intubation and occurrence of air leaks were considered as secondary outcomes.

Results.—Infants showed similar characteristics at birth (group A vs group B: GA 30.3 ± 2 vs 30.2 ± 2 weeks, birth weight 1429 ± 545 vs 1411 ± 560 g) and showed similar serum cytokine levels at all times. Group A underwent longer respiratory support (6.2 ± 2 days vs 3.8 ± 1 days, p = 0.025), longer O_2 dependency (13.8 ± 8 days vs 6.5 ± 4 days, p = 0.027) and was discharged later (GA at discharge 36.7 ± 2.5 weeks vs 35.6 ± 1.2 weeks, p = 0.02). All infants survived. No bronchopulmonary dysplasia (BPD) or neurological disorders occurred.

Conclusions.—Bi-level NCPAP was associated with better respiratory outcomes versus NCPAP, and allowed earlier discharge, inducing the same changes in the cytokine levels. It was found to be well tolerated and safe in the study population.

▶ Bronchopulmonary dysplasia (BPD) remains a major cause of mortality and morbidity in very preterm infants despite steroid treatment, mechanical ventilation, and surfactant replacement therapy. With assisted ventilation, however, outcomes have improved over the decades. Assisted ventilation can be in the form of nasal continuous positive airway pressure (NCPAP), ventilation, and, as we see in this report, bilevel NCPAP. Before reading this report, I was not very familiar with the latter. Bilevel NCPAP is a noninvasive respiratory support that is much more similar to CPAP than to nasal intermittent positive pressure ventilation. It provides 2 alternating levels of CPAP to switch the functional residual capacity of the newborn between 2 different levels. The theoretical benefits of bilevel NCPAP are that the functional residual capacity switching may recruit unstable alveoli (or prevent their collapse) with the generation of a tidal volume between 2 levels of CPAP, offloading some of the respiratory work. This report from Milan, Italy, is important because there have been no previous published reports comparing NCPAP with bilevel NCPAP looking at all outcome variables.

In this study, a group of preterm infants were treated with either CPAP (at a level of 6 cm H_2O) or bilevel CPAP with a lower level of pressure of 4.5 cm H_2O and an upper level of 8 cm H_2O, with a pressure exchange rate of 30 times per minute. The choice of the settings was empirical because the effect of different settings during bilevel NCPAP on the success of the respiratory outcomes has not been investigated previously. The study ultimately demonstrated that the use of bilevel NCPAP did allow for adequate gas exchange and seemed to decrease levels of inflammatory markers, inflammation being one of the major reasons why BPD develops in ventilated babies. This new ventilatory strategy seems to be more efficacious when used in preterm babies in the acute phase of respiratory distress syndrome.

Needless to say, more studies will be needed to see if bilevel NCPAP ventilatory methods are accepted by nurseries at large. At least for now, the data from Italy look very promising in that there was a significantly shorter period of need for respiratory support and lesser O_2 dependency in the bilevel NCPAP-treated preterm infants.

Accompanying this report in the same journal was a summary of information from an investigation carried out in the United Kingdom that examined the role of antenatal steroids when used for extremely preterm babies.[1] These investigators showed that the overall mortality among babies born between 24 and 29 weeks with maternal steroids was lower (19.4%) as compared with their counterparts whose mothers did not receive steroids (35.1%). The gestational-specific mortality figures (percentage) in the steroid-treated group between 24 and 29 weeks' gestation were 61.5, 36.9, 28.5, 17.5, 10.2, and 5.1, by week, respectively, and these were significantly lower than the group without steroid treatment. There was a 9.9% reduction in mortality among babies born at 23 weeks' gestation in the steroid-treated group (79.4% mortality compared with 89.3%). Among survivors, there was no significant effect of antenatal steroid treatment on length of stay, duration of respiratory support, and evidence of chronic lung disease.

J. A. Stockman III, MD

Reference

1. Manktelow BN, Lal MK, Field DJ, Sinha SK. Antenatal corticosteroids and neonatal outcomes according to gestational age: a cohort study. *Arch Dis Child Fetal Neonatal Ed.* 2010;95:F95-F98.

Target Ranges of Oxygen Saturation in Extremely Preterm Infants

SUPPORT Study Group of the Eunice Kennedy Shriver NICHD Neonatal Research Network (Univ of Alabama at Birmingham; Univ of California at San Diego; Case Western Reserve Univ, Cleveland, OH; et al)
N Engl J Med 362:1959-1969, 2010

Background.—Previous studies have suggested that the incidence of retinopathy is lower in preterm infants with exposure to reduced levels of oxygenation than in those exposed to higher levels of oxygenation. However, it is unclear what range of oxygen saturation is appropriate to minimize retinopathy without increasing adverse outcomes.

Methods.—We performed a randomized trial with a 2-by-2 factorial design to compare target ranges of oxygen saturation of 85 to 89% or 91 to 95% among 1316 infants who were born between 24 weeks 0 days and 27 weeks 6 days of gestation. The primary outcome was a composite of severe retinopathy of prematurity (defined as the presence of threshold retinopathy, the need for surgical ophthalmologic intervention, or the use of bevacizumab), death before discharge from the hospital, or both. All infants were also randomly assigned to continuous positive airway pressure or intubation and surfactant.

Results.—The rates of severe retinopathy or death did not differ significantly between the lower-oxygen-saturation group and the higher-oxygen-saturation group (28.3% and 32.1%, respectively; relative risk with lower oxygen saturation, 0.90; 95% confidence interval [CI], 0.76 to 1.06; P = 0.21). Death before discharge occurred more frequently in the lower-oxygen-saturation group (in 19.9% of infants vs. 16.2%; relative risk, 1.27; 95% CI, 1.01 to 1.60; P = 0.04), whereas severe retinopathy among survivors occurred less often in this group (8.6% vs. 17.9%; relative risk, 0.52; 95% CI, 0.37 to 0.73; P<0.001). There were no significant differences in the rates of other adverse events.

Conclusions.—A lower target range of oxygenation (85 to 89%), as compared with a higher range (91 to 95%), did not significantly decrease the composite outcome of severe retinopathy or death, but it resulted in an increase in mortality and a substantial decrease in severe retinopathy among survivors. The increase in mortality is a major concern, since a lower target range of oxygen saturation is increasingly being advocated to prevent retinopathy of prematurity. (ClinicalTrials.gov number, NCT00233324.)

▶ The abstract by Lista et al describes the Surfactant, Positive Pressure, and Pulse Oximetry Randomized Trial Study Group results examining the use of early continuous positive airway pressure (CPAP) in the management of extremely preterm infants.[1] In that study, in addition to looking at the value of early use of CPAP versus surfactant therapy followed by ventilation (if needed), premature infants age 24 weeks 0 days to 27 weeks 6 days of gestation were additionally managed to keep oxygen levels in 2 different target ranges (a lower target range of oxygen saturation, 85% to 89%, compared with a higher range, 91% to 95%). The primary outcome with respect to the oxygen saturation component of the study was a composite of severe retinopathy of prematurity (defined as the presence of threshold retinopathy, the need for surgical ophthalmologic intervention, or the use of bevacizumab), death before discharge from the hospital, or both.

When the study data were looked at, it was clear that the distribution of oxygen saturations was within or above target range in the higher oxygen-saturation group, but in the lower oxygen-saturation group, it was about 90% to 95% (ie, above the target range). The difference in oxygen levels between the groups was about 3 percentage points instead of the intended 6 percentage points that had been planned. Therefore, the study actually compared saturation levels of about 89% to 97% with saturation levels of 91% to 97%. Any conclusions from this study should be ascribed to the latter oxygen saturation ranges. It is not clear why the target ranges were achieved. There was evidence that the nurses in the neonatal intensive care units tended to keep a baby's oxygen saturation toward the higher end of the target range, which may account for the shift of both groups toward higher saturation levels than those targeted. It was observed that there were no significant differences between the oxygen saturation groups and the primary outcome of severe retinopathy of prematurity or death at discharge. However, even with the relatively modest difference in oxygen saturation levels between the groups, the rate of severe retinopathy of prematurity was lower in the lower oxygen-saturation group than in the higher oxygen-saturation group (8.6% vs 17.9%, C < 0.001). The rate of needed treatment with supplemental oxygen at 36 weeks among survivors was lower in the lower oxygen-saturation group than in the higher oxygen-saturation group. There was weak evidence of an increased rate of death before discharge in the lower oxygen-saturation group ($P = .04$). An association between lower oxygen-saturation targets and increased mortality has been reported previously in some but not all nonrandomized trials and has not been observed in the only previous randomized trial that has looked at this.[2]

It is difficult to draw firm conclusions from this study. Targeting oxygen saturation is difficult, as this study proved, and a recommended oxygen saturation range that is effective yet safe remains elusive. We see in this study that a lower oxygen-saturation level significantly reduces the incidence of severe retinopathy of prematurity but may at the same time increase the rate of death before discharge. Presumably, the infants in this study are being followed for a long period of time to determine whether the low-oxygen saturation versus the high-oxygen saturation randomization is associated with any increase in neurodevelopmental problems.

J. A. Stockman III, MD

References

1. Lista G, Castoldi F, Fontana P, et al. Nasal continuous positive airway pressure (CPAP) versus bi-level nasal CPAP in preterm babies with respiratory distress syndrome: A randomized control trial. *Arch Dis Child Fetal Neonatal Ed.* 2010; 95:F85-F89.
2. Askie LM, Henderson-Smart DJ, Irwig GL, Simpson JM. Oxygen-saturation targets and outcomes in extremely premature infants. *N Engl J Med.* 2003;349:959-967.

Early CPAP versus Surfactant in Extremely Preterm Infants

SUPPORT Study Group of the Eunice Kennedy Shriver NICHD Neonatal Research Network (Univ of California at San Diego; Univ of Alabama at Birmingham; Case Western Reserve Univ, Cleveland, OH; et al)
N Engl J Med 362:1970-1979, 2010

Background.—There are limited data to inform the choice between early treatment with continuous positive airway pressure (CPAP) and early surfactant treatment as the initial support for extremely-low-birth-weight infants.

Methods.—We performed a randomized, multicenter trial, with a 2-by-2 factorial design, involving infants who were born between 24 weeks 0 days and 27 weeks 6 days of gestation. Infants were randomly assigned to intubation and surfactant treatment (within 1 hour after birth) or to CPAP treatment initiated in the delivery room, with subsequent use of a protocol-driven limited ventilation strategy. Infants were also randomly assigned to one of two target ranges of oxygen saturation. The primary outcome was death or bronchopulmonary dysplasia as defined by the requirement for supplemental oxygen at 36 weeks (with an attempt at withdrawal of supplemental oxygen in neonates who were receiving less than 30% oxygen).

Results.—A total of 1316 infants were enrolled in the study. The rates of the primary outcome did not differ significantly between the CPAP group and the surfactant group (47.8% and 51.0%, respectively; relative risk with CPAP, 0.95; 95% confidence interval [CI], 0.85 to 1.05) after adjustment for gestational age, center, and familial clustering. The results were similar when bronchopulmonary dysplasia was defined according to the need for any supplemental oxygen at 36 weeks (rates of primary outcome, 48.7% and 54.1%, respectively; relative risk with CPAP, 0.91; 95% CI, 0.83 to 1.01). Infants who received CPAP treatment, as compared with infants who received surfactant treatment, less frequently required intubation or postnatal corticosteroids for bronchopulmonary dysplasia (P<0.001), required fewer days of mechanical ventilation (P = 0.03), and were more likely to be alive and free from the need for mechanical ventilation by day 7 (P = 0.01). The rates of other adverse neonatal outcomes did not differ significantly between the two groups.

Conclusions.—The results of this study support consideration of CPAP as an alternative to intubation and surfactant in preterm infants. (ClinicalTrials.gov number, NCT00233324.)

▶ If you are not familiar with the work of the SUPPORT Study Group, you should try to learn about it. This study group has made a number of contributions to the literature dealing with the tiny premature infant. SUPPORT stands for Surfactant, Positive Pressure, and Oxygenation Randomized Trial. In the report on the use of early continuous positive airway pressure (CPAP) versus surfactant in extremely premature infants, we see the results of a randomized multicenter trial in which newborns who were 24 weeks to 27 weeks and

6 days gestation were randomly assigned to intubation and surfactant treatment within 1 hour after birth or to CPAP treatment initiated in the delivery room with subsequent use of ventilation therapy only as needed. In addition, these newborns were randomly assigned to 1 of 2 target ranges of oxygen saturation. In the study of early CPAP, the primary outcome that was looked for was a decreased probability of developing bronchopulmonary dysplasia as determined by the need for supplemental oxygen at 30 weeks of age. The rates of primary outcome of death or bronchopulmonary dysplasia did not differ significantly between the CPAP group or the surfactant group (47.8% vs 51%). However, the CPAP group as compared with the surfactant group less frequently required intubation in the delivery room (34.4% vs 93.4%) or postnatal corticosteroids for treatment of bronchopulmonary dysplasia (7.2% vs 13.2%) and required ventilation for an average of 3 days less. These results are similar to those of the Continuous Positive Airway Pressure or Intubation at Birth Trial (Australian New Zealand Clinical Trials registry number 12606000258550).

So the question is how do the results of this trial help neonatologists manage newborns and the generalist pediatrician to understand what the neonatologist is up to in the nursery? The data show that starting CPAP at birth in very preterm infants, even if it fails in some, has important benefits and no serious side effects. However, we cannot predict which babies will not have an adequate response to the treatment with CPAP ahead of time and therefore should receive early ventilation and surfactant therapy. This will require additional studies. That having been said, the CPAP strategy as compared with early surfactant treatment did result in a lower rate of intubation both in the delivery room and in the neonatal intensive care unit, a reduced rate of postnatal steroid use, and a shorter duration of ventilation without an increased risk of any adverse neonatal outcome. All of these are important and good findings, particularly in light of the safety of CPAP. It will be interesting to see how long it takes, if at all, for our neonatologist colleagues to embrace this shift in the approach to the tiny preterm infant.

J. A. Stockman III, MD

Early Surgical Ligation Versus a Conservative Approach for Management of Patent Ductus Arteriosus That Fails to Close after Indomethacin Treatment

Jhaveri N, Moon-Grady A, Clyman RI (Univ of California, San Francisco)
J Pediatr 157:381-387, 2010

Objective.—To examine whether a more conservative approach to treating patent ductus arteriosus (PDA) is associated with an increase or decrease in morbidity compared with an approach involving early PDA ligation.

Study Design.—In January 2005, we changed our approach to infants born at age ≤27 weeks gestation who failed indomethacin treatment. We changed from an early surgical approach, in which feedings were stopped and all PDAs were ligated (period 1: January 1999 to December 2004; n = 216) to a more conservative approach in which feedings continued and PDAs were ligated only if cardiopulmonary compromise developed (period 2: January 2005 to August 2009; n = 180). All infants in both periods received prophylactic indomethacin therapy.

Results.—The 2 periods had similar rates of perinatal/neonatal risk factors and indomethacin failure (24%), as well as ventilator management and feeding advance protocols. The conservative approach (period 2) was associated with decreased rates of duct ligation (72% vs 100%; P <.05). Even though infants subjected to this approach were exposed to larger PDA shunts for longer durations, the rates of bronchopulmonry dysplasia, sepsis, retinopathy of prematurity, neurologic injury, and death were similar to those in period 1. The overall rate of necrotizing enterocolitis was significantly lower in period 2 compared with period 1.

Conclusions.—These findings support the need for new controlled, randomized trials to reexamine the benefits and risks of different approaches to PDA treatment.

▶ It was well more than 3 decades ago that a couple of small randomized controlled trials were performed that examined the effects of a persistent symptomatic patent ductus arteriosus (PDA) on neonatal pulmonary morbidity. These studies suggested that surgical closure of a PDA would decrease the need for prolonged ventilatory support and the development of congestive heart failure. It is fairly customary now that if a patient fails to have closure of a PDA with cycles of indomethacin, the PDA will be ligated surgically. Unfortunately, it is not clear whether the findings from studies performed several decades ago are still applicable in the setting of modern neonatal treatment with all the various supportive therapies that can be used to manage tiny infants. It is known that surgical ligation of a PDA, while apparently straightforward in most instances, can have complications associated with it, including pneumothorax, chylothorax, postoperative hypotension, vocal cord paralysis, infection, and scoliosis. Jhaveri et al have examined the impact of adoption of a conservative approach to the ductus that remains patent after 1 or 2 courses of indomethacin therapy. Using a historical cohort study design, these investigators have shown that an aggressive approach (ligation of all PDAs after failure of indomethacin therapy) compared with a conservative approach (watchful waiting and only ligating when signs of cardiopulmonary compromise occur) has no apparent benefit and is associated with an increased risk of necrotizing enterocolitis. The authors conclude that this conservative approach is both safe and beneficial in avoiding immediate ligation of all infants with persistent PDA after failure of medical therapy.

In a commentary on the report of Jhaveri et al, Laughon et al[1] ask the question: what should the next steps be in our approach to ligation of PDA? It is suggested that we should implement what we know and study what we do not know and begin by educating ourselves and our colleagues about the harmful effects of surgical ligation. Clinical trials designed to determine whether any interventions intended to close the PDA reduce mortality and morbidity rates are necessary. If one adheres to the beliefs of Jhaveri et al, surgical ligation of the PDA is, at best, not helpful and, at worse, harmful when undertaken in all patients who have failed indomethacin therapy. It will be interesting to see how our neonatal-perinatal colleagues take up the challenge of figuring all this out.

J. A. Stockman III, MD

Reference

1. Laughon M, Bose C, Benitz WF. Patent ductus arteriosus management: what are the next steps? *J Pediatr.* 2010;157:355-356.

Transfusion-Related Acute Gut Injury: Necrotizing Enterocolitis in Very Low Birth Weight Neonates after Packed Red Blood Cell Transfusion

Blau J, Calo JM, Dozor D, et al (New York Med College, Valhalla)
J Pediatr 158:403-409, 2011

Objective.—This is a repeat cohort study in which we sought to determine whether an association of necrotizing enterocolitis (NEC) <48 hours of a packed red blood cells (PRBC) transfusion was a prior sampling artifact.

Study Design.—All very low birth weight neonates with NEC Stage ≥IIB admitted over an 18-month period were categorized for NEC: (1) <48 hours after a PRBC transfusion; (2) unrelated to the timing of PRBCs; and (3) never transfused.

Results.—Eight hundred eighty-three admissions over 18 months were reviewed; 256 were very low birth weight that resulted in 36 NEC cases and 25% were associated with PRBC (n = 9). PRBC-associated cases had lower birth weight, hematocrit, and rapid onset of signs (<5 hours). The timing of association of PRBC transfusion and NEC differed from random, showing a distribution that was not uniform over time ($\chi^2 = 170.7$, df = 40; $P < .000001$) consistent with the possibility of a causative relationship in certain cases of NEC. Current weight at onset of NEC did not differ; however, the more immature the neonate the later the onset of NEC creating a curious centering of occurrence at a median of 31 weeks postconceptual age.

Conclusions.—We conclude that PRBC-related NEC exists. Transfusion-related acute gut injury is an acronym we propose to characterize a severe neonatal gastrointestinal reaction proximal to a transfusion of PRBCs for anemia. The convergence at 31 weeks postconceptual age approximates the age of presentation of other O_2 delivery and neovascularization syndromes, suggesting a link to a generalized systemic maturational mechanism.

▶ Necrotizing enterocolitis (NEC) is a common problem in any newborn nursery. Overall statistics suggest that NEC occurs in about 10% of the very low birth weight population. Its causes are multiple. Bowel ischemia, infection, mechanical injury, catheter use, excessive enteral feeding, and immunological barrier dysfunction have all been noted to be contributing factors to NEC.

Back in the mid-1980s, the authors of this report noted a spike in the incidence of NEC in their nursery during a 3-month period. During that time, NEC developed in 31% of their very low birth weight newborns and also in 11% of infants with a birth weight greater than 1500 g, a very unexpected finding. The Centers for Disease Control and Prevention was asked to assist the hospital in investigating this NEC outbreak and the only contributory factor that was related was the association with red blood cell transfusion. Infants who had received a red blood cell transfusion, all other risk factors accounted for, had an increased risk of 15.1-fold. No changes in blood bank procedures or blood supply were identified as potentially the culprits. The outbreak ceased without any specific changes in transfusion practice. Another report has suggested an association between transfusion practice and NEC in 12 Boston area neonatal intensive care units.[1]

Blau et al looked at 883 admissions over an 18-month period to attempt to see if there was any correlation with NEC and the timing of packed red blood cell transfusions. They concluded that transfusion-related NEC does exist and that the greatest risk seems to occur at 31 weeks postconceptual age that approximates the age at presentation of neonatal vascularization syndromes, suggesting a link to a more generalized systemic maturational mechanism.

An editorial by Christensen[2] accompanied this report. The editorial proposes 3 plausible explanations for the link between red cell transfusions and NEC. One hypothesis is that proposed by Blau et al that there is a parallel between transfusions and acute lung injury that might involve immunologic mechanisms in organs well beyond the lungs, including the bowel. A second possible explanation is that events occurring before a transfusion are the trigger. For example, anemia can impair blood flow to the intestine triggering NEC and that red cell transfusions themselves are therefore simply a marker of this problem. A third possible explanation involves the well-known storage issues that occur with banked packed red blood cells, including reduced deformability, increased red blood cell adhesion and aggregation, prothrombotic effects of transfusion, and nitric oxide deficiency. Needless to say, these are widely disparate hypotheses. With one hypothesis, one might suspect that withheld red blood cell transfusions would potentially partially address the issue. With another hypothesis, red blood cell transfusions should be given.

Needless to say, transfusion-associated NEC does appear to be a legitimate subtype of NEC but one that most likely accounts for a distinct minority of NEC cases. Few, however, will withhold transfusions when there are other clinical indications for them.

Another commentary referenced the recent decline in birth rates in the United States. That observation now coincides with other reports that in the last decade there has been a decline in overall sexual activity among sexually active individuals in the United States. Specifically, more young Americans in 2006 to 2008 said they had never had sex with anybody than did so in 2002. More also said they had oral sex, but not penile-vaginal sex than in earlier surveys. Across all age groups, more women than men reported same-sex experiences. Data from the National Center for Health Statistics and part of the US

Centers for Disease Control and Prevention (CDC) document this. In the 2006 to 2008 survey, 27% of men and 29% of women aged 15 to 24 years said they had never had any sexual contact with another person, an increase from 22% of men and women in that same age group reporting no sexual contact with another person in 2002. Almost all people aged 25 to 44 (98% of women and 97% of men) reported having had heterosexual sex. In all age groups, same-sex contact was twice as common among women as among men. Among men aged 25 to 44, 97% reported having vaginal intercourse with a woman, 90% reported anal sex with a woman, 44% reported oral sex with a woman and 6% reported any type of sex with a man. Among women aged 25 to 44, 98% reported having had vaginal sex with a man, 89% reported anal sex with a man, 36% reported oral sex with a man and 12% reported any type of sex with a woman. Among teenagers aged 15 to 19 years, 7% of women and 9% of men reported having had oral sex with a partner of the opposite sex, but no vaginal intercourse. More than half of men and women aged 15 to 24 who reported having oral sex said that they had it before penile/vaginal sex.

These data are very important for all those who care for adolescents. The information provided has profound implications for sexually transmitted diseases as well as for pregnancy-related issues.[3]

J. A. Stockman III, MD

References

1. Bednarek FJ, Weisberger S, Richardson DK, Frantz ID 3rd, Shah B, Rubin LP. Variation in blood transfusions among newborn intensive care units. SNAP II Study Group. *J Pediatr.* 1998;133:601-607.
2. Christensen RD. Association between red blood cell transfusions and necrotizing enterocolitis. *J Pediatr.* 2011;158:349-350.
3. Tanne JH. US citizens report slightly less sexual activity than in 2002. *BMJ.* 2011; 342:d1500.

15 Nutrition and Metabolism

Impact of Breast Milk on Intelligence Quotient, Brain Size, and White Matter Development

Isaacs EB, Fischl BR, Quinn BT, et al (Univ College London Inst of Child Health, UK; Harvard Med School, Charlestown, MA; et al)
Pediatr Res 67:357-362, 2010

Although observational findings linking breast milk to higher scores on cognitive tests may be confounded by factors associated with mothers' choice to breastfeed, it has been suggested that one or more constituents of breast milk facilitate cognitive development, particularly in preterms. Because cognitive scores are related to head size, we hypothesized that breast milk mediates cognitive effects by affecting brain growth. We used detailed data from a randomized feeding trial to calculate percentage of expressed maternal breast milk (%EBM) in the infant diet of 50 adolescents. MRI scans were obtained (mean age = 15 y 9 mo), allowing volumes of total brain (TBV) and white and gray matter (WMV, GMV) to be calculated. In the total group, %EBM correlated significantly with verbal intelligence quotient (VIQ); in boys, with all IQ scores, TBV and WMV. VIQ was, in turn, correlated with WMV and, in boys only, additionally with TBV. No significant relationships were seen in girls or with gray matter. These data support the hypothesis that breast milk promotes brain development, particularly white matter growth. The selective effect in males accords with animal and human evidence regarding gender effects of early diet. Our data have important neurobiological and public health implications and identify areas for future mechanistic study.

▶ This report from both Great Britain and the United States is an extremely powerful one underscoring the potential of breast milk feeding to enhance intelligence. There have been a number of reports linking breast feeding with higher scores of tests of neurodevelopment and cognition in later life suggesting that breast milk may impact early brain development with potentially biological, medical, and social implications. At the same time, there have been criticisms of these reports as being poorly adjusted for the higher socioeconomic status seen among many breastfeeding mothers. Studies (pro and con) relating breast milk to intelligence quotient (IQ) have been potentially flawed by lack of experimentation—thus the importance of the report of Isaacs et al.

433

These investigators have been studying members of a cohort of adolescents who participated in a large randomized trial examining the health and developmental effects of early infant nutrition, conducted between 1982 and 1985. The investigators were able to study the effect of breastfeeding very early in the life of these teens who were born preterm. Precise information on the volumes of breast milk consumed (it was given by nasogastric tube) allowed a rare opportunity to explore the potential dose-response effect of breast milk feeding on brain volume and cognition at adolescence. It is important to note that all the neonatal data were recorded in real time rather than retrospectively documented.

So what did Isaacs et al find? They found that subjects born preterm who were receiving breast milk, after adjusting for other confounding factors, had an 8.3-point IQ advantage at 7 to 8 years. A subset of these youngsters were then followed up at 13 to 19 years of age with MRI scanning and cognitive testing. In addition to documenting higher IQ scores, the study documented a higher brain volume and greater amounts of white and gray matter on MRI scanning in those adolescents who had received greater quantities of breast milk in early infancy. The volume of white matter was the strongest correlate with breastfeeding.

These data support the hypothesis that mother's milk is associated with higher cognitive levels, particularly in males. Needless to say, there will be many naysayers who slice and dice this report's methodology, but it is hard to avoid the conclusions reached. It is also hard to believe that these investigators were able to use expensive studies such as MRI in a large number of patients to document the findings.

Interestingly, there are data now emerging about the relationship between obesity and brain performance. This may or may not relate to breast feeding, which is known to forestall the onset of obesity, at least in some studies. In any event, obesity appears to subtly diminish memory and other features of thinking and reasoning even among seemingly healthy people.[1] At least some of these impairments appear reversible through weight loss. One likely mechanism for such cognitive deficits appears to be damage to the wiring that links the brain's information-processing regions. Studies long ago showed that individuals with diseases linked to obesity, including cardiovascular disease, hypertension, and type 2 diabetes, do not score as well on cognitive testing. Investigators have decided to examine whether weight alone, and not related disease, might be partially responsible. Investigators pursued this by giving a series of cognitive tests to 150 obese volunteers. These participants weighed on average just under 300 pounds although some were much heavier. On average, obese participants initially performed on the low end of the normal range for healthy people, but nearly one-quarter of the obese participants' scores on memory and learning actually fell within the impaired range. Tested 12 weeks after bariatric surgery when a minimum of 50 pounds had been lost, the patients scored substantially better. It is not entirely clear what the mechanism might be linking obesity and impaired brain performance. Investigators have speculated that low-grade inflammation, strongly correlated with obesity, could be an important mediator.

J. A. Stockman III, MD

Reference

1. Raloff J. Obesity impairs brain performance. *Science News.* April 23, 2011;8.

Maternal and Neonatal Vitamin B12 Deficiency Detected through Expanded Newborn Screening—United States, 2003–2007
Hinton CF, Ojodu JA, Fernhoff PM, et al (Emory Univ School of Medicine, Atlanta, GA; Association of Public Health Laboratories, Silver Spring, MD)
J Pediatr 157:162-163, 2010

The incidence of neonatal vitamin B_{12} (cobalamin) deficiency because of maternal deficiency was determined by surveying state newborn screening programs. Thirty-two infants with nutritional vitamin B_{12} deficiency were identified (0.88/100 000 newborns). Pregnant women should be assessed for their risk of inadequate intake/malabsorption of vitamin B_{12}.

▶ Maternal vitamin D deficiency is no laughing matter, particularly when that deficiency is capable of affecting a baby in utero. The most common causes of maternal vitamin B_{12} deficiency include adherence to a diet that excludes or has limited amounts of animal products, pernicious anemia, or gastric bypass surgery, which effectively removes intrinsic factor, thus limiting the absorption of vitamin B_{12} in the terminal ilium. Babies born of vitamin B_{12}—deficient mothers are vitamin B_{12} deficient themselves. Unrecognized neonatal vitamin B_{12} deficiency will worsen if the infant is fed without vitamin B_{12} supplementation. Unfortunately, the clinical findings suggestive of vitamin B_{12} deficiency in the neonatal or infant period are quite nonspecific. B_{12} deficiency may result in developmental delay and, occasionally, failure to thrive. Given the nonspecific nature of the symptoms, delay in diagnosis is frequent and can result in irreversible neurologic damage. Early detection and intervention is critical, something that we pediatric providers rarely think about.

It should be noted that newborn state screening programs can help us with the detection of vitamin B_{12} deficiency. Newborn screening involving tandem mass spectrometry will detect many metabolic disorders, including those that result in methylmalonic acidemia. Currently, every state and the District of Columbia screen newborns with tandem mass spectrometry. Studies have shown that this method of screening has the potential to identify B_{12} deficiency in the newborn. This can also lead to the identification of maternal B_{12} nutritional deficiency and its correction before the onset of neurologic symptoms.

What we see from the report of Hinton et al is that newborn screening can indeed detect B_{12} deficiency. A survey of 50 states and 2 territories documented the presence of B_{12} deficiency in 32 infants. Unfortunately, in many cases there was little or no follow-up of these babies since they did not have evidence of any inherited metabolic disorder, the purpose of the newborn screening.

The bottom line here is that B_{12} deficiency should be considered in infants who exhibit failure to thrive, developmental delay, neurologic or behavioral disorders, and those born at risk to mothers for this deficiency. A positive newborn screen for methylmalonic acidemia should not be considered a false-positive if the infant turns out not to have this disorder. One should automatically then think of vitamin B_{12} deficiency as a cause of the false-positive. If a deficiency is suspected, then both the mother and infant should be promptly evaluated for vitamin B_{12} deficiency.

This commentary ends with a fast fact: eating breakfast is truly good for you! An Australian study reports that skipping breakfast over a long period may have detrimental effects on cardiometabolic health. After adjustment for age, sex, and lifestyle factors, those who skipped breakfast in both childhood and adulthood had a larger waist circumference and higher fasting insulin, total cholesterol, and low density lipoprotein cholesterol compared with those who ate breakfast at both points in time.[1] I paid very special attention to this report since I am a firm believer in not eating breakfast. If man's best pal, the canine, can do with one meal a day, so can his keeper. To say this differently, I am as likely to have breakfast in the morning as one is likely to see a picture of Tonya Harding on a box of Wheaties.

J. A. Stockman III, MD

Reference

1. Smith KJ, Gall SL, McNaughton SA, Blizzard L, Dwyer T, Venn AJ. Skipping breakfast: longitudinal associations with cardiometabolic risk factors in the Childhood Determinants of Adult Health Study. *Am J Clin Nutr.* 2010;92:1316-1325.

Infant Obesity: Are We Ready to Make this Diagnosis?
McCormick DP, Sarpong K, Jordan L, et al (Univ of Texas Med Branch at Galveston)
J Pediatr 157:15-19, 2010

Objectives.—To assess the prevalence, risk factors, diagnosis and treatment of infant obesity (weight-for-length) in a pediatric practice.

Study Design.—This was a retrospective nested case-control design. The investigators reviewed and abstracted data from the records of the mothers (while pregnant) and their offspring.

Results.—The prevalence of infant obesity was 16%. Children who were obese at age 24 months were highly likely to have been obese at age 6 months (odds ratio = 13.3, 95% CI = 4.50-39.53). Mothers of obese infants gained more weight during pregnancy (+6.9 kg, $P < .05$) than mothers of healthy weight infants. Obese infants were more likely to have been large for gestational age (Odds ratio = 2.81, 95% CI = 1.27-6.22). However, only 14% and 23% of obese infants aged 6 and 24 months were diagnosed with obesity.

Conclusion.—Infant obesity was common in our practice. Infant obesity strongly predicted obesity at age 24 months. Risk factors included excessive intrapartum weight gain or being born large for gestational age. Clinicians diagnosed obesity in only a minority of children. Primary care providers need to diagnose obesity in infants and work to develop effective interventions.

▶ This is a fascinating report that teaches us one simple lesson, and that is that we should read what we put down on our medical records. To improve the identification and possible treatment of high-risk infants, a group of primary care practitioners in Galveston undertook a study reviewing the electronic medical records of children and their mothers. They looked at the weight status of infants in their practice. They defined obesity as a weight for length ≥95th percentile for age and sex. The investigators found that as many as 16% of infants in the Galveston area are obese, a prevalence significantly higher than the 10% generally accepted at the national level. Unfortunately, despite their obesity, only one-third were diagnosed by their pediatricians as being obese during well child visits.

It is unclear why, at least in Galveston, infants with obesity were not uniformly diagnosed. In an editorial that accompanied this report, it was suggested that there may be a reluctance to label infants as obese and delay this diagnosis in the hope that infants will outgrow their baby fat as they become toddlers.[1] Unfortunately, even if the subject of obesity is raised during infancy, many parents of overweight/obese youngsters may not perceive their child's overweight as a particular health concern at this early age. Compounding this set of issues is the fact that there is little time to discuss such a complex problem as infant obesity during a well baby visit.

In the same issue of the *Journal of Pediatrics*, there appeared a report of Koebnick et al that undertook the challenge of estimating the prevalence of extreme pediatric obesity.[2] The study analyzed records of over 700 000 patients between the ages of 2 and 19 years in Southern California. Some 6.4% of the patients met the criteria for extreme obesity, defined as 120% of the 95th percentile or body mass index $> 35 \, kg/m^2$. Strikingly, the prevalence in Hispanic boys and African American girls was 11% and 12%, respectively. For boys, prevalence peaked at 8% at 10 years of age, and in girls there was a bimodal distribution with peaks at 12 and 18 years. This report suggests that prevalence-wise, serious obesity may be more common in children than in adults.

There is a great deal of emphasis these days on trying to deal with the problems associated with child obesity. Michelle Obama's national call to action, "Let's Move!" campaign, is just one example of a major initiative in this regard. A multifaceted approach that goes well beyond dieticians, psychologists, pediatricians, surgeons, etc, is needed. Please read the commentary by Inge and Xanthakos[1] on this subject. The commentary begins with the opening thoughts of Henri Bergson, the French philosopher (1859-1941), who remarked that "the eyes only see what the mind is prepared to comprehend." The first step in the war on obesity is to identify the enemy, and often it is us because of our failure to recognize the magnitude of the problem.

J. A. Stockman III, MD

References

1. Inge T, Xanthakos S. Obesity at the extremes: the eyes only see what the mind is prepared to comprehend. *J Pediatr.* 2010;157:3-4.
2. Koebnick C, Smith N, Coleman KJ, et al. Prevalence of extreme obesity in a multi-ethnic cohort of children and adolescents. *J Pediatr.* 2010;157:26-31.

Infant Overweight Is Associated with Delayed Motor Development
Slining M, Adair LS, Goldman BD, et al (Univ of North Carolina at Chapel Hill; et al)
J Pediatr 157:20-25, 2010

Objective.—To examine how infant overweight and high subcutaneous fat relate to infant motor development.

Study Design.—Participants were from the Infant Care, Feeding, and Risk of Obesity Project, a prospective, longitudinal study of low-income African-American mother-infant dyads assessed from 3 to 18 months of age (836 observations on 217 infants). Exposures were overweight (weight-for-length z-score ≥90th percentile of 2000 Centers for Disease Control/National Center for Health Statistics growth reference) and high subcutaneous fat (sum of 3 skinfold measurements >90th percentile of our sample). Motor development was assessed by using the Bayley Scales of Infant Development-II. Developmental delay was characterized as a standardized Psychomotor Development Index score <85. Longitudinal models estimated developmental outcomes as functions of time-varying overweight and subcutaneous fat, controlling for age and sex. Alternate models tested concurrent and lagged relationships (earlier weight or subcutaneous fat predicting current motor development).

Results.—Motor delay was 1.80 times as likely in overweight infants compared with non-overweight infants (95% CI, 1.09-2.97) and 2.32 times as likely in infants with high subcutaneous fat compared with infants with lower subcutaneous fat (95% CI, 1.26-4.29). High subcutaneous fat was also associated with delay in subsequent motor development (odds ratio, 2.27; 95% CI, 1.08-4.76).

Conclusions.—Pediatric overweight and high subcutaneous fat are associated with delayed infant motor development.

▶ The conclusions of this report are intuitively obvious. Being overweight as an infant and having a large amount of subcutaneous fat are incompatible with normal motor milestone development. Slining et al documented this finding in more than 200 babies documenting significant delay in motor development in overweight infants as compared with normal-weight infants. The results suggest that infant fatness, as compared with infant relative weight, has a more consistent relationship with motor development. Specifically, high subcutaneous fat seems to be the culprit.

At the other end of the pediatric age spectrum, adolescence, weight may also have some impact on developmental milestones, this related to cognitive performance. Ruiz et al showed that youngsters who were overweight, but who participated in physical sports activity during leisure time, had better cognitive performance.[1] The authors of this report suggest that adolescence is a period of life when the brain has profound plasticity because of changes in both structure and function and that engagement in physical sports activity, no matter what one's weight is, can increase intellectual performance. These authors did not observe an association between weight status and cognitive performance per se. Studies have shown that overweight children and adolescents have lower cognitive performance than those with normal weight after adjusting for a number of potential confounders.

Because cognitive performance is potentially modifiable during teen years, it would be of interest to investigate whether targeted physical activity interventions, especially in individuals with cognitive impairment, might influence cognitive performance during adolescence and later also in life.

This commentary closes with an interesting observation about feeding, self-regulation, and method of early infant feeding. The question raised is whether babies who are bottle fed lack self regulation of milk intake later in life compared with breast-fed babies. A study involving 1250 infants indicates that babies who were bottle fed intensively in early life turn out to be twice as likely to empty a bottle or cup later in life as those who were breast fed.[2] Psychologists will have to figure out what the difference is between the 2 different containers (the bottle and the breast) that account for this disparity.

J. A. Stockman III, MD

References

1. Ruiz JR, Ortega FB, Castillo R, et al. Physical activity, fitness, weight status, and cognitive performance in adolescence. *J Pediatr.* 2010;157:917-922.
2. Li R, Fein SB, Grummer-Strawn LM. Do infants fed from bottles lack self-regulation of milk intake compared with directly breastfed infants? *Pediatrics.* 2010;125:e1386-e1393.

Adolescent BMI Trajectory and Risk of Diabetes versus Coronary Disease
Tirosh A, Shai I, Afek A, et al (Brigham and Women's Hosp, Boston, MA; Ben-Gurion Univ of the Negev, Beer-Sheva; Chaim Sheba Med Ctr, Tel-Hashomer; et al)
N Engl J Med 364:1315-1325, 2011

Background.—The association of body-mass index (BMI) from adolescence to adulthood with obesity-related diseases in young adults has not been completely delineated.

Methods.—We conducted a prospective study in which we followed 37,674 apparently healthy young men for incident angiography-proven coronary heart disease and diabetes through the Staff Periodic Examination Center of the Israeli Army Medical Corps. The height and weight of participants were measured at regular intervals, with the first measurements taken when they were 17 years of age.

Results.—During approximately 650,000 person-years of follow-up (mean follow-up, 17.4 years), we documented 1173 incident cases of type 2 diabetes and 327 of coronary heart disease. In multivariate models adjusted for age, family history, blood pressure, lifestyle factors, and biomarkers in blood, elevated adolescent BMI (the weight in kilograms divided by the square of the height in meters; mean range for the first through last deciles, 17.3 to 27.6) was a significant predictor of both diabetes (hazard ratio for the highest vs. the lowest decile, 2.76; 95% confidence interval [CI], 2.11 to 3.58) and angiography-proven coronary heart disease (hazard ratio, 5.43; 95% CI, 2.77 to 10.62). Further adjustment for BMI at adulthood completely ablated the association of adolescent BMI with diabetes (hazard ratio, 1.01; 95% CI, 0.75 to 1.37) but not the association with coronary heart disease (hazard ratio, 6.85; 95% CI, 3.30 to 14.21). After adjustment of the BMI values as continuous variables in multivariate models, only elevated BMI in adulthood was significantly associated with diabetes ($\beta = 1.115$, P = 0.003; P = 0.89 for interaction). In contrast, elevated BMI in both adolescence ($\beta = 1.355$, P = 0.004) and adulthood ($\beta = 1.207$, P = 0.03) were independently associated with angiography-proven coronary heart disease (P = 0.048 for interaction).

Conclusions.—An elevated BMI in adolescence — one that is well within the range currently considered to be normal — constitutes a substantial risk factor for obesity-related disorders in midlife. Although the risk of diabetes is mainly associated with increased BMI close to the time of diagnosis, the risk of coronary heart disease is associated with an elevated BMI both in adolescence and in adulthood, supporting the hypothesis that the processes causing incident coronary heart disease, particularly atherosclerosis, are more gradual than those resulting in incident diabetes. (Funded by the Chaim Sheba Medical Center and the Israel Defense Forces Medical Corps.)

▶ Everyone knows that obese adults are at high risk for the development of coronary artery disease as well as type 2 diabetes. It is also well known that teenagers with the metabolic syndrome related to obesity have a greater proclivity to the development of type 2 diabetes. What is not known is whether a long history of relative overweight, starting earlier in life, poses a risk later in adulthood of type 2 diabetes and coronary heart disease.

Most data to date show that there is a direct trajectory of weight and height from birth to adolescence with progression of body mass index (BMI) from adolescence into adulthood, although the latter is less well described. Most do believe that obese children probably have higher odds of becoming obese adults. Some studies, but not all, have shown that elevated BMI in childhood and adolescence is associated with an increased risk of disease or death later in life. Not well understood is how BMI interacts with the particular pathologic mechanisms of obesity-related diseases and whether it does so even within the BMI range that is now considered normal.

To address these issues, Tirosh et al used data from the Metabolic Lifestyle and Nutrition Assessment in Young Adults study of the Israel Defense Forces Medical Corps and followed up more than 37 000 apparently healthy young men whose BMI was measured in adolescence and into young adulthood to identify the incidence of onset of type 2 diabetes and coronary heart disease documented by angiography. The study of the Israel Defense Forces Medical Corps data looked at the BMI during adolescence (17.44 ± 0.46 years) and again at multiple points later in life. The BMI during adolescence ranged from 17.3 in the bottom decile to 27.6 at the upper decile, corresponding to a mean weight ranging from 51.9 kg to 83.8 kg. During 650 000 person-years of follow-up (mean follow-up, 17.4 ± 7.4 years), 1173 cases of type 2 diabetes and 327 cases of angiography-proven coronary heart disease were diagnosed between 25 and 45 years of age (ie, young adulthood). BMI as measured in adolescence was a predictor of diabetes in adulthood, with a significantly increased risk observed for the 3 highest BMI deciles (hazard ratio in the highest decile vs the lowest decile, 2.76; 95% confidence interval, 2.11-3.58). The risk of diabetes increased 9.8% for each increment in 1 BMI unit. BMI in adolescence was also a significant predictor of the incidence of angiography-proven coronary heart disease in young men across the entire BMI range (hazard ratio 5.43 between the highest and lowest deciles). When adolescent BMI was modeled as a continuous variable in a multivariate model, the risk of coronary heart disease increased by 12% for each increment in 1 BMI unit (hazard ratio, 1.12).

This large-scale long-term follow-up study clearly indicates the clinical importance of considering a history of one's BMI during adolescence when assessing the risk of coronary heart disease and diabetes in overweight or obese young adults. It is bad to be overweight as an adult, but it is really bad to have begun this problem earlier in life. We finally have data to unequivocally document the relationship between adolescent obesity and adult type 2 diabetes and coronary heart disease.

As an aside, a recent perspective appearing in the journal *Science* tells us that eosinophils in fatty tissue may in fact forestall obesity.[1] Most human fat is stored in the adipose tissue, and, under healthy conditions, it provides a balanced exchange of triglycerides in response to energy demands. It has been documented that adipose tissue is dynamically linked to the immune system. The activity of macrophage cells has a key role in the progression to immunity. It is now documented that eosinophils, an immune cell typically associated with allergic and parasitic infections, regulate the macrophage activation state in mammalian adipose tissue and may have an important role in metabolic homeostasis. As a person's body fat increases, the number of macrophages embedded in the adipose tissue increases. These classically activated macrophages produce proinflammatory cytokines that act systemically and affect metabolism by decreasing the sensitivity of other cells to insulin. Adipose tissue itself releases a hormone into the circulation called adiponectin that regulates glucose and fatty acid metabolism. However, in obesity, adiponectin production drops and macrophages produce resistin, which acts systemically to increase insulin resistance and glucose tolerance, leading to the onset of diabetes. It has now been established that eosinophils promote adipose tissue to produce alternatively activated macrophages, which in turn provide control of glucose metabolism. In mice infected with a parasite designed to increase eosinophils in tissue, fatty mass actually declines, causing the mice to become less obese.

The perspective that appeared in *Science* raises the interesting question, "can the rising incidence of metabolic syndrome, like the prevalence of allergies and autoimmunity, be exacerbated by the absence of certain parasites with which many millennia of humans have been previously exposed to, but we are not now?" Unfortunately, the question remains unanswered.

J. A. Stockman III, MD

Reference

1. Maizels RM, Allen JE. Immunology. Eosinophils forestall obesity. *Science.* 2011; 332:186-187.

Association of Adolescent Obesity With Risk of Severe Obesity in Adulthood

The NS, Suchindran C, North KE, et al (Univ of North Carolina, Chapel Hill)
JAMA 304:2042-2047, 2010

Context.—Although the prevalence of obesity has increased in recent years, individuals who are obese early in life have not been studied over time to determine whether they develop severe obesity in adulthood, thus limiting effective interventions to reduce severe obesity incidence and its potentially life-threatening associated conditions.

Objective.—To determine incidence and risk of severe obesity in adulthood by adolescent weight status.

Design, Setting, and Participants.—A cohort of 8834 individuals aged 12 to 21 years enrolled in 1996 in wave II of the US National Longitudinal Study of Adolescent Health, followed up into adulthood (ages 18-27 years during wave III [2001-2002] and ages 24-33 years during wave IV [2007-2009]). Height and weight were obtained via anthropometry and surveys administered in study participants' homes using standardized procedures.

Main Outcome Measures.—New cases of adult-onset severe obesity were calculated by sex, race/ethnicity, and adolescent weight status. Sex-stratified, discrete time hazard models estimated the net effect of adolescent obesity (aged <20 years; body mass index [BMI] ≥95th percentile of the sex-specific BMI-for-age growth chart or BMI ≥30.0) on risk of severe obesity incidence in adulthood (aged ≥20 years; BMI ≥40.0), adjusting for race/ethnicity and age and weighted for national representation.

Results.—In 1996, 79 (1.0%; 95% confidence interval [CI], 0.7%-1.4%) adolescents were severely obese; 60 (70.5%; 95% CI, 57.2%-83.9%) remained severely obese in adulthood. By 2009, 703 (7.9%; 95% CI, 7.4%-8.5%) non−severely obese adolescents had become severely obese in adulthood, with the highest rates for non-Hispanic black women. Obese adolescents were significantly more likely to develop severe obesity in young adulthood than normal-weight or overweight adolescents (hazard ratio, 16.0; 95% CI, 12.4-20.5).

Conclusion.—In this cohort, obesity in adolescence was significantly associated with increased risk of incident severe obesity in adulthood, with variations by sex and race/ethnicity.

▶ It probably comes as no surprise that those who are obese as teens are likely to be obese as adults. Strangely enough, although observational studies have reported that the prevalences of overweight, obesity, and severe obesity have increased in recent years, individuals who are obese early in life have not been studied longitudinally to determine their risk of developing severe obesity in adulthood. The authors have looked at this problem using a US nationally representative longitudinal cohort to determine the incidence and risk of severe obesity in adulthood among individuals who were obese during adolescence. The correlation was extremely strong with the highest correlation being seen in women (vs men), with the highest risk being for black women.

It appears that obesity rates have increased across all age groups. Data from 2008 show that for those aged 20 to 39 years, the prevalence of severe obesity was running 4.2% for men and 7.6% for women. The same data indicate that severe obesity is actually increasing at a faster rate than mild obesity.[1] The data from the report of The et al show that there is a strong persistence of severe obesity from adolescence into young adulthood, that there is a relatively high incidence rate of severe obesity during the transition from adolescence to adulthood, and that individuals who are obese in adolescence were significantly more likely to become severely obese in adulthood, highlighting the need for primary and secondary prevention of severe obesity early in life.

On a related note, 2010 saw literature suggesting that children exposed to adenovirus 36 were more likely to be obese than children who have had no evidence of infection.[2] Obese children have been shown to be significantly more likely to have antibodies against adenovirus 36 in comparison with their nonobese peers. This information is consistent with previous studies in animals and humans showing that adenovirus 36 is associated with obesity. Chickens, mice, rats, and monkeys infected with the virus all get fat even though the animals do not eat more or exercise less than they did before they were infected.[3] Obviously there is an issue of true causality when it comes to the theory that obesity may in part be an infectious disease. A betting person would better put their money down on McDonald's, GameBoys, and Lazy Boys.

Clearly a family that dines together is a more healthy family than one where everyone eats on the fly. There are beneficial effects of family dinner on diet quality and possibly on body weight. This study of The et al also showed that consumption of cooked meals was an eating behavior included in the healthful lifestyle pattern that was negatively associated with obesity. A cooked meal, in this report, was defined as any eating episode, warm or cold, that includes a combination of food items that go through some type of food preparation to constitute a more or less traditional meal, in contrast to sandwich meals, snacks, or breakfast-like meals. It is likely that cooked meals contain more vegetable content, contributing to a better diet quality and regulation of weight.

While on the topic of overweight, we are beginning to see data suggesting that nonsurgical approaches to obesity may be beginning to work. A recent US Preventive Services Task Force systematic review of weight management interventions published since 2005 for obese children aged 6 years and more concluded that comprehensive moderate- to high-intensity interventions addressing diet, activity, and behavioral management techniques do result in modest, but significant, weight change and that these improvements are sustained in the first 12 months following completion of active treatment.[4] At least in adults, there is growing evidence suggesting that some forms of obesity are associated with dysregulation of central nervous system reward pathways and that bupropion and naltrexone, which are commonly used to manage addictive disorders, may in fact benefit some obese individuals. Treatment with sustained-release naltrexone plus bupropion does offer in one study a new approach to the management of obesity that might improve the ability to control eating behavior and response to food cravings.[5] It will be interesting to see if any of this adult literature trickles down into studies performed on children.

We close this commentary with an update of the long-debated issue of whether obesity and infection might be intertwined. A recent study suggests that children exposed to adenovirus 36 are more likely to be obese than children who have no evidence of such an exposure. Studies of Korean children and Italian adults have shown that obese people are more likely to have antibodies against this particular virus, presumably a sign of prior infection than normal-weight people. Not only are obese children more likely to have antibodies to the virus—22% of obese children had the antibodies compared with 7% of normal-weight kids—but obese kids with evidence of previous adenovirus 36 infections were about 35 pounds heavier on average than obese children who had not caught the virus. To read more about this interesting, but highly speculative, relationship between obesity and a common cold virus, see the editorial that appeared in *Science News*.[2]

J. A. Stockman III, MD

References

1. Flegal KM, Carroll MD, Ogden CL, et al. Prevalence and trends in obesity among US adults, 1999–2008. *JAMA*. 2010;303:235-241.
2. Saey TH. Exposure to cold virus linked to obesity epidemic among children. *Science News*. October 9, 2010:5.
3. Virus boosts fat in chickens and mice. *Science News*. August 5, 2000:87.
4. Whitlock EP, O'Conner EA, Williams SB, Beil TL, Lutz KW. Effectiveness of weight management intervention in children: a targeted systematic review for the USPSTF. *Pediatrics*. 2010;125:e396-e418.
5. Greenway FL, Fujioka K, Plodkowski RA, et al. COR-1 Study Group. Effect of naltrexone plus bupropion on weight loss in overweight and obese adults (COR-1): a multicenter, randomized, double-blind, placebo-controlled phase III trial. *Lancet*. 2010;376:595-605.

Comorbidities of overweight/obesity experienced in adolescence: longitudinal study
Wake M, Canterford L, Patton GC, et al (Royal Children's Hosp, Melbourne, Australia; Murdoch Childrens Res Inst, Melbourne, Australia; et al)
Arch Dis Child 95:162-168, 2010

Objectives.—Adolescent obesity is linked to metabolic and cardiovascular risk, but its associations with adolescents' experienced health and morbidity are less clear. Morbidities experienced by overweight/obese adolescents and associations between morbidities and timing of overweight/obesity were examined.

Methods.—Data were from the Health of Young Victorians Study (HOYVS; 1997, 2000, 2005), a school-based longitudinal study. Outcomes were blood pressure, health status (Pediatric Quality of Life Inventory 4.0 (PedsQL), global health), mental health (Strengths and Difficulties Questionnaire), psychological distress (Kessler-10), physical symptoms, sleep, asthma, dieting, and healthcare needs and visits. Regression methods assessed associations with body mass index status and timing of overweight/obesity.

Results.—Of the 923 adolescents (20.2% overweight, 6.1% obese), 63.5% were classified as "never" overweight/obese, 8.5% as "childhood only", 7.3% as "adolescence only" and 20.8% as "persistent". Compared to non-overweight, current obesity was associated with lower PedsQL physical summary scores (mean −6.58, 95% CI −9.52 to −3.63) and good/fair/poor global health (OR 3.52, 95% CI 1.95 to 6.36), hypertension (systolic 8.86, 95% CI 4.70 to 16.71; diastolic 5.29, 95% CI 2.74 to 10.20) and dieting (OR 5.79, 95% CI 3.28 to 10.23), with intermediate associations for overweight. Associations with psychosocial morbidity were weaker and inconsistent and there were few associations with health symptoms and problems. Only dieting (OR 2.30, 95% CI 1.36 to 3.89) was associated with resolved childhood overweight/obesity.

Conclusions.—Despite poorer overall health, overweight/obese adolescents were not more likely to report specific problems that might prompt health intervention. Morbidity was mainly associated with concurrent, rather than earlier, overweight/obesity.

▶ Surprisingly little has been reported about the health of overweight and obese adolescents—thus the value of this report by Wake et al. The report represents findings from a study that draws on the 3 waves (1997, 2000, and 2005) of the Health Of Young Victorians Study. Briefly, 24 elementary schools from across the state of Victoria, Australia (population 4.6 million in 1997), were selected to have children surveyed over time to determine a number of characteristics of that patient population, including weight and various medical conditions. It was observed that overweight/obese adolescents did experience poorer physical health than their nonoverweight peers but do not report specific health problems that might prompt intervention to reduce their body mass index. Thus, many of these youngsters had unrecognized medical problems that could have readily been addressed.

Regarding physical health, adolescent obesity without a doubt is associated with a number of medical conditions, including high blood pressure, higher fasting insulin levels, adverse lipid profiles, and abnormal glucose tolerance tests, all of which are more often than not asymptomatic at this age and detected only if surveillance is undertaken. Obesity is believed to also cause a range of more overt physical problems. A recent systematic review cited symptoms such as heat intolerance, excessive sweating, intertrigo, heat rash, lethargy, shortness of breath on exercise, joint pain, and headaches.[1] There are also a number of psychosocial impacts of adolescent obesity described.

Current data on obesity in school-age children in the United States are sobering. Almost one-third of US children older than 2 years are already obese or overweight according to the 2007-2008 National Health and Nutrition Examination Survey, and among low-income children of 2 to 5 years of age who are enrolled in federally funded health programs, the proportions range as high as 39%. In as early as 3 years of age, obese children have elevated levels of inflammatory markers that have been linked to heart disease that is manifested later in life. Interventions such as the Let's Move Campaign against childhood obesity as announced by First Lady Michelle Obama on February 9, 2010, must address the problem of obesity even at these very young ages. The Let's Move Campaign may well help to improve the health of Americans through its multilevel comprehensive approach, but pregnant women, infants, and preschool-age children could benefit from being more explicitly incorporated into the campaign.

To read more about Let's Move, see the excellent editorial by Wojcicki and Heyman.[2]

J. A. Stockman III, MD

References

1. National Health and Medical Research Council, Commonwealth of Australia. *Overweight and Obesity in Adults and Children and Adolescence — a Guide for General Practitioners.* Appendix-Weight Management Plan. Canberra, Australia: National Health and Medical Research Council; 2003.
2. Wojcicki JM, Heyman MB. Let's move — childhood obesity prevention from pregnancy and infancy onward. *N Engl J Med.* 2010;362:1457-1459.

Caloric Sweetener Consumption and Dyslipidemia Among US Adults
Welsh JA, Sharma A, Abramson JL, et al (Emory Univ, Atlanta, GA; et al)
JAMA 303:1490-1497, 2010

Context.—Dietary carbohydrates have been associated with dyslipidemia, a lipid profile known to increase cardiovascular disease risk. Added sugars (caloric sweeteners used as ingredients in processed or prepared foods) are an increasing and potentially modifiable component in the US diet. No known studies have examined the association between the consumption of added sugars and lipid measures.

Objective.—To assess the association between consumption of added sugars and blood lipid levels in US adults.

Design, Setting, and Participants.—Cross-sectional study among US adults (n=6113) from the National Health and Nutrition Examination Survey (NHANES) 1999-2006. Respondents were grouped by intake of added sugars using limits specified in dietary recommendations (<5% [reference group], 5%-<10%, 10%-<17.5%, 17.5%-<25%, and ≥25% of total calories). Linear regression was used to estimate adjusted mean lipid levels. Logistic regression was used to determine adjusted odds ratios of dyslipidemia. Interactions between added sugars and sex were evaluated.

Main Outcome Measures.—Adjusted mean high-density lipoprotein cholesterol (HDL-C), geometric mean triglycerides, and mean low-density lipoprotein cholesterol (LDL-C) levels and adjusted odds ratios of dyslipidemia, including low HDL-C levels (<40 mg/dL for men; <50 mg/dL for women), high triglyceride levels (≥150 mg/dL), high LDL-C levels (≥130 mg/dL), or high ratio of triglycerides to HDL-C (>3.8). Results were weighted to be representative of the US population.

Results.—A mean of 15.8% of consumed calories was from added sugars. Among participants consuming less than 5%, 5% to less than 17.5%, 17.5% to less than 25%, and 25% or greater of total energy as added sugars, adjusted mean HDL-C levels were, respectively, 58.7, 57.5, 53.7, 51.0, and 47.7 mg/dL (*P*<.001 for linear trend), geometric mean triglyceride levels were 105, 102, 111, 113, and 114 mg/dL (*P*<.001 for linear trend), and LDL-C levels modified by sex were 116, 115, 118, 121, and 123 mg/dL among women (*P*=.047 for linear trend). There were no significant trends in LDL-C levels among men. Among higher consumers (≥10% added sugars) the odds of low HDL-C levels were 50% to more than 300% greater compared with the reference group (<5% added sugars).

Conclusion.—In this study, there was a statistically significant correlation between dietary added sugars and blood lipid levels among US adults.

▶ In the United States, the consumption of sugar in the diet has increased substantially in recent decades. Most of this increase has not been the result of the ingestion of food products that naturally contain sugars. The increase is largely because of an increased intake of added sugars defined as caloric sweeteners used by the food industry and consumers as ingredients in processed or prepared foods to increase the desirability of these foods. Dietary data suggest that US individuals aged 2 years or older consume nearly 16% of their dietary energy as added sugars. Today, the most commonly consumed added sugars are refined beet or cane sugar (sucrose) and high-fructose corn syrup. The concern about added sugars began to mount in the early part of this past decade when in 2000 the US Dietary Guidelines began to use the term added sugars to help consumers identify foods that provide energy but few micronutrients or phytochemicals. Consumption of foods high in added sugars has been associated with increased obesity, diabetes, and dental caries and with an overall decreased diet quality. Increased carbohydrate consumption also will lower high-density lipoprotein cholesterol (HDL-C) levels, will raise triglyceride levels, and will also raise low-density lipoprotein cholesterol levels—a lipid profile associated with a cardiovascular disease risk.

Unfortunately, there is currently no standard by which individuals can decide how much sugar in their diet is too much sugar with respect to added sugars. Dietary guidelines for added sugar vary widely. The Institute of Medicine suggests a limit of 25% of total energy, the World Health Organization advises less than 10% of total energy, and recent recommendations from the American Heart Association advise limiting added sugars to fewer than 100 calories daily for women and 150 calories daily for men, which would approximate to 5% of total energy. Based on the fact that no known studies have been done to examine the correlation between consumption of added sugars and lipid profiles, Welsh et al decided to assess the association between consumption of added sugars and blood lipid levels in adults in the United States. The data from this study clearly support the importance of dietary guidelines that encourage consumers to limit their intake of added sugars. The more sugar in the diet, the lower the levels of HDL-C, the higher the levels of triglycerides, and increased odds of developing a dyslipidemia.

Our current consumption of large amounts of added sugars as a prominent source of low-nutrient calories is a relatively new phenomenon that did not begin until the mid-19th century when these sweeteners became more widely available and consumption began to increase dramatically. On average here in the United States, one-sixth of daily calories come from these added sugars. Exactly how they cause dysmetabolic effects is not completely understood. Some of the effects could be mediated by fructose found in large quantities in nearly all added sugars. Fructose has been shown to increase lipogenesis in the liver, hepatic triglyceride synthesis, and secretion of very low-density lipoproteins. Fructose also appears to decrease peripheral clearance of lipids.

Now that we have clear data showing precisely the relationship between increasing amounts of added sugars in the diet and adverse lipid profiles, it is time to get specific, even more so than in the past, about a ceiling amount of these in the average American diet. It is time to put pen to paper and get these new recommendations promulgated.

This commentary closes with an observation on a form of cooking that may be a bit healthier for you. If you have not heard of it before, it is called sous vide, a method of cooking that involves vacuum packaging food and immersing it in hot water over a prolonged period of time. This changes the physics of cooking more than one might think. The usual goal in cooking is to bring the food to a specific temperature at which it is perfectly "done." For many foods, such as fish and certain vegetables, the margin of error is quite narrow. In traditional cooking, the high temperature of the pan, oven, or grill pushes heat into the exterior of the food so quickly, that a large temperature gradient forms between the surface and the core. A charbroiled steak, for example, soon becomes boiling hot just under the surface where the water in the meat is flashing to steam; that boiling zone can be a good 86°F hotter than the medium-rare center and conduction keeps transmitting the heat there even after the steak is pulled from the broiler. When cooking sous vide, in contrast, chefs typically set the water bath temperature just 1 or 2 degrees higher than the core temperature they wish to achieve. A computer-controlled heater can hold the water bath within half a degree of that temperature while the food slowly equilibrates. Because the temperature cannot go very high, overcooking is not possible so timing then is much less critical. The vacuum packing prevents air from insulating food, improves food safety and greatly slows oxidation reactions that lead to unwanted color changes or off flavors. Low temperatures will not brown food, but a quick sweep with a blow torch or a fast sear on a griddle can apply the final color and crust. Above all, such food is said to be more nutritious and certainly can be done to the chef's specification virtually every time! To read more about the science of sous vide and how underwater cooking differs from the broiler method, see the editorial comment by Gibbs and Myhrvold.[1]

J. A. Stockman III, MD

Reference

1. Gibbs WW, Myhrvold N. The science of sous vide. *Scientific American.* January 2011;24.

Association of Maternal Stature With Offspring Mortality, Underweight, and Stunting in Low- to Middle-Income Countries

Özaltin E, Hill K, Subramanian SV (Harvard School of Public Health, Boston, MA)
JAMA 303:1507-1516, 2010

Context.—Although maternal stature has been associated with offspring mortality and health, the extent to which this association is universal across developing countries is unclear.

Objective.—To examine the association between maternal stature and offspring mortality, underweight, stunting, and wasting in infancy and early childhood in 54 low- to middle-income countries.

Design, Setting, and Participants.—Analysis of 109 Demographic and Health Surveys in 54 countries conducted between 1991 and 2008. Study population consisted of a nationally representative cross-sectional sample of children aged 0 to 59 months born to mothers aged 15 to 49 years. Sample sizes were 2 661 519 (mortality), 587 096 (underweight), 558 347 (stunting), and 568 609 (wasting) children.

Main Outcome Measures.—Likelihood of mortality, underweight, stunting, or wasting in children younger than 5 years.

Results.—The mean response rate across surveys in the mortality data set was 92.8%. In adjusted models, a 1-cm increase in maternal height was associated with a decreased risk of child mortality (absolute risk difference [ARD], 0.0014; relative risk [RR], 0.988; 95% confidence interval [CI], 0.987-0.988), underweight (ARD, 0.0068; RR, 0.968; 95% CI, 0.968-0.969), stunting (ARD, 0.0126; RR, 0.968; 95% CI, 0.967-0.968), and wasting (ARD, 0.0005; RR, 0.994; 95% CI, 0.993-0.995). Absolute risk of dying among children born to the tallest mothers (≥160 cm) was 0.073 (95% CI, 0.072-0.074) and to those born to the shortest mothers (<145 cm) was 0.128 (95% CI, 0.126-0.130). Country-specific decrease in the risk for child mortality associated with a 1-cm increase in maternal height varied between 0.978 and 1.011, with the decreased risk being statistically significant in 46 of 54 countries (85%) ($\alpha=.05$).

Conclusion.—Among 54 low- to middle-income countries, maternal stature was inversely associated with offspring mortality, underweight, and stunting in infancy and childhood.

▶ Most people in the United States are not familiar with the fact that maternal height is a strong predictor of birth size, completely independent of prepregnancy body mass index (BMI) and weight gain during pregnancy. Short maternal stature is highly associated with uterine volume and blood flow and is associated with risks of fetal growth restriction, cesarean delivery, and cephalopelvic disproportion, the risk of which is likely modified by newborn size. In most instances, short stature is related to maternal undernutrition caused by chronic energy and micronutrient deficiencies, highly prevalent in many developing countries. In Southeast Asia, for example, short stature (less than 145 cm) is present in 10% of women of reproductive age. When looking at short stature and BMI, final adult height in women largely reflects a cumulative outcome measure of environmental exposures from fetal to adult life encompassing nutritional, infectious, sociocultural, and economic influences. Final adult height is largely based on several critical windows for linear growth. These include the fetal period, the early childhood (0 to 24 months), and pubertal and adolescent periods. The problem once in place is likely to span several generations. The long-described theory of intergenerational cycle of growth failure posits that a small woman will deliver a small baby with fetal growth restriction, who will subsequently experience faltering growth as a child and low stature and body weight as an adolescent, ultimately leading to a small adult who will then reproduce small children all over again. There is some basis to the underlying theory of this intergenerational problem.

Özaltin et al do show that maternal height is inversely associated with risks of childhood mortality, underweight, stunting, and wasting. They demonstrate that with every 1-centimeter increase in height, the relative and absolute risk of each of these adverse outcomes is significantly decreased. If one compares a woman with short stature, as defined by a height of less than 145 cm, with a woman in the highest maternal height category of 160 cm, the woman with short stature has a 40% greater risk of any of her offspring dying, after adjusting for other confounding factors. The risks of stunting and underweight in offspring of such short mothers are 2-fold greater in comparison to these problems in infants born of women at the other end of the height spectrum.

Needless to say, the solution to the problem of short stature as described in this report is not singular. The solutions include better nutrition, better economic development in the countries where this is a problem, and better infection control as well as the management of indigenous disease. These solutions will not be easy to come by.

J. A. Stockman III, MD

Effect of DHA Supplementation During Pregnancy on Maternal Depression and Neurodevelopment of Young Children: A Randomized Controlled Trial
Makrides M, the DOMInO Investigative Team (Women's and Children's Hosp, North Adelaide, South Australia, Australia; et al)
JAMA 304:1675-1683, 2010

Context.—Uncertainty about the benefits of dietary docosahexaenoic acid (DHA) for pregnant women and their children exists, despite international recommendations that pregnant women increase their DHA intakes.

Objective.—To determine whether increasing DHA during the last half of pregnancy will result in fewer women with high levels of depressive symptoms and enhance the neurodevelopmental outcome of their children.

Design, Setting, and Participants.—A double-blind, multicenter, randomized controlled trial (DHA to Optimize Mother Infant Outcome [DOMInO] trial) in 5 Australian maternity hospitals of 2399 women who were less than 21 weeks' gestation with singleton pregnancies and who were recruited between October 31, 2005, and January 11, 2008. Follow-up of children (n = 726) was completed December 16, 2009.

Intervention.—Docosahexaenoic acid—rich fish oil capsules (providing 800 mg/d of DHA) or matched vegetable oil capsules without DHA from study entry to birth.

Main Outcome Measures.—High levels of depressive symptoms in mothers as indicated by a score of more than 12 on the Edinburgh Postnatal Depression Scale at 6 weeks or 6 months postpartum. Cognitive and language development in children as assessed by the Bayley Scales of Infant and Toddler Development, Third Edition, at 18 months.

Results.—Of 2399 women enrolled, 96.7% completed the trial. The percentage of women with high levels of depressive symptoms during the first 6 months postpartum did not differ between the DHA and control groups (9.67% vs 11.19%; adjusted relative risk, 0.85; 95% confidence interval [CI], 0.70-1.02; $P = .09$). Mean cognitive composite scores (adjusted mean difference, 0.01; 95% CI, -1.36 to 1.37; $P = .99$) and mean language composite scores (adjusted mean difference, -1.42; 95% CI, -3.07 to 0.22; $P = .09$) of children in the DHA group did not differ from children in the control group.

Conclusion.—The use of DHA-rich fish oil capsules compared with vegetable oil capsules during pregnancy did not result in lower levels of postpartum depression in mothers or improved cognitive and language development in their offspring during early childhood.

Trial Registration.—anzctr.org.au Identifier: ACTRN12605000569606.

▶ This important report from Australia tells us the results from the DOMInO (DHA to Optimize Mother Infant Outcome) study, a large randomized trial of fish oil supplementation during pregnancy. The primary trial outcomes were maternal postpartum depressive symptoms and infant development. Women in the intervention group were asked to consume 3 daily capsules of fish oil that contained a total of 800 mg of docosahexaenoic acid (DHA) and 100 mg of eicosapentaenoic acid (EPA), whereas control women were asked to consume similar supplements of vegetable oil. The purpose of this study was to determine whether fish oil might in some way benefit pregnant women and their offspring.

Fish are a rich source of long-chain n-3 (omega-3) polyunsaturated fatty acids (PUFA), essential nutrients that have important structural and physiological roles in several body systems, including neurological, immunologic, and cardiovascular systems. Because humans cannot synthesize PUFA, these nutrients must be consumed in the diet. Conversion from the parent n-3 PUFA, alpha-linolenic acid, to the more biologically available long-chain n-3 PUFA, DHA and EPA, is insufficient, and therefore, consumption of some preformed long-chain n-3 PUFA is important for optimal health. In the United States and elsewhere, fish is the main dietary source of both DHA and EPA.

n-3 PUFA status is critical during pregnancy. DHA is a necessary structural component of the brain and retina, and DHA uptake into these tissues is rapidly occurring during the second half of gestation and early infancy. Experiments have taken place over the years to show that among offspring of mothers deprived of n-3 PUFA, one can expect deficits in vision and behavior that are not reversible with subsequent supplementation. There is concern that infants born of mothers who consume little or no fish or who are born preterm may not receive enough DHA during the critical early months of brain development. In addition, fish oil may benefit mothers themselves, lowering the risk of postpartum depression and certain other pregnancy complications.

Current guidelines recommend that women consume an average of 200 mg/d of DHA during pregnancy. Absent supplementation, most women in the United States and many other countries eat so little fish that they do not meet these recommended levels. Simply encouraging pregnant women to eat more fish has not proven very successful, especially given all the scares about contamination of fish with methylmercury. For all these reasons, the report of Makrides et al comes none too soon.

The results of the large randomized trial by Makrides et al suggest that the consumption of DHA-rich fish oil supplements during pregnancy does not reduce postpartum depression in mothers or improve cognitive or language outcomes in their children up to 18 months of life. It was expected that the trial of fish oil supplementation during pregnancy would have beneficial effects. It did not.

I grew up in an Irish family in which fish was considered brain food. Everyone got a reasonable amount of it because of religious reasons, where Fridays were meatless. It was that versus scrambled eggs or grilled cheese for dinner. Gosh knows whether it made anyone any smarter, but it was nice to think so. Unfortunately, there is no substitute for fish. DHA alone simply does not cut it, at least not in pregnant women.

J. A. Stockman III, MD

Low 25-Hydroxyvitamin D Levels in Adolescents: Race, Season, Adiposity, Physical Activity, and Fitness

Dong Y, Pollock N, Stallmann-Jorgensen IS, et al (Med College of Georgia, Augusta, GA; et al)
Pediatrics 125:1104-1111, 2010

Objectives.—The objectives were to characterize the vitamin D status of black and white adolescents residing in the southeastern United States (latitude: ~33°N) and to investigate relationships with adiposity.

Methods.—Plasma 25-hydroxyvitamin D levels were measured with liquid chromatography-tandem mass spectroscopy for 559 adolescents 14 to 18 years of age (45% black and 49% female). Fat tissues, physical activity, and cardiovascular fitness also were measured.

Results.—The overall prevalences of vitamin D insufficiency (<75 nmol/L) and deficiency ($\geq$50 nmol/L) were 56.4% and 28.8%, respectively. Black versus white subjects had significantly lower plasma 25-hydroxyvitamin D levels in every season (winter, 35.9 $\pm$ 2.5 vs 77.4 $\pm$ 2.7 nmol/L; spring, 46.4 $\pm$ 3.5 vs 101.3 $\pm$ 3.5 nmol/L; summer, 50.7 $\pm$ 4.0 vs 104.3 $\pm$ 4.0 nmol/L; autumn, 54.4 $\pm$ 4.0 vs 96.8 $\pm$ 2.7 nmol/L). With adjustment for age, gender, race, season, height, and sexual maturation, there were significant inverse correlations between 25-hydroxyvitamin D levels and all adiposity measurements, including BMI percentile ($P = .02$), waist circumference ($P < .01$), total fat mass ($P < .01$), percentage of body fat ($P < .01$), visceral adipose tissue ($P = .015$), and subcutaneous abdominal adipose tissue ($P < .039$). There were significant positive associations between 25-hydroxyvitamin D levels and vigorous physical activity ($P < .01$) and cardiovascular fitness ($P = .025$).

Conclusions.—Low vitamin D status is prevalent among adolescents living in a year-round sunny climate, particularly among black youths. The relationships between 25-hydroxyvitamin D levels, adiposity, physical activity, and fitness seem to be present in adolescence.

▶ There has been a great deal of concern in recent years about an increasingly emergent problem related to vitamin D deficiency in our teen population in the United States. This concern is based on the sedentary nature of much of the teen population, sedentary meaning that these youngsters are spending more time indoors and are not getting much sun exposure. The report of Dong et al from the Georgia Prevention Institute and the Section of Endocrinology in the Department of Medicine, School of Medicine, Boston University, confirms our worst fears in this regard, which is that low vitamin D status is indeed prevalent among adolescents, even in the deep south where you would think the sun shines a good bit of the year. This prevalence is highest among black youth and those teens who are overweight, presumably partly as a result of little physical activity. The study of Dong et al is one of the few studies investigating vitamin D status in the pediatric population in the southern regions of the United States and is the first to address 25-hydroxyvitamin D levels over 4 seasons in a group of black and white adolescents living at southern US latitudes. These youths are at risk for low vitamin D status not only in winter but also throughout the entire year. Obesity and/or body fatness was associated with decreased 25-hydroxyvitamin D levels.

The more we learn about vitamin D deficiency, the more we uncover some of the not so obvious consequences of this vitamin deficiency. For example, researchers recently added serious cognitive decline to the long list of conditions already associated with low levels of vitamin D. In a cohort study, older Italian adults with serum concentrations of 25-hydroxyvitamin D below 25 nmol/L were 60% more likely to experience substantial decline in their cognitive abilities than those with concentrations above 75 nmol/L (adjusted risk ratio 1.60). Insufficient vitamin D has also been linked to a higher risk of cancer, cardiovascular disease, certain infections, autoimmune diseases, osteoporosis, diabetes, and obesity. It isn't clear how vitamin D status affects such a diverse list of health problems. Vitamin D deficiency simply may be a marker for lifestyle issues that put one at risk for these problems. To read more about these associations, see the editorial note in *Archives of Internal Medicine.*[1]

One final comment: we now know that variants near genes involved in cholesterol synthesis, hydroxylation, and vitamin D transport affect vitamin D status, and variation in these loci can be used to identify individuals who have substantially raised risk of vitamin D deficiency. For more on this interesting new finding, see the report below by Wang et al.[2]

J. A. Stockman III, MD

References

1. Editorial note: vitamin D again? *Arch Intern Med.* 2010;170:1135-1141.
2. Wang TJ, Zhang F, Richards JB, et al. Common genetic determinants of vitamin D insufficiency, a genome-wide association study. *Lancet.* 2010;376:180-188.

Common genetic determinants of vitamin D insufficiency: a genome-wide association study

Wang TJ, Zhang F, Richards JB, et al (Massachusetts General Hosp, Boston; King's College London, UK; Jewish General Hosp, Montreal, Quebec, Canada; et al)

Lancet 376:180-188, 2010

Background.—Vitamin D is crucial for maintenance of musculoskeletal health, and might also have a role in extraskeletal tissues. Determinants of circulating 25-hydroxyvitamin D concentrations include sun exposure and diet, but high heritability suggests that genetic factors could also play a part. We aimed to identify common genetic variants affecting vitamin D concentrations and risk of insufficiency.

Methods.—We undertook a genome-wide association study of 25-hydroxyvitamin D concentrations in 33 996 individuals of European descent from 15 cohorts. Five epidemiological cohorts were designated as discovery cohorts (n=16 125), five as in-silico replication cohorts (n=9367), and five as de-novo replication cohorts (n=8504). 25-hydroxyvitamin D concentrations were measured by radioimmunoassay, chemiluminescent assay, ELISA, or mass spectrometry. Vitamin D insufficiency was defined as concentrations lower than 75 nmol/L or 50 nmol/L. We combined results of genome-wide analyses across cohorts using Z-score-weighted meta-analysis. Genotype scores were constructed for confirmed variants.

Findings.—Variants at three loci reached genome-wide significance in discovery cohorts for association with 25-hydroxyvitamin D concentrations, and were confirmed in replication cohorts: 4p12 (overall $p=1\cdot9\times10^{-109}$ for rs2282679, in *GC*); 11q12 ($p=2\cdot1\times10^{-27}$ for rs12785878, near *DHCR7*); and 11p15 ($p=3\cdot3\times10^{-20}$ for rs10741657, near *CYP2R1*). Variants at an additional locus (20q13, *CYP24A1*) were genome-wide significant in the pooled sample ($p=6\cdot0\times10^{-10}$ for rs6013897). Participants with a genotype score (combining the three confirmed variants) in the highest quartile were at increased risk of having 25-hydroxyvitamin D concentrations lower than 75 nmol/L (OR 2·47, 95% CI 2·20—2·78, $p=2\cdot3\times10^{-48}$) or lower than 50 nmol/L (1·92, 1·70—2·16, $p=1\cdot0\times10^{-26}$) compared with those in the lowest quartile.

Interpretation.—Variants near genes involved in cholesterol synthesis, hydroxylation, and vitamin D transport affect vitamin D status. Genetic variation at these loci identifies individuals who have substantially raised risk of vitamin D insufficiency.

▶ Currently, vitamin D deficiency or insufficiency probably affects about half our population. As mentioned elsewhere, sedentary teens, particularly those who are sedentary enough to become obese, are at quite high risk for the development of vitamin D deficiency. Vitamin D deficiency has been associated with a range of disorders other than those associated with bones. Important among the list of disorders is diabetes (both type 1 and type 2). An increased risk of falls, cardiovascular disease, and cancer of the breast, colon, and prostate has also been documented to be associated with low vitamin D levels. Not all vitamin D deficiency can be solely accounted for by the lack of exposure to sun or reported vitamin D intake. Genetic factors may substantially contribute to the variability in vitamin D status as well. Although several rare Mendelian disorders cause functional vitamin D insufficiency, data for the effect of common genetic variations on vitamin D status are quite scarce. The report abstracted represents the work of the Study of Underlying Genetic Determinants of Vitamin D and Highly related to Traits (SUNLIGHT) consortium. This consortium represents a collaboration of a number of nations and was formed in 2008 to help identify common genetic variants affecting vitamin D concentrations and the risk of vitamin D insufficiency.

What we see from the SUNLIGHT consortium are data establishing a role for common genetic variants in the regulation of circulating 25-hydroxyvitamin D concentrations. The presence of harmful alleles at 3 confirmed loci more than doubled the risk of vitamin D insufficiency. A determination of these 3 genes and their status helps to identify those at higher risk for the development of vitamin D deficiency. The bottom line is that the story of vitamin D deficiency, when it comes to its cause, is not as straightforward as too little sunshine/too little vitamin D. Our genes play a very important role as well.

It should be noted that ultraviolet B radiation produces 90% of vitamin D in human beings; only a very small proportion can be obtained through diet. The current trend of avoiding sun exposure to prevent an increased risk of melanoma clearly is likely to result in more vitamin D insufficiency. Avoidance of the sun's rays by covering up or use of sunscreen can compound the problem of a high prevalence of vitamin D insufficiency in the population at large and is thought to have contributed to a recent increase in metabolic bone disease. Given all the rhetoric about vitamin D deficiency and its many side effects, a major concern is that the population at large might seek prolonged sun exposure without protection to boost vitamin D synthesis. Indeed, the American Academy of Dermatology argues that the risks of sun exposure far outweigh the benefits, advocating instead for dietary supplementation as a safe source of vitamin D. Despite the simmering debate about sun exposure surrounding vitamin D, the SUNLIGHT consortium's genome-wide association study does add to our understanding of the genetic basis of interindividual variability in the synthesis of vitamin D, helping to identify who is most at risk of vitamin D insufficiency and related diseases.

J. A. Stockman III, MD

Effects of vitamin D supplementation on bone density in healthy children: systematic review and meta-analysis

Winzenberg T, Powell S, Shaw KA, et al (Univ of Tasmania, Australia; Royal Hobart Hosp, Tasmania, Australia)
BMJ 342:c7254, 2011

Objective.—To determine the effectiveness of vitamin D supplementation for improving bone mineral density in children and adolescents and if effects vary with factors such as vitamin D dose and vitamin D status.

Design.—Systematic review and meta-analysis.

Data Sources.—Cochrane Central Register of Controlled Trials, Medline (1966 to present), Embase (1980 to present), CINAHL (1982 to present), AMED (1985 to present), and ISI Web of Science (1945 to present), last updated on 9 August 2009, and hand searching of conference abstracts from key journals.

Study Selection.—Placebo controlled randomised controlled trials of vitamin D supplementation for at least three months in healthy children and adolescents (aged 1 month to <20 years) with bone density outcomes.

Two authors independently assessed references for inclusion and study quality and extracted data.

Data Synthesis.—Standardised mean differences of the percentage change from baseline in bone mineral density of the forearm, hip, and lumbar spine and total body bone mineral content in treatment and control groups. Subgroup analyses were carried out by sex, pubertal stage, dose of vitamin D, and baseline serum vitamin D concentration. Compliance and allocation concealment were also considered as possible sources of heterogeneity.

Results.—From 1653 potential references, six studies, totalling 343 participants receiving placebo and 541 receiving vitamin D, contributed data to meta-analyses. Vitamin D supplementation had no statistically significant effects on total body bone mineral content or on bone mineral density of the hip or forearm. There was a trend to a small effect on lumbar spine bone mineral density (standardised mean difference 0.15, 95% confidence interval -0.01 to 0.31; P=0.07). Effects were similar in studies of participants with high compared with low serum vitamin D levels, although there was a trend towards a larger effect with low vitamin D for total body bone mineral content (P=0.09 for difference). In studies with low serum vitamin D, significant effects on total body bone mineral content and lumbar spine bone mineral density were roughly equivalent to a 2.6% and 1.7% percentage point greater change from baseline in the supplemented group.

Conclusions.—It is unlikely that vitamin D supplements are beneficial in children and adolescents with normal vitamin D levels. The planned subgroup analyses by baseline serum vitamin D level suggest that vitamin D supplementation of deficient children and adolescents could result in clinically useful improvements, particularly in lumbar spine bone mineral density and total body bone mineral content, but this requires confirmation.

▶ The consequences of not having enough vitamin D can be disastrous to one's health. For example, osteoporotic fractures in adults are a substantial cause of morbidity and mortality resulting in expenditures of as much as $30 billion in the United States. Prevention, which includes manipulation of the development of bone mass during childhood and adolescence, is therefore important. It is a little appreciated fact that if one lays down good quantities of bone early in life, one is largely protected against the consequences of osteoporosis in adulthood.

Winzenberg et al have assessed the impact of vitamin D supplementation on bone density in children. They show that in the population of children at large, vitamin D supplementation has little effect on bone density in the whole body, hip, or forearm. However, in children with low serum vitamin D, supplements had a significant effect on whole body bone mineral content. The authors conclude that supplements are unlikely to be beneficial in children with normal vitamin D concentrations but could result in clinically useful improvements in children who are vitamin D deficient or borderline deficient.

Unfortunately, there is no firm definition of vitamin D deficiency in clinical practice. The definition has been hotly debated, particularly recently given the interest in the potential extraskeletal benefits of vitamin D. Currently, most individuals define vitamin D deficiency as a serum concentration less than 25 nmol/L. Unfortunately, at this value, vitamin D deficiency is fairly prevalent in children on a worldwide basis. For example, a study of adolescent girls in Beijing showed a 45% prevalence of vitamin D concentrations of less than 12.5 nmol/L during the winter months.[1]

The conclusion of the Winzenberg et al report suggests that adequate vitamin D status is needed throughout childhood and adolescence, but this is unlikely to be achieved solely by vitamin D supplementation. Advice on sensible sun exposure and more extensive food fortification needs to be considered.

We close this commentary with an unrelated topic having to do with nutrition. It turns out that purple potatoes may make a healthier meal than plain old Idaho potatoes. A randomized trial recently assessed the effects of eating purple or yellow potatoes, compared with white ones, on markers of inflammation and oxidative stress in healthy men. Blood sampling at baseline and at 6 weeks indicated reduced inflammation and genetic damage in those who ate pigmented potatoes. These possible benefits are attributed to higher concentrations of antioxidants, including phenolic acids and carotenoids in pigmented potatoes.[2] It will be interesting to see if the data from this report can be reproduced. If not, this report was a spud dud.

J. A. Stockman III, MD

References

1. Du X, Greenfield H, Fraser DR, Ge K, Trube A, Wang Y. Vitamin D deficiency and associated factors in adolescent girls in Beijing. *Am J Clin Nutr.* 2005;74:494-500.
2. Kaspar KL, Park JS, Brown CR, Mathison BD, Navarre DA, Chew BP. Pigmented potato consumption alters oxidative stress and inflammatory damage in men. *J Nutr.* 2011;141:108-111.

Effect of Vitamin E or Metformin for Treatment of Nonalcoholic Fatty Liver Disease in Children and Adolescents: The TONIC Randomized Controlled Trial

Lavine JE, for the Nonalcoholic Steatohepatitis Clinical Research Network (Columbia Univ, NY; et al)
JAMA 305:1659-1668, 2011

Context.—Nonalcoholic fatty liver disease (NAFLD) is the most common chronic liver disease in US children and adolescents and can present with advanced fibrosis or nonalcoholic steatohepatitis (NASH). No treatment has been established.

Objective.—To determine whether children with NAFLD would improve from therapeutic intervention with vitamin E or metformin.

Design, Setting, and Patients.—Randomized, double-blind, double-dummy, placebo-controlled clinical trial conducted at 10 university clinical research centers in 173 patients (aged 8-17 years) with biopsy-confirmed NAFLD conducted between September 2005 and March 2010.

Interventions.—Daily dosing of 800 IU of vitamin E (58 patients), 1000 mg of metformin (57 patients), or placebo (58 patients) for 96 weeks.

Main Outcome Measures.—The primary outcome was sustained reduction in alanine aminotransferase (ALT) defined as 50% or less of the baseline level or 40 U/L or less at visits every 12 weeks from 48 to 96 weeks of treatment. Improvements in histological features of NAFLD and resolution of NASH were secondary outcome measures.

Results.—Sustained reduction in ALT level was similar to placebo (10/58; 17%; 95% CI, 9% to 29%) in both the vitamin E (15/58; 26%; 95% CI, 15% to 39%; $P=.26$) and metformin treatment groups (9/57; 16%; 95% CI, 7% to 28%; $P=.83$). The mean change in ALT level from baseline to 96 weeks was -35.2 U/L (95% CI, -56.9 to -13.5) with placebo vs -48.3 U/L (95% CI, -66.8 to -29.8) with vitamin E ($P=.07$) and -41.7 U/L (95% CI, -62.9 to -20.5) with metformin ($P=.40$). The mean change at 96 weeks in hepatocellular ballooning scores was 0.1 with placebo (95% CI, -0.2 to 0.3) vs -0.5 with vitamin E (95% CI, -0.8 to -0.3; $P=.006$) and -0.3 with metformin (95% CI, -0.6 to -0.0; $P=.04$); and in NAFLD activity score, -0.7 with placebo (95% CI, -1.3 to -0.2) vs -1.8 with vitamin E (95% CI, -2.4 to -1.2; $P=.02$) and -1.1 with metformin (95% CI, -1.7 to -0.5; $P=.25$). Among children with NASH, the proportion who resolved at 96 weeks was 28% with placebo (95% CI, 15% to 45%; 11/39) vs 58% with vitamin E (95% CI, 42% to 73%; 25/43; $P=.006$) and 41% with metformin (95% CI, 26% to 58%; 16/39; $P=.23$). Compared with placebo, neither therapy demonstrated significant improvements in other histological features.

Conclusion.—Neither vitamin E nor metformin was superior to placebo in attaining the primary outcome of sustained reduction in ALT level in patients with pediatric NAFLD.

Trial Registration.—clinicaltrials.gov Identifier: NCT00063635.

► Twenty years ago, no one would have thought that nonalcoholic fatty liver disease would become the most common cause of chronic liver disease in children in the United States. Those affected can have a relatively mild fatty infiltration of the liver. This ultimately can lead to advanced fibrosis, cirrhosis, and hepatocellular carcinoma. Cirrhosis due to nonalcoholic fatty liver disease has been described in children. The definition of nonalcoholic fatty liver disease is made on pathologic examination in which more than 5% of hepatocytes demonstrate macrovesicular steatosis in an individual who has no history of alcohol intake. Although many children exhibit this pattern, a subset will demonstrate unique features regarding location or presence of fat, inflammation, and fibrosis. Insulin resistance is frequently identified in both adults and children with nonalcoholic fatty liver disease.

Treatment approaches to nonalcoholic fatty liver disease in adults and children are largely targeted to a reduction in insulin resistance and oxidant stress. The only recognized management strategies so far have been dietary modification and exercise. No randomized controlled trials have been performed in children using liver histology, which is regarded as the gold standard assessment. The nonalcoholic steatohepatitis Clinical Research Network, which has been supported by the National Institutes of Health, has initiated a phase 3, multicenter, randomized, double-blinded, placebo-controlled trial evaluating vitamin E or metformin for the treatment of nonalcoholic fatty liver disease in children. Results of the trial are reported by Lavine et al. Unfortunately, neither vitamin E, given as an antioxidant, nor metformin, given to improve insulin resistance, were any better than placebo in reducing liver transaminase levels in patients with childhood onset of nonalcoholic fatty liver disease. The data do, however, suggest that children treated with vitamin E who had biopsy-proven liver involvement will have some improvement in secondary histologic outcomes with vitamin E treatment. Those children who showed improvement over placebo were those with initial hepatocellular ballooning degeneration. Unfortunately, the risk of biopsy might outweigh the benefits of therapy, so the development of noninvasive markers for identification and monitoring of those who may benefit would be highly desirable. In the meantime, it is critical that such children undergo lifestyle modification while the role of treatment with vitamin E in those who have a biopsy demonstrating abnormal findings is ultimately determined.

J. A. Stockman III, MD

Metabolic Syndrome and Altered Gut Microbiota in Mice Lacking Toll-Like Receptor 5

Vijay-Kumar M, Aitken JD, Carvalho FA, et al (Emory Univ, Atlanta, GA; et al)
Science 328:228-231, 2010

Metabolic syndrome is a group of obesity-related metabolic abnormalities that increase an individual's risk of developing type 2 diabetes and cardiovascular disease. Here, we show that mice genetically deficient in Toll-like receptor 5 (TLR5), a component of the innate immune system that is expressed in the gut mucosa and that helps defend against infection, exhibit hyperphagia and develop hallmark features of metabolic syndrome, including hyperlipidemia, hypertension, insulin resistance, and increased adiposity. These metabolic changes correlated with changes in the composition of the gut microbiota, and transfer of the gut microbiota from TLR5-deficient mice to wild-type germ-free mice conferred many features of metabolic syndrome to the recipients. Food restriction prevented obesity, but not insulin resistance, in the TLR5-deficient mice. These results support the emerging view that the gut microbiota contributes to metabolic disease and suggest that malfunction of the innate immune system may promote the development of metabolic syndrome.

▶ Most of us have thought that obesity is simply a matter of too many calories in and not enough calories out...or is it? This interesting report, obviously dealing with mice, not men, gives us some insight, however, that obesity as a medical condition is perhaps more than a matter of simply living beyond one's seams.

It is quite clear that humanity is facing an epidemic of interrelated metabolic diseases collectively referred to as the metabolic syndrome, the hallmarks of which include hyperglycemia, hyperlipidemia, insulin resistance, obesity and hepatic steatosis. The increasing incidence of metabolic syndrome is widely thought to result from nutrient excess because of increased food consumption and/or reduced levels of physical activity. This nutrient excess results not only in obesity but also activates endoplasmic reticulum stress pathways resulting in chronic activation of proinflammatory kinase cascades that desensitize the metabolic response to insulin. Such insulin resistance results in hyperglycemia and, in some cases, type 2 diabetes. Recent work, however, suggests a possible role for gut bacteria in causing obesity and consequently other aspects of the metabolic syndrome. In both humans and mice, the development of obesity correlates with shifts in the abundance of the 2 dominant bacteria in the gut, the *Bacteroidetes* and the *Firmicutes* phyla. Interestingly, it has been shown that the transfer of gut bacteria from obese mice to germ-free mice recipients leads to an increase in fat mass in the recipients, also lending credence to the speculation that gut bacteria promote obesity by increasing the capacity of the host to extract energy (calories) from ingested food.

Gut bacteria are shaped both by environment and host genetics, in particular, the innate immune system, long appreciated for its role in defending against infection by pathogenic bacteria. In addition to its role in infection/inflammation, immunity may play a key role in promoting metabolic health. Toll-like receptor (TLR) 5 is a transmembrane protein that is specifically expressed in high amounts in intestinal mucosa. The TLR is a component of the immune system response in the gut. Obesity is associated with triggering an increase in immune system activity and thus may contribute to a range of other symptoms associated with obesity, including an elevated risk for cardiovascular disease and type 2 diabetes. Vijay-Kumar et al now show that mice lacking TLR 5, as expressed by intestinal cells, are obese and have many characteristics of the metabolic syndrome that are further exacerbated when mice are put on a high-fat diet. When such mice are treated with antibiotics to kill their intestinal bacteria, the metabolic syndrome is reversed. The bottom line is that gut microbiota in the obese mice were both necessary and sufficient for the resulting obesity.

So what is thought to be going on here? The suggestion is that gut microbes can extract a small amount of calories from what would normally be undigested food and that these calories contribute to weight gain. At the same time, gut flora can trigger immune responses that can affect insulin resistance. The study by Vijay-Kumar et al falls under a growing set of theories that obesity is the result of infection. Needless to say, all this is speculation as of this time, but it is very interesting speculation indeed.

This commentary ends with an observation having to do with blueberry smoothies and the relationship with insulin sensitivity. It turns out that blueberry smoothie drinks are better than nonblueberry smoothies at improving insulin sensitivity in obese adults with insulin.[1] A study was undertaken that involved drinking smoothies twice daily for 6 weeks. By the end of the trial, insulin sensitivity was enhanced in the blueberry group without significant changes, however, in weight, energy intake, and inflammatory markers. Amazing results. How about them apples!

J. A. Stockman III, MD

Reference

1. Stull AJ, Cash KC, Johnson WD, Champagne CM, Cefalu WT. Bioactives in blueberries improve insulin sensitivity in obese, insulin-resistant men and women. *J Nutr.* 2010;140:1764-1768. Epub 2010 Aug 19.

Dietary Intervention in Infancy and Later Signs of Beta-Cell Autoimmunity
Knip M, for the Finnish TRIGR Study Group (Univ of Helsinki and Helsinki Univ Central Hosp, Finland; et al)
N Engl J Med 363:1900-1908, 2010

Background.—Early exposure to complex dietary proteins may increase the risk of beta-cell auto-immunity and type 1 diabetes in children with genetic susceptibility. We tested the hypothesis that supplementing breast milk with highly hydrolyzed milk formula would decrease the cumulative incidence of diabetes-associated autoantibodies in such children.

Methods.—In this double-blind, randomized trial, we assigned 230 infants with HLA-conferred susceptibility to type 1 diabetes and at least one family member with type 1 diabetes to receive either a casein hydrolysate formula or a conventional, cow's-milk—based formula (control) whenever breast milk was not available during the first 6 to 8 months of life. Autoantibodies to insulin, glutamic acid decarboxylase (GAD), the insulinoma-associated 2 molecule (IA-2), and zinc transporter 8 were analyzed with the use of radiobinding assays, and islet-cell antibodies were analyzed with the use of immunofluorescence, during a median observation period of 10 years (mean, 7.5). The children were monitored for incident type 1 diabetes until they were 10 years of age.

Results.—The unadjusted hazard ratio for positivity for one or more autoantibodies in the casein hydrolysate group, as compared with the control group, was 0.54 (95% confidence interval [CI], 0.29 to 0.95), and the hazard ratio adjusted for an observed difference in the duration of exposure to the study formula was 0.51 (95% CI, 0.28 to 0.91). The unadjusted hazard ratio for positivity for two or more autoantibodies was 0.52 (95% CI, 0.21 to 1.17), and the adjusted hazard ratio was 0.47 (95% CI, 0.19 to 1.07). The rate of reported adverse events was similar in the two groups.

Conclusions.—Dietary intervention during infancy appears to have a long-lasting effect on markers of beta-cell autoimmunity—markers that may reflect an autoimmune process leading to type 1 diabetes.

(Funded by the European Commission and others; ClinicalTrials.gov number, NCT00570102.)

▶ This is a fascinating report, and it proposes that what you eat early in life may alter your risk for the development of type 1 diabetes mellitus. The latter condition, of course, is associated with the loss of insulin-producing beta cells in the pancreatic islets in genetically susceptible individuals. In such individuals, preceding the onset of diabetes is the development of diabetes-associated autoantibodies. These appear in the peripheral circulation as markers of emerging beta cell autoimmunity. There are 5 such disease-related autoantibodies that predict the clinical manifestation of type 1 diabetes. Positivity for 2 or more autoantibodies signals a risk of 50% to 100% for the development of type 1 diabetes over the course of 5 to 10 years. It has been long suspected that beta cell autoimmunity begins to be triggered very early in life and that food types in early childhood may modify the risk of type 1 diabetes later in life. Breast feeding for only a short period and early exposure to complex dietary protein have been thought to be risk factors for advanced beta cell autoimmunity or clinical type 1 diabetes. In experimental models of autoimmune diabetes, early nutritional modifications have decreased the likelihood of developing the disease.

Knip et al report findings from a pilot study in which newborns were randomized in a double-blind manner to receive either a casein hydrolysate formula or a conventional cow's milk—based formula whenever breast milk was not available during the first 6 to 9 months of life. All the newborns studied had a first-degree relative with type 1 diabetes. The infants were then followed for up to 10 years. The study showed that among children with an human leukocyte antigen genotype conferring increased risk for type 1 diabetes and a first-degree relative with type 1 diabetes, weaning to a highly hydrolyzed formula during infancy was associated with fewer signs of beta cell autoimmunity up to 10 years of age. The actual development of type 1 diabetes was not able to be assessed since there were insufficient numbers of patients in the report to show differences.

The conclusions of this report are pretty straightforward. The results indicate that a preventive dietary intervention aimed at decreasing the risk of type 1 diabetes may be feasible and important. Such intervention would have to be initiated very early in life because the first signs of beta cell autoimmunity can appear before a child is even 3 months of age. Since most children with type 1 diabetes come from the general population (without a strong family history) a much larger study will need to be undertaken to determine whether it is reasonable to place all infants on such hydrolyzed formula who are not being exclusively breast fed.

Recent data suggest that if there are going to be targeted dietary interventions to prevent the onset of diabetes, certain parts of the United States would be high on the list of places to start with such interventions first. Two swaths spanning the Deep South and Appalachia have emerged as the US diabetes belt. County-by-county mapping shows that the belt also touches parts of North Carolina, Virginia, Florida, Texas, Arkansas, Ohio, and Pennsylvania, according to information from the Centers for Disease Control and Prevention. High diabetes pockets also crop up in Oklahoma, Michigan, Arizona, and the Dakotas. The data do not distinguish between types of diabetes, but nationally more than 90% of diabetes cases are type 2 or adult-onset diabetes. The mapped areas overlap considerably with the "stroke belt." To read more about mapping of diseases such as diabetes and stroke, see the editorial comment appearing in *Science News.*[1]

J. A. Stockman III, MD

Reference

1. Seppa N. Diabetes belt cinches the south: Highest rates in areas with greatest obesity and stroke risk. *Science News.* April 9, 2011;14.

Functional Variants of the *HMGA1* Gene and Type 2 Diabetes Mellitus

Chiefari E, Tanyolaç S, Paonessa F, et al (Università di Catanzaro "Magna Græcia," Catanzaro, Italy; Univ of California, San Francisco; et al)

JAMA 305:903-912, 2011

Context.—High-mobility group A1 (HMGA1) protein is a key regulator of insulin receptor (*INSR*) gene expression. We previously identified a functional *HMGA1* gene variant in 2 insulin-resistant patients with decreased INSR expression and type 2 diabetes mellitus (DM).

Objective.—To examine the association of *HMGA1* gene variants with type 2 DM.

Design, Settings, and Participants.—Case-control study that analyzed the *HMGA1* gene in patients with type 2 DM and controls from 3 populations of white European ancestry. Italian patients with type 2 DM (n = 3278) and 2 groups of controls (n = 3328) were attending the University of Catanzaro outpatient clinics and other health care sites in Calabria, Italy, during 2003-2009; US patients with type 2 DM (n = 970) were recruited in Northern California clinics between 1994 and 2005 and controls (n = 958) were senior athletes without DM collected in 2004 and 2009; and French patients with type 2 DM (n = 354) and healthy controls (n = 50) were enrolled at the University of Reims in 1992. Genomic DNA was either directly sequenced or analyzed for specific *HMGA1* mutations. Messenger RNA and protein expression for HMGA1 and INSR were measured in both peripheral lymphomonocytes and cultured Epstein-Barr virus—transformed lymphoblasts from patients with type 2 DM and controls.

Main Outcome Measures.—The frequency of *HMGA1* gene variants among cases and controls. Odds ratios (ORs) for type 2DM were estimated by logistic regression analysis.

Results.—The most frequent functional *HMGA1* variant, IVS5-13insC, was present in 7% to 8% of patients with type 2 DM in all 3 populations. The prevalence of IVS5-13insC variant was higher among patients with type 2 DM than among controls in the Italian population (7.23% vs 0.43% in one control group; OR, 15.77 [95% confidence interval {CI}, 8.57-29.03]; $P < .001$ and 7.23% vs 3.32% in the other control group; OR, 2.03 [95% CI, 1.51-3.43]; $P < .001$). In the US population, the prevalence of IVS5-13insC variant was 7.7% among patients with type 2 DM vs 4.7% among controls (OR, 1.64 [95% CI, 1.05-2.57]; $P = .03$). In the French population, the prevalence of IVS5-13insC variant was 7.6% among patients with type 2 DM and 0% among controls ($P = .046$). In the Italian population, 3 other functional variants were observed. When all 4 variants were analyzed, *HMGA1* defects were present in 9.8% of Italian patients with type 2 DM and 0.6% of controls. In addition to the IVS5 Cinsertion, the c.310G>T (p.E104X) variant was found in 14 patients and no controls (Bonferroni-adjusted $P = .01$); the c.*82G>A variant (rs2780219) was found in 46 patients and 5 controls (Bonferroni-adjusted $P < .001$); the c.*369del variant was found in 24 patients and no controls (Bonferroni-adjusted $P < .001$). In circulating monocytes and Epstein-Barr virus—transformed lymphoblasts from patients with type 2 DM and the IVS5-13insC variant, the messenger RNA levels and protein content of both HMGA1 and the INSR were decreased by 40% to 50%, and these defects were corrected by transfection with *HMGA1* complementary DNA.

Conclusions.—Compared with healthy controls, the presence of functional *HMGA1* gene variants in individuals of white European ancestry was associated with type 2 DM.

▶ It has been long suspected, and indeed accepted, that the development of type 2 diabetes mellitus is a consequence of both our environment (including eating habits) and our genes. The report of Chiefari et al gives us information about the latter. Linkage analysis and genome-wide association studies have revealed 34 common variants (also called single-nucleotide polymorphisms) associated with type 2 diabetes mellitus. Most of these loci relate to abnormal insulin processing or secretion. Some loci, however, indicate ineffective insulin action or insulin resistance as a contributor. In addition, some genes have been identified that are associated with fasting insulin levels and obesity that contribute to type 2 diabetes mellitus.

Chiefari et al have conducted a study looking for an association between rare variants related to type 2 diabetes mellitus and then sequenced the genes involved. They have confirmed an increased prevalence of another locus to the list of previously known loci.

We have thus discovered more novel loci for type 2 diabetes mellitus and have a better understanding of the molecular mechanisms by which these variants affect the susceptibility to diabetes. This information is able to be combined with other more sophisticated metabolic phenotyping related to beta cell dysfunction, insulin resistance, incretin hormone, hepatic glucose, and lipid metabolism. These understandings will lead to the identification of distinct subtypes of type 2 diabetes mellitus. The idea would be to take this new information as it is unfolding and target specific therapies for various subtypes of type 2 diabetes mellitus. In this regard, common loci variants near the ataxia-telangiectasia mutated gene have been recently associated with diabetes treatment success with metformin. It is anticipated that the discoveries of novel loci, such as high-mobility group A1, will soon be translated into therapeutic decision making, thereby improving the health of patients with type 2 diabetes mellitus.

To read more about the rapidly evolving story related to our genes and the development of type 2 diabetes mellitus, see the excellent editorial by Garg.[1] Also, see the report[2] that follows that tells us more about metformin in the management of nonalcoholic fatty liver disease in children and adolescents, a disorder largely related to obesity and the potential for the development of type 2 diabetes mellitus.

J. A. Stockman III, MD

References

1. Garg A. HMGA1, a novel locus for type 2 diabetes mellitus. *JAMA*. 2011;305:938-939.
2. Tirosh A, Shai I, Afek A, et al. Adolescent BMI trajectory and risk of diabetes versus coronary disease. *N Engl J Med*. 2011;364:1315-1325.

Celiac Autoimmunity in Children with Type 1 Diabetes: A Two-Year Follow-Up

Simmons JH, Klingensmith GJ, McFann K, et al (Vanderbilt Children's Hosp, Nashville, TN; Univ of Colorado Denver, Aurora)
J Pediatr 158:276-281, 2011

Objective.—To determine the benefits of screening for celiac autoimmunity via immunoglobulin A transglutaminase autoantibodies (TG) in children with type 1 diabetes (T1D).

Study Design.—We followed up 79 screening-identified TG+ and 56 matched TG- children with T1D for 2 years to evaluate growth, bone mineral density, nutritional status, and diabetes control. TG+ subjects self-selected to gluten-free or gluten-containing diet.

Results.—Of the initial cohort, 80% were available for reexamination after 2 years. TG+ subjects had consistently lower weight z-scores and higher urine N-telopeptides than TG- subjects, but similar measures of bone density and diabetes outcomes. TG+ children who remained on a gluten-containing diet had lower insulin-like growth factor binding protein 3 z-scores compared with TG+ subjects who reported following a gluten-free diet. Children who continued with high TG index throughout the study had lower bone mineral density z-scores, ferritin, and vitamin D 25OH levels, compared with the TG- group.

Conclusions.—No significant adverse outcomes were identified in children with T1D with screening-identified TG+ who delay therapy with a gluten-free diet for 2 years. Children with persistently high levels of

TG may be at greater risk. The optimal timing of screening and treatment for celiac disease in children with T1D requires further investigation.

▶ It is well known that certain populations have a higher than expected prevalence of celiac disease in comparison to the general pediatric population at large. For example, the prevalence of biopsy-proven celiac disease in Down syndrome has been reported to be as high as 16%. In Turner syndrome, the prevalence of celiac disease has been reported to be as high as 6.5%. Even prior to the report of Simmons et al, it was well recognized that those with type 1 diabetes mellitus will have a significantly elevated probability of biopsy-proven celiac disease. Indeed, routine screening with immunoglobulin A transglutaminase autoantibody (TG) has been recommended in those with type 1 diabetes mellitus. An unanswered question remains regarding the benefit of a gluten-free diet (GFD) in children with type 1 diabetes mellitus who have TG+ antibodies but no symptoms of celiac disease.

Simmons et al followed 79 screening-identified TG+ and 56 matched TG− children with type 1 diabetes for 2 years to evaluate growth, bone mineral density, nutritional status, and diabetes control. The TG+ subjects were self-selected to GFD or gluten-containing diet. No significant adverse outcomes were identified in children with type 1 diabetes mellitus who had screening-identified TG+ who delayed therapy with a GFD for 2 years. Children with persistently high levels of TG, however, might be at greater risk. Needless to say, the optimal timing of screening and treatment for celiac autoimmunity in those with type 1 diabetes mellitus remains to be determined, but a nonaggressive approach does not seem to be all that harmful in asymptomatic children.

Another commentary in this section referenced that there was a possible relationship between adenovirus 36 and obesity. Data are now emerging that there is a relationship between certain enteroviruses and type 1 diabetes mellitus. The incidence rate of type 1 diabetes has increased over the past 25 years at an annual rate of about 3%. This increase cannot be explained only by genetic modifications in the population. It has therefore been suggested that environmental factors such as drugs, toxins, nutrients, and viruses may play a role in the pathogenesis of this form of diabetes mellitus. Viruses of the enterovirus genus, which have an RNA genome, are the most likely candidates, especially serotypes like coxsackie B virus belonging to the human enterovirus B species. The first report of a possible association between enteroviruses and type 1 diabetes was published back in 1969 and scientists have been following the trail of the link between enteroviruses and type 1 diabetes ever since. A recent systematic review and meta-analysis of molecular studies based on detection of viral protein and RNA finds a strong association between enterovirus infection and type 1 diabetes (odds ratio 9.77).[1] If there is a link here, it probably involves an interplay between viruses, pancreatic beta cells, the innate and adaptive immune systems, and the genotype of the patient. Further studies are needed to tease out the association of these factors and to establish the pathogenic mechanisms of enterovirus infections.

J. A. Stockman III, MD

Reference

1. Yeung WC, Rawlinson WD, Craig ME. Enterovirus infection and type 1 diabetes mellitus: Systematic review and meta-analysis of observational molecular studies. *BMJ*. 2011;342:d35.

16 Oncology

Attitudes and Practices of Oncologists Toward Fertility Preservation

Arafa MA, Rabah DM (King Saud Univ, Saudi Arabia)
J Pediatr Hematol Oncol 33:203-207, 2011

Cancer is a life-threatening diagnosis. Fortunately, life-saving treatments are available to increase the chance of survival in many patients. Yet, many of these treatments are damaging to the reproductive organs and the patients' fertility. A cross-sectional study addressing the knowledge and practices of oncologists toward fertility preservation for male and female patients with cancer was conducted in Saudi Arabia. In 3 different regions of the country, oncologists were invited to participate in the study, through a self-administered questionnaire which was handed to them inquiring about their knowledge, attitude, and referral practices for sperm cryopreservation. Only one-half knew about intracytoplasmic sperm injection, oncologists rated their perception of the importance of cryopreservation as 7.8 ± 1.8. Their referral practice was very poor; less than 20% refer their patients to a specialist. Factors that were considered important to start discussion of cryopreservation were type of cancer, age of patient, number of children, marital status, and cost. Religion was not deemed as important as was anticipated. With regards to female fertility preservation, oncologists showed a positive attitude as revealed from their positive perception, however, their referral practices was very poor. Several gaps were present in the knowledge of oncologists, which could influence their attitude and in turn was reflected on their poor practice. Future training session should be organized to the oncologists for increasing their knowledge and enhancing their attitude.

▶ Many years ago, when I was a fellow in pediatric hematology-oncology, I cared for a young male teen with a solid tumor malignancy that required treatment with high-dose cyclophosphamide. This was in amounts that were highly likely to produce problems with long-term fertility. The teen was well along enough in terms of sexual development to have fully mature spermatogenesis. I strongly suggested the possibility of cryopreservation of semen for this youngster before treatment began. Neither the parents nor the urologist responsible for the handling of the semen was supportive of this concept, which was in fact perhaps years before its time. The report of Arafa and Rabah shows us just how far along we have come, or perhaps have not come, in terms of our attitudes and practices about fertility preservation.

The best way to preserve the reproductive potential for men is to cryopreserve and store semen. The preservation of fertility in female cancer survivors is an equally important health issue. The different cryopreservation options available for women for fertility preservation are embryo, oocyte, and ovarian tissue cryopreservation. Such approaches will need to be considered as early as possible during treatment planning before initiating any therapy that might permanently destroy the opportunity to have children in the future. In 2009 at the American Society of Clinical Oncology annual meeting, researchers presented data from a national survey of physician practice patterns to determine whether oncologists communicate the risk of infertility with patients undergoing cancer treatment. Although most oncologists discussed fertility preservation with their patients, less than 25% reported referring patients to reproductive specialists for fertility preservation.[1] Arafa and Rabah have looked at the attitudes of oncologists in Saudi Arabia, a country typical of many in parts of the world where religious and traditional factors could impact the application and feasibility of fertility preservation. In that country, oncologists caring for adults as well as children and adolescents were invited to participate in a self-administered questionnaire inquiring them about the knowledge, attitude, and referral practices for sperm cryopreservation. Interestingly, only about half even were aware of intracytoplasmic sperm injection and hardly any knew about cryopreservation of semen. Fewer than 1 in 5 had referred a patient to a fertility specialist prior to cancer treatment that would possibly alter long-term fertility.

It is hard to say what those practicing in regions of the world where religious perspectives and long-standing traditional beliefs exist would do with this information. The information, however, is a first step in making what the issues are more transparent. It would be interesting to see a timely study of this same nature done in the United States focused only on those who practice pediatric hematology and oncology.

There is a word of caution, however, when it comes to cryopreservation of ovarian tissue. For example, it has been shown that reimplanting cryopreserved ovarian tissue taken from young women embarking on treatment for acute leukemia may be unsafe. Researchers have found that ovarian contamination by malignant cells occurs in acute and chronic leukemia. Polymerase chain reaction has demonstrated the presence of leukemic markers in such samples, although routine histology did not identify these malignant cells. Undergoing chemotherapy before cryopreservation also did not completely exclude contamination of ovarian tissue. Thus the story using cryopreservation for women may be very different than for men.[2]

J. A. Stockman III, MD

References

1. Quinn GP, Vadaparampil ST, Gwede CK, et al. Discussion of fertility preservation with newly diagnosed patients: oncologists' views. *J Cancer Surviv.* 2007;1: 146-155.
2. Dolmans MM, Marinescu C, Saussoy P, Van Langendonckt A, Amorim C, Donnez J. Reimplantation of cryopreserved ovarian tissue from patients with acute lymphoblastic leukemia is potentially unsafe. *Blood.* 2010;116:2908-2914. Epub 2010 Jul 1.

Single-Dose Palifermin Prevents Severe Oral Mucositis During Multicycle Chemotherapy in Patients With Cancer: A Randomized Trial

Vadhan-Raj S, Trent J, Patel S, et al (Univ of Texas M D Anderson Cancer Ctr, Houston)

Ann Intern Med 153:358-367, 2010

Background.—Mucositis can be a serious complication of cancer treatment. Palifermin reduces mucositis when given in multiple doses to patients undergoing hematopoietic stem-cell transplantation.

Objective.—To evaluate the efficacy of palifermin given as a single dose before each cycle in patients receiving multicycle chemotherapy.

Design.—Randomized, double-blind, placebo-controlled trial. (Clinical Trials.gov registration number: NCT00267046)

Setting.—The University of Texas M.D. Anderson Cancer Center, Houston, Texas.

Patients.—48 patients with sarcoma were randomly assigned in a 2:1 ratio to receive palifermin or placebo. All patients received doxorubicin-based chemotherapy (90 mg per m^2 of body surface area over 3 days, by infusion).

Intervention.—Palifermin (180 μg per kg of body weight) or placebo was administered intravenously as a single dose 3 days before each chemotherapy cycle (maximum, 6 cycles). Patients who had severe mucositis received open-label palifermin in subsequent cycles.

Measurements.—Oral assessment of mucositis by using World Health Organization (WHO) oral toxicity scale (grades 0 to 4), with moderate to severe mucositis (grades 2 to 4) as the main outcomes; patient-reported outcome questionnaire; and daily symptom record diary.

Results.—A median of 6 blinded cycles (range, 1 to 6) were completed by the palifermin group and 2 (range, 1 to 6) by the placebo group. Compared with placebo, palifermin reduced the cumulative incidence of moderate to severe (grade 2 or higher) mucositis (44% vs. 88%; $P < 0.001$; difference, −44 percentage points [95% CI, −71 to −16 percentage points) and severe (grade 3 or 4) mucositis (13% vs. 51%; $P = 0.002$; difference, −38 percentage points [CI, −67 to −9 percentage points]). The main adverse effects were thickening of oral mucosa (72% in the palifermin group vs. 31% in the placebo group; $P = 0.007$) and altered taste. Seven of the 8 patients who had severe mucositis in the placebo group received open-label palifermin. None of these patients had severe mucositis in the subsequent cycles (a total of 17) with open-label palifermin.

Limitations.—Study limitations include smaller sample size for the control group, inclusion of only patients with sarcoma, and perceived unblinding of the treatment because of notable differences between the biologic effects of palifermin and placebo.

Conclusion.—A single dose of palifermin before each cycle reduced the incidence and severity of mucositis. The drug was generally well tolerated, but most patients experienced thickening of oral mucosa. Further investigation is needed to determine whether palifermin use will facilitate greater adherence to chemotherapy regimens by reducing mucositis.

▶ There is a lot to be learned from this report of 48 adult patients with sarcoma randomly assigned to receive an agent, palifermin, designed to prevent or minimize oral mucositis or a placebo. These patients were receiving doxorubicin-based chemotherapy, amounts similar in quantity per kilogram to those used for the management of childhood cancer.

Oral mucositis is a frequent and debilitating complication of cancer chemotherapy and radiation therapy in both adults and children. Its symptoms range from mild odynophagia to severe tissue inflammation, edema, and mucosal bleeding that can make eating impossible and, in its most severe form, necessitates intubation to protect a patient's airway. Subsequent administration of cycles of chemotherapy often causes a progressively worse mucositis. Oral ulcers also increase the risk for bacterial and fungal colonization and for systemic infection in immunocompromised patients.

The current management of mucositis is hardly perfect. Good oral hygiene, aggressive use of narcotic analgesics, and frequent physician evaluations are critical to reduce the severity of oral mucositis. Additional interventions that have been studied include cryotherapy (ie, using ice chips) and drugs such as benzydamine, amifostine, and more recently palifermin.

Palifermin is a recombinant human keratinocyte growth factor (KGF) that targets the KGF/FGFR2b receptor. Stimulating this growth factor receptor can have a potent effect on epithelial cell proliferation. Palifermin has been found to be useful as part of the management of autologous hematopoietic stem cell therapy and has been approved for such use by the US Food and Drug Administration. Vadhan-Raj et al describe the effects of palifermin on mucositis in patients receiving intensive treatment for cancer. In a randomized placebo-controlled trial, they found that patients who received doxorubicin-based chemotherapy for sarcoma had a significant improvement in the severity and duration of severe mucositis with palifermin. These patients received a single dose of 180 μg/kg of body weight. The drug was given intravenously.

Given that mucositis can be the most severe complication of some forms of cancer treatment and that mucositis can be a dose-limiting toxicity of some cytotoxic therapy regimens, it will be important to define the role, if any, for this drug as part of the management of children with cancer. Interestingly, the cost of this drug is more than offset by the savings created by limiting the expenses associated with the related management of mucositis.

Stay tuned to learn more about this interesting new form of supportive therapy. Some worry that KGF agonists might initiate cell signals that lead to tumor proliferation or therapeutic resistance. Although this has not been shown to date, it is something that needs to be carefully looked at before everyone jumps on the palifermin bandwagon.

While on issues related to cancer and things about the mouth and face, please recognize that there is a new etiology for facial cancer that has been recently described. It is "arc welder's basal cell carcinoma." Recently, a 36-year-old arc welder presented with a persistent nodular lesion overlying his left nasal alar. Excision biopsy confirmed a basal cell carcinoma with evidence of severe solar damage in the surrounding skin. The patient denied frequent or prolonged sun exposure. He should have been aware that arc welding produces considerable amounts of ultraviolet radiation. The dosage for radiation exposure is related to the proximity of the individual to the arc, duration of exposure, arc current, and welding substrate used. All those involved in welding and their assistants should beware of this problem and take appropriate precautions to minimize their exposure to this nonsolar ultraviolet radiation.[1]

J. A. Stockman III, MD

Reference

1. Bhatt YM, Nigam A, Sissons MCJ. Arc welder's basal cell carcinoma. *BMJ*. 2010; 341:c4222.

Effect of mitoxantrone on outcome of children with first relapse of acute lymphoblastic leukaemia (ALL R3): an open-label randomised trial
Parker C, Waters R, Leighton C, et al (Univ of Manchester, UK; Univ of Oxford, UK; et al)
Lancet 376:2009-2017, 2010

Background.—Although survival of children with acute lymphoblastic leukaemia has improved greatly in the past two decades, the outcome of those who relapse has remained static. We investigated the outcome of children with acute lymphoblastic leukaemia who relapsed on present therapeutic regimens.

Methods.—This open-label randomised trial was undertaken in 22 centres in the UK and Ireland and nine in Australia and New Zealand. Patients aged 1–18 years with first relapse of acute lymphoblastic leukaemia were stratified into high-risk, intermediate-risk, and standard-risk groups on the basis of duration of first complete remission, site of relapse, and immunophenotype. All patients were allocated to receive either idarubicin or mitoxantrone in induction by stratified concealed randomisation. Neither patients nor those giving interventions were masked. After three blocks of therapy, all high-risk group patients and those from the intermediate group with postinduction high minimal residual disease ($\geq 10^{-4}$ cells) received an allogenic stem-cell transplant. Standard-risk and intermediate-risk patients with postinduction low minimal residual disease ($< 10^{-4}$ cells) continued chemotherapy. The primary outcome was progression-free survival and the method of analysis was intention-to-treat. Randomisation was stopped in December, 2007 because of differences in progression-free and overall survival between the two groups. This trial is registered, reference number ISCRTN45724312.

Findings.—Of 239 registered patients, 216 were randomly assigned to either idarubicin (109 analysed) or mitoxantrone (103 analysed). Estimated

3-year progression-free survival was 35·9% (95% CI 25·9—45·9) in the idarubicin group versus 64·6% (54·2—73·2) in the mitoxantrone group (p=0·0004), and 3-year overall survival was 45·2% (34·5—55·3) versus 69·0% (58·5—77·3; p=0·004). Differences in progression-free survival between groups were mainly related to a decrease in disease events (progression, second relapse, disease-related deaths; HR 0·56, 0·34—0·92, p=0·007) rather than an increase in adverse treatment effects (treatment death, second malignancy; HR 0·52, 0·24—1·11, p=0·11).

Interpretation.—As compared with idarubicin, mitoxantrone conferred a significant benefit in progression-free and overall survival in children with relapsed acute lymphobastic leukaemia, a potentially useful clinical finding that warrants further investigation.

▶ We seem to have reached a plateau in terms of success with the management of childhood acute lymphoblastic leukemia (ALL). The overall probability of 5-year event survival now is approximately 80% for the various forms of ALL. It is pretty clear that further improvement might require either novel drugs (which are not available or suitable for most pediatric patients) or further intensification of existing chemotherapies. The experience with ALL over the past 30 years clearly indicates that overtreatment can be somewhat efficacious if high-risk patients are adequately identified. Any further unselected intensification of frontline therapy would be disadvantageous because of severe toxic effects (mostly unpredictable) that can occur in many patients. Late relevant effects are well known. At least for now, effective retrieval therapy that targets the patient truly at risk of failure is therefore needed. Up to now, the chance of cure after systemic relapse has been small, particularly if the disease recurs while the patient is still being treated or within 6 months after the end of treatment. The efficacy of allogenic stem cell transplantation in the prevention of subsequent relapse can be limited because of residual albeit sometimes very minimal and refractory disease at the time of transplant, which often results in early secondary recurrence.

What Parker et al have done is to describe an interesting new approach in something called the ALL R3 study. They have attempted to find novel drug combinations that can improve the chance of a cure after a first relapse. They report a randomized trial for patients with ALL in first relapse who were stratified into high-risk, intermediate-risk, and standard-risk groups on the basis of duration of first complete remission, site of relapse, and immunophenotype. Patients were given 1 of 2 drugs: idarubicin or mitoxantrone. All high-risk patients and those from the intermediate-risk group with postinduction high minimal residual disease then went to allogenic stem cell transplant. Standard-risk and intermediate-risk patients with low postinduction minimal residual disease continued on their chemotherapy.

This report showed that a new agent, mitoxantrone, showed significant benefit in progression-free and overall survival in children with relapsed leukemia. The differences between the 2 therapies were significant enough that the trial had to be stopped partway through because the differences between treatments became so clear. The estimated 3-year progression-free survival of the entire group overall was 50.3% and overall survival was 57.1%. Progression-free survival and overall survival were significantly better for mitoxantrone than for idarubicin. The former drug almost halved the hazard of an event at any given time point for both progression-free and overall survival in comparison to idarubicin. Even if the 2 drugs failed, some patients were able to enter a third remission or to undergo bone marrow transplant. The results of this trial show that, compared with idarubicin, mitoxantrone significantly improves the outcome of children with relapsed ALL.

It should be noted that mitoxantrone has been used in previous trials for the management of childhood acute myeloid leukemia. In the latter disease, there was improved disease-free survival but no differences in survival overall in comparison with standard therapies. With respect to ALL, we will probably see more and more use of mitoxantrone, which, unlike many new drugs, is cheap and readily available.

J. A. Stockman III, MD

MHC variation and risk of childhood B-cell precursor acute lymphoblastic leukemia

Hosking FJ, Leslie S, Dilthey A, et al (Inst of Cancer Res, Sutton, Surrey, UK; Dept of Statistics, Oxford, UK; et al)
Blood 117:1633-1640, 2011

A role for specific human leukocyte antigen (HLA) variants in the etiology of childhood acute lymphoblastic leukemia (ALL) has been extensively studied over the last 30 years, but no unambiguous association has been identified. To comprehensively study the relationship between genetic variation within the 4.5 Mb major histocompatibility complex genomic region and precursor B-cell (BCP) ALL risk, we analyzed 1075 observed and 8176 imputed single nucleotide polymorphisms and their related haplotypes in 824 BCP-ALL cases and 4737 controls. Using these genotypes we also imputed both common and rare alleles at class I (*HLA-A, HLA-B,* and *HLA-C*) and class II (*HLA-DRB1, HLA-DQA1,* and *HLA-DQB1*) HLA loci. Overall, we found no statistically significant association between variants and BCP-ALL risk. We conclude that major histocompatibility complex-defined variation in immune-mediated response is unlikely to be a major risk factor for BCP-ALL.

▶ Acute lymphoblastic leukemia (ALL) remains the most common pediatric cancer. This malignancy is a biologically heterogeneous disease with B-cell precursor ALL as the most common subtype accounting for about 70% of childhood ALL. There is now conclusive evidence that the risk of ALL has an inherited genetic component. There has been considerable interest in the major histocompatibility complex (MHC) locus on chromosome 6p21 because of the proposition that immune dysfunction or delayed infection has a role in ALL etiology. Hosking et al, using existing genotype data, evaluated more than 8000 single nucleotide polymorphisms (SNPs) in the MHC region in

B-cell precursor ALL cases and in 4737 controls. They found no association between HLA alleles from the SNP genotypes and an association with B-cell precursor ALL risk.

Although the reported findings here are negative, they are in fact extremely important. First, with more than 800 cases and 4700 controls, the study is sufficiently powered to identify common variants with modest effects. Second, this study focused only on 1 ALL subtype, B-cell precursor ALL. Although this limits the generalizability of the findings of other subtypes, it reduces heterogeneity and therefore strengthens statistical power. Finally, the study was able to rule out other confounding factors related to the diversity of the population studied.

In an editorial that accompanied this report, Susan Slager from the Mayo Clinic asked the question: do the results of the Hosking et al report mean that we can rule out any role of the MHC region on the risk of B-cell precursor ALL?[1] She says, unfortunately, the answer is no. This study touches on only 1 aspect of the genomic complexity in the region by providing conclusive evidence that common genetic variants within the region lack any association with risk. However, other possible mechanisms, she points out, may still exist including interactions between MHC variants and variants located on other chromosomes, epigenetics, or structural changes (eg, insertions or deletions of chromosomal regions). Further work still needs to be done to determine what role, if any, the MHC region has in ALL risk, but the reporting of negative results from strong studies such as this is a positive thing indeed.

While on the topic of cancer in children, Bonneau et al point out that the chance of repeating a grade is 50% higher in comparison with control groups for childhood cancer survivors.[2] Risk factors for repeating a grade included an older age at diagnosis, attending a secondary school, low educational level of parents, bone marrow transplantation, brain surgery, and physical sequelae. Overall, 1 in 3 childhood cancer survivors had to repeat a grade.

J. A. Stockman III, MD

References

1. Slager SL. When the negative is positive. *Blood.* 2011;117:1441-1442.
2. Bonneau J, Lebreton J, Taque S, et al. School performance of childhood cancer survivors: mind the teenagers! *J Pediatr.* 2011;158:135-141.

Postrelapse survival in childhood acute lymphoblastic leukemia is independent of initial treatment intensity: a report from the Children's Oncology Group
Freyer DR, Devidas M, La M, et al (Univ of Southern California, Los Angeles; Univ of Florida, Gainesville; Children's Oncology Group, Arcadia, CA; et al)
Blood 117:3010-3015, 2011

While intensification of therapy has improved event-free survival (EFS) and survival in newly diagnosed children with acute lymphoblastic leukemia (ALL), postrelapse outcomes remain poor. It might be expected that patients relapsing after inferior initial therapy would have a higher retrieval rate than after superior therapy. In the Children's Oncology Group Study CCG-1961, significantly superior EFS and survival were achieved with an augmented (stronger) versus standard intensity regimen of postinduction intensification (PII) for children with newly diagnosed high-risk ALL and rapid day 7 marrow response (EFS/survival 81.2%/ 88.7% vs 71.7%/83.4%, respectively). This provided an opportunity to evaluate postrelapse survival (PRS) in 272 relapsed patients who had received randomly allocated initial treatment with augmented or standard intensity PII. As expected, PRS was worse for early versus late relapse, marrow versus extramedullary site, adolescent versus younger age and T versus B lineage. However, no difference in 3-year PRS was detected for having received augmented versus standard intensity PII (36.4% ± 5.7% vs 39.2% ± 4.1%; log rank $P = .72$). Similar findings were noted within subanalyses by timing and site of relapse, age, and immunophenotype. These findings provide insight into mechanisms of relapse in ALL, and are consistent with emergence of a resistant subclone that has acquired spontaneous mutations largely independent of initial therapy. This study is registered at www.clinicaltrials.gov as NCT00002812.

▶ All of us know that acute lymphoblastic leukemia (ALL) is the most common malignancy in children. We have had many successes over the last several decades with this disease, with long-term survival now approaching 85% (defined as surviving 5 years or longer after diagnosis). Unfortunately, about 20% of children with ALL, however, will relapse. Certain risk factors have been identified for higher chance of relapse, including age at diagnosis, the presenting white blood cell count, hematopoietic lineage of the disease, and cytogenic abnormalities. Most children who relapse will not survive; thus it is extremely important that a solid first remission take place. Intensification of antileukemia treatment regimens is thought to be a major contributor to the improvement in event-free survival.

Intuitively, it might be expected that patients who relapse would be patients who have received an inferior initial treatment regimen and that these would be the youngsters who would have greater success in retrieval of a solid second remission and possible cure. Presumably, this would occur because the leukemia clone at relapse is less resistant because it was treated with less effective (usually less intense) therapy. Freyer et al evaluated postrelapse survival in almost 300 relapsed ALL patients who had received randomly allocated initial treatment with more intensive or standard initial therapy. The authors hypothesized that relapsed patients who had received the more intensive of 2 initial treatment regimens would have lower postrelapse survival rate than those initially treated with the inferior regimen. Their results, however, indicate that there was no such difference in 3-year survival. Intensification of initial therapy for ALL does not seem simply to prevent soft or marginal relapses that could otherwise be salvaged with good retrieval therapy. This suggests that malignant cells responsible for relapse are present at diagnosis and mutate to a resistant phenotype through the acquisition of spontaneous mutations that are dependent on intrinsic genomic instability rather than treatment exposures. The theory is that the diagnosis and relapse malignant clones come from a common ancestral clone and that distinct mutations emerge at the predominant clones for those who relapse. This means that the initial treatment may not have been a failure as such or that drug resistance has occurred, rather a new malignant clone has evolved from the ancestral malignancy that these children have had.

It is not clear what pediatric oncologists will be able to do with this important new information from the report by Freyer et al. Clearly novel approaches are needed to detect and monitor low-level persistence or reemergence of distinct leukemia subclones. Whether the emergence of such new malignant clones can be prevented during initial therapy remains to be seen.

This commentary closes with a nonrelated observation that scientists have used genetic tracking to prove that an infant who developed leukemia received the cancer cells via transmission across the placenta. The mother of this infant was diagnosed with leukemia just after delivery. Genetic analysis of the 11-month-old child showed a clonal match with her mother's cancer cells. Cancer cells were subsequently detected in a blood sample taken from the baby at birth. These maternally derived cells were missing a section of DNA that ordinarily might have prompted the baby's immune system to eliminate them.[1] The latter finding accounted for the infant developing full-blown leukemia.

J. A. Stockman III, MD

Reference

1. Isoda T, Ford AM, Tomizawa D, et al. Immunologically silent cancer clone transmission from mother to offspring. *Proc Natl Acad Sci U S A.* 2009;106: 17882-17885. Epub 2009 Oct 12.

Hematopoietic Stem Cell Transplantation: A Global Perspective
Gratwohl A, for the Worldwide Network of Blood and Marrow Transplantation (Univ Hosp Basel, Switzerland; et al)
JAMA 303:1617-1624, 2010

Context.—Hematopoietic stem cell transplantation (HSCT) requires significant infrastructure. Little is known about HSCT use and the factors associated with it on a global level.

Objectives.—To determine current use of HSCT to assess differences in its application and to explore associations of macroeconomic factors with transplant rates on a global level.

Design, Setting, and Patients.—Retrospective survey study of patients receiving allogeneic and autologous HSCTs for 2006 collected by 1327 centers in 71 participating countries of the Worldwide Network for Blood and Marrow Transplantation. The regional areas used herein are (1) the Americas (the corresponding World Health Organization regions are North and South America); (2) Asia (Southeast Asia and the Western Pacific Region, which includes Australia and New Zealand); (3) Europe (includes Turkey and Israel); and (4) the Eastern Mediterranean and Africa.

Main Outcome Measures.—Transplant rates (number of HSCTs per 10 million inhabitants) by indication, donor type, and country; description of main differences in HSCT use; and macroeconomic factors of reporting countries associated with HSCT rates.

Results.—There were 50 417 first HSCTs; 21 516 allogeneic (43%) and 28 901 autologous (57%). The median HSCT rates varied between regions and countries from 48.5 (range, 2.5-505.4) in the Americas, 184 (range, 0.6-488.5) in Asia, 268.9 (range, 5.7-792.1) in Europe, and 47.7 (range, 2.8-95.3) in the Eastern Mediterranean and Africa. No HSCTs were performed in countries with less than 300 000 inhabitants, smaller than 960 km², or having less than US $680 gross national income per capita. Use of allogeneic or autologous HSCT, unrelated or family donors for allogeneic HSCT, and proportions of disease indications varied significantly between countries and regions. In linear regression analyses, government health care expenditures ($r^2 = 77.33$), HSCT team density (indicates the number of transplant teams per 1 million inhabitants; $r^2 = 76.28$), human development index ($r^2 = 74.36$), and gross national income per capita ($r^2 = 74.04$) showed the highest associations with HSCT rates.

Conclusion.—Hematopoietic stem cell transplantation is used for a broad spectrum of indications worldwide, but most frequently in countries with higher gross national incomes, higher governmental health care expenditures, and higher team densities.

▶ Hematopoietic stem cell transplantation (HSCT) therapy use has exploded worldwide. HSCT has been used for congenital and acquired disorders of the hematopoietic system as well as for certain chemosensitive, radiosensitive, and immunosensitive malignancies. Earlier on HSCT had bone marrow as its source, but increasingly, stem cells are being sourced from peripheral blood or cord blood. More than 14 million typed volunteer donors or cord blood units from registries worldwide provide these stem cells for patients without family donors. Recent advances have allowed HSCT therapy to be applied to older patients. However, HSCT does not come at a modest cost. It is associated with significant morbidity and mortality and requires a huge infrastructure to support its facilitated use. Despite these costs, HSCT is no longer limited to countries with abundant resources. In fact, for selected indications, HSCT might represent the most cost-effective therapy in some countries, eliminating many years of chemotherapeutic treatment, which in itself would be costly.

Despite the amazingly rapid growth of HSCTs, there has been little coordinated oversight of this therapy worldwide, thus the value of the report of Gratwohl et al. The recently founded Worldwide Network for Blood and Marrow Transplantation undertook a study to collect standardized HSCT activity data on a global level. The report abstracted presents the results of the worldwide HSCT survey. Some 50 417 HSCTs were reported for 2006.

Of these, 21 516 were allogeneic transplants and 20 901 were autologous transplants. The main indications were lymphoproliferative disorders (54.5%), leukemias (33.8%), solid tumors (5.8%), nonmalignant disorders (5.1%), and other nonspecified disorders (1.0%). The most frequent malignant disease for which an allogeneic transplant was given was myeloid leukemia. The most frequent nonmalignant disease was bone marrow failure syndrome, while the most frequent indication for autologous HSCT was a plasma cell disorder. Interestingly, significantly more HSCTs were performed in Europe than in the Americas. There is a close link of HSCT rates with gross national income per capita throughout the world. No HSCTs were performed in countries with less than $700 (US) gross income per capita.

Without question we will likely see more and more use of HSCT. In 2008, for the first time, more unrelated donor HSCTs than family donor HSCTs were reported, with increasing numbers of donor sources coming from across borders. We are also seeing an increase in stem cell tourism.

If there are any firm conclusions drawn from this report, those conclusions include the observation that transplant activity is concentrated in countries with higher health care expenditures, higher gross national income per capita, and higher transplant team density. The availability of such resources and governmental support continues to determine the level of regional HSCT activity.

While on the topic of treatment of cancer, recent information from Northwestern University suggests that nanodiamonds may become a very useful tool in the management of various forms of malignancy. One of the major challenges of chemotherapy relates to tumor cells developing mechanisms to pump drugs right back out after the chemotherapy has entered the cell. When a drug, however, is bound to a nanoparticle, the combination of the drug and the nanoparticle may be too large for the cellular pumps to extract the chemotherapeutic agent so tumors would have a hard time evolving resistance. The value of using nanoparticles made of diamond is multifaceted. Made of carbon, they are nontoxic, and the body's immune system does not attack them. They can bind tightly to a variety of molecules and deliver them right into a tumor. Because they are only 2 to 8 nanometers in diameter, they can be passed by the kidney. Investigators at Northwestern attached nanodiamonds to doxorubicin, a standard chemotherapy drug, and injected them into mice with drug-resistant breast cancer and liver cancer. With the help of the nanodiamonds, the drug stayed in the circulation many times longer than usual, making it significantly more effective. The approach also seemed to result in less toxicity. The mice did not activate enzymatic functions they normally would in response to high levels of such a toxic agent. Needless to say, this has a long way to go before it is tried in humans, but the approach is quite fascinating and very hopeful.[1,2]

J. A. Stockman III, MD

References

1. Merkel TJ, DeSimone JM. Dodging drug-resistant cancer with diamonds. *Sci Transl Med*. 2011;3:73ps8.
2. Chow, Zhang XQ, Chen M, et al. Nanodiamond therapeutic delivery agents mediate enhanced chemoresistant tumor treatment. *Sci Transl Med*. 2011;3:73ra21.

Morbidity and mortality in long-term survivors of Hodgkin lymphoma: a report from the Childhood Cancer Survivor Study
Castellino SM, Geiger AM, Mertens AC, et al (Wake Forest Univ Health Sciences, Winston-Salem, NC; Emory Univ School of Medicine, Atlanta, GA; Fred Hutchinson Cancer Res Ctr, Seattle, WA; et al)
Blood 117:1806-1816, 2011

The contribution of specific cancer therapies, comorbid medical conditions, and host factors to mortality risk after pediatric Hodgkin lymphoma (HL) is unclear. We assessed leading morbidities, overall and cause-specific mortality, and mortality risks among 2742 survivors of HL in the Childhood Cancer Survivor Study, a multi-institutional retrospective cohort study of survivors diagnosed from 1970 to 1986. Excess absolute risk for leading causes of death and cumulative incidence and standardized incidence ratios of key medical morbidities were calculated. Cox regression models were used to estimate hazard ratios (HRs) and 95% confidence intervals (CIs) of risks for overall and cause-specific mortality. Substantial excess absolute risk of mortality per 10,000 person-years was identified: overall 95.5; death due to HL 38.3, second malignant neoplasms 23.9, and cardiovascular disease 13.1. Risks for overall mortality included radiation dose $\geq$ 3000 rad ($\geq$ 30 Gy; supra-diaphragm: HR, 3.8; 95% CI, 1.1-12.6; infradiaphragm + supradiaphragm: HR, 7.8; 95% CI, 2.4-25.1), exposure to anthracycline (HR, 2.6; 95% CI, 1.6-4.3) or alkylating agents (HR, 1.7; 95% CI, 1.2-2.5), non—breast second malignant neoplasm (HR, 2.6; 95% CI 1.4-5.1), or a serious cardiovascular condition (HR, 4.4; 95% CI 2.7-7.3). Excess mortality from second neoplasms and cardiovascular disease vary by sex and persist >20 years of follow-up in childhood HL survivors.

▶ Long-term survivors of Hodgkin lymphoma (HL) are a subset of children with cancer who are at particularly high risk for the late effects of therapy. High cure rates mean that survivors can live for many decades after surgery, and nodular sclerosis, the most common subtype of HL and preferentially afflicts girls and has mediastinal involvement in a large percentage of cases, is treated with radiation therapy. The latter is a well-known risk factor for secondary cancers. This interaction of disease characteristics has led to extremely high rates of solid tumors, particularly breast cancer, and ischemic heart disease in this population of survivors.

What Castellino et al have done is report on morbidity and mortality in almost 3000 survivors of HL from the Childhood Cancer Survivor Study. This report represents the largest available study of survivors of HL who were diagnosed in childhood or adolescence. All the patients in this report were treated before 1986, and the long-term follow-up is therefore truly long. We learn from this report that despite excellent survival rates, beyond 10 years of survivorship there is significant excess mortality from secondary malignancies and cardiovascular disease with no plateau in the latter's occurrence. At 20 years after initial treatment for HL, the excess risk of cardiovascular disease actually rivals that of secondary solid tumors.

If one looks at the information from this report in detail, one sees that the scale of breast cancer morbidity is quite remarkable. The cumulative incidence at 30 years after diagnosis is almost 20%. Breast cancer, cardiovascular disease, and thyroid cancer were the principal morbidities identified in this report, and as 94% of patients received supradiaphragmatic radiation, it is probable that radiation therapy was the cause of the excess morbidity. The authors of this report identified a radiation dose greater than 30 Gy as a risk factor for overall mortality, but it is important to recognize that lower doses of radiation were also linked to morbidity. A recent survivorship report evaluated the long-term outcome of pediatric patients with HL who received low-dose radiation. This study demonstrated that secondary tumors occurred with similar frequency and latency as in studies where patients with HL received high-dose radiation.[1]

For more on the topic of long-term sequelae of HL, see the report of Dunleavy and Bollard.[2] It is not clear what we can do with the information that has been provided from these studies other than to consider the long-term toxicity of the treatments we provide when selecting therapy for newly diagnosed patients. The trick obviously is to target therapies that maintain high cure rates while obviating the need for combination radiation and chemotherapy that may cause unacceptable long-term effects. Alternative approaches such as using immune-based therapies involving monoclonal antibodies and tumor-specific T cells are examples of targeted approaches already being evaluated in clinical trials for youngsters with HL. Needless to say, we need to learn fast whether these alternative therapies are just as effective on the short haul, but it will be decades before we know how much sparing of morbidity these agents will provide.

This commentary concludes with a suggestion: If you would like an extremely interesting book on cancer to read, pick up a copy of *The Emperor of All Maladies: A Biography of Cancer* by Siddhartha Mukherjee.[3] This wonderful book provides a snapshot of stories about cancer throughout the years. You will learn that the first to describe cancer was the Egyptian physician Imhotep around 2625 BCE. He described in some detail breast cancer in 48 cases. The author offers a superb sketch of the scant record of cancer from antiquity before leaping over a long interval when not much happened and then delving into the late 19th century recounting Paul Ehrlich's discovery of the principle of specific affinity and his fruitless search for a discriminating anticancer drug as well as William Halsted's introduction of the radical mastectomy (obviously before Halsted became a full-time cocaine addict). This book is tremendously enjoyable reading for any physician.

J. A. Stockman III, MD

References

1. O'Brian MM, Donaldson SS, Balise RR, Whittemore AS, Link MP. Second malignant neoplasms in survivors of pediatric Hodgkin's lymphoma treated with low-dose radiation and chemotherapy. *J Clin Oncol.* 2010;28:1232-1239.

2. Dunleavy K, Bollard CM. Sobering realities of surviving Hodgkin lymphoma. *Blood.* 2011;117:1772-1773.
3. Mukherjee S. *The emperor of all maladies: a biography of* cancer. New York, NY: Scribner; 2010.

Outcome after Reduced Chemotherapy for Intermediate-Risk Neuroblastoma

Baker DL, for the Children's Oncology Group (Princess Margaret Hosp for Children, Perth, Western Australia, Australia; et al)

N Engl J Med 363:1313-1323, 2010

Background.—The survival rate among patients with intermediate-risk neuroblastoma who receive dose-intensive chemotherapy is excellent, but the survival rate among patients who receive reduced doses of chemotherapy for shorter periods of time is not known.

Methods.—We conducted a prospective, phase 3, nonrandomized trial to determine whether a 3-year estimated overall survival of more than 90% could be maintained with reductions in the duration of therapy and drug doses, using a tumor biology–based therapy assignment. Eligible patients had newly diagnosed, intermediate-risk neuroblastoma without MYCN amplification; these patients included infants (<365 days of age) who had stage 3 or 4 disease, children (≥365 days of age) who had stage 3 tumors with favorable histopathological features, and infants who had stage 4S disease with a diploid DNA index or unfavorable histopathological features. Patients who had disease with favorable histopathological features and hyperdiploidy were assigned to four cycles of chemotherapy, and those with an incomplete response or either unfavorable feature were assigned to eight cycles.

Results.—Between 1997 and 2005, a total of 479 eligible patients were enrolled in this trial (270 patients with stage 3 disease, 178 with stage 4 disease, and 31 with stage 4S disease). A total of 323 patients had tumors with favorable biologic features, and 141 had tumors with unfavorable biologic features. Ploidy, but not histopathological features, was significantly predictive of the outcome. Severe adverse events without disease progression occurred in 10 patients (2.1%), including secondary leukemia (in 3 patients), death from infection (in 3 patients), and death at surgery (in 4 patients). The 3-year estimate (±SE) of overall survival for the entire group was 96±1%, with an overall survival rate of 98±1% among patients who had tumors with favorable biologic features and 93±2% among patients who had tumors with unfavorable biologic features.

Conclusions.—A very high rate of survival among patients with intermediate-risk neuroblastoma was achieved with a biologically based treatment assignment involving a substantially reduced duration of chemotherapy and reduced doses of chemotherapeutic agents as compared with the regimens used in earlier trials. These data provide support for further reduction in chemotherapy with more refined risk stratification.

(Funded by the National Cancer Institute; ClinicalTrials.gov number, NCT00003093.)

▶ Some things have not changed when it comes to statistics related to neuroblastoma. Neuroblastoma remains the most common extracranial solid tumor in childhood. This one malignancy accounts for 50% of all cancers diagnosed in the first year of life. Neuroblastoma remains a difficult-to-predict cancer in terms of its clinical course that ranges from spontaneous regression to rapid progression and death depending on age and a number of biologic features of the tumor. Given the variable clinical course of the malignancy, it is incumbent upon us to figure out ways to maximize outcomes while minimizing the risk of deleterious consequences of therapy. This report from several cancer research centers tells us what we can safely do with the management of intermediate-risk neuroblastoma.

Intermediate-risk neuroblastoma is generally defined as stage 3 or 4 disease without *MYCN* amplification in an infant (younger than 365 days); stage 3 disease and favorable histological features in a child (aged ≥365 days); and stage 4S disease with a diploid tumor-cell DNA index, unfavorable histological features, or both. Stage 4S is defined as a special metastatic stage of neuroblastoma in infants with a primary tumor restricted to one side of the midline and with metastatic sites limited to the liver, skin, bone marrow, or a combination of these sites (with <10% of marrow cells replaced by tumor). We know that the rate of overall survival among patients with intermediate-risk disease exceeds 80% with the use of moderately aggressive chemotherapy. The report of Baker et al tells us about the outcomes of infants and children with intermediate-risk neuroblastoma who have been managed with the use of reduced outpatient-based chemotherapy. Eligible patients had newly diagnosed intermediate-risk neuroblastoma without *MYCN* amplification. Patients who had tumors with favorable biological features received 4 cycles of chemotherapy, and those who had tumors with unfavorable biological features received 8 cycles of chemotherapy with carboplatin, etoposide, cyclophosphamide, and doxorubicin administered at 3-week intervals followed by surgical excision of the primary tumor to achieve a complete response or a very good partial response. Among all the patients eligible for follow-up, the 3-year estimates of event-free and overall survival were 88% ± 2% and 96% ± 1%, respectively.

This study shows that less is more. Most infants and some children with advanced neuroblastoma without *MYCN* amplification can be cured with substantially reduced cytotoxic therapy as compared with the regimens that have been used in previous pediatric cooperative cancer study group trials. Using the same drug combinations, the duration of therapy can be reduced somewhere between 40% and 70%. Thus, high cure rates can be achieved with a minimization of exposure to cancer agents that can have long-term late effects. Less, indeed, is more.

J. A. Stockman III, MD

Papillary Thyroid Cancer in Children and Adolescents Does Not Differ in Growth Pattern and Metastatic Behavior

Machens A, Lorenz K, Thanh PN, et al (Martin Luther Univ, Halle (Saale), Germany)
J Pediatr 157:648-652, 2010

Objective.—To provide comprehensive clinicopathologic data, comparing the growth pattern and metastatic behavior of papillary thyroid cancer between children and adolescents.

Study Design.—This clinicopathologic investigation included 83 consecutive patients ages 6 to 18 years operated on for papillary thyroid cancer at a tertiary referral center in Germany (1994 to 2009).

Results.—There was no difference in sex distribution, re-operation rate, medical history of external radiation, multifocal tumor growth, number of thyroid cancers, extrathyroidal tumor growth, lymph node metastasis, numbers of involved and removed nodes or distant metastasis among patients ages 6 to 11, 12 to 15, and 16 to 18 years. Patients with extrathyroidal growth, unlike those with intrathyroidal growth, had larger tumors, especially in the oldest age group (means of 20, 26, and 44 mm for patients ages 6 to 11, 12 to 15, and 16 to 18 years; $P = .015$); the statistical significance was lost after correction for multiple testing.

Conclusion.—Having comparable extent of disease, children should not undergo less extensive neck operations than adolescents for papillary thyroid cancer.

▶ This report, like so many others, reminds us that children are not small adults. This is true when it comes to infrequent diseases such as papillary thyroid cancer. Thyroid cancer is uncommon in childhood and adolescence with an estimated frequency of 0.7 per 1 million. If someone in the pediatric population does get thyroid cancer, it is most likely a papillary thyroid malignancy. If you look at a comparison between children/adolescents and adults, the former group has significantly larger papillary thyroid cancers (usually at least 50% larger in various series compared with adults) and more likely spread to regional lymph nodes and distant organs by the time a diagnosis is made. It has also been suggested that there are higher recurrence rates of cervical lymph node metastases in children versus adults. Despite these apparently adverse factors, papillary thyroid cancer has a better prognosis in children than in adults, with 98%, 97%, and 91% of pediatric patients surviving 5, 15, and 30 years, respectively. Part of this added survival could be because therapeutic doses of radioactive iodine may more effectively eradicate malignant thyroid tissue since children have more active iodine metabolism.

Unfortunately, there is not a great deal written about papillary thyroid cancer in children and adolescents, most likely because of its relative infrequency. The report of Machens et al from Germany adds a lot to our understanding about this disorder. The center from which this study is reported is well known throughout Europe for the care of children with various thyroid diseases, including cancer. The investigators were able to look at the records of 83 consecutive patients aged 18 years and younger who were operated on for papillary thyroid cancer over a 15-year period between 1994 and 2009. Their observations show that in young children, the tumor more frequently breached the thyroid capsule, presumably because thyroid volumes are smaller than those in adults. Almost all children and adolescents harbored lymph node metastases in addition to extrathyroidal tumor extension. As often as not, these regional metastases were the trigger for a work up rather than the thyroid gland finding themselves. With these findings, the authors indicate that children should not have less extensive neck operations than adolescents unless one is prepared to accept a high rate of regional recurrence in young children.

It is quite clear that the management of thyroid cancer should be handled in tertiary centers that have excellent track records in both surgical management as well as other forms of treatment. A feel of the thyroid should be part of every well-child visit. A recent report from Italy tells us how frequently, when a thyroid nodule is detected, various causes will be found.[1] The Italian investigators did a retrospective study on 120 patients with thyroid nodules diagnosed in childhood and adolescence accumulating data from 9 Italian centers. Of children and adolescents presenting with thyroid nodules, 53% were shown to have a goitrous nodule (all were euthyroid). Twenty-two percent of the youngsters had a papillary carcinoma (all were euthyroid). Some 13% had a follicular adenoma. Most of the latter children were hyperthyroid. Five percent of youngsters had a follicular carcinoma, all of whom were euthyroid. Smaller percentages of youngsters with nodules had other forms of adenoma and carcinoma.

J. A. Stockman III, MD

Reference

1. Corrias A, Mussa A, Baronio F, et al. Diagnostic features of thyroid nodules in pediatrics. *Arch Pediatr Adolesc Med.* 2010;164:714-719.

Everolimus for Subependymal Giant-Cell Astrocytomas in Tuberous Sclerosis

Krueger DA, Care MM, Holland K, et al (Cincinnati Children's Hosp Med Ctr, OH; et al)
N Engl J Med 363:1801-1811, 2010

Background.—Neurosurgical resection is the standard treatment for subependymal giant-cell astrocytomas in patients with the tuberous sclerosis complex. An alternative may be the use of everolimus, which inhibits the mammalian target of rapamycin, a protein regulated by gene products involved in the tuberous sclerosis complex.

Methods.—Patients 3 years of age or older with serial growth of subependymal giant-cell astrocytomas were eligible for this open-label study. The primary efficacy end point was the change in volume of subependymal giant-cell astrocytomas between baseline and 6 months. We gave everolimus orally, at a dose of 3.0 mg per square meter of body-surface area, to achieve a trough concentration of 5 to 15 ng per milliliter.

Results.—We enrolled 28 patients. Everolimus therapy was associated with a clinically meaningful reduction in volume of the primary subependymal giant-cell astrocytoma, as assessed on independent central review (P<0.001 for baseline vs. 6 months), with a reduction of at least 30% in 21 patients (75%) and at least 50% in 9 patients (32%). Marked reductions were seen within 3 months and were sustained. There were no new lesions, worsening hydrocephalus, evidence of increased intracranial pressure, or necessity for surgical resection or other therapy for subependymal giant-cell astrocytoma. Of the 16 patients for whom 24-hour video electroencephalography data were available, seizure frequency for the 6-month study period (vs. the previous 6-month period) decreased in 9, did not change in 6, and increased in 1 (median change, −1 seizure; P=0.02). The mean (±SD) score on the validated Quality-of-Life in Childhood Epilepsy questionnaire (on which scores can range from 0 to 100, with higher scores indicating a better quality of life) was improved at 3 months (63.4 ± 12.4) and 6 months (62.1 ± 14.2) over the baseline score (57.8 ± 14.0). Single cases of grade 3 treatment-related sinusitis, pneumonia, viral bronchitis, tooth infection, stomatitis, and leukopenia were reported.

Conclusions.—Everolimus therapy was associated with marked reduction in the volume of subependymal giant-cell astrocytomas and seizure frequency and may be a potential alternative to neurosurgical resection in some cases, though long-term studies are needed. (Funded by Novartis; ClinicalTrials.gov number, NCT00411619.)

▶ Most every pediatrician has seen or is currently involved with the care of a child with tuberous sclerosis. This is why this report from Cincinnati is so important. Its prevalence runs about 1 in 6000 live births. It can have devastating effects on affected youngsters. It is characterized by benign tumors (hamartomas) in multiple organ systems, including the brain, kidney, skin, lung, heart, and retina. Most patients have mutations in either of 2 tuberous sclerosis genes: TSC1 or TSC2. Unfortunately, many children will have developmental delay and seizures. Subependymal giant-cell astrocytomas, slow-growing glioneuronal tumors, commonly develop in as many as 20% of patients with tuberous sclerosis. These astrocytomas are associated with a clinically significant risk of illness and death, including sudden death from acute hydrocephalous, the risk of which is directly proportionate to the volume of the subependymal giant-cell astrocytoma. These tumors do not regress spontaneously; and the volume of the tumor, once present, increases progressively.

Subependymal giant-cell astrocytomas are best managed with surgery; but, unfortunately, the deep location of these tumors can make resection difficult. Surgery carries a high risk of perioperative and postoperative complications. Incompletely resected subependymal giant-cell astrocytomas will invariably reoccur, necessitating repeat surgeries. To date, no effective alternative to surgery has been identified, and that is where the report of Krueger et al comes in.

Krueger et al have undertaken a study to determine if everolimus may help to reduce the volume of subependymal giant-cell astrocytomas. Everolimus inhibits the byproduct of the tuberous sclerosis gene, a substance known as mTOR complex 1. This substance leads to abnormal cellular growth, proliferation, and protein synthesis. Several prior case reports have suggested that mTOR inhibition will lead to the shrinkage or stabilization of renal angiomyolipomas, lymphangioleiomyomatosis, facial angiofibromas, and subependymal giant-cell astrocytomas. What Krueger et al have done is to design a major study to examine the effect of everolimus on subependymal giant-cell astrocytomas and seizures in patients with tuberous sclerosis complex. Studies included patients 3 years of age or older with a definitive diagnosis of tuberous sclerosis complex. The drug, everolimus, was administered orally. Follow-up was for a 6-month period. It was clear that everolimus did result in a marked reduction in the volume of subependymal giant-cell astrocytomas and also the frequency of seizures.

It is clear that there very well may be a role for everolimus in the management of subependymal giant-cell astrocytomas. Children who die as a result of these astrocytomas tend to experience rapid growth of the tumor that is usually not associated with symptoms until the tumors obstruct the foramen of Monro. From beginning to end, these tumors can cause death from acute hydrocephalus in as little as 18 months. A reduction in the volume of subependymal giant-cell astrocytomas by as little as 30% is generally sufficient to alleviate or reduce the risk of hydrocephalus or invasion into other brain tissue. Everolimus may accomplish this goal without the need for surgery.

In summary, this study of patients with subependymal giant-cell astrocytomas associated with tuberous sclerosis complex showed that 75% of patients will have a reduction by 30% or more in the volume of their tumors at 6 month's treatment. This suggests that medical treatment with everolimus may be a potential alternative to neurosurgical resection in some cases, although long-term studies will be needed to confirm this possibility.

J. A. Stockman III, MD

Everolimus for Advanced Pancreatic Neuroendocrine Tumors
Yao JC, for the RAD001 in Advanced Neuroendocrine Tumors, Third Trial (RADIANT-3) Study Group (Univ of Texas M D Anderson Cancer Ctr, Houston; et al)
N Engl J Med 364:514-523, 2011

Background.—Everolimus, an oral inhibitor of mammalian target of rapamycin (mTOR), has shown antitumor activity in patients with advanced pancreatic neuroendocrine tumors, in two phase 2 studies. We evaluated the agent in a prospective, randomized, phase 3 study.

Methods.—We randomly assigned 410 patients who had advanced, low-grade or intermediate-grade pancreatic neuroendocrine tumors with radiologic progression within the previous 12 months to receive everolimus, at a dose of 10 mg once daily (207 patients), or placebo (203 patients), both in conjunction with best supportive care. The primary end point was progression-free survival in an intention-to-treat analysis. In the case of patients in whom radiologic progression occurred during the study, the treatment assignments could be revealed, and patients who had been randomly assigned to placebo were offered open-label everolimus.

Results.—The median progression-free survival was 11.0 months with everolimus as compared with 4.6 months with placebo (hazard ratio for disease progression or death from any cause with everolimus, 0.35; 95% confidence interval [CI], 0.27 to 0.45; P<0.001), representing a 65% reduction in the estimated risk of progression or death. Estimates of the proportion of patients who were alive and progression-free at 18 months were 34% (95% CI, 26 to 43) with everolimus as compared with 9% (95% CI, 4 to 16) with placebo. Drug-related adverse events were mostly grade 1 or 2 and included stomatitis (in 64% of patients in the everolimus group vs. 17% in the placebo group), rash (49% vs. 10%), diarrhea (34% vs. 10%), fatigue (31% vs. 14%), and infections (23% vs. 6%), which were primarily upper respiratory. Grade 3 or 4 events that were more frequent with everolimus than with placebo included anemia (6% vs. 0%) and hyperglycemia (5% vs. 2%). The median exposure to everolimus was longer than exposure to placebo by a factor of 2.3 (38 weeks vs. 16 weeks).

Conclusions.—Everolimus, as compared with placebo, significantly prolonged progression-free survival among patients with progressive advanced pancreatic neuroendocrine tumors and was associated with a low rate of severe adverse events. (Funded by Novartis Oncology; RADIANT-3 ClinicalTrials.gov number, NCT00510068.)

▶ Pancreatic endocrine tumors are infrequent in children, but they do occur. The report of Yao et al included adults as young as 20 years, making this report and the one that appeared in the *New England Journal of Medicine* of relevance to the pediatric population.[1]

Pediatric endocrine tumors are classified as functional (10%-30% of tumors) or nonfunctional. Functional pancreatic neuroendocrine tumors have long fascinated us because they produce florid syndromes, owing to the secretion of various biologically active hormones such as insulin and gastrin. In the past, the hormone excess syndrome was the leading cause of death, not tumor progression. With advances in surgical and medical treatments, the natural history of the spread of pancreatic neuroendocrine tumors is becoming the major determinant of death in patients with functional tumors, similar to patients with nonfunctional tumors. This is occurring because more than 50% of all pancreatic neuroendocrine tumors, except insulinomas, are malignant and may pursue an aggressive course. The 5-year survival rate of patients with metastatic pancreatic cancer is low and has not changed for the last 2 decades. The reason is that no new specific treatments for malignant pancreatic neuroendocrine tumors have been developed in recent times. While many patients will have a subjective response to chemotherapy, responses are rarely complete, and such treatment is associated with considerable side effects.

Also, the development of new treatments is complicated by the fact that the pathogenesis of pancreatic neuroendocrine tumors is poorly understood and appears to differ from that of the more common adenocarcinoma.

What Yao et al and Raymond et al have reported are results that hold promise for patients with malignant pancreatic neuroendocrine tumors.[1] One group studied the tyrosine kinase inhibitor sunitinib and the other the mammalian target of rapamycin inhibitor everolimus. Sunitinib as compared with placebo caused a more than doubling of progression-free survival (11.4 vs 5.5 months), an increase in the rate of objective tumor response, and an increase in overall survival. Everolimus caused a 65% reduction in the estimated risk of progression (progression-free survival of 11.0 months with everolimus vs 4.6 months with placebo) and an increase by a factor of 3.7 in estimates of the proportion of patients with progression-free survival at 18 months (34% with everolimus vs 9% with placebo). Sunitinib malate works by delaying tumor growth, diminishing tumor angiogenesis via inhibition of vascular endothelial growth factor. Everolimus via a different mechanism of action also inhibits angiogenesis.

Thus now we have 2 studies that provide optimism regarding the treatment of malignant pancreatic neuroendocrine tumors, rare in children but nonetheless present. The 2 drugs reported are effective at improving disease-free survival, even in patients in whom other treatments have failed, and thus offer effective therapies where there were none before. Unfortunately, both drugs have some side effects that cause patients to withdraw their use. Needless to say, neither drug appears to be a magic bullet, but at least now we have new hope that a novel form of tumor treatment will open up avenues of therapy not seen before with these rare tumors.

J. A. Stockman III, MD

Reference

1. Raymond E, Dahan L, Raoul J-L, et al. Sunitinib malate for the treatment of pancreatic neuroendocrine tumors. *N Engl J Med.* 2011;364:501-513.

Human Papillomavirus and Survival of Patients with Oropharyngeal Cancer

Ang KK, Harris J, Wheeler R, et al (Univ of Texas M D Anderson Cancer Ctr, Houston; Radiation Therapy Oncology Group Statistical Ctr, Philadelphia, PA; Huntsman Cancer Inst, Salt Lake City, UT; et al)
N Engl J Med 363:24-35, 2010

Background.—Oropharyngeal squamous-cell carcinomas caused by human papillomavirus (HPV) are associated with favorable survival, but the independent prognostic significance of tumor HPV status remains unknown.

Methods.—We performed a retrospective analysis of the association between tumor HPV status and survival among patients with stage III or IV oropharyngeal squamous-cell carcinoma who were enrolled in a randomized trial comparing accelerated-fractionation radiotherapy (with acceleration by means of concomitant boost radiotherapy) with standard-fractionation radiotherapy, each combined with cisplatin therapy, in patients with squamous-cell carcinoma of the head and neck. Proportional-hazards models were used to compare the risk of death among patients with HPV-positive cancer and those with HPV-negative cancer.

Results.—The median follow-up period was 4.8 years. The 3-year rate of overall survival was similar in the group receiving accelerated-fractionation radiotherapy and the group receiving standard-fractionation radiotherapy (70.3% vs. 64.3%; P=0.18; hazard ratio for death with accelerated-fractionation radiotherapy, 0.90; 95% confidence interval [CI], 0.72 to 1.13), as were the rates of high-grade acute and late toxic events. A total of 63.8% of patients with oropharyngeal cancer (206 of 323) had HPV-positive tumors; these patients had better 3-year rates of overall survival (82.4%, vs. 57.1% among patients with HPV-negative tumors; P<0.001 by the log-rank test) and, after adjustment for age, race, tumor and nodal stage, tobacco exposure, and treatment assignment, had a 58% reduction in the risk of death (hazard ratio, 0.42; 95% CI, 0.27 to 0.66). The risk of death significantly increased with each additional pack-year of tobacco smoking. Using recursive-partitioning analysis, we classified our patients as having a low, intermediate, or high risk of death on the basis of four factors: HPV status, pack-years of tobacco smoking, tumor stage, and nodal stage.

Conclusions.—Tumor HPV status is a strong and independent prognostic factor for survival among patients with oropharyngeal cancer. (ClinicalTrials.gov number, NCT00047008.)

▶ We now know a lot about the link between human papillomavirus (HPV) and cervical cancer. The literature is growing rapidly with respect to the linkage of this virus with oropharyngeal squamous cell carcinoma. Ang et al report findings from their collaborative study that contribute to the body of literature documenting that HPV-positive oropharyngeal squamous cell carcinoma represents a distinct clinical pathological entity associated with a better prognosis than HPV-negative oropharyngeal squamous cell carcinoma.

It appears now that oropharyngeal squamous cell carcinoma can be divided into 2 distinct causes. HPV-positive cases are associated with sex-related risk factors that have been linked to cervical cancer and an increased likelihood of orogenital findings, whereas tobacco and alcohol consumption are the key risk factors for HPV-negative cases. Classic epidemiologic studies suggest that there is actually little interaction between the 2 sets of risk factors, suggesting that HPV-positive cancer and HPV-negative cancer may each have a distinct pathogenesis. The predominant HPV type to cause oropharyngeal carcinoma is type 16. Expression of viral E6 and E7 oncoproteins that inactivate the tumor-suppressor protein (p53) and the retinoblastoma protein (pRb), respectively, is necessary for malignant behavior of these tumors.

This report underscores the rationale for immunizing both male and female teens against HPV. Both men and women can develop oropharyngeal squamous cell carcinoma as a result of transmission of HPV during sexual activity at a young or very young age. Currently, surgery is the only treatment provided for oropharyngeal squamous cell carcinoma even though p16-positive tumors have a better prognosis than p16-negative tumors. Because these 2 cancers seem to be distinct entities, one can speculate that their treatment or prevention might benefit from different approaches. With respect to prevention, approximately 90% of HPV-positive cancers contain HPV type 16, and another 5% have HPV type 18. Both HPV types are targeted by the 2 preventive HPV vaccines approved by the Food and Drug Administration. Vaccination, if performed before exposure to the virus, might prevent a large number of HPV-positive cases of oropharyngeal squamous cell carcinoma. As of now, these vaccines have been documented to prevent persistent genital infection with these types of HPV and precancerous lesions, but it is not yet totally known whether they can prevent oropharyngeal HPV infection, although it is highly likely that they can.

This commentary closes with a neat observation about the use of smart phones. Might you want to know whether you have cancer? There soon may be an app for that. Cancer researchers have come up with a small device that—with the aid of a smart phone—could allow physicians to find out within 60 minutes whether a suspicious lump in a patient is cancerous or benign. Investigators at Massachusetts General Hospital have developed a miniature version of a nuclear magnetic resonance (NMR) machine—the workhorse tool that allows researchers to identify chemical compounds by the way their nuclei react in magnetic fields. The researchers found a way to match magnetic nanoparticles to proteins so the machine could pick up these specific proteins and separate them out from a gemisch of chemicals, like those found in a tumor cell sample. A standard laboratory NMR approaches the size of a filing cabinet, but the new devices are about just a fraction of that size. The scientists did thin needle biopsies of malignant tumors, then labeled the cells with various magnetic nanoparticles designed to attach to known cancer-associated proteins and injected the cells into a miniature NMR machine. The device, whose data can be read with a smart phone app instead of a computer, detected varying levels of cancer cells very handily. The technique accurately diagnosed biopsy specimens 96% of the time in less than 1 hour per patient. The micro-NMR diagnosis was correct 100% of the time. This could allow surgeons and oncologists to provide the results of a needle biopsy literally as soon as the patient is waking up from a procedure. To learn more about this, see the summary by Kaiser.[1]

J. A. Stockman III, MD

Reference

1. Kaiser J. Cancer diagnosis by smartphone. *Science.* http://news.sciencemag.org/sciencenow/2011/02/cancer-diagnosis-by-smart-phone.html. Published February 23, 2011. Accessed August 24, 2011.

Late Onset Hearing Loss: A Significant Complication of Cancer Survivors Treated With Cisplatin Containing Chemotherapy Regimens

Kolinsky DC, Hayashi SS, Karzon R, et al (Washington Univ School of Medicine, St Louis, MO; St Louis Children's Hosp, MO)
J Pediatr Hematol Oncol 32:119-123, 2010

Cisplatin is a known ototoxic agent and has been associated with late onset hearing loss (LOHL) in children beyond completion of treatment. We completed a retrospective review of 160 patients yielding 59 who received cisplatin and had sufficient data to determine the presence of LOHL. LOHL was defined as a significant change in hearing thresholds 6 months past the last cisplatin therapy. A significant change was defined as a decrease of > 15 dB in a frequency from 1 to 8 kHz in either ear, or a decrease of 10 dB at 2 or more frequencies in the same ear, compared with the previously entered audiogram. Hearing loss was classified using the Brock grading system for each ear. Of the 59 patients evaluated, 51% exhibited LOHL. Univariate analysis indicated LOHL was significantly associated with age of diagnosis ($P = 0.031$), diagnosis of medulloblastoma ($P = 0.035$), hearing aids ($P = 0.010$), and cranial radiation ($P = 0.044$), particularly to the posterior fossa ($P = 0.023$). Multivariate analysis revealed only radiation to the posterior fossa ($P = 0.02$) and the use of hearing aids ($P = 0.01$) were significantly associated with LOHL. LOHL is a significant complication in childhood cancer survivors who receive cisplatin. Long-term audiologic monitoring after therapy is needed to identify the affected patients.

▶ We are seeing more and more use of platinum-containing analogs used these days as chemotherapeutic agents, mostly for treatment of solid tumors. These agents are particularly commonly used for pediatric malignancies. Platinum-containing analogs have a number of adverse effects, including nausea and vomiting, nephrotoxicity, neurotoxicity, and ototoxicity. The incidence of the latter has been reported to be as low as 11% and as high as 91% depending on the dose of cisplatin used. Not only does it depend on the individual doses of cisplatin but also on the cumulative dosage that has been used, the method of drug administration, and the intervals between treatment. Unfortunately, cisplatin ototoxicity is characterized by an irreversible, bilateral, sensorineural, high-frequency hearing loss. Decreases in hearing thresholds have been noted within 48 hours after treatment. While the decrement in hearing sensitivity first occurs at high frequencies, gradually this can progress to lower frequencies with subsequent doses. When hearing loss progresses into the frequencies associated with speech recognition, profound detrimental effects on speech and language development can occur in younger children. The psychosocial and school performance consequences therefore are quite significant. Another problem with cisplatin ototoxicity is that it can have delayed manifestations. In 1 study, progressive hearing loss was observed only 136 months after the completion of cisplatin therapy.[1]

The report of Kolinsky et al represents data from a study designed to assess the incidence of delayed-onset hearing loss from cisplatin and to characterize the risk factors associated with developing late-onset hearing loss in childhood cancer survivors. The study was a retrospective one looking at 160 patients of whom 59 had received cisplatin. Of these 59 patients, 51% exhibited late-onset hearing loss as defined by a decrease in hearing of greater than 15 dB in a frequency from 1 kHz to 8 kHz in either ear or a decrease of 10 dB at 2 or more frequencies in the same ear, compared with baseline audiograms. These data indicate that late-onset hearing loss resulting from cisplatin administration is a significant problem in childhood cancer survivors. The data also seem to indicate that patients diagnosed at a younger age seem to be more at risk for developing this problem. Certain diagnoses had an even higher prevalence of hearing loss. For example, of 9 patients diagnosed with medulloblastoma, 8 (88%) in this report experienced a late-onset hearing loss after cisplatin administration. Radiation to the head proved to be an additional risk factor associated with this late outcome problem, particularly in patients who receive radiation to the posterior fossa. Because medulloblastoma is commonly localized to the posterior fossa, the findings of posterior fossa radiation may in fact be a surrogate for neuroblastoma. It was not possible in this study to separate radiation to the posterior fossa from a diagnosis of neuroblastoma because of this strong association.

The findings from this report and the findings from earlier reports indicate that childhood cancer survivors are indeed at risk for hearing deterioration years after completion of therapy. Thus, one of the long-term surveillance studies that should be performed is a periodic hearing examination. At-risk patients should be protected from further exposure to ototoxic agents including antibiotics that can further damage hearing. As young patients enter their teen years and adult years, noise exposure (from recreational activities, rock concerts, amplified headsets, etc) and/or occupational duties involving noise from machinery can be expected to increase the risk of additional hearing loss. Patients and their parents should be forewarned about these additional hazards.

This commentary closes with an unrelated observation having to do with a new way of detecting a cancer. A portable sensor that uses gold nanoparticles coated with specific organic compounds to detect levels of certain exhaled volatile substances can distinguish between the breath of patients with lung cancer and the breath of healthy controls. Using gas chromatography and mass spectroscopy to analyze breath samples from 56 patients with lung cancer and 40 healthy controls, researchers were able to successfully identify "signature" biomarkers for the malignancy. What an easy way to sniff out cancer![2]

J. A. Stockman III, MD

References

1. Bertolini P, Lasalle M, Mercier G, et al. Platinum compound related to ototoxicity in children: long-term follow-up reveals continuous worsening of hearing loss. *J Pediatr Hematol Oncol.* 2004;26:649-655.
2. Stephenson J. Sniffing out lung cancer? *JAMA.* 2009;302:1640.

Long-term Cause-Specific Mortality Among Survivors of Childhood Cancer
Reulen RC, for the British Childhood Cancer Survivor Study Steering Group
(Univ of Birmingham, Edgbaston, UK; et al)
JAMA 304:172-179, 2010

Context.—Survivors of childhood cancer are at increased risk of premature mortality compared with the general population, but little is known about the long-term risks of specific causes of death, particularly beyond 25 years from diagnosis at ages when background mortality in the general population starts to increase substantially.

Objective.—To investigate long-term cause-specific mortality among 5-year survivors of childhood cancer in a large-scale population-based cohort.

Design, Setting, and Patients.—British Childhood Cancer Survivor Study, a populationbased cohort of 17 981 5-year survivors of childhood cancer diagnosed with cancer before age 15 years between 1940 and 1991 in Britain and followed up until the end of 2006.

Main Outcome Measures.—Cause-specific standardized mortality ratios (SMRs) and absolute excess risks (AERs).

Results.—Overall, 3049 deaths were observed, which was 11 times the number expected (SMR, 10.7; 95% confidence interval [CI], 10.3-11.1). The SMR declined with follow-up but was still 3-fold higher than expected (95% CI, 2.5-3.9) 45 years from diagnosis. The AER for deaths from recurrence declined from 97 extra deaths (95% CI, 92-101) per 10 000 person-years at 5 to 14 years from diagnosis, to 8 extra deaths (95% CI, 3-22) beyond 45 years from diagnosis. In contrast, during the same periods of follow-up, the AER for deaths from second primary cancers and circulatory causes increased from 8 extra deaths (95% CI, 7-10) and 2 extra deaths (95% CI, 2-3) to 58 extra deaths (95% CI, 38-90) and 29 extra deaths (95% CI, 16-56), respectively. Beyond 45 years from diagnosis, recurrence accounted for 7% of the excess number of deaths observed while second primary cancers and circulatory deaths together accounted for 77%.

Conclusion.—Among a cohort of British survivors of childhood cancer, excess mortality from second primary cancers and circulatory diseases continued to occur beyond 25 years from diagnosis.

▶ There has been much written about the long-term complications related to the management of childhood cancer, but this report by Reulen et al tells us about the really long follow-up of childhood cancer survivors when it comes to ultimate mortality risk from second cancers, circulatory disease, and pulmonary disease. It appears that there is a persistent elevated risk of mortality even beyond 25 years from the diagnosis of childhood cancer relative to the general population. While the absolute excess risk (AER) of mortality due to recurrence of the original disease declined from 97 extra deaths per 10 000 person-years at 5 to 14 years from diagnosis to just 8 extra deaths beyond 45 years from diagnosis, the AER for deaths from secondary primary tumor, circulatory deaths, and cardiac deaths increased from 8, 2, and 1 extra deaths to 58, 28, and 15 extra deaths, respectively. Beyond 45 years from diagnosis, recurrence accounted for 7% of the excess number of deaths observed, while secondary primary cancers and circulatory deaths together accounted for 77%. It is interesting to note that there was no increase in deaths from suicide or other mental disorders.

It seems clear that the excess mortality due to second primary cancer and circulatory disease is likely attributable to late complications of treatment. Second primary cancers are a well-recognized late complication of childhood cancer, largely due to exposure to radiation during treatment, but specific cytotoxic drugs have also been implicated in the development of second primary cancers. Buried within these second primary cancers is a small proportion of all secondary primary cancer deaths that might be related to familial cancerous syndromes such as Li Fraumeni and heritable retinoblastoma. Exposure to cranial irradiation does increase the risk of stroke, and exposure to chest irradiation has been associated with heart disease, which can also result from the use of certain chemotherapeutic agents such as anthracyclines.

The findings of this report underscore the need for survivors of childhood cancer to be regularly examined and carefully followed up decades out from their initial cure. The principal clinical message from these data is stated in the concluding paragraph of this report, and the message is very straightforward: "77% of excess numbers of death observed among those surviving beyond 45 years from diagnosis of childhood cancer are due to secondary primary cancers and circulatory deaths." The trick will be to find ways to successfully intervene to reduce these untoward outcomes.

J. A. Stockman III, MD

Growth Hormone Treatment in Children is not Associated with an Increase in the Incidence of Cancer: Experience from KIGS (Pfizer International Growth Database)

Wilton P, Mattsson AF, Darendeliler F (Pfizer Endocrine Care, NY; Pfizer Endocrine Care, Sollentuna, Sweden; Istanbul Univ, Turkey)
J Pediatr 157:265-270, 2010

Objective.—To assess the incidence of cancer in patients treated with growth hormone (GH) in KIGS—the Pfizer International Growth Database—without cancer or any other condition in medical history known to increase the risk of cancer.

Study Design.—Data were analyzed from patients with growth disorders enrolled in an observational survey KIGS who had no known increased risk of developing cancer before starting recombinant human GH treatment. The incidence of cancer in this patient cohort (overall, site-specific, and according to etiology of growth disorder) was compared with the incidence in the general population by using the standardized incidence ratio (ie, relating the observed to expected number of cases with stratification for age, sex, and country).

Results.—A total of 32 new malignant neoplasms were reported in 58 603 patients, versus the 25.3 expected (incidence, 16.4 per 100 000 patient-years; standardized incidence ratio, 1.26; 95% confidence interval, 0.86-1.78). No category of growth disorder showed a statistically significant difference in observed compared with the expected number of cases.

Conclusion.—There is no evidence in this series that GH treatment in young patients with growth disorders results in an increased risk of developing cancer relative to that expected in the normal population. However, surveillance for an extended time should continue to allow further assessment.

▶ When I was on faculty at Northwestern University Medical School more than 20 years ago, the first data began to appear suggesting that there might be a link between an increased risk of malignancy and the administration of growth hormone. It was in 1988 that the first report of leukemia in a growth hormone–deficient child undergoing growth hormone therapy was reported.[1] This report of a potential association between leukemia and growth hormone treatment started a small flurry of interest in looking at the potential relationship between this form of therapy and the development of cancer. In the interval period of time, we have seen a tiny number of reports suggesting the possibility of such a relationship, including the identification of 2 cases of colorectal cancer in a long-term cohort study of children and adolescents treated with pituitary-derived growth hormone.[2] Needless to say, the relationship between growth hormone and cancer development has been a controversial one, and this is why the report by Wilton et al is so important. It uses information from the Pfizer International Growth Database (KIGS) to address the controversy.

KIGS is a large international pharmacoepidemiological database that was established in 1987 to monitor long-term clinical and safety outcomes in children with growth disorders who had been receiving recombinant human growth hormone (Genotropin; Pfizer, New York, NY). The database protocol requires that physicians report all adverse events in patients followed up in KIGS, regardless of whether they are associated with growth hormone treatment or not. The database now has information on almost 59 000 patients covering almost 200 000 patient-years of follow-up for analysis. The reasons for growth hormone treatment included idiopathic growth hormone deficiency (54% of patients), Turner syndrome (11%), congenital growth hormone deficiency (5%), being born small for gestational age (7%), and acquired growth hormone deficiency (3%). A small number of other conditions, including chronic renal insufficiency and Prader-Willi syndrome, were responsible for short stature, requiring treatment in the remaining patients. Over the recent 20-year period, new malignant neoplasms were reported in 32 patients in KIGS who had no known factors conveying an a priori increased risk. Cancer was diagnosed at a mean age of 11.9 years. The mean duration of growth hormone therapy before the diagnosis of cancer was 3.6 years. In 6 patients, a malignant neoplasm was reported for as long as 3.1 years after stopping growth hormone. The types of malignancies reported cover the entire spectrum of cancers/leukemias seen in children with no one malignancy standing out among the others.

The findings from this report when calculated against the age-matched population of non–growth hormone treatment show that the overall incidence of cancer in the growth hormone–treated population was similar to that of the general population. In fact, for leukemia diagnosis, there were fewer children than expected with this form of malignancy in comparison with the general population, albeit the numbers being quite small to begin with. The data, however, are sufficiently rigorous to exclude a large increase in a cancer incidence in patients treated with growth hormone, if one excludes children with known risk factors for cancer development. These youngsters will need to be followed up for some time to confirm these findings. If there is an association between growth hormone therapy and cancer, it is likely that the development of a tumor would take some time. Thus far, however, there is no evidence that tumor incidence is increased with time in the analysis of the KIGS study data.

J. A. Stockman III, MD

References

1. Watannabe S, Tsunematsu Y, Fujimoto J, et al. Leukemia in patients treated with growth hormone. *Lancet.* 1988;331:1159-1160.
2. Swerdlow AJ, Higgins CD, Adlard P, Preece MA. Risk of cancer in patients treated with human pituitary growth hormone in the UK 1959-85: a cohort study. *Lancet.* 2002;360:273-277.

Screening and Surveillance for Second Malignant Neoplasms in Adult Survivors of Childhood Cancer: A Report From the Childhood Cancer Survivor Study
Nathan PC, Ness KK, Mahoney MC, et al (Hosp for Sick Children, Toronto, Ontario, Canada; St Jude Children's Res Hosp, Memphis, TN; Memorial Sloan-Kettering Cancer Ctr, NY; et al)
Ann Intern Med 153:442-451, 2010

Background.—Survivors of childhood cancer may develop a second malignant neoplasm during adulthood and therefore require regular surveillance.

Objective.—To examine adherence to population cancer screening guidelines by survivors at average risk for a second malignant neoplasm and adherence to cancer surveillance guidelines by survivors at high risk for a second malignant neoplasm.

Design.—Retrospective cohort study.

Setting.—The Childhood Cancer Survivor Study (CCSS), a 26-center study of long-term survivors of childhood cancer that was diagnosed between 1970 and 1986.

Patients.—4329 male and 4018 female survivors of childhood cancer who completed a CCSS questionnaire assessing screening and surveillance for new cases of cancer.

Measurements.—Patient-reported receipt and timing of mammography, Papanicolaou smear, colonoscopy, or skin examination was categorized as adherent to the U.S. Preventive Services Task Force guidelines for survivors at average risk for breast or cervical cancer or the Children's Oncology Group guidelines for survivors at high risk for breast, colorectal, or skin cancer as a result of cancer therapy.

Results.—In average-risk female survivors, 2743 of 3392 (80.9%) reported having a Papanicolaou smear within the recommended period, and 140 of 209 (67.0%) reported mammography within the recommended period. In high-risk survivors, rates of recommended mammography among women were only 241 of 522 (46.2%) and the rates of colonoscopy and complete skin examinations among both sexes were 91 of 794 (11.5%) and 1290 of 4850 (26.6%), respectively.

Limitations.—Data were self-reported. Participants in the CCSS are a selected group of survivors, and their adherence may not be representative of all survivors of childhood cancer.

Conclusion.—Female survivors at average risk for a second malignant neoplasm show reasonable rates of screening for cervical and breast cancer. However, surveillance for new cases of cancer is very low in survivors at the highest risk for colon, breast, or skin cancer, suggesting that survivors and their physicians need education about their risks and recommended surveillance.

▶ This report reminds us that there are more than 325 000 individuals who had childhood cancer and who are alive now in the United States. These are the adult survivors of childhood cancer, many of whom are at an increased risk of a second malignancy as a result of the therapy for their primary cancer. Statistics show that approximately 10% of adult survivors of childhood cancer will develop a second malignancy within 30 years of initial cancer diagnosis and that such malignancies are the major cause of mortality in such individuals. Depending on the type of second cancer, the latter's treatment may be somewhat compromised by the initial therapy used in childhood. For example, a female survivor who develops invasive node-positive breast cancer during adulthood may not be able to receive adjuvant doxorubicin if she had anthracycline chemotherapy for her childhood cancer. For these and other reasons, adhering to strict screening protocol for breast or cervical cancer and other forms of cancer in adulthood is imperative to detect disease at its earliest and most readily treatable stages. Secondary cancers with high prevalence include breast cancer, colorectal and other types of gastrointestinal cancer, malignant melanoma, and nonmelanoma skin cancer. All these occur at a younger age and with an increased frequency in survivors of childhood cancer when compared with the general population.

What Nathan et al have done is to evaluate adherence to recommended screening and surveillance in survivors of childhood cancer at average or high risk for a second malignant neoplasm during adulthood. The Children's Oncology Group has developed guidelines for screening survivors of childhood cancers whose treatment put them at elevated risk for breast, colorectal, and skin cancer. Nathan et al surveyed more than 8000 survivors of childhood cancer and found that most patients who were eligible for breast, colorectal, and skin cancer screening in fact did not report having been screened within the recommended interval. Reported screening rates were worse for colorectal cancer (just 11.5%), followed by skin cancer (26.6%) and breast cancer (46.2%).

It is clear that the rates of surveillance for secondary malignancies for those at high risk for a therapy-related second malignant neoplasm are alarmingly low. One can easily recognize what such a deficiency can cause in terms of morbidity and mortality. Women who have had radiation therapy to the chest during childhood have a 13% to 20% cumulative incidence of breast cancer by age 40 to 45 years, a risk that is similar to that observed in women with breast cancer susceptibility gene mutations. The chance of developing colorectal cancer if abdominal or pelvic radiation was given as part of primary therapy in childhood results in a 3.9- to 4.7-fold increased risk compared with the general population. Similar statistics exist for melanoma and nonmelanoma skin cancers.

There are several take-home messages from this National Cancer Institute report. One message is that it is incumbent upon us as pediatric care providers to instill in those patients who leave our care the necessity of careful surveil-lance follow-up. Second, we must be sure that the transition of these patients into adult care is smooth, seamless, and with a road map describing what type of surveillance is needed and when it should be delivered. Last, patients and families need to be aware of the need to minimize, to the extent possible, addi-tional risk factors imposed by things such as radiation from medical imaging. There has been a lot written about the latter recently. Although the average dose from natural background sources has not changed, the average radiation dose from medical imaging has increased more than 6-fold. Medical imaging now contributes about 50% of overall radiation dose to the US population compared with just 15% 3 decades ago. The largest contributor to this dramatic increase in population radiation exposure is the CT scan. In 1980, fewer than 3 million CT scans were performed in the United States, but the annual number now approaches 80 million and is increasing by approximately 10% per year. CT scanning is not the only culprit here. Newer radiographic imaging modalities such as positron emission tomography/CT, single-photon emission CT, and CT screening of asymptomatic individuals are likely to increase the population radi-ation exposure still further. A recent survey of Massachusetts physicians shows that 28% of diagnostic imaging referrals represent defensive practices.[1] Radia-tion doses from CT scans are 100 to 500 times those from conventional radiog-raphy, depending on what part of the body is imaged. There are projections that in the United States alone, CT scans may contribute to about 29 000 new cancers each year.[2]

J. A. Stockman III, MD

References

1. Hillman BJ, Goldsmith FC. The uncritical use of high-tech medical imaging. *N Engl J Med.* 2010;363:4-6.
2. Berrington de González A, Mahesh M, Kim KP, et al. Projected cancer risks from computed tomographic scans performed in the United States in 2007. *Arch Intern Med.* 2009;169:2071-2077.

Stillbirth and neonatal death in relation to radiation exposure before conception: a retrospective cohort study
Signorello LB, Mulvihill JJ, Green DM, et al (International Epidemiology Inst, Rockville, MD; Univ of Oklahoma; St Jude Children's Res Hosp, Memphis, TN; et al)
Lancet 376:624-630, 2010

Background.—The reproductive implications of mutagenic treatments given to children with cancer are not clear. By studying the risk of untoward pregnancy outcomes, we indirectly assessed the risk of transmission of germline damage to the offspring of survivors of childhood cancer who were given radiotherapy and chemotherapy.

Methods.—We did a retrospective cohort analysis, within the Childhood Cancer Survivor Study (CCSS), of the risk of stillbirth and neonatal death among the offspring of men and women who had survived childhood cancer. Patients in CCSS were younger than 21 years at initial diagnosis of an eligible cancer, were treated at 25 US institutions and one Canadian institution, and had survived for at least 5 years after diagnosis. We quantified the chemotherapy given to patients, and the preconception radiation doses to the testes, ovaries, uterus, and pituitary gland, and related these to the risk of stillbirth or neonatal death using Poisson regression analysis.

Findings.—Among 1148 men and 1657 women who had survived childhood cancer, there were 4946 pregnancies. Irradiation of the testes (16 [1] of 1270; adjusted relative risk 0·8 [95 CI 0·4−1·6]; mean dose 0·53 Gy [SD 1·40]) and pituitary gland (17 [3] of 510, 1·1 [0·5−2·4] for more than 20·00 Gy; mean dose 10·20 Gy [13·0] for women), and chemotherapy with alkylating drugs (26 [2] of 1195 women, 0·9 [0·5−1·5]; ten [1] of 732 men, 1·2 [0·5−2·5]) were not associated with an increased risk of stillbirth or neonatal death. Uterine and ovarian irradiation significantly increased risk of stillbirth and neonatal death at doses greater than 10·00 Gy (five [18] of 28, 9·1 [3·4−24·6]). For girls treated before menarche, irradiation of the uterus and ovaries at doses as low as 1·00−2·49 Gy significantly increased the risk of stillbirth or neonatal death (three [4] of 69, 4·7 [1·2−19·0]).

Interpretation.—Our findings do not support concern about heritable genetic changes affecting the risk of stillbirth and neonatal death in the offspring of men exposed to gonadal irradiation. However, uterine and ovarian irradiation had serious adverse effects on the offspring that were probably related to uterine damage. Careful management is warranted of pregnancies in women given high doses of pelvic irradiation before puberty.

▶ Signorello et al report a retrospective cohort analysis of the Childhood Cancer Survivor Study looking at rates of stillbirth and neonatal death in adult survivors of childhood cancer. In this report, enrolled participants were diagnosed between 1970 and 1986 and had diagnoses of leukemia, lymphoma, sarcoma, central nervous system cancer, Wilms tumor, kidney cancer, or neuro-blastoma. The study reports the risk of stillbirth (defined as fetal death after the 20th gestational week) and neonatal death (defined as death within the first 28 days after birth).

The findings of this report showed no effect of childhood cancer treatment on the ability of male survivors to contribute to a successful pregnancy, although the radiation doses received directly by the testes were lower than the uterine/ovarian doses of the women in this study. Female survivors, however, had a significantly increased risk (relative risk, 12.3) of having a stillbirth and neonatal death if they had received a radiation dose greater than 2.5 Gy before menarche because of the direct effects of irradiation to the uterus/ovaries. By contrast, postmenarchal girls treated with greater than 2.5 Gy had a relative risk of 0.2. The reasons for the difference between premenarchal and postmenarchal sensitivity to radiation are unclear.

The bottom line from this report is that when it comes to stillbirth and neonatal death, a history of irradiation to the pelvic area is of significant concern to childhood cancer survivors. Should uterine irradiation be unavoidable, parents should be informed that their daughter's offspring might be at risk of stillbirth and neonatal death when their daughter reaches adulthood. For childhood cancer survivors, reproductive counseling and testing in a specialized center to assess the feasibility and potential risks associated with pregnancy provide the best opportunities for families to deal with this complex issue.

The concern that CT scan radiation causes cancer is mounting. The number of CT scans administered continues to soar. In 1980, 3 million scans were given in the United States. In 2006, this number had increased to 67 million. It should be noted that the Radiology Department of Massachusetts General Hospital in Boston now uses software to actually help physicians determine whether a CT scan is truly necessary in specific medical circumstances. They have published a report showing that the rate of rise in CT scan ordering which was 3% per quarter dropped to just 0.25% as a result of the implementation of this software as part of the decision-making process.[1]

J. A. Stockman III, MD

Reference

1. Schenkman L. Second thoughts about CT imaging. *Science.* 2011;331:1002-1004.

Early life exposure to diagnostic radiation and ultrasound scans and risk of childhood cancer: case-control study
Rajaraman P, Simpson J, Neta G, et al (Natl Cancer Inst, Bethesda, MD; Univ of York, UK)
BMJ 342:d472, 2011

Objective.—To examine childhood cancer risks associated with exposure to diagnostic radiation and ultrasound scans in utero and in early infancy (age 0-100 days).

Design.—Case-control study.

Setting.—England and Wales.

Participants.—2690 childhood cancer cases and 4858 age, sex, and region matched controls from the United Kingdom Childhood Cancer Study (UKCCS), born 1976-96.

Main Outcome Measures.—Risk of all childhood cancer, leukaemia, lymphoma, and central nervous system tumours, measured by odds ratios.

Results.—Logistic regression models conditioned on matching factors, with adjustment for maternal age and child's birth weight, showed no evidence of increased risk of childhood cancer with in utero exposure to ultrasound scans. Some indication existed of a slight increase in risk after in utero exposure to x rays for all cancers (odds ratio 1.14, 95% confidence interval 0.90 to 1.45) and leukaemia (1.36, 0.91 to 2.02), but this was not statistically significant. Exposure to diagnostic x rays in early infancy (0-100 days) was associated with small, non-significant excess risks for all cancers and leukaemia, as well as increased risk of lymphoma (odds ratio 5.14, 1.27 to 20.78) on the basis of small numbers.

Conclusions.—Although the results for lymphoma need to be replicated, all of the findings indicate possible risks of cancer from radiation at doses lower than those associated with commonly used procedures such as computed tomography scans, suggesting the need for cautious use of diagnostic radiation imaging procedures to the abdomen/pelvis of the mother during pregnancy and in children at very young ages.

▶ In the article by Fuchs et al,[1] you will see a discussion regarding the long-term potential risk associated with the use of radiologic imaging as part of the evaluation and/or management of patients with inflammatory bowel disease. Such patients unfortunately have to undergo frequent diagnostic imaging. In this report, we see the concerns expressed about total lifetime exposure to diagnostic radiation that is part of the cancer surveillance for children with malignancies. For patients recovering from cancer, some cancer surveillance protocols call for several CT scans per year for many years. A survey of CT scanning, for example, at the University of California Davis Medical Center has shown that about 5% of patients with a malignancy have had more than 20 CT scans.[2] At the same institution, the average patient with a pediatric malignancy had 2.88 scans and the median was 4 scans per patient. Certain cancer surveillance protocols, however, require 20, 30, or even 40 or more scans over a number of years.

A typical abdominal CT scan would lead to a dose of about 5 to 10 mGy to the abdomen, and smaller doses are deposited to tissues away from the scanned area by x-ray scattered radiation. Radiation-absorbed dose in the units of milligray represents a physically measurable quantity (energy/mass), and medical physicists typically use computer modeling techniques to compute the radiation dose deposited to a number of organs during a given CT scan or other x-ray imaging procedure. The effective dose (ED) is used by the medical community to assess the relative risk associated from a given x-ray imaging procedure such as a CT scan. Determining ED requires that the radiation dose (expressed as mGy) be computed to a number of different organs and tissues, and then a weighting factor is applied to these doses. The unit of ED is the sievert (Sv). It is generally accepted that a lifetime exposure of 50 mSv is the break point for an increase in the risk of the development of cancer of some significance.

The report of Rajaraman et al tells us about what exposure to x-rays in utero and in early infancy can do to the otherwise healthy infant. For example, the authors found no increased risk of childhood cancer with in utero exposure to ultrasound scans and some indication of an elevated risk after in utero exposure to x-rays for all cancers (odds ratio, 1.14) and leukemia (odds ratio, 1.36). Exposure to diagnostic x-rays in early infancy was associated with a small nonsignificant excess risk for all cancers and leukemias as well as an increased risk of lymphoma (odds ratio, 5.14, 1.27 to 20.78 on the basis of small numbers). The bottom line is that exposures to x-rays in utero and in early infancy are associated with a small increase in risk of all childhood cancers and leukemia. Others have reported that in utero exposure to radiation from diagnostic radiography is associated with an increased risk of childhood cancer. The findings from this report add to these earlier understandings.

If you want to read more about the risk of exposure to radiological imaging and how to minimize this risk, see the excellent clinical review by Davies et al.[3] You will learn that CT coronary angiography exposes the human breast to 51 mSv. Even a simple barium enema results in a radiation dose to the colon of 15 mSv. A CT of the brain is the equivalent of 150 chest x-rays. An intravenous pyelogram is the equivalent of 150 chest x-rays. A CT coronary angiogram is worth 800 chest x-rays or the equivalent of 2433 days of natural background radiation exposure.

J. A. Stockman III, MD

References

1. Fuchs Y, Markowitz J, Weinstein T, et al. Pediatric inflammatory bowel disease and imaging-related radiation: Are we increasing the likelihood of malignancy? *J Pediatr Gastroenterol Nutr.* 2011;52:280-285.
2. Lam D, Wootton-Torges SL, McGahan JP, et al. Abdominal pediatric cancer surveillance using serial computed tomography: evaluation of organ absorbed dose and effective dose. *Semin Oncol.* 2011;38:128-135.
3. Davies AG, Wathen CG, Gleeson FV. Risks of exposure to radiological imaging and how to minimize them. *BMJ.* 2011;342:589-593.

Mobile phone base stations and early childhood cancers: case-control study
Elliott P, Toledano MB, Bennett J, et al (Imperial College London, UK)
BMJ 340:c3077, 2010

Objective.—To investigate the risk of early childhood cancers associated with the mother's exposure to radiofrequency from and proximity to macrocell mobile phone base stations (masts) during pregnancy.

Design.—Case-control study.

Setting.—Cancer registry and national birth register data in Great Britain.

Participants.—1397 cases of cancer in children aged 0-4 from national cancer registry 1999-2001 and 5588 birth controls from national birth register, individually matched by sex and date of birth (four controls per case).

Main Outcome Measures.—Incidence of cancers of the brain and central nervous system, leukaemia, and non-Hodgkin's lymphomas, and all cancers combined, adjusted for small area measures of education level, socioeconomic deprivation, population density, and population mixing.

Results.—Mean distance of registered address at birth from a macrocell base station, based on a national database of 76,890 base station antennas in 1996-2001, was similar for cases and controls (1107 (SD 1131) m v 1073 (SD 1130) m, P=0.31), as was total power output of base stations within 700 m of the address (2.89 (SD 5.9) kW v 3.00 (SD 6.0) kW, P=0.54) and modelled power density (−30.3 (SD 21.7) dBm v −29.7 (SD 21.5) dBm, P=0.41). For modelled power density at the address at birth, compared with the lowest exposure category the adjusted odds ratios were 1.01 (95% confidence interval 0.87 to 1.18) in the intermediate and 1.02 (0.88 to 1.20) in the highest exposure category for all cancers (P=0.79 for trend), 0.97 (0.69 to 1.37) and 0.76 (0.51 to 1.12), respectively, for brain and central nervous system cancers (P=0.33 for trend), and 1.16 (0.90 to 1.48) and 1.03 (0.79 to 1.34) for leukaemia and non-Hodgkin's lymphoma (P=0.51 for trend).

Conclusions.—There is no association between risk of early childhood cancers and estimates of the mother's exposure to mobile phone base stations during pregnancy.

▶ There seems to be no end of belief to the possibility that exposure to transmission lines will increase a child's risk of the development of cancer. Radiofrequency fields are now ubiquitous. Several studies have assessed the potential of radiofrequency fields having adverse health effects, but most studies have been predominantly negative with respect to their results. The 2 main areas of research have been exposure associated with the use of mobile phones and the risk associated with transmitters, including mobile phone masts. The study by Elliott et al assesses whether proximity to mobile phone masts during pregnancy raises the risk of children developing leukemia or a tumor in the brain or other parts of the central nervous system. The study identified almost 14 000 British children registered with leukemia or a tumor in the central nervous system between 1999 and 2001 and compared each of these children with 4 controls sampled from national birth registries, matched for sex and date of birth. The study found no association between the risk of cancer in early childhood and exposure to a mobile phone base station during pregnancy.

The importance of the report of Elliott et al is that it is the largest study to date in terms of numbers of individuals studied. The study would have had a > 90% probability of detecting a doubled risk of brain cancer between the 85th and 15th centiles of the modeled power density of the study. For childhood leukemia, which has a higher incidence, the figure is over 99%.

The study of Elliott et al is the first to focus on the risk of brain tumors and leukemia after exposure during pregnancy. Radiofrequency field studies mostly consider broadcast transmitters and cancers in adults. The highest incidence of childhood cancer occurs in the first 5 years of life, so it is less necessary to conduct long-term studies. Just running the math, with malignant disease being so rare in children, it is unlikely that more than a few cases could ever be attributed to proximity to radiofrequency transmitters even if there was an association, which has not yet been and probably never will be documented.

If there is 1 conclusion from this report, it is that radio transmitters are not a significant cause of death, certainly not so in comparison with the number of deaths caused from distraction while using mobile phones while driving. The scare tactics used by some who just do not want a radiofrequency transmitter in their neighborhood has caused more than one family to relocate, with all of its stresses and costs. There are lots of things to worry about in life; this is not one of them. Radiation exposure from medical imaging is an entirely different story.

The report by Elliott et al tells us about mobile phone base stations. If you are interested in hearing about cell phones and their effects on the brain, see the article by Volkow et al.[1] This report is the first investigation in humans of glucose metabolism in the brain after cell phone use. The investigators placed cell phones on the right and left ears of 147 health participants and used positron emission tomography with the injection of radio-labeled glucose to determine whether brain glucose metabolism was altered when using a cell phone over a 50-minute period. Exposure to radiofrequency radiation emitted from a cell phone for 50 minutes did increase glucose metabolic rates in very selected cortical regions of the brain. A significant linear correlation was observed between enhanced neural metabolic rate and the estimated rate of radiofrequency energy absorption expected in brain regions. Even though the health consequences of these effects on brain glucose metabolism are unknown, the results point to a conclusion that cell phone use can possibly affect brain function. It is not yet known whether this phenomenon is mediated by an increase in temperature. It is known that temperature of the skin on the head in contact with the cell phone can increase by more than 2°C after 10 minutes of cell phone use. The increase in temperature is mainly attributable to the heat generated by the operating phone and to a much lesser extent by the radiofrequency energy emitted. The results of this study add to concern about the possible acute and long-term effects of radiofrequency emissions from wireless phones, including both mobile and cordless desktop phones. Although the biological significance, if any, of increased glucose metabolism from acute cell phone exposure is unknown, the results do warrant further investigation. To read more about cell phone radiofrequency radiation, see the excellent editorial by Lai and Hardell.[2] Reading all this stuff makes one want to go out, get a couple of tin cans, and string them together as a way of communicating as this editor once did growing up in Philadelphia with his friend across the alleyway.

J. A. Stockman III, MD

References

1. Volkow ND, Tomasi D, Wang GJ, et al. Effects of cell phone radiofrequency signal exposure on brain glucose metabolism. *JAMA*. 2011;305:808-814.
2. Lai H, Hardell L. Cell phone radiofrequency radiation exposure and brain glucose metabolism. *JAMA*. 2011;305:828-829.

17 Ophthalmology

Perinatal Systemic Inflammatory Response Syndrome and Retinopathy of Prematurity
Sood BG, on Behalf of the NICHD neonatal research network (Wayne State Univ, Detroit, MI; et al)
Pediatr Res 67:394-400, 2010

Fetal and neonatal inflammation is associated with several morbidities of prematurity. Its relationship to retinopathy of prematurity (ROP) has not been investigated. Our objective was to determine the relationship between cytokine levels and ROP in the first 3 postnatal wks. Data for this study were derived from the NICHD Cytokine Study. Dried blood spots (DBS) were obtained from infants <1000 g on days 0–1, 3 ± 1, 7 ± 2, 14 ± 3, and 21 ± 3. Infants were classified into three groups—no, mild, and severe ROP. Multiplex Luminex assay was used to quantify 20 cytokines. Temporal profiles of cytokines were evaluated using mixed-effects models after controlling for covariates. Of 1074 infants enrolled, 890 were examined for ROP and 877 included in the analysis. ROP was associated with several clinical characteristics on unadjusted analyses. Eight cytokines remained significantly different across ROP groups in adjusted analyses. IL-6 and IL-17 showed significant effects in early time periods (D0–3); TGF-β, brain-derived neurotrophic factor (BDNF), and regulated on activation, normal T cell expressed and secreted (RANTES) in later time periods (D7–21) and IL-18, C-reactive protein (CRP), and neurotrophin-4 (NT-4) in both early and later time periods. We conclude that perinatal inflammation may be involved in the pathogenesis of ROP.

▶ There is a rapidly emerging body of literature to suggest that retinopathy of prematurity (ROP), the major cause of blindness in infancy, is either caused by or made significantly worse by the presence of inflammatory mediators in the circulation. ROP, of course, is a vasoproliferative disorder of the developing retina. It is a biphasic disease consisting of an initial period of blunted vascular growth followed by a second period of vasoproliferation recognized with careful eye examination 4 weeks to 6 weeks after birth. The proliferation of blood vessels, better known as angiogenesis, is affected and regulated by a complex network of cytokines, extracellular matrix components, and growth factors. Little is known about the actual effect of inflammatory cytokines and their ability to modulate angiogenesis, particularly in the newborn as related to the development of ROP. This is the importance of this report by Sood et al.

What Sood et al have now documented is that there is a clear association between perinatal inflammation as evaluated by cytokine levels and ROP. In preterm infants, the development of ROP is associated with elevated levels of interleukin (IL)-6 and lower levels of IL-17 and IL-18. It appears that cytokines do affect angiogenesis in the retina. In this study, the investigators found a panel of 6 inflammatory markers and 2 growth factors that were significantly associated with ROP in the first 6 weeks of life. Careful analysis of the data suggests that documenting cytokine dysregulation in ROP may offer a window of opportunity to diagnose and treat ROP medically earlier than current standards of ROP screening examinations.

While on the topic of oxidative stress, a recent report reinforces my belief that exercise is not good for you. Nasca et al tell us that acute exercise (a session of short duration and progressive intensity) induces oxidative stress in children aged 8 to 10 years.[1] These investigators looked at the effect of real-life exercise programs on systemic oxidative stress as measured by urinary concentrations of certain prostaglandins, a noninvasive index of lipid peroxidation. The bottom line is that this pilot study showed that even in healthy children, exercise programs as frequently recommended may significantly increase in vivo lipid peroxidation. Needless to say, this study, which included only 18 youngsters, should not be a prescription to be a couch potato. It does make one wonder whether young children, especially if unfit and/or overweight, should be exposed to exercise in a more gradual, enjoyable, and noncompetitive manner.

This commentary closes with a brief case report that documents the 809th reason not to exercise. An 18-year-old man presented with sudden painless blurring of the vision of his right eye after a few rounds of push-up exercises. A college student, he had no history of vascular disease or blood dyscrasias. On examination, vision in his right eye was 20/200. Vision in his left eye was 20/20. Retinal examination of the right eye showed a crescent-shaped subhyaloid hemorrhage overlying the macula. Coagulation tests were normal. Three months after laser therapy, the vision in the right eye had improved to 20/40. This patient demonstrated evidence of what is known as "Valsalva retinopathy." This occurs because of a sudden rise in intraocular venous pressure, causing retinal capillaries to spontaneously rupture. Push-up exercises typically cause a Valsalva maneuver. The outcome of Valsalva hemorrhagic retinopathy is generally good with laser therapy, although not necessarily perfect.[2] If there is basic learning from this case report it is that performing push-ups is a dangerous exercise, unless you are willing to turn a "blind eye" to the consequences thereof, including becoming a cyclops.

J. A. Stockman III, MD

References

1. Nasca MM, Zhang R, Super DM, Hazen SL, Hall HR. Increased oxidative stress in healthy children following an exercise program: a pilot study. *J Dev Behav Pediatr.* 2010;31:386-392.
2. Hassan M, Tajunisah I. Valsalva hemorrhagic retinopathy after push-ups. *Lancet.* 2011;337:504.

Efficacy of Intravitreal Bevacizumab for Stage 3+ Retinopathy of Prematurity

Mintz-Hittner HA, for the BEAT-ROP Cooperative Group (Univ of Texas Health Science Ctr at Houston—Med School)

N Engl J Med 364:603-615, 2011

Background.—Retinopathy of prematurity is a leading cause of childhood blindness worldwide. Peripheral retinal ablation with conventional (confluent) laser therapy is destructive, causes complications, and does not prevent all vision loss, especially in cases of retinopathy of prematurity affecting zone I of the eye. Case series in which patients were treated with vascular endothelial growth factor inhibitors suggest that these agents may be useful in treating retinopathy of prematurity.

Methods.—We conducted a prospective, controlled, randomized, stratified, multicenter trial to assess intravitreal bevacizumab monotherapy for zone I or zone II posterior stage 3+ (i.e., stage 3 with plus disease) retinopathy of prematurity. Infants were randomly assigned to receive intravitreal bevacizumab (0.625 mg in 0.025 ml of solution) or conventional laser therapy, bilaterally. The primary ocular outcome was recurrence of retinopathy of prematurity in one or both eyes requiring retreatment before 54 weeks' postmenstrual age.

Results.—We enrolled 150 infants (total sample of 300 eyes); 143 infants survived to 54 weeks' postmenstrual age, and the 7 infants who died were not included in the primary-outcome analyses. Retinopathy of prematurity recurred in 4 infants in the bevacizumab group (6 of 140 eyes [4%]) and 19 infants in the laser-therapy group (32 of 146 eyes [22%], $P = 0.002$). A significant treatment effect was found for zone I retinopathy of prematurity ($P = 0.003$) but not for zone II disease ($P = 0.27$).

Conclusions.—Intravitreal bevacizumab monotherapy, as compared with conventional laser therapy, in infants with stage 3+ retinopathy of prematurity showed a significant benefit for zone I but not zone II disease. Development of peripheral retinal vessels continued after treatment with intravitreal bevacizumab, but conventional laser therapy led to permanent destruction of the peripheral retina. This trial was too small to assess safety. (Funded by Research to Prevent Blindness and others; ClinicalTrials.gov number, NCT00622726.)

▶ Retinopathy of prematurity (ROP) is a neovascular retinal disorder of childhood that causes loss of vision by means of macular dragging and retinal detachment. It generally occurs in infants born before 31 weeks' gestational age, results in variable episodes of tissue hyperoxia and tissue hypoxia and consequent induction of vascular endothelial growth factor (VEGF). ROP is the leading cause of childhood blindness in our country and in other developed nations. The incidence of blindness in infants because of ROP is relatively low (about 1 case in 820 infants) because of excellent neonatal care and appropriate screening and treatment. Nonetheless, the disorder is a major cause of childhood blindness in developing countries, manifesting in larger premature infants (birth weights ≤2000 g; mean 1400 g). The worldwide prevalence of blindness because of ROP is about 50 000.

The pathogenesis of ROP involves 2 discrete phases: phase I occurs roughly from 22 to 30 weeks postmenstrual age and phase II from roughly 31 to 44 weeks postmenstrual age. It is now understood that phase I involves relative hyperoxia and decreased VEGF levels, whereas phase II involves relative hypoxia and increased VEGF levels. The use of anti-VEGF agents, primarily intravitreal bevacizumab, is an emerging treatment for acute ROP. The Food and Drug Administration approved intravenous bevacizumab in 2004 for treatment of metastatic colon cancer. The drug works by reducing the size and number of new blood vessels feeding metastases. Off-label use of intravitreal bevacizumab therapy for ophthalmologic neovascular disorders began shortly thereafter. The off-label use of bevacizumab has increased rapidly because it is readily available, quite inexpensive, and offers patients positive results in certain conditions such as age-related macular degeneration for which there are no other good treatment options.

Mintz-Hittner et al describe a multicenter randomized trial with the potential to stimulate a dramatic shift in the treatment of acute ROP. The investigators found that among infants with zone 1 disease, the recurrence rate was just 6% with intravitreal bevacizumab but 42% with conventional laser therapy. Moreover, intravitreal bevacizumab therapy resulted in mild anatomical retinal abnormality in just 1 eye of 31 infants, whereas conventional laser treatment resulted in a mild structural abnormality in 16 eyes and severe abnormality in 2 eyes of 33 infants (Fig 3 in the original article). Although the differences in outcomes were not significant among infants with posterior zone II ROP, data nonetheless suggest the same pattern. Thus, this important report of Mintz-Hittner et al shows superior efficacy of intravitreal bevacizumab over laser therapy as measured by means of disease recurrence and abnormal structural outcomes. This is a true breakthrough in disease management.

With data provided to date, it seems reasonable to assume that intravitreal bevacizumab is safe. However, it is well known that intravitreal bevacizumab in adults reaches the systemic circulation. This will raise concern of untoward effects on an infant's developing organs. Such an effect has not been documented to date. The dose of intravitreal bevacizumab is a fraction of the dose used for treatment of colon cancer, and the amount of circulating bevacizumab would be expected to be extraordinarily small unless there is some breakdown of the blood-retinal barrier that might theoretically increase the level of the drug in the circulation. To determine systemic safety with statistical assurance would require a huge sample size. Continued vigilance will be important as the use of this drug in tiny babies continues.

The bottom line is that bevacizumab has distinct advantages with respect to simplicity of administration (requiring no intubation); a rapid effect; a high likelihood of decreased loss of visual field (especially for zone I disease); continued normal retinal vascularization; use in patients with an opaque cornea or lens (which makes laser therapy very difficult); ocular safety when used appropriately; and a demonstrated superior efficacy in zone I disease. There are disadvantages. These include the critical issue of timing, the possibility of late recurrence, which will require prolonged weekly observation (ie, until 54 weeks postmenstrual age), and the possibility of systemic effects.

In a commentary that accompanied this report, James Reynolds from the Department of Ophthalmology at the University of Buffalo commented that "as our experience with bevacizumab grows, its indications and relative contraindications will be refined. In the meantime, intravitreal bevacizumab should become the treatment of choice for zone I ROP."[1] Dr Reynolds' comments appear to be right on the mark!

This commentary closes with a fast fact having to do with video games and their ability to help treat eye disorders. It has now been documented that playing video games can help improve the vision of adults with amblyopia. Researchers have found that subjects who play video games for 40 hours while wearing a patch over their good eye have a 30% improvement in visual acuity![2]

J. A. Stockman III, MD

References

1. Reynolds JD. Bevacizumab for retinopathy of prematurity. *N Engl J Med.* 2011; 364:677-678.
2. Editorial comment. Video game watching and amblyopia. *Science Medicine.* 2010; 16:1061.

A Higher Incidence of Intermittent Hypoxemic Episodes Is Associated with Severe Retinopathy of Prematurity

Di Fiore JM, Bloom JN, Orge F, et al (Case Western Reserve Univ and Rainbow Babies and Children's Hosp, Cleveland, OH; et al)
J Pediatr 157:69-73, 2010

Objective.—Retinopathy of prematurity (ROP), a vasoproliferative disorder of the retina in preterm infants, is associated with multiple factors, including oxygenation level. We explored whether the common intermittent hypoxemic events in preterm infants are associated with the development of ROP.

Study Design.—Oxygen desaturation events were quantified in 79 preterm infants (gestational age, 24 to 27-6/7 weeks) during the first 8 weeks of life. Infants were classified as requiring laser treatment for ROP versus having less severe or no ROP. A linear mixed model was used to study the association between the incidence of intermittent hypoxia and laser treatment of ROP, controlling for gestational age, sex, race, multiple births, and initial severity of illness.

Results.—For all infants, hypoxemic events increased with postnatal age ($P < .001$). Controlling for all covariates, a higher incidence of oxygen desaturation events was found in the infants undergoing laser therapy for ROP ($P < .001$), males ($P < .02$), and infants of younger gestational age ($P < .003$).

Conclusions.—The incidence of hypoxemic events was higher in infants with ROP requiring laser therapy. Therapeutic strategies to optimize oxygenation in preterm infants should include minimization of desaturation episodes, which may in turn decrease serious morbidity in this high-risk population.

▶ Di Fiore et al tell us that a greater frequency of hypoxic occurrences in premature infants is associated with the development of retinopathy of prematurity (ROP). The study design that reached these conclusions used high-resolution pulse oximetry to determine the frequency and pattern of hypoxemic events during the first 2 months of life in preterms born at gestational ages 24.5 to 27.6 weeks. These findings are consistent with other reports that oxygenation fluctuations in the early newborn period are independent risk factors for the development of severe ROP. Prolonged hyperoxia suppresses production of vascular endothelial growth factor (VEGF) and induces vasoconstriction and vaso-obliteration of existing immature retinal blood vessels. Hypoxia, on the other hand, upregulates VEGF leading to neovascularization. Either of these 2 combinations alters the normal balance between proangiogenic and antiangiogenic factors, leading to an increased probability of the development of ROP. Thus the influence of oxygen or oxygenation on the development or healing of ROP is a function of multiple factors at multiple levels. Too high or too little oxygen represent important variables as does male sex (an independent risk factor).

We are seeing more and more written about the availability of oxygen controllers that minimize the fluctuations in oxygenation status of preterm infants.[1] Variations in oxygen levels also relate to ambient noise, unnecessary disturbances, including suctioning, and blood draws. These too can be controlled to some degree.

For more on the topic of ROP and the topic of the interrelationship between it and oxidative stress and inflammation, see the excellent commentary by Dammann.[2] Oxidative stress that can be a consequence of inflammation has long been implicated in the etiology of ROP. Evidence is just beginning to accumulate that markers of inflammation appear to be associated with ROP in human studies. Needless to say, the more we learn about ROP, the more complicated the story gets.

J. A. Stockman III, MD

References

1. Urschitz MS, Horn W, Seyfang A, et al. Automatic control of the inspired oxygen fraction in preterm infants: a randomized crossover trial. *Am J Respir Crit Care.* 2004;170:1095-1100.
2. Dammann O. Inflammation and retinopathy of prematurity. *Acta Paediatr.* 2010; 99:975-977.

Complications and Visual Prognosis in Children With Aniridia

Lee H, Meyers K, Lanigan B, et al (Children's Univ Hosp, Dublin, Ireland)
J Pediatr Ophthalmol Strabismus 47:205-210, 2010

Purpose.—To characterize the ophthalmological findings, assess surgical outcomes, and review visual outcomes in aniridia.

Methods.—A retrospective case review was performed and data were collected, including patient demographics, incidence of aniridia-associated keratopathy, glaucoma, cataract, retinal breaks or detachments, optic nerve hypoplasia, macular hypoplasia, poor vision, and nystagmus. All outcomes from surgery, including penetrating keratoplasty, trabeculectomy, Ahmed valve insertion, and cataract extraction, were recorded.

Results.—Six children (12 eyes) had corneal abnormalities, 4 had optic nerve hypoplasia, 9 had nystagmus, and 2 had retinal detachments. Four patients (7 eyes) required penetrating keratoplasty. Five patients (9 eyes) developed glaucoma and only 1 of the 4 trabeculectomies performed succeeded. Of the 6 Ahmed valve procedures performed, all succeeded in maintaining a satisfactory intraocular pressure but some required needling and 5-fluorouracil. Eight patients developed cataract and 7 required surgery. Visual outcomes were poor despite treatment. Nine patients had Snellen acuity of 6/60 or less and required low visual aids to function.

Conclusion.—Aniridia is a disorder that requires multiple surgeries. It has a poor visual prognosis despite early diagnosis and aggressive management. Newer techniques such as Ahmed valves and Boston keratoprostheses offer hope, but its proliferative nature makes treatment difficult.

▶ Most pediatricians know something about aniridia, namely that it is associated with partial or complete absence of the irises of the eye (Fig 1). What few of us know, however, is the full scope of the other manifestations of this disorder whose incidence varies from between 1:64 000 and 1:100 000. Yes, it is an autosomal dominant entity, but it can occur sporadically. Two out of 3 cases are familial and one-third are sporadic. We now know that the disorder is due to mutations in the *PAX6* gene on 11p13. The report of Lee et al helps us understand more about the overall disorder.

What Lee et al have done is to summarize the findings in 11 patients (22 eyes) with aniridia who have been seen at Temple Street Children's Hospital between 1985 and 2007. This particular children's hospital is in Dublin, Ireland. The investigators reported that the mean age at first presentation was 30 months. Four patients presented at younger than 1 month, 4 at younger than 2 years of age, and the remainder were older than 2 years at presentation. Four had autosomal dominant aniridia, 3 had sporadic aniridia, and 2 had the Wilms tumor, aniridia, genitourinary malformations, and mental retardation complex. One had aniridia associated with Peters anomaly, and 1 is currently being observed for Rieger syndrome. One of the common findings in aniridia, besides the iris deficiency, was the presence of corneal

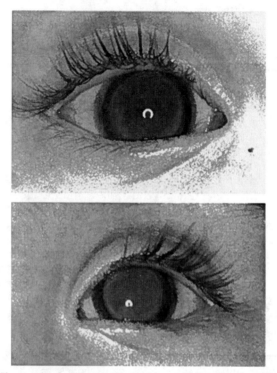

FIGURE 1.—Photographs of a 10-month-old male infant with bilateral total aniridia. Top = right eye. Bottom = left eye. Each eye demonstrates an absent iris and only a rudimentary iris root and zonules are visible. (Reprinted with permission from SLACK Incorporated: Lee H, Meyers K, Lanigan B, et al. Complications and visual prognosis in children with aniridia. *J Pediatr Ophthalmol Strabismus.* 2010;47:205-210.)

abnormalities. Keratopathy was quite common leading to corneal ulcers and in some cases the need for stem cell transplant. Five of the children developed glaucoma and 8 patients developed cataracts. Optic nerve hypoplasia was found in 4 children and macular hypoplasia in 6, with nystagmus in 8. Two patients actually had retinal detachments. Nine patients had visual impairment with a Snellen visual acuity of 6/60 or less and required low vision aids such as telescopes, magnifiers, and Braille. Only 2 patients had useful functioning vision without low visual aids.

What this report is telling us is that aniridia is a severe panocular disorder. This means that more than the iris is involved as an ocular manifestation in a significant proportion of children. We also know that about two-thirds of cases of aniridia are associated with Wilms tumor since both abnormalities are due to deletions of 11p13. Some patients with aniridia also have Gillespie syndrome, ring chromosome 6 syndrome, Rieger syndrome, Smith-Lemli-Opitz syndrome, Biemond syndrome, and XXXY syndrome.

The ocular management of aniridia depends on what its associated findings are. For example, management of mild aniridia-associated keratopathy involves preservative-free lubricants and dark glasses that aid against photophobia. In moderate keratopathy, the use of serum drops and amniotic membrane transplants may aid the survival and promote the growth of limbal stem cells of the cornea. In severe disease, limbal cell transplant is recommended. Penetrating keratoplasty tends to result in failure of a transplant. Data seem to show that corneal tissue removed from donors under the age of 50 years work best. There is also a corneal prosthesis known as the Boston keratoprosthesis that may be helpful. The management of glaucoma is the same as in virtually anyone with glaucoma. Unfortunately, treatment of the latter condition in those with aniridia is often difficult. Only about 1 in 3 patients will respond satisfactorily to medical treatment alone such as with oral carbonic anhydrase inhibitors. Most patients will ultimately require surgical intervention and will also require cataract treatment, performed in the usual way. The major causes of visual impairment, optic nerve hypoplasia, and macular hypoplasia, needless to say, are not managed easily.

If there is a bottom line having to do with the management of aniridia, it is to be aware of its presence by looking for it. Since two-thirds will have the genetic form associated with the Wilms tumor, one does not want to miss the diagnosis. Every child must be followed by a competent ophthalmologist, preferably a pediatric ophthalmologist, well versed in managing all of the ocular complications of the disorder.

This commentary closes with an observation related to hereditary blindness. An international group of investigators from Switzerland, France, Germany, Ireland, and the United States has successfully used a gene therapy strategy to treat retinitis pigmentosa in mice. This disease, which causes incurable blindness, is a form of inherited retinal degeneration resulting from diverse mutations in more than 44 genes expressed in rod photoreceptors. To restore responsiveness to light in mice with the disorder, investigators used an adeno-associated virus to insert a gene from a light-sensitive bacterium into the animal's cone cell DNA. The inserted gene encodes a protein that is a light-activated chloride pump. Expression of this ion pump protein restored damaged and nonfunctional cone photoreceptors in the retinas of mice with the disorder. Also, using human in vitro retinas, the investigators showed that upregulation of the ion pump would reactivate light-insensitive human photoreceptors.[1]

J. A. Stockman III, MD

Reference

1. Hampton T. Treating hereditary blindness. *JAMA*. 2010;304:733.

Is a 6-Week Course of Ganciclovir Therapy Effective for Chorioretinitis in Infants with Congenital Cytomegalovirus Infection?

Shoji K, Ito N, Ito Y, et al (Natl Ctr for Child Health and Development, Tokyo, Japan; et al)
J Pediatr 157:331-333, 2010

Effective treatment for chorioretinitis caused by congenital cytomegalovirus (CMV) infection remains unknown. We report an infant with congenital CMV infection, who required a 6-month course of antiviral therapy to control his chorioretinitis. Long-term treatment may be necessary for managing congenital CMV-associated chorioretinitis.

▶ This case of a newborn with chorioretinitis secondary to congenital cytomegalovirus (CMV) is highly illustrative of the pitfalls associated with treatment for congenital CMV infection. Treatment of symptomatic congenital CMV historically has been done with the use of intravenous ganciclovir for a 6-week period. For infants with hearing and developmental problems, some improvement has been noted with such therapy. In addition to intravenous ganciclovir, valganciclovir has been used. This is the monovalyl ester prodrug of ganciclovir and has good oral bioavailability and is converted to ganciclovir after absorption. Given in appropriate dosing, valganciclovir administered orally can achieve similar blood concentrations to ganciclovir administered intravenously. What we are seeing now in practice is the transition from the use of intravenous ganciclovir to oral valganciclovir as the preferred treatment for infants with symptomatic congenital CMV infection.

The report by Shoji et al documents a well-known fact that congenital CMV does result in shedding of virus for long periods of time. This virus can be detected in congenitally infected infants in urine for years. Viruria can be suppressed by ganciclovir treatment, but it returns promptly after a 6-week treatment regimen. It is reasonable to expect that longer treatment for congenital CMV infection could produce more sustained suppression of the virus and in fact improve outcome compared with the traditional use of this drug for just 6 weeks. That is exactly what Shoji et al describe in an infant with congenital CMV chorioretinitis. In this infant, response was seen with a 6-week treatment schedule of intravenous ganciclovir, but the ocular disease reoccurred shortly after the completion of the scheduled treatment. Subsequent therapy brought the chorioretinitis under control. This documents the need for careful follow-up examinations after cessation of antiviral treatment. The availability of valganciclovir oral solution would make a longer treatment schedule easier to administer.

It has been suggested that a multicenter, randomized, placebo-controlled clinical trial comparing 6 weeks versus 6 months of oral valganciclovir would help to define the benefits and risks of longer treatment of symptomatic congenital CMV infection. Such a trial is currently under way (NCT00466817, www.clinicaltrials.gov). Whether children with congenital CMV infection who are symptom free at birth but have hearing loss would benefit from such antiviral treatment also remains to be determined with a long-term clinical study.

On a somewhat related note, please be aware that there are almost 20 infants who have now been reported since the 1970s who have developed CMV infection as a result of breast milk feeding from a mother who is CMV positive.[1] Little is known, however, about the actual acquiring of clinical disease and disability as a result of breast milk feeding in such circumstances. The only way to prevent this problem, if one is aware of its possibility, is pasteurization, the preferred procedure to inactivate human milk CMV because freezing does not completely eliminate the virus.

This commentary closes with a clinical curio. Have you ever wondered why the old 3D glasses that were used many years ago that relied on red-cyan lenses went the way of Godzilla? What has replaced them? It turns out that when 3D movies returned to theaters 6 years ago with the opening of Chicken Little, they came with new specs. Instead of the old dark red-cyan lenses, we now have new eye gear that a variety of sophisticated methods that bring sharp, full color, 3D images to the viewer's eyes without limiting the spectrum of colors that one can see. Dolby, one of the major players in the 3D movie market, just received a patent for these lenses (patent number 7 784 938). The Dolby glasses rely on a phenomenon called spectral separation. A projector breaks up each of the 3 primary colors into multiple spectra and beams 2 different images—one meant for the left eye, one meant for the right eye—to the screen in rapid succession, one right after another. The images are projected at a rate of 144 frames per second so you do not notice the trick. Multilayer filters on the Dolby glasses allow the left eye to see shorter wavelength bands of blue, green and red than the right eye. Both eyes get the same full spectrum of color, but it is not the exact same frequency that the other eye is getting, allowing the impression of depth. To read more about this fascinating ophthalmologic technology, see the editorial by Kuchment, which contains a diagram of how this works.[2]

J. A. Stockman III, MD

References

1. Kurath S, Resch B. Cytomegalovirus in transmission via breast milk: how to support breast milk to premature infants and prevent severe infection? *Pediatr Infect Dis J*. 2010;29:680-681.
2. Kuchment A. Patient watch. *Scientific American*. 2010;30.

18 Respiratory Tract

Normal ranges of heart rate and respiratory rate in children from birth to 18 years of age: a systematic review of observational studies

Fleming S, Thompson M, Stevens R, et al (Oxford Univ, Headington, UK; et al)
Lancet 377:1011-1018, 2011

Background.—Although heart rate and respiratory rate in children are measured routinely in acute settings, current reference ranges are not based on evidence. We aimed to derive new centile charts for these vital signs and to compare these centiles with existing international ranges.

Methods.—We searched Medline, Embase, CINAHL, and reference lists for studies that reported heart rate or respiratory rate of healthy children between birth and 18 years of age. We used non-parametric kernel regression to create centile charts for heart rate and respiratory rate in relation to age. We compared existing reference ranges with those derived from our centile charts.

Findings.—We identified 69 studies with heart rate data for 143 346 children and respiratory rate data for 3881 children. Our centile charts show decline in respiratory rate from birth to early adolescence, with the steepest fall apparent in infants under 2 years of age; decreasing from a median of 44 breaths per min at birth to 26 breaths per min at 2 years. Heart rate shows a small peak at age 1 month. Median heart rate increases from 127 beats per min at birth to a maximum of 145 beats per min at about 1 month, before decreasing to 113 beats per min by 2 years of age. Comparison of our centile charts with existing published reference ranges for heart rate and respiratory rate show striking disagreement, with limits from published ranges frequently exceeding the 99th and 1st centiles, or crossing the median.

Interpretation.—Our evidence-based centile charts for children from birth to 18 years should help clinicians to update clinical and resuscitation guidelines.

▶ Measurements of heart rate and respiratory rate are extraordinarily fundamental to the assessment of the physiologic status of both well and unwell children. Infancy and childhood are periods of enormous physiological and developmental changes, particularly in the early months and years of life. Over the years, investigators have attempted to establish what constitutes normal heart and respiratory rates at different ages, but these investigations have taken place in various populations, settings, and geographical locations using different measurement techniques. The result is that evidence for what

521

is normal for these measurements at different ages and the ability to identify that which is clearly abnormal is, at best, hardly perfect. Thus far, there have been no attempts made to systematically aggregate these data to provide normal reference ranges for vital signs in children at different ages.

Fleming et al have accepted the challenge of looking at the literature to systematically review and synthesize data from about 150 healthy children to create new centile charts for heart rate and respiratory rate. They provide us important evidence to underpin future clinical guidelines and recommendations. They found 69 studies that obtained high-quality data on both heart rate and respiratory rate. The figures illustrate the data that they have derived from their systematic review of the literature.

Needless to say, the data from this report, while important, must always be placed into the context of the situation in which you are seeing a youngster. Heart rate may be raised by various factors unrelated to illness (by distress or agitation). Heart rate can be influenced, of course, by temperature or pain. The effects of these external factors will probably differ among age ranges. Nonetheless, the data provided by the centile charts of Fleming et al are valuable and can be used to initiate important new studies to establish where the clinical boundaries should be set for different ages to assist clinicians in distinguishing between normal and abnormal heart and respiratory rates. One can bet that the information provided by Fleming et al will lead to revised algorithms, risk scores, and treatment guidelines. Figs 2 and 4 are worth copying and placing in every examination room.

This commentary closes with a question. Have you ever heard of the term mulch pneumonitis? Recently described was the case of a 16-year-old girl with a mutation of gp47phox who died following exposure to mulch. This mutation is one of the several causing autosomal recessive presentations of chronic granulomatous disease (CGD), a disorder first recognized in the 1950s that has an estimated prevalence of 1:250 000 in the general population.

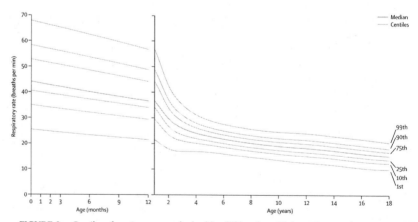

FIGURE 2.—Centiles of respiratory rate for healthy children from birth to 18 years of age. (Reprinted from The Lancet, Fleming S, Thompson M, Stevens R, et al. Normal ranges of heart rate and respiratory rate in children from birth to 18 years of age: a systematic review of observational studies. *Lancet.* 2011;377:1011-1018. Copyright 2011, with permission from Elsevier.)

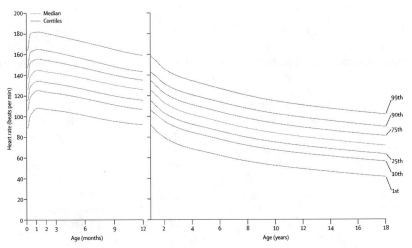

FIGURE 4.—Centiles of heart rate for healthy children from birth to 18 years of age. (Reprinted from The Lancet, Fleming S, Thompson M, Stevens R, et al. Normal ranges of heart rate and respiratory rate in children from birth to 18 years of age: a systematic review of observational studies. *Lancet.* 2011;377: 1011-1018. Copyright 2011, with permission from Elsevier.)

This youngster's history indicates she suffered from respiratory tract infections beginning in early infancy. Over the years she had a history of respiratory problems, but at age 16 came to hospital with increasing breathlessness within hours of exposure to mulch. She underwent a bronchoscopy with various tissue samplings that established a diagnosis of CGD. Despite massive ventilatory support and ECMO, she died. It appears that overwhelming exposure to large numbers of *Aspergillus* spores was the likely explanation for her fatal mulch pneumonitis. Given the rapid onset of symptoms in this patient, it is likely that the therapeutic window to commence aggressive treatment was measured just in hours.[1]

J. A. Stockman III, MD

Reference

1. Ameratonga R, Woon ST, Vyas J, Roberts S. Fulminant mulch pneumonitis in undiagnosed chronic granulomatous disease: a medical emergency. *Clin Pediatr.* 2010;49:1143-1146.

Maternal Vitamin A Supplementation and Lung Function in Offspring

Checkley W, West KP Jr, Wise RA, et al (Johns Hopkins Univ, Baltimore, MD; et al)
N Engl J Med 362:1784-1794, 2010

Background.—Vitamin A is important in regulating early lung development and alveolar formation. Maternal vitamin A status may be an important determinant of embryonic alveolar formation, and vitamin A deficiency in a mother during pregnancy could have lasting adverse effects on the lung health of her offspring. We tested this hypothesis by examining the long-term effects of supplementation with vitamin A or beta carotene in women before, during, and after pregnancy on the lung function of their offspring, in a population with chronic vitamin A deficiency.

Methods.—We examined a cohort of rural Nepali children 9 to 13 years of age whose mothers had participated in a placebo-controlled, double-blind, cluster-randomized trial of vitamin A or beta-carotene supplementation between 1994 and 1997.

Results.—Of 1894 children who were alive at the end of the original trial, 1658 (88%) were eligible to participate in the follow-up trial. We performed spirometry in 1371 of the children (83% of those eligible) between October 2006 and March 2008. Children whose mothers had received vitamin A had a forced expiratory volume in 1 second (FEV_1) and a forced vital capacity (FVC) that were significantly higher than those of children whose mothers had received placebo (FEV_1, 46 ml higher with vitamin A; 95% confidence interval [CI], 6 to 86; FVC, 46 ml higher with vitamin A; 95% CI, 8 to 84), after adjustment for height, age, sex, body-mass index, calendar month, caste, and individual spirometer used. Children whose mothers had received beta carotene had adjusted FEV_1 and FVC values that were similar to those of children whose mothers had received placebo (FEV_1, 14 ml higher with beta carotene; 95% CI, −24 to 54; FVC, 17 ml higher with beta carotene, 95% CI, −21 to 55).

Conclusions.—In a chronically undernourished population, maternal repletion with vitamin A at recommended dietary levels before, during, and after pregnancy improved lung function in offspring. This public health benefit was apparent in the preadolescent years.

▶ Many of us have not been aware of the relationship between lung development, lung function, and retinoids. Checkley et al report that, in a region with endemic vitamin A (retinol) deficiency, children whose mothers had received vitamin A supplementation before, during, and for 6 months after pregnancy have better lung function when they were tested at 9 to 11 years of age, than children whose mothers had received β-carotene supplementation or placebo. The extent of the increased lung function is linearly related to the mothers' postpartum serum retinol concentration. Because of a local ordinance, all children received supplemental vitamin A beginning at 6 months of age. Thus, the period during which supplementation with vitamin A was most relevant was from gestation through a postnatal age of 6 months. The key lung function measured was the volume of gas forcefully expired in the first second after full inspiration (FEV_1). It is well known that the determinants of FEV_1 are primarily the diameter of the conducting airways (bronchi and bronchioles), the number of alveolar attachments to the bronchioles, and the elastic recoil of alveoli with the latter 2 helping to keep bronchioles open as lung volume diminishes during expiration. The issue, of course, is how might maternal administration of vitamin A during pregnancy actually influence the lung function of children a decade after they are born. To learn more about this, see the interesting editorial of Massaro et al.[1] In this editorial, we are reminded that the formation of alveoli in humans begins during the fetal period and has been thought to end when the child is about 8 years of age. However, the formation of alveoli in Old World monkeys, which are related to humans, continues until early adulthood, making it likely that the same is true in humans; if so, the period during which environmental events could adversely influence the formation of alveoli is quite lengthy.

Except in the case of vision, enzymatically produced metabolites of vitamin A (eg, all-trans retinoic acid), not vitamin A itself, are the physiologically active retinoids. In mice, retinoic acid stabilizes conducting airways that have been formed already and prevents excess branching. Thus, vitamin A deficiency during gestation might be expected to result in abnormal conducting airways with suboptimal function, manifesting as low FEV_1. It is suspected that it is all-trans retinoic acid that induces the formation of alveoli.

It is obvious from the study of Checkley et al that all pregnant women should have ample access to adequate amounts of vitamin A to prevent vitamin A deficiency. Those especially at risk are those in underdeveloped countries and women who have had multiple full-term pregnancies with a relatively short interval between pregnancies. The problems noted at the end of the first decade of life are sufficiently problematic in those born of mothers who are vitamin A deficient that routine supplementation seems entirely appropriate.

J. A. Stockman III, MD

Reference

1. Massaro D, Massaro GD. Lung development, lung function and retinoids. *N Engl J Med.* 2010;362:1829-1839.

A Large-Scale, Consortium-Based Genomewide Association Study of Asthma

Moffatt MF, for the GABRIEL Consortium (Imperial College, London, UK; et al)
N Engl J Med 363:1211-1221, 2010

Background.—Susceptibility to asthma is influenced by genes and environment; implicated genes may indicate pathways for therapeutic intervention. Genetic risk factors may be useful in identifying subtypes of asthma and determining whether intermediate phenotypes, such as elevation of the total serum IgE level, are causally linked to disease.

Methods.—We carried out a genomewide association study by genotyping 10,365 persons with physician-diagnosed asthma and 16,110 unaffected persons, all of whom were matched for ancestry. We used random-effects pooled analysis to test for association in the overall study population and in subgroups of subjects with childhood-onset asthma (defined as asthma developing before 16 years of age), later-onset asthma, severe asthma, and occupational asthma.

Results.—We observed associations of genomewide significance between asthma and the following single-nucleotide polymorphisms: rs3771166 on chromosome 2, implicating *IL1RL1/IL18R1* ($P = 3 \times 10^{-9}$); rs9273349 on chromosome 6, implicating *HLA-DQ* ($P = 7 \times 10^{-14}$); rs1342326 on chromosome 9, flanking IL33 ($P = 9 \times 10^{-10}$); rs744910 on chromosome 15 in *SMAD3* ($P = 4 \times 10^{-9}$); and rs2284033 on chromosome 22 in *IL2RB* ($P = 1.1 \times 10^{-8}$). Association with the *ORMDL3/GSDMB* locus on chromosome 17q21 was specific to childhood-onset disease (rs2305480, $P = 6 \times 10^{-23}$). Only *HLA-DR* showed a significant genomewide association with the total serum IgE concentration, and loci strongly associated with IgE levels were not associated with asthma.

Conclusions.—Asthma is genetically heterogeneous. A few common alleles are associated with disease risk at all ages. Implicated genes suggest a role for communication of epithelial damage to the adaptive immune system and activation of airway inflammation. Variants at the *ORMDL3/GSDMB* locus are associated only with childhood-onset disease. Elevation of total serum IgE levels has a minor role in the development of asthma. (Funded by the European Commission and others.)

▶ This report reminds us that not all asthma is the same, thus the importance of trying to find out the implications of our genes on the expression of asthma. Asthma in childhood differs from the asthma that begins in adulthood. Childhood asthma, for example, is more common in boys than in girls and certainly can persist throughout life. It is frequently associated with atopy, although the link between atopic sensitization and asthma symptoms in children is absent in many populations, calling into question the potential role of IgE production in the disease. When it comes to adult-onset asthma, this typically does not begin until at least middle age, is definitely more common in women than in men, is much less likely to be associated with a history of allergy, and often is very resistant to treatment. In adulthood, asthma appears to be occupationally related in many following exposures to dust and chemicals.

To study the potential relationship between one's gene makeup and the expression of asthma, the GABRIEL (a Multidisciplinary Study to Identify the Genetic and Environmental Causes of Asthma) in Europe has conducted genomewide association studies that have identified multiple markers on chromosome 17q21 that are strongly associated with childhood-onset asthma. This report from the GABRIEL Consortium includes information not only on childhood-onset asthma but on later-onset and occupational asthma. More than 10 000 subjects were evaluated with appropriate equal numbers of controls. Studies were undertaken of single nucleotide polymorphisms (SNPs). The study identified likely genes in a pathway that initiates type 2 helper T-cell inflammation response to epithelial damage and points to candidate genes that may act in a pathway that downregulates airway inflammation and remodeling. The studies confirm the strong and specific effect of chromosome 17q on childhood-onset asthma, although the results cannot be used to determine any one individual's risk of asthma. Also observed was an association between SNPs flanking *IL33* on chromosome 9 and atopic asthma. There were suggestive data pointing to 2 other genes that have been associated with Crohn disease. The authors speculate that asthma and Crohn disease may have shared mechanisms, perhaps involving a modulation of microbial interactions with mucosal surfaces. Interestingly, the authors found very little overlap with the principal loci that confer susceptibility to asthma and those that regulate total serum levels of IgE. It is speculated that the elevation of IgE levels seen in many asthmatic patients may be an inconsistent secondary effect of asthma rather than its cause.

Although this report has no specific implications for the direct care of asthmatic patients, the more we learn about our genes and the susceptibility to certain diseases, the closer we are to learning about the pathophysiology of these diseases.

J. A. Stockman III, MD

Smoke-free Legislation and Hospitalizations for Childhood Asthma
Mackay D, Haw S, Ayres JG, et al (Univ of Glasgow, UK; Scottish Collaboration on Public Health Res Policy, Edinburgh, UK; Univ of Birmingham, UK; et al)
N Engl J Med 363:1139-1145, 2010

Background.—Previous studies have shown that after the adoption of comprehensive smoke-free legislation, there is a reduction in respiratory symptoms among workers in bars. However, it is not known whether respiratory disease is also reduced among people who do not have occupational exposure to environmental tobacco smoke. The aim of our study was to determine whether the ban on smoking in public places in Scotland, which was initiated in March 2006, influenced the rate of hospital admissions for childhood asthma.

Methods.—Routine hospital administrative data were used to identify all hospital admissions for asthma in Scotland from January 2000 through October 2009 among children younger than 15 years of age. A negative binomial regression model was fitted, with adjustment for age group, sex, quintile of socioeconomic status, urban or rural residence, month, and year. Tests for interactions were also performed.

Results.—Before the legislation was implemented, admissions for asthma were increasing at a mean rate of 5.2% per year (95% confidence interval [CI], 3.9 to 6.6). After implementation of the legislation, there was a mean reduction in the rate of admissions of 18.2% per year relative to the rate on March 26, 2006 (95% CI, 14.7 to 21.8; P<0.001). The reduction was apparent among both preschool and school-age children. There were no significant interactions between hospital admissions for asthma and age group, sex, urban or rural residence, region, or quintile of socioeconomic status.

Conclusions.—In Scotland, passage of smoke-free legislation in 2006 was associated with a subsequent reduction in the rate of respiratory disease in populations other than those with occupational exposure to environmental tobacco smoke. (Funded by NHS Health Scotland.)

▶ The data from this report are a powerful vindication of any politician who stood up for the rights of nonsmokers and children in signing of local or state bills banning smoking in public places. The information in this report comes from Scotland. In Scotland, the Smoking, Health and Social Care (Scotland) Act banned smoking in all enclosed public places and workplaces as of March 26, 2006. Since then, it has been documented that the legislation has been extraordinarily successful in its primary goal of reducing exposure to environmental tobacco smoke in public places such as bars. There has been in the interim a reduction in respiratory symptoms among workers in bars, for example, and, astoundingly, even among workers who continue to smoke themselves. One of the fears of such legislation was that banning smoking in public places and the workplace might result in increased smoking within the home, currently one of the few havens for smokers. On the contrary, in Scotland, the legislation has resulted in a greater adoption of voluntary bans on smoking in homes and a reduction in the overall exposure of children to environmental tobacco smoke. What has not been looked at, at least until this report appeared, was whether the risk of hospital admission for childhood asthma would in any way be influenced by the introduction of comprehensive smoke-free legislation. This is what the report of Mackay et al is all about.

The study from Scotland examined hospital admissions for asthma for the periods January 1, 2000 (well before the legislation banning smoking was in place), through 2009 (almost 4 years after the smoking legislation was implemented). After adjusting for all reasonable confounding variables, the study showed that after the introduction of comprehensive smoke-free legislation there was a reduction in the incidence of asthma among people who did not have occupational exposure to environmental tobacco smoke. The analysis was limited to data on children, and the reduction in the incidence of asthma was observed among both preschool- and school-aged children. Before the legislation, admissions for asthma were increasing at slightly more than 5% per year, but after implementation of the legislation there was an average reduction in the rate of admissions of just over 18% per year (Fig 1 in the original article).

The data from this report are similar to information provided from Arizona where overall admissions for asthma have also fallen since the implementation of restrictions on smoking in public places, with the greatest reductions observed in counties that had no preexisting partial bans.[1] The information from Scotland shows no evidence of displacement of smoking into the home as a result of smoking bans in public places. Rather the legislation has resulted in an increase in voluntary restrictions in the home. The overall exposure of children to environmental tobacco smoke, measured objectively with the use of salivary cotinine concentrations, has actually fallen since the implementation of the Scottish legislation.

The report from Scotland is not a perfect one. The study included only asthma requiring admission to hospital. There were no available data on less severe exacerbations of asthma that did not require hospitalization. It is possible that some unknown intervention may have occurred during the study period resulting in a reduction in admissions for asthma. The authors did examine whether there were any other interventions that might have produced such a profound decrease in asthma admissions and found none.

The bottom line is that efforts to reduce exposure to secondhand smoke are worth undertaking anytime, anyplace, and in any manner. Such efforts, for whatever reason, will have the epiphenomenon of benefiting children in indirect ways such as was documented in Scotland.

This commentary closes with a few fast curios from the literature regarding smoking:

- A Buddhist monk has become the first person to be arrested under Bhutan's stringent anti-tobacco law. This monk was charged with smuggling 72 packs of chewing tobacco into Bhutan from an Indian-bordered town. Bhutan, with a population of around 700 000, has vowed to become the first tobacco-free country in the world.[2]

- In an effort to cut costs, the government of Cuba announced that it will no longer offer state-subsidized cigarettes for the elderly. Cubans age 55 or older had been allowed to purchase 4 packs a month for about $0.30 total.[3]

- The Japanese government has introduced tax increases of 35% on the price of cigarettes, increasing the price of a pack of a typical domestic brand to almost $5. The proportion of men who smoke has fallen from 54% in 2000 to 37% in 2010. Among women in Japan, it has remained unchanged at around 12%.[4]

- Statistics now show that more than 300 million Chinese people currently smoke (53% of men and 2% of women). More than 60% of adults are exposed to secondhand tobacco smoke in the workplace, yet less than a quarter are aware that exposure to tobacco smoke causes life-threatening illness.[5]

- Last, most are not aware that tobacco smoke contains very tiny amounts of radioactive polonium-210. This isotope in November 2006 killed former KGB operative Alexander Litvinenko, who died in a London hospital after being assassinated with this radioactive substance. In smokers, the polonium-210 builds up to the equivalent radiation dosage of 300 chest X-rays a year for a person who smokes 1½ packs a day...a little-known fact.[6]

J. A. Stockman III, MD

References

1. Herman PM, Walsh ME. Hospital admissions for acute myocardial infarction, angina, stroke and asthma after implementation of Arizona's comprehensive statewide smoking ban. *Am J Public Health*. 2010;101:491-496.
2. Editorial comment. Bhutan tobacco ban. *Lancet*. 2011;377:281.
3. Editorial comment. Policy playback. *Nat Med*. 2010;10:1060.
4. Editorial comment. Japan imposes large tax hike on tobacco. *BMJ*. 2010;341:750.
5. Editorial comment. Smoking in China. *Lancet*. 2010;376:2280.
6. Rego B. Radioactive smoke. *Scientific American*. January 2011:79.

Global burden of acute lower respiratory infections due to respiratory syncytial virus in young children: a systematic review and meta-analysis

Nair H, Nokes DJ, Gessner BD, et al (The Univ of Edinburgh, UK; Kenya Med Res Inst [KEMRI], Kilifi; Agence de Médecine Préventive, Paris, Frane; et al)
Lancet 375:1545-1555, 2010

Background.—The global burden of disease attributable to respiratory syncytial virus (RSV) remains unknown. We aimed to estimate the global incidence of and mortality from episodes of acute lower respiratory infection (ALRI) due to RSV in children younger than 5 years in 2005.

Methods.—We estimated the incidence of RSV-associated ALRI in children younger than 5 years, stratified by age, using data from a systematic review of studies published between January, 1995, and June, 2009, and ten unpublished population-based studies. We estimated possible boundaries for RSV-associated ALRI mortality by combining case fatality ratios with incidence estimates from hospital-based reports from published and unpublished studies and identifying studies with population-based data for RSV seasonality and monthly ALRI mortality.

Findings.—In 2005, an estimated 33·8 (95% CI 19·3—46·2) million new episodes of RSV-associated ALRI occurred worldwide in children younger than 5 years (22% of ALRI episodes), with at least 3·4 (2·8—4·3) million episodes representing severe RSV-associated ALRI necessitating hospital admission. We estimated that 66 000—199 000 children younger than 5 years died from RSV-associated ALRI in 2005, with 99% of these deaths occurring in developing countries. Incidence and mortality can vary substantially from year to year in any one setting.

Interpretation.—Globally, RSV is the most common cause of childhood ALRI and a major cause of admission to hospital as a result of severe ALRI. Mortality data suggest that RSV is an important cause of death in childhood from ALRI, after pneumococcal pneumonia and *Haemophilus influenzae* type b. The development of novel prevention and treatment strategies should be accelerated as a priority.

▶ By now most of us should be more than familiar with Millennium Development Goal 4. The goal is to reduce under-5 mortality by two-thirds by 2015. One of the challenges in meeting this goal is the current prevalence of acute serious lower respiratory tract infections throughout the world. Respiratory syncytial virus (RSV) is 1 of the 3 major leading causes of death from lower respiratory tract infection worldwide. It is also the only agent of the 3 major organisms that causes death from respiratory tract infections—RSV, *Streptococcus pneumoniae*, and *Haemophilus influenzae*—for which no vaccine is available. The current burden of RSV in young children indicates the potential of an effective vaccine. However, information from developing countries—where most of the world's children live—is scarce, making estimation of childhood disease mortality a challenge, at least until the report of Nair et al appeared. These investigators aimed to quantify the burden of RSV (in 2005) by a systematic review of articles published from 1995 through 2009. The investigators examined rates of

RSV-associated lower respiratory tract infections, serious (leading to hospital admission) infections of this type, and deaths in children younger than 5 years. The article itself is important in its use of several analytical approaches and by inclusion of unpublished data from an additional 10 published studies.

Nair et al estimate that in 2005 RSV caused almost 34 million cases of lower respiratory tract infection in children younger than 5 years, accounting for 22% of all infections of this type and 3% to 9% of deaths in this age group. The data also seem to indicate that the global burden of RSV is increasing. The burden is especially great in developing countries where the birth rates are highest. A 43% increase in the world's population has been noted since the 1980s. The RSV mortality throughout the world is difficult to estimate but according to the Nair et al report it might be running as high as 155 000 deaths per year. The data from the Millennium study and others seem to indicate that the RSV organism is the foremost cause of lower respiratory tract infections in children worldwide. The current increase in predominance of the burden of RSV in nations with limited resources gives us information about where strategies to focus the control of this virus are best emphasized. To read more about RSV infection worldwide, see the excellent commentary by Caroline Brese Hall on this topic.[1] Dr Hall reminds us of a quotation from Charles Dickens: "There should be nothing so preventable...as the death of a little child."[2]

This commentary closes with an unrelated observation that echinacea is not a good treatment for the common cold. Barrett et al studied 719 patients aged 12 to 80 years with a new onset cold in a blinded, open-label study using echinacea pills versus placebo.[3] Illness duration and severity were not statistically significant with echinacea compared with placebo and the results clearly do not support the ability of the dose of echinacea used to substantively change the course of the common cold. It looks like we are back to vitamin C and zinc lozenges.

J. A. Stockman III, MD

References

1. Hall CB. Respiratory syncytial virus in young children. *Lancet.* 2010;375: 1500-1502.
2. Dickens C. *One Other Hospital for Children.* London, UK: Bradbury and Evans; 1858:379-380.
3. Barrett B, Brown R, Rakel D, et al. Echinacea for treating a common cold: a randomized trial. *Ann Intern Med.* 2010;153:769-777.

Steroids and bronchodilators for acute bronchiolitis in the first two years of life: systematic review and meta-analysis

Hartling L, Fernandes RM, Bialy L, et al (Univ of Alberta, Edmonton, Canada; Inst of Molecular Medicine, Lisbon, Portugal; et al)
BMJ 342:d1714, 2011

Objective.—To evaluate and compare the efficacy and safety of bronchodilators and steroids, alone or combined, for the acute management of bronchiolitis in children aged less than 2 years.

Design.—Systematic review and meta-analysis.

Data Sources.—Medline, Embase, Central, Scopus, PubMed, LILACS, IranMedEx, conference proceedings, and trial registers.

Inclusion Criteria.—Randomised controlled trials of children aged 24 months or less with a first episode of bronchiolitis with wheezing comparing any bronchodilator or steroid, alone or combined, with placebo or another intervention (other bronchodilator, other steroid, standard care).

Review Methods.—Two reviewers assessed studies for inclusion and risk of bias and extracted data. Primary outcomes were selected by clinicians a priori based on clinical relevance: rate of admission for outpatients (day 1 and up to day 7) and length of stay for inpatients. Direct meta-analyses were carried out using random effects models. A mixed treatment comparison using a Bayesian network model was used to compare all interventions simultaneously.

Results.—48 trials (4897 patients, 13 comparisons) were included. Risk of bias was low in 17% (n=8), unclear in 52% (n=25), and high in 31% (n=15). Only adrenaline (epinephrine) reduced admissions on day 1 (compared with placebo: pooled risk ratio 0.67, 95% confidence interval 0.50 to 0.89; number needed to treat 15, 95% confidence interval 10 to 45 for a baseline risk of 20%; 920 patients). Unadjusted results from a single large trial with low risk of bias showed that combined dexamethasone and adrenaline reduced admissions on day 7 (risk ratio 0.65, 0.44 to 0.95; number needed to treat 11, 7 to 76 for a baseline risk of 26%; 400 patients). A mixed treatment comparison supported adrenaline alone or combined with steroids as the preferred treatments for outpatients (probability of being the best treatment based on admissions at day 1 were 45% and 39%, respectively). The incidence of reported harms did not differ. None of the interventions examined showed clear efficacy for length of stay among inpatients.

Conclusions.—Evidence shows the effectiveness and superiority of adrenaline for outcomes of most clinical relevance among outpatients with acute bronchiolitis, and evidence from a single precise trial for combined adrenaline and dexamethasone.

▶ In a brief commentary that accompanied this report, it was noted that doctors of patients often need to consider a wide range of treatments with different outcomes and that searching for robust evidence of which one is best will often yield only a single meta-analysis of treatment A versus treatment B versus placebo, which may not do much to guide decision making in the real world.[1] Hartling et al use a complex method to combine several systematic reviews on the same condition to analyze outcome data for all relevant treatment comparisons. Specifically, they look at meta-analyses of bronchodilators and steroids, alone or combined, in the acute management of bronchiolitis in patients aged 24 months or younger.

Hartling et al document that evidence shows a benefit of a bronchodilator and steroids for reducing admission rates for youngsters presenting with bronchiolitis. Unless further information comes in the not so distant future, this meta-analysis will stand as the holy grail of those who believe that bronchodilators and steroids do alter the course of acute bronchiolitis in infants and toddlers. Please note that high-risk infants have been generally excluded from studies looking at the effectiveness of bronchodilators and steroids, and thus, there is no available evidence to guide the outpatient or inpatient management of those at greatest risk of morbidity and mortality. To read more about the management of acute bronchiolitis, see the editorial by Ducharme.[2]

J. A. Stockman III, MD

References

1. Editorial comment. Steroids and bronchodilators for acute bronchiolitis in babies and toddlers. *BMJ.* 2011;342:807.
2. Ducharme FM. Management of acute bronchiolitis: inhaled adrenaline shows promise in outpatients, but treatment for inpatients remains unclear. *BMJ.* 2011; 342:773-774.

Lack of Predictive Value of Tachypnea in the Diagnosis of Pneumonia in Children

Shah S, Bachur R, Kim D, et al (Boston Univ School of Medicine, MA; Children's Hosp Boston, MA)
Pediatr Infect Dis J 29:406-409, 2010

Background.—The World Health Organization (WHO) recommends the use of tachypnea as a proxy to the diagnosis of pneumonia in resource poor settings.

Objective.—To assess the relation between tachypnea and radiographic pneumonia among children evaluated in a pediatric emergency department (ED).

Methods.—Prospective study of children less than 5 years of age undergoing chest radiography (CXR) for possible pneumonia was conducted in an academic pediatric ED. Tachypnea was defined using 3 different measurements: (1) mean triage respiratory rate (RR) by age group, (2) age-defined tachypnea based on WHO guidelines (<2 months [RR ≥60/min], 2 to 12 months [RR ≥50], 1 to 5 years [RR ≥40]), and (3) physician-assessed tachypnea based on clinical impression assessed before CXR. The presence of pneumonia on CXR was determined by an attending radiologist.

Results.—A total of 1622 patients were studied, of whom, 235 (14.5%) had radiographic pneumonia. Mean triage RR among children with pneumonia (RR = 39/min) did not differ from children without pneumonia (RR = 38/min). Twenty percent of children with tachypnea as defined by WHO age-specific cut-points had pneumonia, compared with 12% of children without tachypnea ($P < 0.001$). Seventeen percent of children who were assessed to be tachypneic by the treating physician had pneumonia, compared with 13% of children without tachypnea ($P = 0.07$).

Conclusion.—Among an ED population of children who have a CXR performed to assess for pneumonia, RR alone, and subjective clinical impression of tachypnea did not discriminate children with and without radiographic pneumonia. However, children with tachypnea as defined by WHO RR thresholds were more likely to have pneumonia than children without tachypnea.

▶ Going back to the days of Sir William Osler, a rapid respiratory rate has been held as one of the hallmarks of the possible diagnosis of pneumonia. The World Health Organization has provided a protocol that is helpful in the diagnosis of pneumonia. The entry criterion for the algorithm used with this protocol is the presence of either cough or difficulty in breathing. If a child presents with either of these symptoms, the World Health Organization protocol suggests that the child be assessed for pneumonia. The subsequent identification of pneumonia is based on the child's age and respiratory rate.[1] The rationale for developing such a protocol is fairly simple. Such protocols are believed to detect more than 80% of children in the developing world who would require antibiotic treatment for bacterial pneumonia. The difficulty is, however, that although tachypnea has been previously used to identify children at risk for pneumonia, the actual value of tachypnea in the diagnosis of pneumonia is not based on any firm body of literature. Thus the importance of this study by Shah et al.

Shah et al conducted a prospective study of more than 1600 children younger than 5 years of age who had chest X-rays taken for the suspicion of pneumonia. Respiratory rates were measured using age-defined definitions for tachypnea (less than 2 months of age: respiratory rate ≥60/mn; 2-12 months: respiratory rate ≥50; 1-5 years: respiratory rate ≥40). The data from this report show that 20% of children with tachypnea as defined by the World Health Organization age-specific cutoffs had pneumonia, compared with 12% of children without tachypnea. The bottom line is that respiratory rate alone does not discriminate children with and without radiographic evidence of pneumonia. Tachypnea therefore is not a sensitive indicator of pneumonia, but it does increase the likelihood of having radiographic findings consistent with pneumonia.

So how can a care provider determine whether a child presenting with a fever has a serious bacterial infection like pneumonia? Craig et al have developed a computerized diagnostic model that provides an estimate of the risk of serious bacterial infection in children with febrile illnesses.[2]

J. A. Stockman III, MD

References

1. Mulhollend EK, Simoes EA, Costales MO, McGrath EJ, Manalac EM, Gove S. Standardized diagnosis of pneumonia in developing countries. *Pediatr Infect Dis J.* 1992;11:77-81.
2. Craig JC, Williams GJ, Jones M, et al. The accuracy of clinical and symptoms signs for the diagnosis of serious bacterial infection in young febrile children: prospective cohort study of 15 781 febrile illnesses. *BMJ.* 2010;340:c1594.

Ambulatory Visit Rates and Antibiotic Prescribing for Children With Pneumonia, 1994–2007

Kronman MP, Hersh AL, Feng R, et al (The Children's Hosp of Philadelphia, PA; Univ of California, San Francisco; Univ of Pennsylvania School of Medicine, Philadelphia)

Pediatrics 127:411-418, 2011

Background.—The incidence of pediatric hospitalizations for community-acquired pneumonia (CAP) has declined after the widespread use of the heptavalent pneumococcal conjugate vaccine. The national incidence of outpatient visits for CAP, however, is not well established. Although no pediatric CAP treatment guidelines are available, current data support narrow-spectrum antibiotics as the first-line treatment for most patients with CAP.

Objective.—To estimate the incidence rates of outpatient CAP, examine time trends in antibiotics prescribed for CAP, and determine factors associated with broad-spectrum antibiotic prescribing for CAP.

Patients and Methods.—The National Ambulatory and National Hospital Ambulatory Medical Care Surveys (1994–2007) were used to identify children aged 1 to 18 years with CAP using a validated algorithm. We determined age group–specific rates of outpatient CAP and examined trends in antibiotic prescribing for CAP. Data from 2006–2007 were used to study factors associated with broad-spectrum antibiotic prescribing.

Results.—Overall, annual CAP visit rates ranged from 16.9 to 22.4 per 1000 population, with the highest rates occurring in children aged 1 to 5 years (range: 32.3–49.6 per 1000). Ambulatory CAP visit rates did not change between 1994 and 2007. Antibiotics commonly prescribed for CAP included macrolides (34% of patients overall), cephalosporins (22% overall), and penicillins (14% overall). Cephalosporin use increased significantly between 2000 and 2007 ($P = .002$). Increasing age, a visit to a nonemergency department office, and obtaining a radiograph or complete blood count were associated with broad-spectrum antibiotic prescribing.

Conclusions.—The incidence of pediatric ambulatory CAP visits has not changed significantly between 1994 and 2007, despite the introduction of heptavalent pneumococcal conjugate vaccine in 2000. Broad-spectrum antibiotics, particularly macrolides, were frequently prescribed despite evidence that they provide little benefit over penicillins.

▶ It is nice to see an article on an old-fashioned disease such as pneumonia. This report interestingly observed that despite the introduction of the pneumococcal vaccine more than 10 years ago, there has been no decline in the overall incidence of ambulatory visits for community-acquired pneumonia, but the incidence of pediatric hospitalizations for community-acquired pneumonia has in fact declined significantly. When I was growing up quite a few decades ago, our family doctor would assign a diagnosis of walking pneumonia to anyone diagnosed with pneumonia who did not require hospitalization. If he heard bilateral rales, the term double pneumonia was applied.

The diagnosis of pneumonia in the pediatric population can be a challenge for clinicians. Obviously an x-ray provides the definitive diagnosis, but indications for a chest x-ray vary. For patients who exhibit signs of respiratory distress or who have lower respiratory signs, the decision to obtain a radiograph is somewhat straightforward. However, many children have a chest x-ray obtained as part of their evaluation of a febrile illness. Many of the latter have fever and cough but no specific findings of pneumonia by examination. Recently, Shah et al[1] examined the question of whether there is any role for a chest x-ray in a child with a high fever and cough. These investigators enrolled almost 2000 patients into a prospective observational study of children undergoing a chest x-ray for possible pneumonia. Of 1866 patients enrolled, 308 had no physical findings of respiratory distress or lower respiratory tract findings but had a chest x-ray obtained to determine whether an occult pneumonia was present. Statistically, 1 in 15 patients presenting with a fever and cough in such circumstances had radiographic evidence of pneumonia. Not a single child with fever for less than 1 day and without any cough or without worsening cough had radiographic evidence of pneumonia. The authors concluded that obtaining a chest x-ray for the detection of occult pneumonia in children without cough and fever for less than 1 day in duration should be discouraged.

To read more about national hospitalization trends for pediatric pneumonia and related complications, see the report of Lee et al.[2] While the rates of community-acquired hospitalization for pneumonia have declined as a result of the introduction of the pneumococcal vaccine, rates of local complications are increasing in all pediatric age groups. This is particularly true of empyema, which accounts for more than 97% of all local complications. The highest rates of complications appear to be occurring among preschool-aged children. It is unclear whether trend can be attributed to changing epidemiological features of pneumonia that have occurred after the introduction of the pneumococcal vaccine. Rates of local complications may also be influenced by the increasing prevalence of community-acquired methicillin-resistant *Staphylococcus aureus*, which has become the pathogen most commonly associated with empyema in recent years.

J. A. Stockman III, MD

References

1. Shah S, Mathews B, Neuman MI, Bachur R. Detection of occult pneumonia in a pediatric emergency department. *Pediatr Emerg Care*. 2010;26:615-621.
2. Lee GE, Lorch SA, Sheffler-Collins S, Kronman MP, Shah SS. National hospitalization trends for pediatric pneumonia and associated complications. *Pediatrics*. 2010;126:204-213.

Does sweat volume influence the sweat test result?

Goldberg S, Schwartz S, Francis M, et al (Hebrew Univ Med School, Jerusalem, Israel)
Arch Dis Child 95:377-381, 2010

Objective.—Low volume sweat samples are considered unreliable for the diagnosis of cystic fibrosis, based on the assertion that sweat conductivity and chloride are reduced at lower sweating rates. We aimed to re-evaluate the relationship between sweat volume and test results.

Design.—We reviewed all sweat tests performed in our institution to assess the relationship between sweat volume and conductivity, and between sweat volume and sweat chloride. We also compared results between pairs of sweat tests taken simultaneously from a single patient, one with sweat volume below and the other above the currently accepted minimum volume (15 μl).

Results.—A weak inverse relationship between sweat volume and sweat conductivity was found (n=1500, R^2=0.105, p<0.001). There was no correlation between sweat volume and sweat chloride (n=463, R^2=0.002, p>0.05). In discordant pairs (one below and one exceeding the accepted minimum volume), the mean test result in the low volume sample was slightly higher than its counterpart. In 76 such pairs, mean conductivity was 41.1 ± 14.6 mmol/l in the lower volume sample, compared with 36.8 ± 16.0 mmol/l in the higher volume sample (p<0.001). Similarly, in 33 of the pairs, mean sweat chloride was 28.4 ± 15.7 mmol/l in the lower volume sample compared with 25.1 ± 15.2 mmol/l in the higher volume sample (p=0.004).

Conclusion.—A normal sweat conductivity and/or chloride value from a sweat volume <15 μl in a patient whose clinical symptoms are not very suggestive of cystic fibrosis, renders this diagnosis unlikely. In contrast, elevated sweat chloride or conductivity measured from a sample whose volume is <15 μl may represent an artefact related to the low volume.

▶ Quantitative sweat chloride testing is the only method of sweat testing approved for the diagnosis of cystic fibrosis across many centers. For individuals older than 6 months, sweat chloride concentration greater than 60 mmol/L is consistent with cystic fibrosis with values between 40 mmol/L and 60 mmol/L being borderline and values of less than 40 mmol/L being considered normal. Early studies noted an association between low sweating rate and decreased sweat electrolyte concentration, and since these early reports, it has been recommended that a normal sweat test result obtained from a low volume of sweat should not be accepted, as it may be falsely negative. The minimum accepted sweat volume is related to the collecting system used. For many of these systems, a minimum sweat volume required for accurate sampling is 15 μl of sweat collected in 30 minutes. In such circumstances, if the sweat volume is less than 15 μl, repeat testing is recommended or expensive investigations such as genetic testing are then used.

In the report of Goldberg et al, the question "Does sweat volume really influence the sweat test result?" is addressed. The authors of this report had the opportunity to study this since in their institution in Israel, 2 simultaneous sweat tests are routinely performed on every patient (1 in each forearm). The investigators therefore had an ideal database with which to reevaluate the effect of low-sweat volume on test results. They could examine discordant sample volumes—one of 15 μl or more and the other of less than 15 μl in the same patient. The investigators found no significant relationship between sweat volume and chloride concentration. There was a negative correlation between sweat volume and conductivity, but this was statistically a very weak relationship.

Needless to say, the results of this study are in striking contrast to several studies that have reported lower sweat chloride results with insufficient volume samples. If confirmed by further studies, the authors of this report state that their findings have important ramifications. Current recommendations advise against accepting the results of a low-volume sweat test and suggest repeat testing in such instances. This policy is widely accepted and the vast majority of sweat chloride laboratories in the United States do not report the results of low-volume sweat samples. The authors of this report suggest that such a policy has 2 important implications. First, a delay in diagnosis may generate parent and/or patient anxiety. Repeat sweat testing incurs additional health care cost. The Israeli data do in fact suggest that accepting the test result of a low-volume sample will not cause the diagnosis of cystic fibrosis to be missed. One can suspect that further studies including clinical correlates and a larger group of patients with cystic fibrosis will be needed before new recommendations would be accepted based on data from the study in Israel. That having been said, the authors of this report suggest that when only a single low-volume sweat sample is available, the decision to repeat the test should depend on the results. Obviously every abnormal test will need to be repeated. If the result is within the normal range and the patient has a high index of clinical suspicion for cystic fibrosis, repeated testing is also warranted. However, when the index of suspicion is low, it is very likely that repeated testing will only confirm that the patient is not affected by cystic fibrosis. Despite this statement, the authors still conclude that further studies are warranted.

J. A. Stockman III, MD

Effect of Azithromycin on Pulmonary Function in Patients With Cystic Fibrosis Uninfected With *Pseudomonas aeruginosa*: A Randomized Controlled Trial

Saiman L, for the AZ0004 Azithromycin Study Group (Columbia Univ, NY; et al)

JAMA 303:1707-1715, 2010

Context.—Azithromycin is recommended as therapy for cystic fibrosis (CF) patients with chronic *Pseudomonas aeruginosa* infection, but there has not been sufficient evidence to support the benefit of azithromycin in other patients with CF.

Objective.—To determine if azithromycin treatment improves lung function and reduces pulmonary exacerbations in pediatric CF patients uninfected with *P aeruginosa*.

Design, Setting, and Participants.—A multicenter, randomized, double-blind placebo-controlled trial was conducted from February 2007 to July 2009 at 40 CF care centers in the United States and Canada. Of the 324 participants screened, 260 were randomized and received study drug. Eligibility criteria included age of 6 to 18 years, a forced expiratory volume in the first second of expiration (FEV_1) of at least 50% predicted, and negative respiratory tract cultures for *P aeruginosa* for at least 1 year. Randomization was stratified by age of 6 to 12 years vs 13 to 18 years and by CF center.

Intervention.—The active group (n=131) received 250 mg (weight 18-35.9 kg) or 500 mg (weight ≥36 kg) of azithromycin 3 days per week (Monday, Wednesday, and Friday) for 168 days. The placebo group (n=129) received identically packaged placebo tablets on the same schedule.

Main Outcome Measures.—The primary outcome was change in FEV_1. Exploratory outcomes included additional pulmonary function end points, pulmonary exacerbations, changes in weight and height, new use of antibiotics, and hospitalizations. Changes in microbiology and adverse events were monitored.

Results.—The mean (SD) age of participants was 10.7 (3.17) years. The mean (SD) FEV_1 at baseline and 168 days were 2.13 (0.85) L and 2.22 (0.86) L for the azithromycin group and 2.12 (0.85) L and 2.20 (0.88) L for the placebo group. The difference in the change in FEV_1 between the azithromycin and placebo groups was 0.02 L (95% confidence interval [CI], −0.05 to 0.08; P=.61). None of the exploratory pulmonary function end points were statistically significant. Pulmonary exacerbations occurred in 21% of the azithromycin group and 39% of the placebo group. Participants in the azithromycin group had a 50% reduction in exacerbations (95% CI, 31%-79%) and an increase in body weight of 0.58 kg (95% CI, 0.14-1.02) compared with placebo participants. There were no significant differences between groups in height, use of intravenous or inhaled antibiotics, or hospitalizations. Participants in the azithromycin group had no increased risk of adverse events, but had less cough (−23% treatment difference; 95% CI, −33% to −11%) and less productive cough (−11% treatment difference; 95% CI, −19% to −3%) compared with placebo participants.

Conclusion.—In children and adolescents with CF uninfected with *P aeruginosa*, treatment with azithromycin for 24 weeks did not result in improved pulmonary function.

Trial Registration.—clinicaltrials.gov Identifier: NCT00431964.

▶ For reasons that are not entirely clear, there is fairly good evidence that azithromycin (an antibiotic with both antimicrobial and anti-inflammatory properties) can be of benefit to children and adults with cystic fibrosis. Four separate randomized placebo-controlled trials have been conducted in adults and children with cystic fibrosis, most of whom had chronic infection with *Pseudomonas aeruginosa*. All 4 studies demonstrated that azithromycin is associated with reduced pulmonary exacerbations, increased weight gain, or both, as well as improved lung function. Based on these studies, most cystic fibrosis centers now recommend azithromycin as an ongoing chronic therapy for patients with cystic fibrosis who are infected with *P aeruginosa*. However, an outstanding question is whether azithromycin would be of any benefit to patients with cystic fibrosis who are uninfected with *P aeruginosa*. To address this question, the AZ0004 Azithromycin Study Group designed a multicenter, randomized, double-blind, placebo-controlled trial at 40 cystic fibrosis centers in the United States and Canada, in which patients either received or did not receive daily azithromycin. None of these patients had been positive for *P aeruginosa* for at least 1 year at the time of entry into the study. The conclusion from this study is very straightforward. In children and adolescents with cystic fibrosis who are not infected with *P aeruginosa*, giving azithromycin daily for 24 weeks did not result in any improvement in pulmonary function.

Although the patients in this study did not in any way appear harmed by the administration of azithromycin, given the lack of clinical efficacy, it seems clear that at least as of now, there is no value in administering this macrolide to patients with cystic fibrosis who are not infected with *P aeruginosa*. Interestingly, a few patients treated with this agent did have fewer than expected pulmonary exacerbations and a significant increase in weight gain. The authors of this report suggest that further studies of azithromycin are warranted to further investigate its potential use in this smaller population of patients.

J. A. Stockman III, MD

Infection With Transmissible Strains of *Pseudomonas aeruginosa* and Clinical Outcomes in Adults With Cystic Fibrosis

Aaron SD, Vandemheen KL, Ramotar K, et al (Univ of Ottawa, Ontario, Canada; et al)
JAMA 304:2145-2153, 2010

Context.—Studies from Australia and the United Kingdom have shown that some patients with cystic fibrosis are infected with common transmissible strains of *Pseudomonas aeruginosa*.

Objectives.—To determine the prevalence and incidence of infection with transmissible strains of *P aeruginosa* and whether presence of the organism was associated with adverse clinical outcomes in Canada.

Design, Setting, and Participants.—Prospective observational cohort study of adult patients cared for at cystic fibrosis clinics in Ontario, Canada, with enrollment from September 2005 to September 2008. Sputum was collected at baseline, 3 months, and yearly thereafter for 3 years; and retrieved *P aeruginosa* isolates were genotyped. Vital status (death or lung transplant) was assessed for all enrolled patients until December 31, 2009.

Main Outcome Measures.—Incidence and prevalence of *P aeruginosa* isolation, rates of decline in lung function, and time to death or lung transplantation.

Results.—Of the 446 patients with cystic fibrosis studied, 102 were discovered to be infected with 1 of 2 common transmissible strains of *P aeruginosa* at study entry. Sixty-seven patients were infected with strain A (15%), 32 were infected with strain B (7%), and 3 were simultaneously infected with both strains (0.6%). Strain A was found to be genetically identical to the Liverpool epidemic strain but strain B has not been previously described as an epidemic strain. The incidence rate of new infections with these 2 transmissible strains was relatively low (7.0 per 1000 person-years; 95% confidence interval [CI], 1.8-12.2 per 1000 person-years). Compared with patients infected with unique strains of *P aeruginosa*, patients infected with the Liverpool epidemic strain (strain A) and strain B had similar declines in lung function (difference in decline in percent predicted forced expiratory volume in the first second of expiration of 0.64% per year [95% CI, -1.52% to 2.80% per year] and 1.66% per year [95% CI, -1.00% to 4.30%], respectively). However, the 3-year rate of death or lung transplantation was greater in those infected with the Liverpool epidemic strain (18.6%) compared with those infected with unique strains (8.7%) (adjusted hazard ratio, 3.26 [95% CI, 1.41 to 7.54]; $P=.01$).

Conclusions.—A common strain of *P aeruginosa* (Liverpool epidemic strain/strain A) infects patients with cystic fibrosis in Canada and the United Kingdom. Infection with this strain in adult Canadian patients with cystic fibrosis was associated with a greater risk of death or lung transplantation.

▶ It is well known that *Pseudomonas aeruginosa* inhabits the bronchopulmonary tree of the significant majority of patients with cystic fibrosis (CF). In general, infection with *P aeruginosa* is associated with increased morbidity and mortality in those so infected. At the same time, there is a wide variation in the clinical outcomes of those infected with *P aeruginosa*. Some will experience a rapid decline in pulmonary function after infection, whereas others simply harbor the organism for long periods without obvious effects. It has been suspected that this marked difference in prognosis relates to differences among infecting strains of *P aeruginosa*.

P aeruginosa transmissible strains are genetically identical strains that infect unrelated patients with CF. Transmissible strains of *P aeruginosa* have not been described in North American patients with CF, while they have been described in the United Kingdom and Australia. What Aaron et al have done is to perform a multiyear prospective study of all adult patients with CF in the province of Ontario, Canada (adult population: 13 million), to determine whether patients with CF are infected with transmissible strains of *P aeruginosa* and if so, to determine the prevalence of infection and the incidence rates of new infections with these strains. They also looked to see if such strains of *P aeruginosa* were associated with clinically important adverse outcomes.

Data from this report indicate that a sizeable minority of adult Canadian patients with CF are infected with 1 of the 2 common strains of *P aeruginosa*. The most prevalent transmissible strain found was the Liverpool epidemic strain, which was found to infect more than 15% of the Canadian patients. This same strain is known to infect approximately 11% of patients with CF receiving care in clinics in England and Wales. It is currently unknown if infection with the Liverpool epidemic strain or other transmissible strains of *P aeruginosa* is prevalent among US patients with CF, including children with CF. Presumably these strains are being passed human to human. Interestingly, spread of the Liverpool epidemic strain from a patient with CF to a pet cat has been described, suggesting that family pets can also serve as reservoirs for transmissible strains within the community.[1] This is proof positive that cats are nothing but trouble. There are data to suggest that harboring transmissible strains of *P aeruginosa* may add to the morbidity seen in patients with CF. For example, the 3-year rate of death or need for lung transplantation was significantly higher in those with the Liverpool epidemic strain than in those infected with unique *P aeruginosa* strains.

The Liverpool strain of transmissible *P aeruginosa* was first identified in Liverpool, England, in 1996 and obviously is spreading. It is hard to believe that it has not crossed the border from Canada to the United States. When it does, this bad organism can be added to the adverse risk factors for outcome in patients with CF. We need to learn a lot more about its impact in childhood to be sure about its potential for creating problems in the young.

J. A. Stockman III, MD

Reference

1. Mohan K, Fothergill JL, Storra RJ, Ledson MJ, Winstanley C, Walshaw MJ. Transmission of *Pseudomonas aeruginosa* epidemic strain from a patient with cystic fibrosis to a pet cat. *Thorax*. 2008;63:839-840.

Effect of VX-770 in Persons with Cystic Fibrosis and the G551D-*CFTR* Mutation

Accurso FJ, Rowe SM, Clancy JP, et al (Univ of Colorado Denver and Children's Hosp, Aurora; Univ of Alabama at Birmingham; et al)
N Engl J Med 363:1991-2003, 2010

Background.—A new approach in the treatment of cystic fibrosis involves improving the function of mutant cystic fibrosis transmembrane conductance regulator (CFTR). VX-770, a CFTR potentiator, has been shown to increase the activity of wild-type and defective cell-surface CFTR in vitro.

Methods.—We randomly assigned 39 adults with cystic fibrosis and at least one G551D-*CFTR* allele to receive oral VX-770 every 12 hours at a dose of 25, 75, or 150 mg or placebo for 14 days (in part 1 of the study) or VX-770 every 12 hours at a dose of 150 or 250 mg or placebo for 28 days (in part 2 of the study).

Results.—At day 28, in the group of subjects who received 150 mg of VX-770, the median change in the nasal potential difference (in response to the administration of a chloride-free isoproterenol solution) from baseline was -3.5 mV (range, -8.3 to 0.5; $P = 0.02$ for the within-subject comparison, $P = 0.13$ vs. placebo), and the median change in the level of sweat chloride was -59.5 mmol per liter (range, -66.0 to -19.0; $P = 0.008$ within-subject, $P = 0.02$ vs. placebo). The median change from baseline in the percent of predicted forced expiratory volume in 1 second was 8.7% (range, 2.3 to 31.3; $P = 0.008$ for the within-subject comparison, $P = 0.56$ vs. placebo). None of the subjects withdrew from the study. Six severe adverse events occurred in two subjects (diffuse macular rash in one subject and five incidents of elevated blood and urine glucose levels in one subject with diabetes). All severe adverse events resolved without the discontinuation of VX-770.

Conclusions.—This study to evaluate the safety and adverse-event profile of VX-770 showed that VX-770 was associated with within-subject improvements in CFTR and lung function. These findings provide support for further studies of pharmacologic potentiation of CFTR as a means to treat cystic fibrosis. (Funded by Vertex Pharmaceuticals and others; ClinicalTrials.gov number, NCT00457821.)

▶ Most therapies for cystic fibrosis attempt to alleviate the clinical signs and symptoms of the disorder without getting to the specific pathophysiology of the disease. Accurso et al have taken a new approach that involves improving the function of the mutant cystic fibrosis transmembrane conductance regulator (CFTR). They do this using a new drug that appears safe and may very well work in vivo.

With financial support and scientific advice from the Cystic Fibrosis Foundation and contributions from the scientific community, scientists from Vertex Pharmaceuticals initiated high-throughput screening and chemical engineering to develop an orally bioavailable drug that would target CFTR in all organs. The goal was to find an agent that would facilitate the opening of the defective channels regulated by CFTR. The drug they found is known as VX-770. This drug affects CFTR channels increasing chlorine and bicarbonate flow across epithelial membranes. Accurso et al have assessed the effect of VX-770 after 14 and 28 days of treatment on 2 outcomes: CFTR function and disease manifestations. They examined CFTR activity in both nasal epithelial and sweat glands. They showed partial restoration of chloride conductance. Similarly, measurement of the sweat chloride concentration (the elevation of which indicates cystic fibrosis) showed partial restoration of chloride transport in sweat glands. With respect to disease manifestations, these investigators found that VX-770 increased the forced expiratory volume in 1 second. It was surprising that VX-770 would improve pulmonary function so rapidly, but it did. These studies were performed on a variant of CF based on a mutation known as

G551D-CFTR, which is not the most prevalent mutation (the prevalent being delta-F508). As compared with G551D, delta-F508 is the 800-lb gorilla because of its much greater prevalence. In vitro experiments have shown that VX-770 increases the activity of CFTR-delta-F508 channels, provided that these channels reach cell surface. Thus, although the precise mechanism by which VX-770 increases channel activity remains uncertain, this drug might have usefulness in patients with other CF mutations.

There is no question that the research of Accurso et al represents a milestone along the pathway of discovery leading to better preventions, treatments, and cures of cystic fibrosis. While all await definitive gene therapy, tinkering with the basic pathophysiologic defect in cystic fibrosis is a worthy undertaking.

This commentary closes with a clinical curio. Were you aware that wind instrument players are at more risk than other musicians for lung diseases, hypersensitivity pneumonitis in particular? The latter condition decreases lung function, making it impossible to continue playing. Infections are a common cause of this problem. Two cases have been reported of hypersensitivity pneumonitis due to the playing of instruments contaminated by bacteria and molds. The affected musicians had specific serum antibodies against the organisms identified in their instruments. Perhaps a periodic cleaning would obviate this medical problem.[1] Also, note that it is far safer to breathe the exhaust coming from the Series 997 Porsche 911 Turbo than to inhale Los Angeles air that enters the automobile's intact manifold, so efficient is the engineering of the vehicle and so polluted is the city's atmosphere.[2]

J. A. Stockman III, MD

References

1. Editorial comment. Musician-associated hypersensitivity pneumonitis. *BMJ.* 2010; 341:786.
2. J Clarkson personal observation. Top Gear, BBC Television.

19 Therapeutics and Toxicology

The Epidemiology of Prescriptions Abandoned at the Pharmacy

Shrank WH, Choudhry NK, Fischer MA, et al (Brigham and Women's Hosp and Harvard Med School, Boston, MA; Harvard Univ, Cambridge, MA; CVS Caremark, Woonsocket, RI; et al)
Ann Intern Med 153:633-640, 2010

Background.—Picking up prescriptions is an essential but previously unstudied component of adherence for patients who use retail pharmacies. Understanding the epidemiology and correlates of prescription abandonment may have an important effect on health care quality.

Objective.—To evaluate the rates and correlates of prescription abandonment.

Design.—Cross-sectional cohort study.

Setting.—One large retail pharmacy chain and one large pharmacy benefits manager (PBM) in the United States.

Measurements.—Prescriptions bottled at the retail pharmacy chain between 1 July 2008 and 30 September 2008 by patients insured by the PBM were identified. Pharmacy data were used to identify medications that were bottled and either dispensed or returned to stock (RTS) or abandoned. Data from the PBM were used to identify previous or subsequent dispensing at any pharmacy. The first (index) prescription in a class for each patient was assigned to 1 of 3 mutually exclusive outcomes: filled, RTS, or RTS with fill (in the 30 days after abandonment, the patient purchased a prescription for a medication in the same medication class at any pharmacy). Outcome rates were assessed by drug class, and generalized estimating equations were used to assess patient, neighborhood, insurance, and prescription characteristics associated with abandonment.

Results.—10 349 139 index prescriptions were filled by 5 249 380 patients. Overall, 3.27% of index prescriptions were abandoned; 1.77% were RTS and 1.50% were RTS with fill. Patients were least likely to abandon opiate prescriptions. Prescriptions with copayments of $40 to $50 and prescriptions costing more than $50 were 3.40 times and 4.68 times more likely, respectively, to be abandoned than prescriptions with no copayment (*P* < 0.001 for both comparisons). New users of medications had a 2.74 times greater probability of abandonment than prevalent users

545

($P < 0.001$), and prescriptions delivered electronically were 1.64 times more likely to be abandoned than those that were not electronic ($P < 0.001$).

Limitation.—The study included mainly insured patients and analyzed data collected during the summer months only.

Conclusion.—Although prescription abandonment represents a small component of medication nonadherence, the correlates to abandonment highlight important opportunities to intervene and thereby improve medication taking.

▶ This report describes the epidemiology of prescriptions that are never picked up at a pharmacy. While the report largely deals with adults, almost 12% of the prescriptions alluded in this report involved children aged 0 to 17 years and the overall information provided by this report therefore becomes critically important to us who provide pediatric care. Several studies indicate that somewhere between 17% and 20% of patients do not collect new prescriptions from pharmacies.[1] In a study representing more than 80% of retail pharmacy prescriptions in the United States, patients abandoned 5.1% and 6.3% of new prescriptions in 2008 and 2009 respectively.[2]

Shrank et al shed light on this issue of prescription abandonment by examining data from a large retail chain pharmacy. The data indicate that 3.27% of all indexed prescriptions were returned to stock. Patients never collected 1.77% of more than 10 million prescriptions received by the study pharmacies. If there is any good news in this, it is that the low proportions of prescriptions abandoned give some reassurance that the system is working reasonably well. Many health care and manufacturing processes would be very pleased to be operating on a variance of less than 2%. Also reassuring is the finding that almost half of prescriptions initially abandoned are subsequently dispensed within 30 days. This may reflect intervention by a pharmacist or physician, successful implementation of a delayed treatment strategy, deliberate coordination of prescriptions supplied by the patient, or an insurance company finally giving approval for a pharmaceutical.

If there is a downside to the data from this report, it is that millions of prescriptions are having to be reshelved. Shrank et al identified several factors associated with abandoned prescriptions, including high prescription copayments, prescription of brand named drug products, receipt of multiple prescribed medications, the use of a particular prescription type, and electronic delivery of prescriptions to the pharmacy. Prescription copayments and brand name products are strong contributors to patients' out-of-pocket expenses. It should come as no surprise that the higher copayments, the more likely it is that a patient will abandon a prescription. Also not surprising is that brand name drugs, with their typically higher copayments, are more frequently abandoned than generic drugs. Patients with several prescribed medications experience a multiplier effect and bear a greater burden of out-of-pocket expenses. Although federal and industry-sponsored programs have provided some relief, particularly for the elderly and indigent patient, out-of-pocket medical costs have affected individuals at all income levels. Interestingly, Shrank et al have found that electronic prescribing increases the risk for abandonment.

Prescriptions delivered to a pharmacy electronically are 1.64 times more likely than hard copy prescriptions to be abandoned. It is likely that these findings are explained by the lack of paper prescription to remind patients. Also, if a patient is not interested in taking a drug or cannot afford it, they simply do not take a paper prescription to the pharmacy, whereas all electronic prescriptions presumably are properly filled by a pharmacist.

Needless to say, abandoned prescriptions and delays in filling critical medications have important clinical implications. It is hard to say what we can do about the problem. In general, we and pharmacists have no control over copayments. What we can do, however, is to be sure to use the most cost-effective medication possible. All too often, we do not pay enough attention to a patient's or family's out-of-pocket costs. This information is readily available in many pharmacy systems.

While this report suggests that prescription abandonment is a small component of adherence, it does identify several factors associated with abandonment and points the way toward solutions. Unfortunately, this report did not break down whether prescriptions written for children were more likely or less likely to be abandoned. This would be useful information, and the authors should have provided it.

This commentary closes with a historical note discussing the origins of the word *formulary* and *pharmacopoeia*. *Formulary* comes from the word *formula*, defined back in 1706 as "a physician's Prescription or Bill appointing medicines to be prepared by an Apothecary." Older than *formulary* is its exact synonym, *pharmacopoeia*, Greek, literally meaning "drug-making." The term *pharmacopoeia* entered the English language at the start of the 17th century and has stuck with us ever since.[3]

J. A. Stockman III, MD

References

1. Shah NR, Hirsch AG, Zacker C, et al. Predictors of first-fill adherence for patients with hypertension. *Am J Hypertens*. 2009;22:392-396.
2. Pharma Insight 2009. *Patients take More Power Over Prescription Decisions [News Release]*. www.wolterskluwerpharma.com. March 16, 2010. Accessed December 27, 2010.
3. Aronson J. Formularies and pharmacopoeias. *BMJ*. 2011;342:d34.

Malicious Use of Pharmaceuticals in Children
Yin S (Rocky Mountain Poison and Drug Ctr, Denver, CO)
J Pediatr 157:832-836, 2010

Objective.—To describe malicious administration of pharmaceutical agents to children.

Study Design.—We performed a retrospective study of all pharmaceutical exposures involving children <7 years old reported to the US National Poison Data System from 2000 to 2008 for which the reason for exposure was coded as "malicious."

TABLE 2.—Most Commonly Reported Major and Generic Drug Categories

Analgesics	176
Acetaminophen alone	50 (28.4%)
Ibuprofen	30 (17.0%)
Acetaminophen in combination with other drug	16 (9.1%)
Stimulants/street drugs	173
Marijuana	42 (24.3%)
Cocaine	30 (17.3%)
Methamphetamine	27 (15.6%)
Sedatives/hypnotics/antipsychotics	158
Benzodiazepines	62 (39.2%)
Atypical antipsychotics	52 (25.0%)
Other type of sedative/hypnotic/antipsychotic	19 (12.0%)
Cold and cough preparations	155
Acetaminophen and dextromethorphan combinations with decongestant and/or antihistamine without phenylpropanolamine	62 (40%)
Antihistamine and/or decongestant with codeine without phenylpropanolamine	27 (17.4%)
Antihistamine and/or decongestant without phenylpropanolamine and opioid	25 (16.1%)
Unknown drug	155
Ethanol (beverage)	111
Topical preparations	106
Other type of topical antiseptic	24 (22.6%)
Diaper care and rash products	13 (12.3%)
Methyl salicylate	13 (12.3%)
Hydrogen peroxide	11 (10.4%)
Gastrointestinal preparations	89
Laxatives	67 (75.3%)
Other type of gastrointestinal preparation	8 (9.0%)
Antihistamines	85
Diphenhydramine alone	60 (70.6%)
Other antihistamines alone	23 (27.1%)
Antidepressants	75
Selective serotonin reuptake inhibitor	33 (44.0%)
Trazodone	17 (22.7%)
Amitriptyline	12 (16.0%)
Cardiovascular	62
Clonidine	38 (61.3%)
β-blockers	6 (9.7%)
Calcium antagonists	6 (9.7%)

Results.—A total of 1439 cases met inclusion criteria. The mean number of cases per year was 160 (range, 124 to 189) that showed an increase over time. The median (IQR) age was 2 (1.5) years. Outcome data were available for 1244 (86.4%) patients. Of these exposures, 172 resulted in moderate or major outcomes or death. 9.7% of cases involved >1 exposed substance. The most common reported major pharmaceutical categories were analgesics, stimulants/street drugs, sedatives/hypnotics/antipsychotics, cough and cold preparations, and ethanol. In 51% of cases there was an exposure to at least one sedating agent. There were 18 (1.2%) deaths. Of these, 17 (94%) were exposed to sedating agents, including antihistamines (8 cases) and opioids (8 cases).

Conclusions.—Malicious administration of pharmaceuticals should be considered an important form of child abuse (Table 2).

▶ Until this report appeared, most of us were not aware of how common drugs were being maliciously used in children. The author of this report expands the definition of child abuse to include the malicious use of pharmaceuticals. The nontherapeutic use of pharmaceuticals does not cleanly fit into the usual definition of child maltreatment, but it should. There are reports of child homicide using pharmaceuticals. Munchausen by proxy syndrome via poisoning is well described.[1] Sadly, drug-facilitated sexual abuse in children has also been described.[2]

Hypothesizing that the malicious use of pharmaceuticals may in fact be an underrecognized form and/or component of child abuse, Yin studied this potential problem, describing patterns of malicious administration of pharmaceuticals to children as reported to US poison control centers. The study looked at children younger than 7 years reported to the National Poison Data System where the system was notified of malicious drug use in a child. Of approximately 21 million exposures reported to the database during the years 2000 through 2008, 1439 (0.007%) cases met inclusion criteria for malicious drug abuse in childhood. Table 2 lists the most commonly reported major and generic drugs maliciously given to children. On average, 160 cases per year are reported to US poison control centers with a documented 2 deaths per year resulting from malicious use of drugs in children. Chances are quite strong that these numbers severely underrepresent the actual exposures that are occurring. So much so that the author of this report suggests that any child suspected of abuse should be screened for malicious drug exposure.

Why children are exposed to the malicious use of pharmaceuticals remains speculative. Infant crying has been demonstrated to be an important precipitant of the shaken baby syndrome, and one can theorize that a care provider may choose to sedate a crying child to get him/her to stop crying. Also, a physically abused baby is likely to be more irritable, and those inflicting harm may wish to sedate after an inflicted injury. For all we know, kids may be given drugs simply to allow a parent a break. In the study of Dart et al, sedation appeared to be the intent of many nontherapeutic uses of over-the-counter cough and cold medications in children.[3] Other reasons hypothesized for nontherapeutic administration of pharmaceuticals may include homicide, punishment, Munchausen by proxy, or amusement.

It is not common that one sees single-author studies appearing in the literature these days. Our hat is off to Dr Yin for taking on the solo task of informing all of us about the malicious use of pharmaceuticals in children.

This commentary closes with the related observation that professional misconduct can be quite expensive for everyone involved. In 2007, research institutions filed 217 allegations of misconduct to the US Office of Research Integrity. A 2009 survey of scientists found that 2% of respondents admitted to committing scientific misconduct. Researchers at the Roswell Park Cancer Center in Buffalo, New York, had to investigate a senior scientist who was accused of fabricating images and other data in a federal grant application. The investigation itself cost in excess of $525 000 (representative of hours spent on the case by salaried faculty, computer forensic personnel, and IT staff time). To read more about the price of misconduct, see the editorial by Palmer.[4]

J. A. Stockman III, MD

References

1. Meadow R. Munchausen syndrome by proxy. *Arch Dis Child.* 1982;57:92-98.
2. Spiller HA, Rogers J, Sawyer TS. Drug facilitated sexual assault using an over-the-counter ocular solution containing tetrahydrozoline (Visine). *Leg Med (Tokyo).* 2007;9:192-195.
3. Dart RC, Paul IM, Bond GR, et al. Pediatric fatalities associated with over the counter (nonprescription) cough and cold medications. *Ann Emerg Med.* 2009; 53:411-417.
4. Palmer TG. Price of misconduct probes can surpass $500,000. *Nat Med.* 2010;16: 939.

Evaluation of Consistency in Dosing Directions and Measuring Devices for Pediatric Nonprescription Liquid Medications

Yin HS, Wolf MS, Dreyer BP, et al (New York Univ School of Medicine and Bellevue Hosp Ctr; Northwestern Univ, Chicago, IL; et al)
JAMA 304:2595-2602, 2010

Context.—In response to reports of unintentional drug overdoses among children given over-the-counter (OTC) liquid medications, in November 2009 the US Food and Drug Administration (FDA) released new voluntary industry guidelines that recommend greater consistency and clarity in OTC medication dosing directions and their accompanying measuring devices.

Objective.—To determine the prevalence of inconsistent dosing directions and measuring devices among popular pediatric OTC medications at the time the FDA's guidance was released.

Design and Setting.—Descriptive study of 200 top-selling pediatric oral liquid OTC medications during the 52 weeks ending October 30, 2009. Sample represents 99% of the US market of analgesic, cough/cold, allergy, and gastrointestinal OTC oral liquid products with dosing information for children younger than 12 years.

Main Outcome Measures.—Inclusion of measuring device, within-product inconsistency between dosing directions on the bottle's label and dose markings on enclosed measuring device, across-product use of nonstandard units and abbreviations, and presence of abbreviation definitions.

Results.—Measuring devices were packaged with 148 of 200 products (74.0%). Within this subset of 148 products, inconsistencies between the medication's dosing directions and markings on the device were found in 146 cases (98.6%). These included missing markings (n = 36, 24.3%) and superfluous markings (n = 120, 81.1%). Across all products, 11 (5.5%) used atypical units of measurement (eg, drams, cc) for doses listed. Milliliter, teaspoon, and tablespoon units were used for doses in 143 (71.5%), 155 (77.5%), and 37 (18.5%) products, respectively. A nonstandard abbreviation for milliliter (not mL) was used by 97 products. Of the products that included an abbreviation, 163 did not define at least 1 abbreviation.

Conclusion.—At the time the FDA released its new guidance, top-selling pediatric OTC liquid medications contained highly variable and inconsistent dosing directions and measuring devices.

▶ It was in November 2009 that the US Food and Drug Administration (FDA) released new voluntary guidelines to industry groups responsible for manufacturing, marketing, and distributing over-the-counter (OTC) liquid medications, particularly those intended for use by children. These recommendations include the following provisions:

- All OTC liquid drug products should include a measuring device.
- A given product's device and directions should use the same abbreviations and units of measurement.
- Devices should bear only necessary markings and should not hold significantly more than the largest dose described.
- Abbreviations should conform to standards and should be defined.
- Decimals or fractions should be used with care.
- Studies should be done to confirm accurate use by consumers.

These guidelines were put into place largely in response to numerous reports of unintentional overdoses that were attributed, in part, to products with inconsistent or confusing labels and measuring devices.

Yin et al attempted to determine whether the FDA recommendations as outlined were in fact being followed and did so by looking at the top selling 200 pediatric oral liquid OTC medications sold in the United States. These constitute almost all of the US market for allergy, cough/cold, pain, and gastrointestinal OTC oral liquid products that would be used for children. Yin et al observed that more than 25% of these products failed to include a measuring device. Virtually all the products had inconsistencies between the medication dosing directions and the actual markings on measuring devices if they were included. Fig 3 in the original article shows the common patterns that were seen with the medication delivery devices. These delivery devices more often than not had missing markings, superfluous markings, and units of measurements people would not ordinarily be familiar with such as drams and cubic centimeters.

This report is worth reading in some detail. It reminds us that even frequently used terms such as teaspoon and tablespoon may be misinterpreted. Errors in understanding teaspoon versus tablespoon have been found in numerous prior reports as causes of under- or overdosing. This is particularly true when these two words are abbreviated—tsp and tbsp, respectively. It should also be noted that when manufacturers do use these terms, it encourages, however subtly, parents to endorse the use of kitchen spoons, which notoriously are associated with measurement error. The use of decimal points without leading zeros may also lead to unintended overdosing, as can the use of nonrecommended fraction formats. Confusion with decimal points has been found to contribute to 10-fold overdose (eg, administration of 5 mL instead of 0.5 mL).

While the FDA guidelines released in 2009 are a clear step toward the goal of providing clear, consistent, and unambiguous medication information to consumers, the findings from this report document quite high levels of variability and inconsistency with medication labeling and measuring devices. Unfortunately, the FDA's guidelines are purely voluntary, and there is no legal obligation on the part of a pharmaceutical company to follow them. Perhaps enough attention to this issue has been generated by this *JAMA* report that those manufacturers who are not following the recommendations will be humbled or embarrassed into doing so.

As an aside, if you want to update yourself with the controversy surrounding orphan drug pricing, see the excellent discussion of this in a recent issue of the *British Medical Journal*.[1] You will see, for example, that the cost of idursulfase to manage Hunter disease (mucopolysaccharidosis II) now runs well over half a million dollars a year per patient.

J. A. Stockman III, MD

Reference

1. Roos JC, Hyry HI, Cox TM. Orphan drug pricing may warrant a competition law investigation. *BMJ*. 2010;341:c6471.

Adverse Events From Cough and Cold Medications After a Market Withdrawal of Products Labeled for Infants
Shehab N, Schaefer MK, Kegler SR, et al (Ctrs for Disease Control and Prevention, Atlanta, GA)
Pediatrics 126:1100-1107, 2010

Objective.—A voluntary market withdrawal of orally administered, over-the-counter, infant cough and cold medications (CCMs) was announced in October 2007. The goal of this study was to assess CCM-related adverse events (AEs) among children after the withdrawal.

Methods.—Emergency department (ED) visits for CCM-related AEs among children <12 years of age were identified from a nationally representative, stratified, probability sample of 63 US EDs, for the 14 months before and after announcement of withdrawal.

Results.—After withdrawal, the number and proportion of estimated ED visits for CCM-related AEs involving children <2 years of age were less than one-half of those in the prewithdrawal period (1248 visits [13.3%] vs 2790 visits [28.7%]; difference: −15.4% [95% confidence interval [CI]: −25.9% to −5.0%]), whereas the overall number of estimated ED visits for CCM-related AEs for children <12 years of age remained unchanged (9408 visits [95% CI: 6874−11 941 visits] vs 9727 visits [95% CI: 6649−12 805 visits]). During both periods, two-thirds of estimated ED visits involved unsupervised ingestions (ie, children finding and ingesting medications).

Conclusions.—ED visits for CCM-related AEs among children <2 years of age were substantially reduced after withdrawal of over-the-counter infant CCMs. Further reductions likely will require packaging improvements to reduce harm from unsupervised ingestions and continued education about avoiding CCM use for young children. Monitoring of CCM-related harm should continue because recommendations were updated in October 2008 to avoid the use of CCMs for children <4 years of age.

▶ It was on October 11, 2007, that the Consumer Healthcare Products Association announced a voluntary market withdrawal on behalf of the leading makers of over-the-counter cough and cold medications of orally administered cough and cold medications labeled or intended for infants.[1] The Food and Drug Administration got into the act in 2008 also recommending the avoidance of use of these products to treat infants and children younger than 2 years, largely based on the risk of life-threatening side effects.[2] What we see in the report of Shehab et al is the first documentation of changes in the number of emergency department visits related to cough- and cold-related medication adverse events since the announcement of the withdrawal of over-the-counter products for infants.

Since over-the-counter cough and cold products have been removed from pharmacy shelves, the numbers of related adverse effects involving children younger than 2 years have been reduced by more than half. Unfortunately, because of the relatively large numbers of unsupervised ingestions of cough and cold medications among children 2 to 5 years of age, the overall numbers of emergency department visits for related adverse events and the contribution of cough and cold medications to the total medication-related emergency visit burden have remained unchanged for children younger than 12 years. The latter findings point to the need for continued interventions targeted at reducing the potential for harm when children find and ingest medications.

The bottom line here is that there is good news in that parents apparently are not plying their young kids with over-the-counter cough and cold medications. This report did not study whether parents were insisting on alternatives from their care providers, such as antibiotics. This seems unlikely. The big winners in all this are the manufacturers of salt water nose drops.

This commentary closes with the observations that 1 of the innocent bystanders these days in the declining arena of pharmaceutical free lunches to doctors turns out to be local restaurants. Banning drug companies from giving away free lunches to doctors is having a severe impact on local catering businesses, at least in Massachusetts, and many restaurants are crying for the ban to be lifted. One journalist in Massachusetts has lamented that the legislature is seriously considering changing its laws to give companies more influence over doctors just to satisfy local fast food franchises. In Los Angeles, a company called Dr Lunch is devoted entirely to providing free drug company lunches for doctors. The local medics sing its praises.[3] Hopefully the New England Legislature mentioned will come to its senses and realize that there is no such thing as a "free lunch."

J. A. Stockman III, MD

References

1. Consumer Healthcare Products Association. Makers of OTC cough and cold medications announce voluntary withdrawal of oral infant medicines. www. chpa-info.org. Accessed October 11, 2007.
2. US Food and Drug Administration, News and events. FDA releases recommendations regarding use of over-the-counter cough and cold products. Products should not be used in children under two years of age; evaluation continues in older populations. www.fda.gov/newsevents/newsroom/pressannouncements/2008/ucm116839.htm. Accessed December 27, 2010.
3. Editorial comment. Banning free lunches. *BMJ*. 2010;341:c3842.

Vapor Rub, Petrolatum, and No Treatment for Children With Nocturnal Cough and Cold Symptoms

Paul IM, Beiler JS, King TS, et al (Penn State College of Medicine, Hershey, PA)
Pediatrics 126:1092-1099, 2010

Objective.—To determine if a single application of a vapor rub (VR) or petrolatum is superior to no treatment for nocturnal cough, congestion, and sleep difficulty caused by upper respiratory tract infection.

Methods.—Surveys were administered to parents on 2 consecutive days—on the day of presentation when no medication had been given the previous evening, and the next day when VR ointment, petrolatum ointment, or no treatment had been applied to their child's chest and neck before bedtime according to a partially double-blinded randomization scheme.

Results.—There were 138 children aged 2 to 11 years who completed the trial. Within each study group, symptoms were improved on the second night. Between treatment groups, significant differences in improvement were detected for outcomes related to cough, congestion, and sleep difficulty; VR consistently scored the best, and no treatment scored the worst. Pairwise comparisons demonstrated the superiority of VR over no treatment for all outcomes except rhinorrhea and over petrolatum for cough severity, child and parent sleep difficulty, and combined symptom score. Petrolatum was not significantly better than no treatment for any outcome. Irritant adverse effects were more common among VR-treated participants.

Conclusions.—In a comparison of VR, petrolatum, and no treatment, parents rated VR most favorably for symptomatic relief of their child's nocturnal cough, congestion, and sleep difficulty caused by upper respiratory tract infection. Despite mild irritant adverse effects, VR provided symptomatic relief for children and allowed them and their parents to have a more restful night than those in the other study groups.

▶ The authors of this report are doing us a service by working through a number of old-time therapies to either debunk or validate their use. One of their earlier studies is already a classic, one that looked at the effects of dextromethorphan, diphenhydramine, and placebo on nocturnal cough and sleep quality for coughing children and their parents.[1] Similarly, the benefits, or lack thereof, of honey on cold symptoms have also been examined.[2] In this report, the clinical benefits of Vicks VapoRub are assessed. Vicks VapoRub contains camphor (4.8%), menthol (2.6%), and eucalyptus oil in a petrolatum base. It is made by Proctor and Gamble at their facilities in Cincinnati, Ohio.

By way of background, it was in 1994 that the American Academy of Pediatrics Committee on Drugs indicated that because alternatives exist for all indications for camphor therapy, other therapeutic agents that do not contain camphor should be considered, such as dextromethorphan. Subsequently, dextromethorphan was no longer recommended for the management of simple upper respiratory infection in children. Unfortunately, when that recommendation was made, nothing was said about the potential reuse of camphor, menthol, eucalyptus oil, or other common cold remedies. Before the report of Paul et al, there have been no contemporary evidence-based studies to support or refute the efficacy of agents such as Vicks VapoRub with respect to the relief of symptoms of common cold.

What these investigators have done is to design a partially blinded study in which parents were asked to evaluate whether cold symptoms were improved with the use of a dollop of Vicks VapoRub versus a similar-looking control product (petrolatum). The study was blinded partially by the fact that parents were required to place Vicks VapoRub under their noses prior to the application of the medications on their child's upper lip. Examined were variables such as duration of cough, duration of congestion, cough frequency, cough severity, congestion severity, runny nose severity, and the effects on both the child's and parent's ability to sleep. With respect to cough severity and cough frequency, Vicks VapoRub fared significantly better than no treatment but only marginally better than petrolatum alone. The most profound effects in the comparisons were for outcomes related to sleep. As rated by parents, children treated with Vicks VapoRub were significantly more able to sleep than were children randomized to receive petrolatum or no treatment. No significant difference was detected between petrolatum and no treatment. Similarly, parents of children treated with Vicks VapoRub rated their own ability to sleep as significantly better than did parents of children randomized to petrolatum or no treatment. Presumably, parents slept better simply because their children slept better.

Thus, it is that Vicks VapoRub is better than nothing when it comes to relief of nighttime cold symptoms. These benefits have to be weighed against the fact that camphor-containing products are not entirely benign. Toxicities have been reported with the ingestion of camphor as a liquid preparation and camphorated oil. Seizures have been documented with the ingestion of illegally sold camphor.[3] Seizures associated with dermal exposure are generally limited to young infants. Vicks VapoRub use is not recommended for infants. It should be noted that the Food and Drug Administration has approved camphor as an effective antitussive but limits its concentrations in preparations to 11%, far above the amount found in Vicks VapoRub. Data suggest that at a concentration of 4.8%, it would take 20 ml of Vicks VapoRub to produce any toxic effect and 40 ml to potentially cause a death in a child younger than 6 years.[4]

J. A. Stockman III, MD

References

1. Paul IM, Yoder KE, Crowell KR, et al. The effect of dextromethorphan, diphen-hydramine, and placebo on nocturnal cough and sleep quality for coughing children and their parents. *Pediatrics.* 2004;114:e85-e90, www.pediatrics.org/cgi/content/full/114/e85.
2. Paul IM, Beiler J, McMonagle A, Shaffer ML, Duda L, Berlin CM Jr. The effect of honey, dextromethorphan, and no treatment on nocturnal cough and sleep quality for coughing children and their parents. *Arch Pediatr Adolesc Med.* 2007;161:1140-1146.
3. Khine H, Weiss D, Graber N, Hoffman RS, Esteban-Cruciani N, Avner JR. A cluster of children with seizures caused by camphor poisoning. *Pediatrics.* 2009;123:1269-1272.
4. Love JN, Sammon M, Smereck J. Are one or two dangerous? Camphor exposure in toddlers. *J Emerg Med.* 2004;27:49-54.

Two Unusual Pediatric Cases of Dilutional Hyponatremia
Boetzkes S, Van Hoeck K, Verbrugghe W, et al (Univ of Antwerp, Belgium)
Pediatr Emerg Care 26:503-505, 2010

Dilutional hyponatremia, although not uncommon, is an underestimated problem in the pediatric population. In most cases, it results from excessive hydration or water retention, also described as the so-called water intoxication.

One of the most known causes is the use of desmopressin in enuretic children. This drug enhances the free water reabsorption in the renal collecting ducts. The addition of the anticholinergic agent oxybutynin aggravated the condition by causing a dry mouth with excessive thirst and water intake in our first case.

Dietary water overconsumption, either voluntary or involuntary, is a phenomenon seen in formula-fed babies. But in our second case, a game involving forced ingestion of large amounts of water had serious consequences including hyponatremia-related coma. An effort should therefore be made to inform caretakers about the risks of these games.

These cases, provoked by rather unusual and peculiar causes, illustrate again that electrolytes and especially serum [Na$^+$] are key points to be determined in a child with diminished consciousness. Moreover, an accurate history including the intake of medication and dietary information should be made.

▶ It is not often that I see a summary of an article presenting just 2 cases. The 2 cases reported by these investigators from Belgium, however, are quite illustrative, and the discussion associated with the cases provides us with a very detailed and up-to-date review of the topic of hyponatremia. Hyponatremia is a disorder that every pediatrician should be familiar with.

The first case reported was that of a 10-year-old girl who was being treated for enuresis with desmopressin nasal spray. Desmopressin is well known to be associated with hyponatremia, but in the case of the 10-year-old, she had been taking desmopressin for the previous 2 years with no difficulty whatsoever. This youngster did, however, eventually develop headache with continuous vomiting and anorexia, followed by deterioration of consciousness and generalized convulsions. Her serum sodium was found to be 118 mmol/L. With the taking of a careful history, it appeared that 5 days before the onset of these symptoms, the management of this youngster's enuresis was modified to include the use of the anticholinergic drug oxybutynin (Ditropan), given at a low dose of 5 mg/d in addition to a continuation of her nasal spray desmopressin. In retrospect, it appears that the dry mouth associated with the use of oxybutynin most likely caused this youngster to take in a fair amount of water, the combination of desmopressin and this excess water producing the profound hyponatremia. With fluid restriction and some hypertonic saline, the youngster recovered.

The second case was of a 12-year-old boy who presented with headache, nausea, and vomiting. When seen in the emergency room, his consciousness deteriorated, leading to profound lethargy. His serum sodium was found to be 120 mmol/L. Various causes of hyponatremia were not found until a careful history was taken. It appears that the boy had participated in a quiz at a boy scouts' meeting called piss-quiz. In the game, approximately lasting 1 hour, he was forced to drink water every time he answered the questions of the quiz incorrectly. It is estimated that he drank a minimum of 4 liters of tap water within that 1-hour period. Correction of the hyponatremia rapidly occurred with fluid restrictions and some intravenous saline.

Hyponatremia has been described after the intake of several drugs either by releasing antidiuretic hormone (ADH), by potentiating the effect of ADH in the kidneys, or by other mechanisms. Hyponatremia in enuretic children treated with medications such as desmopressin have been well described. Overconsumption of water certainly can cause hyponatremia such as noted in the second case of the 12-year-old boy scout. Overconsumption of water can also occur involuntarily, particularly in infants and small children. In the latter situation, this is usually the result of a formula preparation error. Forced water intake has also been reported in a few cases of child abuse. In psychiatric patients, polydipsia is a well-known cause of water intoxication, especially in schizophrenic and anorectic patients. Some years back, a schizophrenic patient was found water intoxicated, sitting in a tub of hot water into which the patient had placed tea bags. She was found freely drinking of the liquid in the largest teapot yet described.

Needless to say, the trick when it comes to delusional hyponatremia is in its prevention. When it comes to piss-games, a word to the wise would be to not be the dumbest kid in the game (or would that be an oxymoron?).

J. A. Stockman III, MD

HLA-A*3101 and Carbamazepine-Induced Hypersensitivity Reactions in Europeans

McCormack M, Alfirevic A, Bourgeois S, et al (Royal College of Surgeons in Ireland, Dublin, UK; Univ of Liverpool, UK; Wellcome Trust Sanger Inst, Hinxton, UK; et al)

N Engl J Med 364:1134-1143, 2011

Background.—Carbamazepine causes various forms of hypersensitivity reactions, ranging from maculopapular exanthema to severe blistering reactions. The HLA-B*1502 allele has been shown to be strongly correlated with carbamazepine-induced Stevens—Johnson syndrome and toxic epidermal necrolysis (SJS—TEN) in the Han Chinese and other Asian populations but not in European populations.

Methods.—We performed a genomewide association study of samples obtained from 22 subjects with carbamazepine-induced hypersensitivity syndrome, 43 subjects with carbamazepine-induced maculopapular exanthema, and 3987 control subjects, all of European descent. We tested for an association between disease and HLA alleles through proxy single-nucleotide polymorphisms and imputation, confirming associations by high-resolution sequence-based HLA typing. We replicated the associations in samples from 145 subjects with carbamazepine-induced hypersensitivity reactions.

Results.—The HLA-A*3101 allele, which has a prevalence of 2 to 5% in Northern European populations, was significantly associated with the hypersensitivity syndrome ($P = 3.5 \times 10^{-8}$). An independent genomewide association study of samples from subjects with maculopapular exanthema also showed an association with the HLA-A*3101 allele ($P = 1.1 \times 10^{-6}$). Follow-up genotyping confirmed the variant as a risk factor for the hypersensitivity syndrome (odds ratio, 12.41; 95% confidence interval [CI], 1.27 to 121.03), maculopapular exanthema (odds ratio, 8.33; 95% CI, 3.59 to 19.36), and SJS—TEN (odds ratio, 25.93; 95% CI, 4.93 to 116.18).

Conclusions.—The presence of the HLA-A*3101 allele was associated with carbamazepine-induced hypersensitivity reactions among subjects of Northern European ancestry. The presence of the allele increased the risk from 5.0% to 26.0%, whereas its absence reduced the risk from 5.0% to 3.8%.(Funded by the U.K. Department of Health and others.)

▶ Carbamazepine is used a fair amount in the treatment of seizure disorders in children as well as in adults. It is also used to manage bipolar disorder and trigeminal neuralgia. The problem with carbamazepine in some patients is the development of hypersensitivity reactions. These can be mild, moderate, or severe. Among individuals of European ancestry, maculopapular exanthema, the mildest form, occurs in 5% to 10% of treated individuals. More severe reactions certainly can occur and can carry with them serious morbidity and mortality. For example, the hypersensitivity syndrome characterized by rash, fever, eosinophilia, hepatitis, and nephritis has an associated mortality of

10%. Other serious side effects include the Stevens-Johnson syndrome (SJS) and toxic epidermal necrolysis (TEN). Although TEN is the most infrequent of these complications, it carries with it the highest mortality (up to 30%).

In those of Asian ancestry, carbamazepine-induced SJS and TEN are strongly associated with the HLA-B*1502 allele, particularly in Han Chinese populations as well as in persons from Hong Kong, Malaysia, Thailand, and India and in descendents of immigrants from Southeast Asia and areas of the world where the HLA-B*1502 allele is prevalent. Needless to say, there are a number of individuals of Asian origin in the United States with this HLA type. This HLA allele type tends to be very specific for the problem. For example, among persons of Han Chinese descent, carbamazepine-induced SJS-TEN almost never occurs in noncarriers of the HLA-B*1502 allele, a true evidence that this allele is directly involved in the pathogenesis of the condition. This strong association between HLA-B*1502 and carbamazepine-induced SJS-TEN was recently documented again in an important report in the *New England Journal of Medicine*.[1]

What McCormack et al have done is examine individuals of Northern European ancestry to see if there is a significant link with HLA typing. They found that the presence of HLA-A*3101 allele was strongly associated with carbamazepine-induced hypersensitivity reactions in the Northern European ancestry population. The presence of the allele increases the risk of serious dermatologic problems from 5% to 26%. The sensitivity and specificity values estimated for Europeans with HLA-A*3101 are 26% and 96%, respectively. If one accepts a conservative estimate of the prevalence of carbamazepine hypersensitivity at 5%, on the basis of the data from the report by McCormack et al, one can calculate that 83 patients would have to be screened with HLA typing to prevent 1 case of carbamazepine hypersensitivity. The prevalence of carbamazepine-induced hypersensitivity that was determined in the context of the Standard and New Antiepileptic Drugs trial was actually found to be 10%. On the basis of the latter prevalence, the number of persons who would need to be screened to prevent 1 instance of carbamazepine-induced hypersensitivity is just 39. On the basis of these statistics, the authors of this report suggest that consideration be given to adding the association with HLA-A*3101 to the drug label for carbamazepine. Indeed, the Food and Drug Administration already has required labeling of carbamazepine, highlighting the problem with SJS-TEN. It seems reasonable that all those starting on this important drug should be screened for their HLA typing.

J. A. Stockman III, MD

Reference

1. Chen P, Lin JJ, Lu CS, et al. Carbamazepine-induced toxic effects and HLA-B*1502 screening in Taiwan. *N Engl J Med.* 2011;364:1126-1133.

Pain-related behaviors and neurochemical alterations in mice expressing sickle hemoglobin: modulation by cannabinoids

Kohli DR, Li Y, Khasabov SG, et al (Univ of Minnesota, Minneapolis; et al)
Blood 116:456-465, 2010

Sickle cell disease causes severe pain. We examined pain-related behaviors, correlative neurochemical changes, and analgesic effects of morphine and cannabinoids in transgenic mice expressing human sickle hemoglobin (HbS). Paw withdrawal threshold and withdrawal latency (to mechanical and thermal stimuli, respectively) and grip force were lower in homozygous and hemizygous Berkley mice (BERK and hBERK1, respectively) compared with control mice expressing human hemoglobin A (HbA-BERK), indicating deep/musculoskeletal and cutaneous hyperalgesia. Peripheral nerves and blood vessels were structurally altered in BERK and hBERK1 skin, with decreased expression of μ opioid receptor and increased calcitonin gene-related peptide and substance P immunoreactivity. Activators of neuropathic and inflammatory pain (p38 mitogen-activated protein kinase, STAT3, and mitogen-activated protein kinase/extracellular signal-regulated kinase) showed increased phosphorylation, with accompanying increase in COX-2, interleukin-6, and Toll-like receptor 4 in the spinal cord of hBERK1 compared with HbA-BERK. These neurochemical changes in the periphery and spinal cord may contribute to hyperalgesia in mice expressing HbS. In BERK and hBERK1, hyperalgesia was markedly attenuated by morphine and cannabinoid receptor agonist CP 55940. We show that mice expressing HbS exhibit characteristics of pain observed in sickle cell disease patients, and neurochemical changes suggestive of nociceptor and glial activation. Importantly, cannabinoids attenuate pain in mice expressing HbS.

▶ All of us know that sickle cell disease (SCD) goes hand in glove with pain. Vasoocclusion is believed to be the root cause of the pain. Damage to tissue supplied by occluded blood vessels may also be responsible for creating a state of chronic vascular inflammation explaining many features of sickle cell pain. This tissue damage and vascular inflammation is capable of generating a number of inflammatory mediators that initiate an electrical pain impulse transmitted along peripheral nerves to the dorsal horn of the spinal cord. This impulse then ascends along the contralateral spinothalamic tract to the thalamus, which interconnects reversibly with other centers, most notably with the limbic system, a mediator of both emotion and memory. Neurologists will also tell you that the central nervous system (CNS) inhibits the transmission of the painful stimulus at the level of the dorsal horn via a descending pathway, with norepinephrine and serotonin as neurotransmitters. Eventually, the modified electrochemical impulse that started at the site of vasoocclusion is sent to the cerebral cortex where it is ultimately perceived as pain. Needless to say, this final pain perception is somewhat subjective and is the result of a highly complex interplay among enhancing and inhibiting factors within the CNS in addition to a host of coexisting psychosocial and environmental factors.

What Kohli et al have done is to take advantage of a transgenic sickle cell mouse model expressing human sickle hemoglobin to characterize the behavioral, neurochemical, and pharmacologic aspects of sickle cell pain as well as to find alternatives to opioid analgesics to treat pain. The mouse strain expressing the sickle gene is known as the Berkley strain (BERK and hBERH1). These mice were able to undergo alterations at the neurochemical level, peripheral nerve level, and blood vessel level and were able to be analyzed for behavioral responses to their pain. The findings from this report suggest that the characteristics and severity of sickle cell pain depend on the location, extent, and chronicity of the neurochemical damage that ensues after vasoocclusion. Thus, depending on whether the damage is peripheral and/or central, the pain may be limited to musculoskeletal and cutaneous hyperalgesia alone or in combination with inflammatory and neuropathic pain. At the pharmacologic level, the hyperalgesia was able to be attenuated by morphine and cannabinoid agonists. These findings imply that the use of medicinal cannabinoids may play an important role in the management of sickle cell pain similar to the reported role in the management of other types of pain. Used in combination with opioids, cannabinoids may decrease the amount of opioids needed to achieve adequate pain relief.

There was a very interesting additional finding in the report of Kohli et al that may relate to what is seen in humans with SCD. One of the observations in this study provides a welcomed explanation for several of the perplexing observations in patients with SCD. It has been noted that some hospitalized patients with acute painful crises become refractory to treatment with opioids after about 3 or 4 days following admission and continue to have severe pain despite the administration of even higher doses of opioids. With no good explanation for this phenomenon, unfortunately some have attributed this refractoriness to narcotics to maladaptive behavior. It is interesting that the study of Kohli et al observed decreased expression of opioid receptors in the SCD mouse model after several days of administration of narcotics. This is a possible explanation for the observed refractoriness to opioids in some patients who may benefit from the use of medicinal cannabinoids. It is unfortunate that the presumed maladaptive behaviors of patients with SCD have a more plausible explanation such as that proposed by Kohli et al. In these patients, the need for additional opioids is not an addiction to the drug but rather a pseudoaddiction resulting from actual undertreatment of pain. Drug-seeking behavior may very well turn out to be pain relief—seeking behavior resulting from intolerance, hyperalgesia, and refractoriness of certain receptors after a period of exposure to opioids.

If there is any good news in the now just over 100-year struggle to understand SCD, it is that we have an excellent animal model that opens the way to a better understanding of the pathophysiology and treatment of sickle cell pain.

J. A. Stockman III, MD

A Family-based Randomized Controlled Trial of Pain Intervention for Adolescents With Sickle Cell Disease

Barakat LP, Schwartz LA, Salamon KS, et al (The Children's Hosp of Philadelphia, PA)

J Pediatr Hematol Oncol 32:540-547, 2010

The study had 2 aims—to determine the efficacy of a family-based cognitive-behavioral pain management intervention for adolescents with sickle cell disease (SCD) in (1) reducing pain and improving health-related variables and (2) improving psychosocial outcomes. Each adolescent and a family support person were randomly assigned to receive a brief pain intervention (PAIN) (n = 27) or a disease education attention control intervention (DISEASE ED) (n = 26) delivered at home. Assessment of primary pain and health-related variables (health service use, pain coping, pain-related hindrance of goals) and secondary psychosocial outcomes (disease knowledge, disease self-efficacy, and family communication) occurred at baseline (before randomization), postintervention, and 1-year follow-up. Change on outcomes did not differ significantly by group at either time point. When groups were combined in exploratory analyses, there was evidence of small to medium effects of intervention on health-related and psychosocial variables. Efforts to address barriers to participation and improve feasibility of psychosocial interventions for pediatric SCD are critical to advancing development of effective treatments for pain. Sample size was insufficient to adequately test efficacy, and analyses did not support this focused cognitive-behavioral pain management intervention in this sample of adolescents with SCD. Exploratory analyses suggest that comprehensive interventions, that address a broad range of skills related to disease management and adolescent health concerns, may be more effective in supporting teens during health-care transition.

▶ Acute and chronic, unpredictable pain remains the most common presenting complaint of patients with sickle cell disease (SCD), frequently requiring hospitalization and capable of interference with daily activities. For whatever reason, the pain associated with painful crises in subjects with SCD often increases during the period of adolescence. Pain relief with medication is often ineffective, raising the issue of whether behavioral interventions might assist the patient in dealing with this problem. Gil et al, for example, have shown that pain coping skills can be taught effectively. Increased practice of pain coping skills is linked to fewer health care contacts, fewer school absences, and less interference with household activities.[1]

Barakat et al designed a study to evaluate a developmentally and culturally appropriate, family- and community-based, cognitive-behavioral intervention for pain control in subjects with SCD. They examined a well-codified brief pain intervention (PAIN) program as well as a disease education attention control intervention (DISEASE ED) delivered at home. Designed as a family-based intervention, this study ultimately included a wide range of family members in its implementation, reflecting the strength of the African American family and its ability to mobilize on behalf of an adolescent with SCD. Both approaches had some significant level of effectiveness without one being remarkably better than the other.

The report that follows is a fascinating one giving us significant new insights to the complexities of the pathogenesis of sickle cell pain and its management.

J. A. Stockman III, MD

Reference

1. Gil KM, Anthony KK, Carson JW, Redding-Lallinger R, Daeschner CW, Ware RE. Daily coping practice predicts treatment effects in children with sickle cell disease. *J Pediatr Psychol.* 2001;26:163-173.

Glowing in the dark: time of day as a determinant of radiographic imaging in the evaluation of abdominal pain in children

Burr A, Renaud EJ, Manno M, et al (UMass Memorial Med Ctr, Worcester, MA)
J Pediatr Surg 46:188-191, 2011

Background/Purpose.—Although ultrasound is often the preferred pediatric imaging study, many institutions lack ultrasound access at night; and computerized tomography (CT) becomes the only radiological method available for evaluation of appendicitis in children. The purpose of this study was to characterize patterns of daytime and nighttime use of ultrasound or CT for evaluation of pediatric appendicitis and to measure consequent differences in radiation exposure and cost.

Methods.—A retrospective chart review of patients evaluated for appendicitis from October 2004 to October 2009 (N = 535) was performed to evaluate daytime and nighttime use of ultrasound and CT for pediatric patients.

Results.—Average age was 10.2 years (range, 3-17 years). During the day, 6 times as many ultrasounds were performed as CTs (230 vs 35). At night, half as many ultrasounds were performed (50 vs 110). Average radiation dose per child during the day was significantly lower than at night (day, 0.52 mSv per patient; night, 2.75 mSv per patient). Average radiology costs were lower for daytime patients ($2491.06 day vs $4045.00 night; $P < .05$).

Conclusions.—Dependence on CT at night results in higher average radiation exposure and cost. Twenty-four—hour ultrasound availability would decrease radiation exposure and cost of evaluation of children presenting with appendicitis.

▶ Timing is everything in life. This is true whether you are a comedian or a patient being admitted to a hospital with abdominal pain. In the latter incidence, if you pop on the doorstep of a hospital at night, chances are statistically significantly higher that someone will place you into a CT scanner rather than calling a technician to do an ultrasound.

Several interesting things happen during the night in hospitals. Many institutions do not have on-call ultrasound support, and this lack of access increases the use of CT at night. Also, CT is preferred by nonradiology clinicians because of its general availability and uniformity of use, in contrast to pediatric ultrasound, which requires highly specialized training for both performance and interpretation. The report from the University of Massachusetts Memorial Medical Center in Worcester dramatically shows us just what happens if you are a pediatric patient (average age, 10.2 years) presenting with abdominal pain and the need for evaluating the differential diagnosis of appendicitis. During the day at that institution, 6 times as many ultrasounds were performed as CTs for such evaluation. At night, half as many ultrasounds were performed as CTs. The average radiation dose exposure during the day was remarkably lower than at night. The cost of radiology services ran 40% less during the day.

The authors of this report chose a very catchy title for the report: "Glowing in the dark." Needless to say, we do not want children to become fireflies. A recent study showed that, excluding dental x-rays, the average US child undergoes nearly 8 diagnostic imaging procedures by 18 years of age.[1] The latter report is based on a large population-based study examining the use of radiography, CT scans, and other imaging procedures in pediatric populations. Its findings are founded on health insurance records of more than 350 000 children in 5 large US health care markets. Overall, the researchers found that 42.5% of the children had undergone an imaging procedure during the 3-year study period ending in 2007. About a quarter had 2 or more procedures, while 16% had 3 or more. Radiography, which typically has low radiation exposure levels, accounted for nearly 85% of the procedures, but the study cautioned that CT scans, fluoroscopy, and other techniques that deliver higher exposures are not infrequent. Nearly 8% of the children had undergone a CT scan, and the use of the latter dramatically increased in older children.

So what can be done about all this? The well-established principles of radiation protection are justification and optimization. The care provider's role is paramount in justification, and the radiology facility has a major role to optimize the technique used during an examination to produce the minimum possible radiation dose without hampering the diagnostic purpose of the study. An editorial that appeared in the *Lancet* in 2010 suggested that one way to address concerns is to track lifetime radiation exposure (radiation history).[2] The International Atomic Energy Agency suggests that all of us carry a smart card that would include this history.[3]

For more on this topic, read the editorial by Brenner and Hricak.[4]

J. A. Stockman III, MD

References

1. Dorfman AL, Fazel R, Einstein AJ, et al. Use of medical imaging procedures with ionizing radiation in children: a population-based study. *Arch Pediatr Adolesc Med*. 2011;165:458-464.
2. Rehani M, Frush D. Tracking radiation exposure of patients. *Lancet*. 2010;376: 754-755.

3. Rehani M. *Smart Protection. IAEA Bull.* 50, http://www.iaea.org/publications/magazine/bulletin/bull502/50205813137.html; 2009. Accessed February 12, 2010.
4. Brenner DJ, Hricak H. Radiation exposure from medical imaging: time to regulate? *JAMA.* 2010;304:208-209.

Inflammatory Effects of Phthalates in Neonatal Neutrophils

Vetrano AM, Laskin DL, Archer F, et al (Univ of Medicine and Dentistry of New Jersey-Robert Wood Johnson Med School, New Brunswick; Rutgers Univ, Piscataway, NJ; et al)
Pediatr Res 68:134-139, 2010

Hospitalized infants are exposed to numerous devices containing the plasticizer di-(2-ethylhexyl) phthalate. Urinary levels of the phthalate metabolite, mono-(2-ethylhexyl) phthalate (MEHP), are markedly elevated in premature infants. Phthalates inactivate peroxisome proliferator-activated receptor-γ (PPAR-γ), a nuclear transcription factor that mediates the resolution of inflammation, a process impaired in neonates. We speculate that this increases their susceptibility to MEHP, and this was analyzed. MEHP inhibited neutrophil apoptosis; neonatal cells were more sensitive than adult cells. In neonatal, but not in adult neutrophils, MEHP also inhibited chemotaxis, stimulated oxidative metabolism, and up-regulated expression of NADPH oxidase-1. In both adult and neonatal neutrophils, MEHP stimulated IL-1β and VEGF production, whereas IL-8 production was stimulated only in adult cells. In contrast, MEHP-inhibited production of MIP-1β by adult cells, and Regulated on Activation Normal T Cell Expressed and Secreted (RANTES) by neonatal neutrophils. The effects of MEHP on apoptosis and oxidative metabolism in neonatal cells were reversed by the PPAR-γ agonist, troglitazone. Whereas troglitazone had no effect on MEHP-induced alterations in inflammatory protein or chemokine production, constitutive IL-8 and MIP-1β production was reduced in adult neutrophils, and RANTES and MIP-1β in neonatal cells. These findings suggest that neonatal neutrophils are more sensitive to phthalate-mediated inhibition of PPAR-γ, which may be related to decreased anti-inflammatory signaling.

▶ When I was growing up, materials made of plastic had only been around for about 20 years or so. I can still remember the slogan of a well-known chemical company that read: Better Living Through Chemistry. Well, plastic materials, particularly their by-products, do not necessarily make for longevity. One of the potential toxicants released from hydrocarbon-derived plastic products includes phthalates (phthalate esters, bisphenol A, and styrene). Phthalate esters are components of many commercial plastic products and are used largely to increase the flexibility of the materials. Phthalates are ubiquitous. One in particular, bis (2-ethylhexyl) phthalate (DEHP), is widely used as a plasticizer in the manufacturing of articles made of polyvinyl chloride plastics. DEHP is the only plasticizer approved by the US Food and Drug Administration for medical use, and it is this form of plasticizer that one sees in intravenous (IV) bags and IV tubing. DEHP is known to have adverse effects on development and reproduction. Its metabolites have been shown to exhibit proinflammatory activity by upregulating proinflammatory expression in neutrophils. Elevated phthalate levels in pregnancy have been reported to cause placental inflammation increasing the risk of preterm delivery.

Vetrano et al present evidence that phthalates like DEHP have immunological promodulatory effects in neonates. Although there have been scattered reports of immune modulation in response to phthalates, this report is the first establishing mechanisms underlying alterations of neutrophil function in human newborns. In fact, newborns seem to be particularly sensitive to this immunomodulatory effect. Unfortunately, hospitalized newborns are among the most at risk for being exposed to phthalates because virtually all the fluids, nutrients, and gases they are exposed to come through phthalate-containing plastic materials.

DEHP and its by-products are known to cause hormonal disruption and to mediate responses as diverse as embryo lethality in rats and obesity and metabolic disorders and asthma exacerbation in humans. Infants are especially susceptible in part because of the slow excretion of plasticizer by-products. One can theorize that since an increased susceptibility exists of newborns to bronchopulmonary dysplasia and other inflammatory diseases, exposure to proinflammatory agents such as plasticizers will only make such conditions worse. High levels of DEHP have been reported in the gastrointestinal tissues of infants who have succumbed to necrotizing enterocolitis.[1]

It is fair to say based on data from the literature that neonatal neutrophils are more sensitive to exposure to plastic material by-products. The consequences of this exposure can theoretically be very widespread. To learn more about this topic, see the excellent commentary on the article by Vetrano et al by Heck.[2]

Last, be aware that new information is emerging that shows that bisphenol A (BPA) can indeed be more harmful than previously thought. BPA is an industrial chemical used to make polycarbonate plastic resins, epoxy resins, and other products. Because of its attributes, it is found in a wide variety of common products, including digital media (eg, CDs, DVDs), electrical and electronic equipment, automobiles, sports safety equipment, and reusable food and drink containers. Some 2.8 million tons of BPA are produced globally each year. The use of polycarbonate plastic resins for food applications is considered safe by the US Food and Drug Administration. It should be noted, however, that there is a lot of literature these days about exposure to BPA in thermal receipt paper that has a heat-sensitive coating containing BPA that can rub off on cashiers' fingers. A recent study has shown that if you take healthy abdominal skin (removed from women during elective surgical procedures), and apply BPA to the surface of the skin, half of the applied BPA will actually migrate well into the tissue.[3] Currently BPA cannot be seen or smelled so no one knows how to identify receipt paper with the chemical, although some paper manufacturers are considering imbedding tiny red fibers to mark paper that contains BPA. The concern about BPA is that it mimics the hormone estrogen and has been tied to health risks ranging from behavior problems in children to obesity and heart ailments, although the medical implications of this are highly controversial.

J. A. Stockman III, MD

References

1. Hillman LS, Goodwin SL, Sherman WR. Identification and measurement of plasticizer in neonatal tissues after umbilical catheters and blood products. *N Engl J Med.* 1975;292:381-386.
2. Heck DE. It's the plastic!: commentary on the article by Vetrano et al. on page 134. *Pediatr Res.* 2010;68:99.
3. Raloff J. Skin is no barrier to BPA, study shows. Science News. http://www.sciencenews.org/view/generic/id/64972/title/Skin_is_no_barrier_to_BPA,_study_shows. Published December 4, 2010 Accessed July 25.

Hair Mercury Levels of Women of Reproductive Age in Ontario, Canada: Implications to Fetal Safety and Fish Consumption

Schoeman K, Tanaka T, Bend JR, et al (Univ of Western Ontario, London, Canada; The Hosp for Sick Children, Toronto, Ontario, Canada)
J Pediatr 157:127-131, 2010

Objective.—To study hair mercury concentrations among women of reproductive age in relation to fish intake in Ontario, Canada.

Study Design.—Three groups were studied: 22 women who had called the Motherisk Program for information on the reproductive safety of consuming fish during pregnancy, a group of Japanese residing in Toronto (n = 23) consuming much larger amounts of fish, and a group of Canadian women of reproductive age (n = 20) not seeking advice, were studied. Mercury concentrations in hair samples were measured using inductively coupled plasma mass spectrometry. Seafood consumption habits were recorded for each participant. Based on the types of fish consumed and consumption frequencies, the estimated monthly intake of mercury was calculated. Hair mercury concentrations were correlated to both the number of monthly seafood servings and the estimated ingested mercury dose.

Results.—There were significant correlations between fish servings and hair mercury (Spearman $r = 0.73$, $P < .0001$) and between amounts of consumed mercury and hair mercury concentrations (Spearman $r = 0.81$, $P < .0001$). Nearly two thirds of the Motherisk callers, all of the Japanese women, and 15% of the Canadian women of reproductive age had hair mercury above 0.3 μg/g, which was shown recently to be the lowest observable adverse effect level in a large systematic review of all perinatal studies.

Conclusions.—Because of very wide variability, general recommendations for a safe number of fish servings may not be sufficient to protect the fetus. Analysis of hair mercury may be warranted before pregnancy in selected groups of women consuming more than 12 ounces of fish per week, as dietary modification can decrease body burden and ensure fetal safety.

▶ Eating fish is good for you in general. Fish are a source of high-quality lean protein and obviously rich in n-3 polyunsaturated fatty acids. The latter are essential for the growth of the developing fetal brain. At the same time, almost all fish contain some mercury. Those who eat a lot of fish have higher mercury levels, and there is a concern that high maternal mercury levels could adversely affect fetal development. At the same time, there is not necessarily a direct correlation between maternal fish ingestion and maternal mercury levels. Given the benefits of n-3 polyunsaturated fatty acids, some have actually suggested that greater maternal fish consumption during pregnancy would be associated with improved child neurodevelopment.[1]

What Schoeman et al have done is to report on hair mercury levels from 3 small convenience samples in Toronto, Canada, including concerned women seeking advice about fish consumption during pregnancy, highly educated middle-class women of childbearing age, and Japanese immigrants, the latter including workers in a fish market and Japanese restaurants. The authors report that many study participants exceeded the lowest observed adverse effect of 0.3 μg/g mercury in hair, a threshold derived from unpublished data. The authors conclude that because of very wide variability, general recommendations for a safe number of fish servings may not be sufficient to protect the fetus. For those worried about mercury in fish, particularly pregnant women, recognize that wild-caught salmon is low in methylmercury (median 0 mg/kg fish) and is an excellent source of n-3 polyunsaturated fatty acids, such that a single weekly serving will provide a pregnant woman with her recommended intake. Canned white (albacore) tuna is also a very good source of fatty acids but may contain substantially more methylmercury (median 0.34 mg/kg fish). Compared with white tuna, canned light tuna on average contains less methylmercury (median 0.08 mg/kg fish) but also less polyunsaturated fatty acid. Other fish commonly consumed in the United States such as shrimp and pollock are low in mercury but also low in n-3 polyunsaturated fatty acid. The trick in all this is to get your n-3 polyunsaturated fatty acid intake at a sufficient level while minimizing your mercury exposure if you are a pregnant woman. To read more about this, see the excellent editorial by Oken.[2]

One final comment about fish and fish oil. Data continue to emerge that fish oil may fend off breast cancer. Women who reported taking fish oil at the start of a large cancer prevention study were determined to be roughly half as likely as nonusers to develop ductal carcinoma of the breasts, the most common form of breast cancer. Fish oil did not influence the risk of lobular breast cancer.[3]

Before leaving this commentary dealing with a toxic heavy metal, recognize that lead poisoning is still with us, at least on a global level if not just locally. Recently reported was a mass lead poisoning in the Northern Nigerian state of Zamfara, the magnitude of which was considered by the World Health Organization as unprecedented. It appears that gold mining activity in Zamfara led to a substantial rise in numbers of deaths of children and hundreds of people needing treatment for dangerously high levels of lead. A total of 161 deaths have been attributed to the incident by the end of 2010 with possibly hundreds and potentially thousands of others having become ill. Investigators suspected lead contamination in ground water and soil when in 1 village 30% of the children under the age of 5 had expired from unknown causes. Samples of soil in the area showed lead concentrations of greater than 100 000 ppm (the limit for residential areas in the United States is 400 ppm). Currently several thousand children in Nigeria are under treatment for lead poisoning as a result of this environmental catastrophe.[4]

J. A. Stockman III, MD

References

1. Oken E, Wright RO, Kleinman KP, et al. Maternal fish consumption, hair mercury, and infant cognition in a US cohort. *Environ Health Perspect.* 2005;113: 1376-1380.
2. Oken E. Fish intake and mercury levels: Only part of the picture. *J Pediatr.* 2010; 157:10-12.
3. Seppa N. Fish oil may fend off breast cancer. *Science News.* July 31, 2010:13, http://www.britannica.com/bps/additionalcontent/18/52540584/Fish-oil-may-fend-off-breast-cancer. Accessed June 30, 2011.
4. Moszynski P. Mass lead poisoning in Nigeria causes "unprecedented" emergency. *BMJ.* 2010;341:c0431.

Acute Ethanol Poisoning in a 4-Year-Old as a Result of Ethanol-Based Hand-Sanitizer Ingestion

Engel JS, Spiller HA (King's Daughters Med Ctr, Ashland, KY; Kentucky Regional Poison Ctr, Louisville)
Pediatr Emerg Care 26:508-509, 2010

Alcohol-based hand sanitizers have become widely available because of widespread usage in schools, hospitals, and workplaces and by consumers. We report what we believe is the first unintentional ingestion in a small child producing significant intoxication. A 4-year-old 14-kg girl was brought to the emergency department with altered mental status after a history of ingesting an alcohol-based hand sanitizer. Physical examination revealed an obtunded child with periods of hypoventilation and a hematoma in the central portion of her forehead from a fall at home that occurred after the ingestion. Abnormal vital signs included a heart rate of 139 beats/min and temperature of 96.3°F, decreasing to 93.6°F. Abnormal laboratory values consisted of potassium of 2.6 mEq/L and a serum alcohol of 243 mg/dL. A computed tomography scan of her brain without contrast showed no acute intracranial abnormality. A urine drug screen for common drugs of abuse was reported as negative. The child was intubated, placed on mechanical ventilation, and admitted for medical care. She recovered over the next day without sequelae. As with other potentially toxic products, we would recommend caution and direct supervision of use when this product is available to young children.

▶ This brief little report reminds us that not all the good things around us are really all that safe. With each of the recent flu seasons, alcohol-based hand sanitizers became ubiquitous in virtually every environment including schools, hospitals, work, and workplaces. Alcohol-based hand sanitizers have been shown to reduce absenteeism in elementary schools and are recommended in classrooms as part of an infection-control program.[1] The same is true of their use in the workplace and in hospitals.

The active ingredient in alcohol-based sanitizers is ethanol and/or isopropanol. These forms of alcohol are present in concentrations of 60% to 95%. The report of Engel et al tells about a 4-year-old who developed ataxia, hyperexcitability, and altered mental status. Emergency medical services (EMS) were called to the family home. The family reported the ingestion of Purell Hand Sanitizer (ethanol 62%, isopropanol 10%; Johnson & Johnson Consumer Products, Skillman, New Jersey). The child was hypoventilating and desaturating. The EMS team could smell alcohol on her breath. Various studies were done on arrival to an emergency department. Serum ethanol levels were reported as 243 mg/dL. No other toxins were found with blood and urine studies. The child was extubated for airway protection and transferred to a tertiary care children's hospital, where after 24 hours she was successfully extubated and discharged without sequelae. The only other complication of the alcohol intoxication was hypothermia. The rectal temperature was documented to be 93.6°F on admission to the emergency room. Hypoglycemia was not observed.

In retrospect, it appears that this child probably consumed between 1.5 and 2 ounces of hand sanitizer, based on the demonstrated alcohol level and the child's body weight. This suggests a relatively large ingestion for this child at her age, given the high concentration of alcohol in the hand sanitizer.

In general, alcohol-based hand sanitizers have been considered safe around children younger than 6 years of age.[2] Given the right circumstances, however, acute ethanol poisoning can occur and can be very serious as evidenced by this case of a 4-year-old.

J. A. Stockman III, MD

References

1. Hammond B, Aly Y, Findler E, Dolan M, Donovan S. Effect of hand sanitizer on elementary school absenteeism. *Am J Infect Control.* 2000;28:340-346.
2. Miller M, Borys D, Morgan D. Alcohol-based hand sanitizers and unintended pediatric exposures: a retrospective review. *Clin Pediatr(Phila).* 2009;48:429-431.

Initial Location Determines Spontaneous Passage of Foreign Bodies From the Gastrointestinal Tract in Children

Lee JH, Lee JS, Kim MJ, et al (Sungkyunkwan Univ School of Medicine, Seoul, South Korea)
Pediatr Emerg Care 27:284-289, 2011

Objective.—The purpose of this study was to follow the natural course of spontaneous passage (SP) of ingested foreign bodies (FBs) in children.

Methods.—The medical records of 249 patients who ingested FBs were reviewed. In addition, they were studied by telephone questionnaires to follow up spontaneously passed FB. The factors associated with SP such as age, the type, size, and initial location of the FBs were analyzed.

Results.—Foreign bodies were spontaneously passed in 145 patients (58.2%), endoscopic removal was performed in 100 patients (40.2%), and operative removal was performed in 4 patients (1.6%). Most SP FBs were passed within 5 days. The SP rates (SPRs) according to the initial location were the following: 12.2% for the esophagus ($P < 0.0001$), 71.4% for the stomach, 85.7% for the small bowel, and 96.4% for the colon. There was no significant difference in the SPR according to age. When coins and disk batteries that required early endoscopic removal were excluded, the SPR was 63.4% for FBs less than 10 mm, 80.4% for FBs 10 to 20 mm, 72.8% for FBs 20 to 30 mm, and 50.0% for FBs more than 30 mm ($P = 0.091$). The initial location of the FB (odds ratio, 33.7; 95% confidence interval, 14.4—79.0) and the size of the FB (odds ratio, 3.5; 95% confidence interval, 1.0—11.6) were independent predictors of SP by multivariate analysis.

Conclusions.—Most FBs in the gastrointestinal tract are spontaneously passed without complication, and the initial location of FBs was found to be the main determining factor for SPR. Ingested FBs, in children, even sharp or relatively large FBs, can be spontaneously passed when they are located below the esophagus.

▶ This report of Lee et al examines the age-old issue of whether one should intervene in removing a foreign body from the gastrointestinal tract that has been inadvertently swallowed by a child. The results of the study showed that the probability of spontaneous passage of ingested foreign bodies found below the esophagus is 77.7%, indicating that it is highly likely that if a foreign body has passed the esophagus, it will be passed spontaneously. Thus the prognosis of ingested foreign bodies is the initial location. Interestingly, when it comes to coins, these investigators did not find that larger coins had more difficulty in being passed than smaller coins, contrary to prior reports. The report also showed that most single magnets are spontaneously passed within 4 days. The management of magnet ingestion has been a topic of much literature. Clearly, the ingestion of 2 magnets, which can cause strong contact between them, can result in mucosal pressure necrosis, intestinal obstruction, intestinal fistula, and perforation. Open surgery is generally needed in such cases.

J. A. Stockman III, MD

Efficacy and safety of scorpion antivenom plus prazosin compared with prazosin alone for venomous scorpion (*Mesobuthus tamulus*) sting: randomised open label clinical trial

Bawaskar HS, Bawaskar PH (Bawaskar Hosp and Res Centre, Maharashtra, India)

BMJ 341:c7136, 2011

Objective.—Envenomation by *Mesobuthus tamulus* scorpion sting can result in serious cardiovascular effects. Scorpion antivenom is a specific treatment for scorpion sting. Evidence for the benefit of scorpion antivenom and its efficacy compared with that of commonly used vasodilators, such as prazosin, is scarce. We assessed the efficacy of prazosin combined with scorpion antivenom, compared with prazosin alone, in individuals with autonomic storm caused by scorpion sting.

Design.—Prospective, open label randomised controlled trial.

Setting.—General hospital inpatients (Bawaskar Hospital and Research Centre Mahad Dist-Raigad Maharashtra, India).

Participants.—Seventy patients with grade 2 scorpion envenomation, older than six months, with no cardiorespiratory or central nervous system abnormalities.

Intervention.—Scorpion antivenom plus prazosin (n = 35) or prazosin alone (n = 35) assigned by block randomisation. Treatment was not masked. Analysis was by intention to treat.

Main Outcome Measures.—The primary end point was the proportion of patients achieving resolution of the clinical syndrome (sweating, salivation, cool extremities, priapism, hypertension or hypotension, tachycardia) 10 hours after administration of study drugs. Secondary end points were time required for complete resolution of clinical syndrome, prevention of deterioration to higher grade, doses of prazosin required overall and within 10 hours, and adverse events. The study protocol was approved by the independent ethics committee of Mumbai.

Results.—Mean (SD) recovery times in hours for the prazosin plus scorpion antivenom group compared with the prazosin alone groups were: sweating 3 (1.1) *v* 6.6 (2.6); salivation 1.9 (0.9) *v* 3 (1.9); priapism 4.7 (1.5) *v* 9.4 (1.5). Mean (SD) doses of prazosin in the groups were 2 (2.3) and 4 (3.5), respectively. 32 patients (91.4%, 95% confidence interval 76.9% to 97.8%) in the prazosin plus antivenom group showed complete resolution of the clinical syndrome within 10 hours of administration of treatment compared with eight patients in the prazosin group (22.9%, 11.8% to 39.3%). Patients from the antivenom plus prazosin group recovered earlier (mean 8 hours, 95% CI 6.5 to 9.5) than those in the control group (17.7 hours, 15.4 to 19.9; mean difference −9.7 hours, −6.9 to −12.4). The number of patients whose condition deteriorated to a higher grade was similar in both groups (antivenom plus prazosin four of 35, prazosin alone five of 35). Hypotension was reported in fewer patients in the antivenom plus prazosin group (12 of 35, 34.3%) than in the prazosin group (19 of 35, 54.3%), but the difference was not statistically significant. No difference was noted in change in blood pressure and pulse rate over time between two groups.

Conclusion.—Recovery from scorpion sting is hastened by simultaneous administration of scorpion antivenom plus prazosin compared with prazosin alone.

Trial Registration Number.—CTRI/2010/091/000584 (Clinical Trials Registry India).

▶ If you live in the eastern part of the United States, you do not tend to think too much about scorpion stings. If you live in the southwest, however, or intend to travel widely throughout the world, you should pay attention to this report. In the linked randomized clinical trial, Bawaskar and Bawaskar compare the effectiveness of scorpion antivenom plus or minus prazosin for treatment of scorpion stings. The trial is a reminder that global health researchers often neglect conditions that matter to large numbers of unique communities. Of the 1500 species of scorpions worldwide, about 30 are potentially very dangerous to humans. About 1.2 million scorpion stings occur worldwide each year, of which roughly 3250 are fatal. The incidence and severity vary geographically, obviously, with reported incidence among the general population varying from 5 per 100 000, for example, in France to almost 7000 per 100 000 in Venezuela. In addition to what we see in the southwest United States, scorpion stings are extremely common in countries such as Algeria, Israel, Tunisia, Mexico, Chile, and Saudi Arabia.

It was back in 2007 that the World Health Organization held the first-ever meeting to define responses to the critical shortage of therapeutic antisera for the treatment of venomous snakebites and scorpion stings. Several manufacturers in developed countries have abandoned antisera production because they find it unprofitable. Even now the few manufacturers that still make the stuff do so cautiously because of uncertainties about market demand and the safety of production, a result of limited regulatory frameworks. An estimated 10 million vials of high-quality potent antisera are needed annually to respond effectively to snakebites and scorpion stings, but the current worldwide production capacity is well below this, and antisera for one region may not be applicable to another.

Bawaskar and Bawaskar found that patients given antivenom plus prazosin for treatment of the Indian red scorpion sting recovered more quickly than those given prazosin alone. The data from the report are important because a great deal of emphasis is being placed now on increasing the production of antisera for snakebites, but little is being spoken about for the management of the sting of the scorpion. For whatever it is worth, I am a Scorpio who has never visited Algeria, Israel, Tunisia, Chile, or Saudi Arabia. However, I do intend to drop into Vegas and Scottsdale every now and then, and if I'm bitten by a scorpion, I hope I will have access to adequate amounts of antisera.

J. A. Stockman III, MD

Inhalant Abuse: Monitoring Trends by Using Poison Control Data, 1993–2008

Marsolek MR, White NC, Litovitz TL (Natl Capital Poison Ctr, Washington, DC; Univ of Virginia School of Medicine, Charlottesville)
Pediatrics 125:906-913, 2010

Purpose.—To demonstrate the value of poison control data as an adjunct to national drug abuse surveys and a source of data to inform and focus prevention efforts.

Methods.—National Poison Data System (NPDS) data are collected and compiled in real time by the 60 US poison centers as callers seek guidance for poison exposures. Demographic, geographic, product, outcome, and treatment-site data for the 35 453 inhalant cases reported between 1993 and 2008 were analyzed.

Results.—The prevalence of inhalant cases reported to US poison control centers decreased 33% from 1993 to 2008. Prevalence was highest among children aged 12 to 17 years and peaked in 14-year-olds. In contrast to national survey data showing nearly equal use of inhalants by both genders, 73.5% of NPDS inhalant cases occurred in boys, which suggests that boys may pursue riskier usage behaviors. Most cases (67.8%) were managed in health care facilities. More than 3400 different products were reported. Propellants, gasoline, and paint were the most frequent product categories. Propellants were the only product category that substantially increased over time. Butane, propane, and air fresheners had the highest fatality rates. Prevalence for all inhalants was highest in western mountain states and West Virginia, but geographic distribution varied according to product type. Gasoline was a proportionately greater problem for younger children; propellants were an issue for older children.

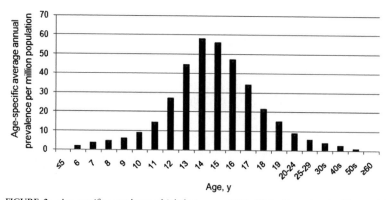

FIGURE 2.—Age-specific prevalence of inhalant cases, 1993–2008. (Reproduced with permission from Pediatrics, Marsolek MR, White NC, Litovitz TL. Inhalant abuse: monitoring trends by using poison control data, 1993–2008. *Pediatrics.* 2010;125:906-913. Copyright © 2010 by the American Academy of Pediatrics.)

TABLE 2.—The 25 Most Frequently Implicated Products Ranked According to Fatality Rate for All Single-Substance Cases

Product	All	Major Effects	Deaths	Hazard Index[a]	Fatality Rate[b]
All substances	30 094	705	167	29.0	5.5
Butane	620	19	36	88.7	58.1
Propane	270	9	7	59.3	25.9
Air fresheners	1239	22	27	39.5	21.8
Nitrous oxide	731	18	10	38.3	13.7
Carburetor cleaners	582	43	5	82.5	8.6
Fluorocarbons/freon	1631	59	14	44.8	8.6
Dusters	2457	69	13	33.4	5.3
Nitrites/nitrates	431	16	2	41.8	4.6
Toluene/xylene	1096	48	5	48.4	4.6
Adhesive/glue	1105	18	4	19.9	3.6
Hair spray	279	2	1	10.8	3.6
Disinfectants	347	4	1	14.4	2.9
Polishes/waxes	350	5	1	17.1	2.9
Paint thinner	458	14	1	32.8	2.2
Typewriter correction fluid	566	4	1	8.8	1.8
Paint	3036	80	5	28.0	1.6
Gasoline	4329	72	7	18.2	1.6
Helium	689	9	1	14.5	1.5
Formalin/formaldehyde	197	6	0	30.5	0.0
Deodorant	302	3	0	9.9	0.0
Ethanol (nonbeverage)	233	2	0	8.6	0.0
Albuterol	415	1	0	2.4	0.0
Marker/ink	419	1	0	2.4	0.0
Nail polish remover	182	0	0	0.0	0.0
Nail polish	160	0	0	0.0	0.0

[a]The hazard index was calculated as the number of cases that resulted in major effects or death per 1000 cases.
[b]The fatality rate was calculated as the number of cases that resulted in death per 1000 cases.

Conclusions.—NPDS should be used to monitor inhalant abuse because it provides unique, timely, and clinically useful information on medical outcomes experienced by users, includes detailed product information (brand and formulation), and can potentially be used to identify real-time demographic, geographic, and product trends. Focusing inhalant prevention efforts on the most hazardous products and most seriously affected users may improve and facilitate strategic prevention, enabling interventions such as targeted education, product reformulation, repackaging, relabeling, or prohibition of sales of especially hazardous inhalant products to youth.

▶ There has been remarkable change in the way youngsters get a "buzz" these days in comparison with even just 10 years ago. As you see in this report, propellants have taken off like rocket propellants in terms of substances of abuse. This is particularly so in the last decade. This study emanates from inhalant cases reported to the US poison control centers over a period of approximately 15 years. For the purposes of the report, intentional abuse was defined as having an exposure resulting from the intentional, improper, or incorrect use of a substance where the victim was likely attempting to achieve a euphoric or psychotropic effect.

As one can see in the figure (Fig 2), inhalant abuse is most common in the teenage years. It takes a pretty hardy 50-year-old to want to breathe in something like typewriter correction fluid fumes. The table (Table 2) lists the 25 most frequently implicated products ranked according to fatality rate for all single-substance cases. By far, butane, propane, and air fresheners lead the pack of most frequently used inhalant substances of abuse. Curiously, some of the inhalants, as noxious as one might think they might be, have no mortality associated with them. It is not possible, therefore, to die embalmed by sniffing formaldehyde nor will you go to your grave as a result of sucking on a can of deodorant aerosol.

If there is one deficiency in the information we are provided from the poison control centers, it is that there is no way to know whether any of the toxic effects reported are the result of an accumulation of many episodes of exposure to toxic inhalants. It only takes one time, however, to potentially kill, but multiple exposures may be necessary to produce brain degeneration.

J. A. Stockman III, MD

Unintentional Child Poisonings Through Ingestion of Conventional and Novel Tobacco Products

Connolly GN, Richter P, Aleguas A Jr, et al (Harvard Univ, Boston, MA; Centers for Disease Control and Prevention, Atlanta, GA; Northern Ohio Poison Control Ctr, Cleveland)
Pediatrics 125:896-899, 2010

Objective.—This study examines child poisonings resulting from ingestion of tobacco products throughout the nation and assesses the potential toxicity of novel smokeless tobacco products, which are of concern with their discreet form, candy-like appearance, and added flavorings that may be attractive to young children.

Methods.—Data representing all single-substance, accidental poisonings resulting from ingestion of tobacco products by children <6 years of age, reported to poison control centers, were examined. Age association with ingestion of smokeless tobacco versus other tobacco products was tested through logistic regression. Total nicotine content, pH, and un-ionized nicotine level were determined, and the latter was compared with values for moist snuff and cigarettes.

Results.—A total of 13 705 tobacco product ingestion cases were reported, >70% of which involved infants < 1 year of age. Smokeless tobacco products were the second most common tobacco products ingested by children, after cigarettes, and represented an increasing proportion of tobacco ingestions with each year of age from 0 to 5 years (odds ratio: 1.94 [95% confidence interval: 1.86–2.03]). A novel, dissolvable, smokeless tobacco product with discreet form, candy-like appearance, and added flavorings was found to contain an average of 0.83 mg of

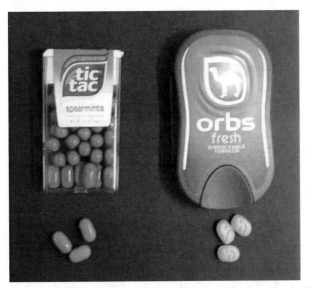

FIGURE 1.—Comparison of Orbs tobacco pellets and Tic Tac candies. (Reproduced with permission from *Pediatrics*, Connolly GN, Richter P, Aleguas A Jr, et al. Unintentional child poisonings through ingestion of conventional and novel tobacco products. *Pediatrics*. 2010;125:896-899. Copyright © 2010 by the American Academy of Pediatrics.)

nicotine per pellet, with an average pH of 7.9, which resulted in an average of 42% of the nicotine in the un-ionized form.

Conclusion.—In light of the novelty and potential harm of dissolvable nicotine products, public health authorities are advised to study these products to determine the appropriate regulatory approach (Fig 1).

▶ Without question, unintentional ingestion of tobacco products remains a major cause of infant and child toxic exposures being reported to poison control centers throughout our country. Ninety percent or more of such accidental poisonings occur in children younger than 6 years of age. Besides conventional smokeless tobacco, novel smokeless tobacco products, including dissolvable compressed tobacco pellets called Camel Orbs (R.J. Reynolds Tobacco Company, Winston-Salem, NC) are now of major concern since this product has a candy-like appearance and added flavorings that may be attractive to young children. Please be aware that the ingestion of as little as one milligram of nicotine by a small child can produce symptoms including nausea and vomiting. Severe toxic effects of nicotine ingestion may include weakness, convulsions, unresponsiveness, and impaired respiration and ultimately may lead to respiratory arrest and death. The estimated minimal lethal pediatric dose is 1.0 mg of nicotine per kilogram of body weight.[1]

Connolly et al inform us with up-to-date information about the potential toxicity of novel smokeless tobacco products based on information derived from the National Poison Data System, compiled by the Association of Poison Control Centers based on reports of 61 regional centers serving the nation. For the period 2006 through 2008, a total of 13 705 cases were reported for all types of tobacco products. Most (>70%) ingestions were in infants less than 1 year of age. Many of the cases related to the ingestion of Camel Orbs. This is a novel, dissolvable, compressed tobacco product put on the market in 2009 by R.J. Reynolds Tobacco Company. The promotional literature on this product indicates that it contains 1 mg of nicotine per pellet that is about the size of a typical Tic Tac® candy (Fig 1). Studies have shown that the average pH of an Orbs pellet is 7.9, which is more alkaline than cigarette tobacco (pH < 6.0) and results in an average 42% of the nicotine in the un-ionized form, compared with averages of 28% to 30% for moist snuff and <10% for cigarettes. Un-ionized nicotine is absorbed more rapidly in the mouth, which might enhance toxicity. Furthermore, the discreet form of Orbs might make the ingestion of nicotine, a highly addictive drug, easy and attractive for adolescents.

It should be noted that the recently introduced Family Smoking Prevention and Tobacco Control Act, which provides the Food and Drug Administration with certain authority to regulate tobacco products, prohibits cigarette constituents or additives that provide a characterizing flavor to the tobacco or tobacco smoke. This prohibition does not, however, apply to other tobacco products. There currently is also no control over the size and quantity of compressed smokeless tobacco products. Thus it is entirely possible for a tiny tyke to get a handful of Orbs into his or her mouth.

This commentary closes with some interesting observations related to regulations restricting smoking, this in large-hub airports. The Centers for Disease Control and Prevention periodically analyzes the smoking policies of airports in the United States, ones characterized as large-hub. A large-hub airport is defined by the Federal Aviation Administration as an airport that accounts for ≥ 1% of total passenger boardings in the United States. Combined, there are 29 large-hub airports in the United States and these account for approximately 70% of total passenger boardings in our country. Smoking regulations in airports are established not by the federal government, but by state statute, county or city ordinance, airport/transit authority rules, regulations, or policies. An airport is described as smoke-free indoors when smoking by anyone is prohibited at all times, in all indoor areas of the airport. In 2010, 7 of the 29 US large-hub airports did allow smoking indoors. These airports were Hartsfield-Jackson Atlanta International, Dallas/Fort Worth International, Denver International, McCarran International (Las Vegas), Charlotte-Douglas International, Washington-Dulles International, and Salt Lake City International. All the airports that reported smoking restricted it to the following areas: public smoking rooms, bars, and private airline clubs. Only time will tell whether these high-volume airports will bite the bullet and do what is right. Thus far, the federal government has laid low on this issue. Perhaps we should put some pressure on our physician congressmen to figure out a way, somehow, of getting the federal government involved with good legislation that deals with this problem. By the way, the national elections held in 2010 added 7 new physician congressmen to the ranks of those on the Hill. They joined 12 physician incumbents in the House and Senate. Combined, this is not an immodest number to move national agendas when it comes to healthcare.

J. A. Stockman III, MD

Reference

1. McGuigan MA. Nicotine. In: Dart RG, ed. *Medical Toxicology.* 3rd ed. Philadelphia, PA: Lippincott Williams and Wilkins; 2003:601-604.

Article Index

Chapter 1: Adolescent Medicine

Chapter 2: Allergy and Dermatology

Chapter 5: Dentistry and Otolaryngology (ENT)

Chapter 6: Endocrinology

Chapter 7: Gastroenterology

Chapter 8: Genitourinary Tract

Chapter 9: Heart and Blood Vessels

Chapter 10: Infectious Diseases and Immunology

Chapter 11: Miscellaneous

Chapter 12: Musculoskeletal

Chapter 13: Neurology and Psychiatry

Chapter 14: Newborn

Chapter 15: Nutrition and Metabolism

Chapter 16: Oncology

Chapter 17: Ophthalmology

Chapter 18: Respiratory Tract

Chapter 19: Therapeutics and Toxicology

Author Index

Edwards Brothers Inc.
Ann Arbor MI. USA
March 19, 2012